Fundamental Approaches to the
Management of Cardiac Arrhythmias

Fundamental Approaches to the Management of Cardiac Arrhythmias

by

Ruey J. Sung, M.D.

Professor of Medicine,
Stanford University School of Medicine, and
Director, Cardiac Electrophysiology & Arrhythmia Service,
Stanford University Medical Center,
Stanford, California, U.S.A.

and

Michael R. Lauer, M.D., Ph. D.

Clinical Assistant Professor of Medicine,
Stanford University School of Medicine,
Stanford, California, U.S.A. and
Attending Cardiac Electrophysiologist,
The Permanente Medical Group,
Assistant Director, Cardiac Electrophysiology Laboratory,
Kaiser-Permanente Medical Center,
San Jose, California, U.S.A.

KLUWER ACADEMIC PUBLISHERS
DORDRECHT / BOSTON / LONDON

A C.I.P. Catalogue record for this book is available from the Library of Congress.

ISBN 0-7923-6559-3

Published by Kluwer Academic Publishers,
P.O. Box 17, 3300 AA Dordrecht, The Netherlands.

Sold and distributed in North, Central and South America
by Kluwer Academic Publishers,
101 Philip Drive, Norwell, MA 02061, U.S.A.

In all other countries, sold and distributed
by Kluwer Academic Publishers,
P.O. Box 322, 3300 AH Dordrecht, The Netherlands.

Printed on acid-free paper

Printed in the Netherlands.

DEDICATION

To my mentor, Professor Agustin Castellanos, Jr., my wife, Kuei, my mother, Ping-Shing Lin, and my children, Janet, Emory, and Tain-Yen.

–RJS

To my wife, Leslie, and my mother, Lillian.

–MRL

"What deserves the most emphasis and what does unite us all in science is our unconflicted and overriding devotion to the culture of science. What is great is the discipline of science not the people doing it. Science *enables* us – ordinary people doing ordinary things, which when assembled reveal the extraordinary and awesome beauties of nature."

Arthur Kornberg, M.D.
Nobel Laureate
Emma Pfeiffer Merner Professor of Biochemistry, Emeritus
Stanford University School of Medicine

PREFACE

Our purpose in writing this book was to produce a clinically-oriented, non-multi-authored textbook of cardiac electrophysiology that would be useful to practicing electrophysiologists, cardiologists, fellows in training as well as associated electrophysiology professionals, including nurses and technologists. While all clinical textbooks risk becoming outdated even before they're published, and few textbooks of a manageable size can claim to be completely comprehensive, our goal was to produce a book that systematically presents a thorough discussion of the *fundamental principles and concepts* important to the practice of clinical electrophysiology. We do not discuss basic cellular electrophysiology for its sake alone, but instead include basic science material only when it is helpful in explaining the overlying clinical principles. Cardiac electrophysiology, as with any subspecialty, behaves as a living organism with continuous evolution of its standards and practices. However, even though the details and tools of management (catheters, drugs, devices, etc.) may change with dazzling speed, the fundamental principles of diagnosis and management generally change very little and they remain the critical underpinning of the day-to-day management of patients with cardiac arrhythmias.

In the first third of the book we present the principles of clinical cardiac electrophysiology as it is currently practiced. We assume the reader has a basic background in the evaluation of patients with cardiac rhythm disturbances, including the history-taking, performance of the physical examination, routine laboratory evaluation, and a comfortable familiarity with surface 12-lead electrocardiography including basic rhythm and arrhythmia analysis. In chapters 1 and 2 our focus is on the arrhythmogenic anatomy and understanding the fundamentals of the diagnostic electrophysiology study in patients with brady- and tachyarrhythmias. In chapters 3 through 6, respectively, we proceed to discuss the basic principles of antiarrhythmic drug therapy, catheter ablation, and device therapy using pacemakers and implantable cardioverter-defibrillators.

In the remaining chapters of the book, we focus on the details of the diagnosis and management of specific brady- and tachyarrhythmias using the principles outlined in the earlier sections of the book applied to clinical material collected over the years. For more advanced readers, most chapters can be read individually as self-contained units assuming an understanding of the diagnostic and therapeutic principles presented in the first portion of the book. In chapters 7 and 8 we briefly discuss the acute management of brady- and tachyarrhythmias, while in chapters 9 and 10 we discuss disorders of sinoatrial node function and atrioventricular function, respectively. In chapters 11 through 14 we present major topics including AV nodal reentrant tachycardia, preexcitation syndromes and their concealed variants, atrial tachycardias and flutter, and finally atrial fibrillation, respectively. Finally, we focus on ventricular tachyarrhythmias, with a discussion of the spectrum of monomorphic ventricular tachycardia in chapter 15, polymorphic ventricular tachycardia and the long QT syndromes in chapter 16, and ventricular fibrillation and sudden arrhythmic death in chapters 17.

As with all authors, we greatly value the input of our readers. Suggestions, corrections, and constructive criticisms of all types are welcomed. We can be contacted by electronic mail at the addresses below.

Ruey J. Sung, M.D.
rsung@cvmed.stanford.edu

Michael R. Lauer, M.D., Ph.D.   Stanford, California
michael.lauer@kp.org   June, 2000

CONTENTS

6 Implantable Cardioverter-Defibrillator Therapy

7 Diagnosis and Acute Management of Patients with Symptomatic Bradyarrhythmias

8 Diagnosis and Acute Management of Patients with Symptomatic Tachyarrhythmias

9 Disturbances of Sinoatrial Node Function

10 Disturbances of Atrioventricular Conduction

11 Atrioventricular Nodal Reentrant Tachycardia

12 Ventricular Preexcitation Syndromes: The Wolff-Parkinson-White Syndrome and Variants

13 Atrial Tachycardias and Atrial Flutter

14 Atrial Fibrillation

15 The Spectrum of Monomorphic Ventricular Tachycardia

16 Polymorphic Ventricular Tachycardia and Long QT Syndromes

17 Ventricular Fibrillation and Sudden Cardiac Death

ACKNOWLEDGMENTS

We extend our deepest gratitude to our clinical electrophysiology fellows, cardiology fellows, nurses, technicians, and support staffs of the electrophysiology laboratories at Jackson Memorial Hospital (University of Miami, Miami, Florida), Moffit Hospital, San Francisco General Hospital, and Veterans Administration Medical Center (University of California, San Francisco, California), Letterman Army Hospital (Presidio at San Francisco, California), Kaiser-Santa Teresa Medical Center (San Jose, California), and the Sen-Tung Sung Memorial Electrophysiology Laboratory at the Stanford University Medical Center (Stanford, California). In particular, we want to thank the late Mr. Francisco Garcia-Montes, Mr. Booker T. Pullen, and Drs. Charlie Young, Edmund Keung, Edward Huycke and Thomas Svinarich for their invaluable inspirational and collaborative support throughout the years. Without the assistance of all these individuals it would not have been possible to complete this book.

CHAPTER 1

FUNCTIONAL ANATOMY AND MECHANISMS OF CARDIAC ARRHYTHMIAS

Fundamentally, clinical cardiac electrophysiology is the study of the normal and abnormal functional properties of the electrically excitable tissues of the heart. While an appreciation for the anatomy of the discrete components of the cardiac conduction system is certainly important, cardiac electrophysiologists are generally less concerned with the precise anatomical details than the *functional* behavior of electrical conduction within and through these structures. The anatomic conduction system is best viewed as a physiological continuum through which electrical current flows within three-dimensional structures. At different points along the course of the conduction system there occur normal variations in conduction pattern, velocity, and direction. Clinically significant disruptions of cardiac rhythm may develop when altered anatomy (structure) leads to abnormal alterations of conduction pattern, velocity, and direction (function).

1.1 Functional Anatomy of the Conduction System

Most, if not all, of the gross anatomical features of the heart and conduction system critical to the study of cardiac electrophysiology are presented in introductory or intermediate level physiology courses. The histological details and specifics of the cellular architecture of the normal and abnormal specialized conducting system continue to emerge and have been reviewed in detail elsewhere [1-18].

Figure 1-1 schematically depicts an overview of the normal conduction system. The heart's normal intrinsic pacemaker termed the *sinoatrial (SA) node*, lies within the sulcus terminalis between the superior vena cava and the right atrial appendage. It measures up to 2-cm in length and 0.5-cm wide. Specialized cells within the SA node generate Ca^{++}-dependent action potentials that spread through the transitional cells at the node's border to activate the atrial myocardium. This wavefront of depolarization conducts through the atria to the *atrioventricular (AV) node*, possibly by preferential *internodal tracts* comprised of cells that are indistinguishable from working atrial myocardium. At least three such preferential approaches to the AV node have been proposed including the superior, inferior, and middle pathways [6,16]. However, other authorities have persuasively argued no such anatomically-definable preferential pathways exist [19]. The superior internodal tract proceeds from the cephalic portion of the SA node to anterior portion of the atrial septum to merge with the anterior and superior approaches to the AV node. The middle pathway arises from the middle portion of the SA node and travels along the limbus fossa ovalis to also merge with the anterior atrial septal approaches to AV node. The inferior tract runs from the caudal portion of the SA node along the lower part of the atrial septum near the opening of the inferior vena cava to reach the posterior approaches to the AV node near the ostium of the coronary sinus. In addition, some authorities believe that an anterosuperiorly directed pathway through the atrial appendage to the anterior/superior approaches to the AV node. Finally, Bachmann's bundle may provide a preferential connection from the SA node to the left atrial septum with a left atrial extension connecting to the anterior approaches to the AV node.

In the absence of an accessory pathway (see "Mechanisms of Cardiac Arrhythmias" on page 7), the AV node/His bundle axis provides the only electrical connection between the atria and ventricles. The gross and microscopic anatomy of the AV junction is complex and the structural definition of the AV node has been the subject of controversy virtually since its original description [20-24]. Based upon histologic examination, three different areas of specialized tissues can be observed connecting the working atrial and

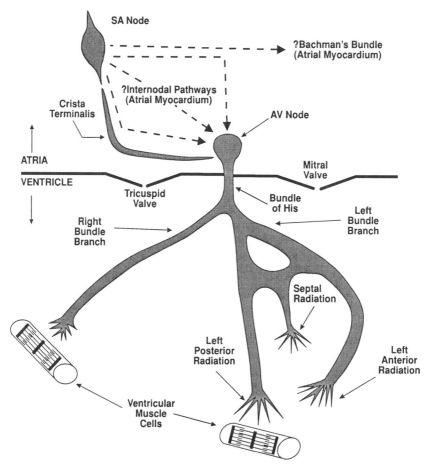

FIGURE 1-1. Schematic diagram of cardiac specialized conduction system, including sinoatrial node, atrioventricular node, His bundle, bundle branches, and arborizing network of Purkinje fibers. See text for details. AV, atrioventricular; SA, sinoatrial.

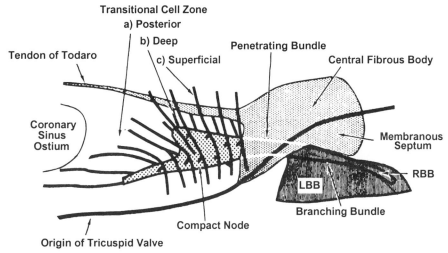

FIGURE 1-2. Diagrammatic representation of the AV junctional area in the human heart. The compact node is composed of leftward and rightward going components and is continuous anteriorly with the penetrating AV bundle. The compact node is continuous with three groups of transitional cells: (1) superficial, passing superficial to the tendon of Todaro and partly extending over the compact node into the tricuspid valve base; (2) deep, connecting with the left side of the septum; and (3) posterior, connecting the atrial myocardium above and below the ostium of the coronary sinus. LBB = left bundle branch; RBB = right bundle branch. Adapted from [3] with permission.

ventricular myocardia at the AV junction: (1) transitional cells (nodal approaches) positioned between the atrial myocardium and the compact node; (2) the compact node proper; and (3) the non-branching part of the His bundle (Figure 1-2) [3]. The atrial components of these specialized tissues at the AV junction are contained within the triangle of Koch, with two of its sides formed by the tendon of Todaro and the tricuspid annulus, and its base marked by the ostium of the coronary sinus (Figure 1-3). In the adult human heart, the mean length of the triangle of Koch (measured from the central fibrous body to the nearest edge of the coronary sinus) is 17±3 (10–24) mm, and the mean width (measured from the tricuspid annulus to the nearest edge of the coronary sinus) is 13±3 (6–21) mm [25]. The compact node has a length of 5–7 mm and a width of 2–5 mm [26].

Lying at the apex of the triangle of Koch, the compact node penetrates the central fibrous body to become the His bundle. Transitional cells can be grouped into three zones: superficial, deep, and posterior. The superficial zone is continuous with the anterior and superior aspect of the compact node, the posterior zone joins the inferior and posterior part of the compact node, and the deep zone connects the left atrial septum to the deep part of the compact node (Figure 1-2) [3]. These transitional cell zones are also referred to as "nodal approaches" [22] or "atrionodal bundles" [27]. In canine heart experiments, these transitional cell zones have been demonstrated to possess functional properties of specialized conduction tissues distinctly different from those of the working atrial myocardium [27].

In the rabbit heart, there is a dual input to the compact node during anterograde conduction [28-32] – an anterior input entering the node as a broad wavefront anterior to the coronary sinus ostium and a posterior input entering the node beneath the coronary sinus ostium via the crista terminalis. During retrograde conduction, the earliest exit to the atrium is in the interatrial septum, anterior to the coronary sinus ostium, at the same location of the anterior input during anterograde conduction; the crista terminalis is activated much later than the interatrial septum (Figure 1-4).

While not all investigators agree, the AV junction appears to consist of histologically distinct cell types, including P cells, and various types of transitional cells [33]. P-cells make up about 5% of the specialized cells in the AV junction, while transitional cells account for approximately 95%. Transitional cells vary in size and morphology, and appear to have an intricate interwoven arrangement displaying various forms of connections (end-to-end, side-to-side, end-to-side, and combinations of these). Connections appear not to be by conventional intercalated disks or gap junctions (i.e., containing mainly connexin 45 and 40 with small or no connexin 43) [34-37]. The highest concentration of P cells is at the distal junction of the AV node and His bundle and are often associated with nerve endings.

Based on cellular electrophysiological properties, the AV node has been divided into the AN, N, and NH cell zones; and even smaller subdivisions [28-32] (Figure 1-4). The AN region consists of large Purkinje-like cells comprising the internodal pathways with a large portion of the slender transitional cells. The N region corresponds primarily to the mass of interweaving and interconnected transitional cells of all types, while the

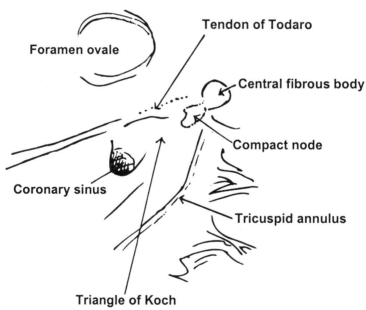

FIGURE 1-3. The central fibrous body at the apex, the tendon of Todaro and the tricuspid annulus at the sides and the coronary sinus at the base demarcate the triangle of Koch. The compact AV node, which penetrates the central fibrous body to become the AV (His) bundle, has an approximate length and width of 5-7 mm and 2-5 mm, respectively. The triangle of Koch has a mean length (measured from the central fibrous body to the nearest edge of the coronary sinus) of approximately 17±3 mm and a mean height (measured from the tricuspid annulus to the nearest edge of the coronary sinus) of approximately 13±3 mm.

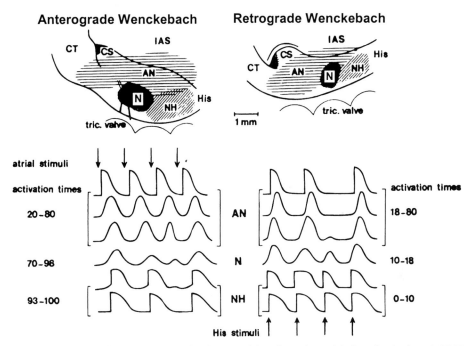

FIGURE 1-4. Schematic representations of action potential configuration and timing of activation of AN, N, and NH cell regions during antegrade and retrograde Wenckebach phenomenonin the rabbit heart. The upper panel illustrates the location of the AV junctional regions (AN, N, and NH zones) in which action potentials are recorded. Note the central position of the relatively small N zone. The lower panel shows the resting potential configuration in these various zones during anterograde stimulation (left side) and during retrograde stimulation (right side). Activation times are pooled from different experiments, and are expressed as a percentage of total A-H or H-A conduction time. From [28] with permission.

NH region appears to be where P cells and some transitional cells connect with large Purkinje-type cells of the His bundle [33]. The disparity in cell types and arrangements accounts for anisotropic conduction demonstrated at the AV junction [38].

The *His* or *AV bundle* begins as the AV node penetrates the central fibrous body. From the penetrating portion of the His bundle soon arises the major branching fascicles of the specialized conducting tissue in the ventricles termed the *His-Purkinje system*. The main *left bundle branch* arborizes into fan-shaped posterior and anterior radiations. Further divisions from the larger *posterior fascicle* combine with contributions from the *anterior fascicle* to produce a septal branch of the left bundle branch. The large *right bundle branch* bifurcates from the continuation of the penetrating segment of the His bundle and ends with a trifurcation supplying the anterolateral papillary muscle, parietal band, and lower septal aspect of the right ventricle. Conduction in the atrial and ventricular muscle and the His-Purkinje system occurs relatively rapidly due to fast Na^+-dependent action potentials. The rapid activation of the working ventricular muscle through the His-Purkinje system triggers the ventricular contraction.

The complex regional endocardial anatomy of the right atrium also plays a crucial role in a number of tachyarrhythmias, including atrial tachycardias and atrial flutter. Orifices of superior and inferior vena cava lie in the superior and inferior aspects of the right atrium, respectively. The tricuspid annulus lies anterior to the cavity of the right atrium. The endocardium of the right atrium is divided into an anterior trabeculated portion (the true embryonic right atrium), and a posterior smooth-walled segment that is derived from the embryonic sinus venosus. Separating these distinct anatomic regions laterally, is the crista terminalis, and inferiorly, the eustachian ridge. The crista terminalis extends from the high inter-atrial septum, anteriorly and superiorly to the orifice of the superior vena cava, and radiates caudally along the posterolateral wall. At its inferior extent, it courses anterior to the orifice of the inferior vena cava. The eustachian ridge is the remnant of the embryonic sinus venosus valve and extends from the orifice of the inferior vena cava, along the floor of the right atrium, to the ostium of the coronary sinus. An isthmus, approximately 1- to 2-cm in width resides between the inferior aspect of the tricuspid valve annulus and the eustachian ridge. The ostium of the coronary sinus lies medial to the orifice of the inferior vena cava, where the floor of the right atrium rises to become the atrial septum.

1.2   Vascular Supply to the Conduction System

The vascular supply to the SA node originates from the right coronary artery in 55% of patients and the left coronary artery in 45%. In approximately 90% of individuals the AV node receives its blood supply from a branch of the right coronary artery. In 10% of cases, an additional or the sole vascular supply, comes from the left coronary artery. In 90% of patients, the His bundle vascular supply comes from branches of the left anterior descending artery. In the remaining 10% of patients, the His bundle receives its blood supply from the right coronary artery. The right and main left bundle branches receives its blood from perforating branches of the anterior and posterior descending arteries (mixed right and left coronary contribution). The left bundle anterior radiation generally receives its vascular supply from anterior perforating branches, while the posterior radiation is supplied by posterior perforating branches.

1.3   Autonomic Innervation & Nervous Control

There is extensive sympathetic and parasympathetic innervation of the SA and AV nodes [39]. The cardiac plexus, formed by sympathetic nerves originating from the upper thoracic spinal cord and parasympathetics from the medulla, surrounds the aortic arch and is the source of the cardiac autonomic innervation. The rate of depolarization and generation of action potentials in the SA node is exquisitely sensitive to the level of sympathetic and parasympathetic tone. Enhanced parasympathetic activity or decreased sympathetic activity results in a decrease in the rate of depolarization in the SA node, decreasing the rate of action potential generation, as well as increased conduction time through the AV node. On the other hand, enhanced sympathetic and reduced parasympathetic tone increases the rate of depolarization and action potential generation and decreases conduction time through the AV node. While the SA and AV node regions receive extensive autonomic innervation, sparse innervation is noted distal to the AV node, including the His bundle and bundle branches.

1.4 Mechanisms of Cardiac Arrhythmias

The three major mechanisms for clinical cardiac arrhythmias, *reentry, abnormal automaticity*, and *triggered activity*, are discussed in more detail elsewhere (see Table 3-10. on page 115 and "Concept of excitable gap" on page 121). Without doubt, *reentry with circus movement* is the most common mechanism responsible for the generation of clinical cardiac arrhythmias. However, triggered activity and abnormal automaticity appear to play a role in some clinical tachyarrhythmias. Much of the discussion in the later chapters of this book will focus on the details of the mechanisms responsible for specific arrhythmias.

1.4.1 REENTRY

The significance of reentry as a mechanism of clinical arrhythmias has been appreciated since the model of Mines in 1913 (Figure 1-5, Panel A) [40]. Implicit to this model is the existence of a fully excitable gap (white part of the circuit) between the crest of the excitation wave and its tail of relative refractoriness (dotted area). The model of Lewis [41,42] (Figure 1-5, Panel B), involves circus movement around two obstacles. A *functional* conduction block is hypothesized in the isthmus region between the two anatomical obstacles. As long as the excitable gap remains shorter than the circumference of the smaller of the two obstacles, "short-circuiting" of the circulating impulse through the isthmus is prevented, and the cycle length is determined by the revolution time around both obstacles.

In Moe's model of intra-atrial reentry [43,44] (Figure 1-5, Panel C), rapidly conducting muscle bundles like the internodal bands and Bachmann's bundle form closed loops that serve as preferential circuits through which flutter waves may circulate.

The leading circle model of reentry of Allessie [45-47] does not require a fixed anatomic obstacle to define the length of a circular pathway (Figure 1-5, Panel D). Instead the reentrant circuit in which the impulse circulates is completely defined by the functional electrophysiologic properties of the fibers composing the circuit. Under these circumstances, the smallest possible pathway in which the impulse can circulate is the circuit in which the "stimulating efficacy" of the impulse is just enough to excite the tissue ahead. Thus, the perimeter of the leading circle is equal to the wavelength of refractoriness of the circulating impulse. In the center of the leading circle, dimensions are too small for sustained circus movement, and the central area of the leading circle is activated by small centripetal wavelets that collide in the middle of the circuit creating a functional site of block which prevents "short-circuiting" of the reentrant wave. This model predicts a small or undetectable excitable gap.

From these various historical and ongoing studies, the picture that emerges is that while the details of reentrant mechanism responsible for clinical arrhythmias may vary from patient-to-patient and from tachyarrhythmia-to-tachyarrhythmia, fundamental prin-

ciples are remarkably consistent and are summarized in Figure 1-6. The fundamental
components of reentry circuits include: 1) an entry-way allowing a premature depolarizing wavefront access to the circuit; 2) an exit-way allowing the reentrant wavefront access to the myocardium at large; 3) at least two conducting limbs of tissue connected at
their distal and proximal ends which are usually separated by; 4) a central and peripheral
anatomic obstacle and/or functional region of conduction block; 5) a region of unidirec-

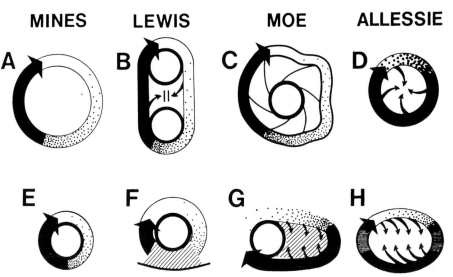

FIGURE 1-5. Models of reentry. Panel A shows the simplest model of reentry, in which the impulse continuously encircles a large anatomic obstacle. Panel B proposes circus movement around two anatomical obstacles, such as the venae cavae, in association with a central area of functional conduction block. Panel C
illustrates Moe's model of intra-atrial reentry in which rapidly conducting muscle bundles form closed loops
that serve as preferential circuits through which reentrant waves circulate. Panel D shows Allessie's leading
circle model of reentry. This model does not require a fixed anatomic obstacle to define the length of a circular
pathway; instead the reentrant circuit in which the impulse circulates is completely defined by the functional
electrophysiologic properties of the fibers composing the circuit. The perimeter of the leading circle is equal to
the wavelength of refractoriness of the circulating impulse. In the lower row of this figure are some additional
variants of intramyocardial circuits are given. In panel E, shortening of the wavelength of the impulse facilitates reentry. Under these conditions, some of the natural openings in the heart may become big enough to
serve as central anatomic obstacles for stable reentry. Conditions that shorten the wavelength also will favor
leading circle reentry, because a smaller arc of functional conduction block may suffice to initiate reentrant
excitation within the myocardium. In panel F, an area of depressed conduction is assumed between two anatomic boundaries. The presence of such an isthmus of depressed conduction will stabilize the re-entrant process
because it produces an excitable gap in the healthy part of the circuit. In panel G, an area of prolonged refractoriness neighbors an anatomic obstacle. The revolution time in such a circular pathway may be long enough to
create an excitable gap in the normal myocardium. Only at the free end of the arc of functional conduction
block in the area with prolonged refractoriness, there is a tight fit between the circulating depolarization wave
and its tail of refractoriness. This functionally determined turning point is the only unstable part of the circuit.
During subsequent cycles the impulse may pivot at slightly different points, resulting in only minor variations
in size and cycle length of the circuit. However, the localization of the circuit will be fixed, and the resulting
re-entrant arrhythmia could last for a long time. Panel H illustrates the concept of anisotropic reentry. The
properties of anisotropic reentry are (1) the central functional arc of conduction block is oriented parallel to the
long axis of the muscle fibers; (2) the circuit is ellipsoid in shape; (3) conduction velocity along the circuit is
not constant but fast along the long axis and slow at either of the two pivoting points; and (4) the anisotropy at
the pivoting points creates an excitable gap. Tissue that is absolutely refractory is signified by full black fill.
Tissue which is relatively reractory is speckled (black dots on white background). Fully excitable tissue is indicated by complete white fill. From [111] with permission.

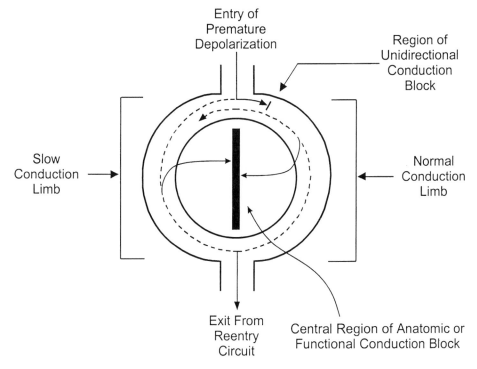

FIGURE 1-6. Schematic diagram illustrating simplified hypothetical reentry circuit. A premature depolarization wavefront blocks in one limb of the circuit and then conducts anterograde in the other. Because conduction is slow, by the time the impulse returns to its original entry point in the reentry circuit, the tissue is no longer refractory and conduction can reenter the circuit leading to a sustained tachycardia. See text for details.

tional conduction block to a premature depolarization in one of the conduction limbs, and finally; and 6) (especially in cases in micro-reentry), a region of slow conduction within the other conduction limb. While not always required, slow conduction enhances the stability of the reentrant circuit and increases the arrhythmia inducibility by shortening the reentrant wavelength (in cm) [= conduction velocity (in cm/ms) x refractory period (in msec)]. The shorter the wavelength, the shorter the anatomic length of myocardial tissue that can support a reentrant circuit. As the reentrant wavelength gets shorter (relative to the length of the anatomic circuit), the excitable gap gets larger, increasing the possibility that a premature depolarization will be able to enter the reentrant circuit at a time that the tissue is excitable. An understanding of these basic concepts will become useful when we discuss the mechanism of antiarrhythmic drugs (see "Termination of Reentry by Antiarrhythmic Drugs" on page 121).

In any model of reentry, the length of the excitation wave plays a crucial role both in the initiation and perpetuation of circulating propagation. When the wavelength (defined as the product of refractory period and conduction velocity) is long, a large area of unidirectional conduction block is required to make the impulse reenter itself. Conversely, when the reentrant wavelength is short, either by depressed conduction or by a short refractory period, small areas of conduction block already may set up reentrant circuits.

Because conduction block is more likely to occur in a small than in a large part of the myocardium, the *inducibility* of reentrant arrhythmias also will be directly related to the length of the cardiac impulse. For the perpetuation of reentrant rhythms, the wavelength is of crucial importance. Interventions that prolong the wavelength will increase the minimal size of intramyocardial circuits. If an excitable gap is present in the reentrant loop, prolongation of the wavelength will first reduce and finally close the excitable gap, leading to instability and a high chance of block of the circulating impulse.

As mentioned above, in order to sustain a stable reentrant circuit, a central boundary and a peripheral boundary are required in order to prevent "short circuiting", thereby maintaining conduction within the reentrant circuit. The classic example of reentry is exhibited in patients with Wolff-Parkinson-White Syndrome. These patients often develop a reentrant tachycardia involving both the atria and ventricles. The critical, protected part of the reentrant circuit involves the accessory AV connection and the normal AV connection (His bundle). Both these AV connections are electrically isolated from surrounding conductive tissues by normal fibrous tissue, including the central fibrous body and the annulus fibrosus, which prevents "short circuiting" and extinction of the circulating reentrant impulse. Other macroreentrant circuits are also possible, including the typical clockwise or counterclockwise atrial flutter circuits, or the circuit responsible for bundle branch reentrant ventricular tachycardia. Microreentry involves a circular reentry impulse traveling within a very small reentry circuit. In this case, a well-protected region of slow conduction generally provides maintenance of the reentry circuit. The reentry circuit can be very small if conduction is slow enough within a particular region. This is because, very slow conduction would allow adjacent, normally-conducting regions of the reentry circuit to recover excitability before the reentrant impulse again encounters that tissue. Microreentry is responsible for AV nodal reentrant tachycardia in which the slow conduction pathway provides the region of protected slow conduction. Microreentry may also be the mechanism responsible for many forms of ventricular tachycardia in patients with a myocardial scar from a previous myocardial infarction. However, the exact mechanism(s) by which microreentry occurs remains to be determined, but it may partially result from *anisotropic conduction* resulting from disparities in conduction velocity of the cardiac impulse depending upon whether it is occurring perpendicular or parallel to the long axis of myocardial fiber orientation.

In the electrophysiology laboratory, reentrant tachycardias are generally inducible with premature extrastimuli that are delivered with appropriate timing to enter the reentrant circuit. Similarly, appropriately timed premature stimuli that enter the reentrant circuit may terminate or reset the tachycardia (see "Mapping Using Concealed Entrainment" on page 147). Overdrive pacing at a rate faster than a reentrant tachycardia may terminate or entrain the tachycardia if the paced impulses succeed in entering the reentrant circuit (see "Mechanism of pacing-induced termination of reentrant tachyarrhythmias" on page 354 and Figure 6-62). While there are exceptions, vagal maneuvers, β-adrenergic blockers, Ca^{++}-channel blockers, or adenosine usually have no effect on the conduction of the tachycardia impulse within a reentrant circuit that does not utilize the AV node as part of the circuit.

1.4.2 ABNORMAL AUTOMATICITY

Abnormal impulse formation may be responsible for some tachyarrhythmias, particularly some focal atrial or ventricular tachycardias. It is assumed that a small cluster of cells demonstrating abnormal automaticity, often responsive to catecholamines, is responsible for tachycardia initiation. This mechanism may be particularly likely if the nest of abnormal cells is poorly-coupled to the adjacent large area of myocardium, protecting the cells from electrotonic interactions from the normal myocardium (i.e., impulses can exit, but not enter, the cluster of abnormal cells). Unlike reentrant tachycardias, automatic tachycardias are generally not provoked using programmed electrical stimulation or rapid pacing protocols. However, these tachycardias may be spontaneously initiated during the administration of exogenous catecholamines. They typically exhibit a "warm-up" phenomenon (progressive acceleration of rate during first few beats after onset) and a "warm-down" phenomenon (progressive deceleration of rate during last few beats before termination). Tachyarrhythmias due to abnormal automaticity often exhibit transient suppression (but not termination) by rapid overdrive pacing, but the arrhythmia quickly resumes after cessation of pacing. Likewise, vagal maneuvers and adenosine may cause transient suppression and, because it may be catecholamine-sensitive, β-adrenergic blocking agents may provide long term suppression.

1.4.3 TRIGGERED ACTIVITY

Rarely, triggered activity due to early or delayed afterdepolarizations may be the mechanism responsible for some cardiac tachyarrhythmias. Possible examples include atrial and ventricular tachyarrhythmias resulting from digitalis intoxication and ventricular tachycardia originating in the right ventricular outflow tract of some patients with structurally normal hearts. In the electrophysiology laboratory, rapid fixed-rate pacing may provoke tachycardias caused by triggered activity, which is often facilitated by catecholamines. Overdrive termination and acceleration may be observed, and vagal maneuvers, adenosine, or β-adrenergic and Ca^{++} channel blocking agents may slow or terminate triggered tachyarrhythmias.

1.5 Arrhythmogenic Anatomy

A number of normal and abnormal anatomical structures (Figure 1-7) have been implicated in the genesis of cardiac arrhythmias (Table 1-1.) These arrhythmias and their anatomical bases will be discussed in more detail later in this book.

Sinoatrial reentrant tachycardia (high cristal focal tachycardia, see "Classification of Atrial Tachycardias" on page 609 & see "Focal Atrial Tachycardia" on page 610) may result from reentry within the SA node or the SA node and adjacent atrial myocardium. Likewise, there is still debate whether the anatomic substrate for AV node reentry lies entirely within the confines of the AV node proper or may also involve adjacent atrial tissue, possibly atrial myocardium or transitional cells.

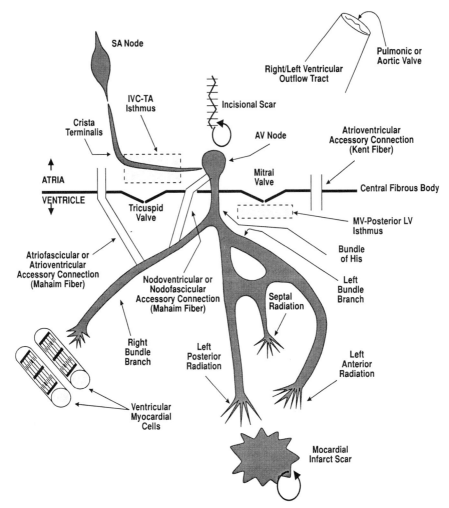

FIGURE 1-7. Schematic illustration summarizing the locations of many of the known anatomical substrates associated with the development of cardiac arrhythmias. Refer to the text for details. AV, atrioventricular; IVC, inferior vena cava; LV, left ventricle; MV, mitral valve; SA, sinoatrial; TA, tricuspid annulus.

In the fully developed human heart, the atrial and ventricular myocardia are almost completely electrically insulated from each other by fibrous atrioventricular rings (*annulus fibrosus*). Only at the AV node-His bundle region is electrical continuity established, permitting cardiac impulse conduction from the atria to the ventricles. As long as the insulation of the annulus fibrosus is not breached, atrial impulses are conducted to the ventricle only by way of the AV node-His-Purkinje system [48,49]. Because of its decremental conduction properties, the AV node functions as a protective barrier [50], delaying AV conduction and preventing an excessive number of atrial impulses from reaching the ventricles. When the annulus fibrosus insulation is disrupted or the normal AV node-His-Purkinje pathway is short-circuited by an accessory AV connection, the

TABLE 1-1. Anatomic substrates associated with the development of cardiac arrhythmias

Anatomic Structure	Type of Arrhythmia	Mechanism of Arrhythmia
SA node + adjacent tissues	SART	Microreentry
AV node + adjacent tissues	AVNRT	Microreentry
Accessory connection (Kent-fiber)	Orthodromic & antidromic AVRT	Macroreentry
Accessory connection (PJRT-type)	Orthodromic AVRT with long R-P' interval	Macroreentry
Accessory connection (Mahaim-fiber)	Antidromic AVRT	Macroreentry
Crista terminalis	AT	Reentry/automaticity/triggered activity?
Atrial isthmus: IVC-TV annulus & crista terminalis	AFL	Macroreentry
Bundle branches (with IVCD)	Bundle branch reentrant VT or fascicular tachycardia	Macroreentry
Myocardial scar (+ isthmus) associated with infarct or cardiomyopathy	AT, AF, VT, VF	Macroreentry or microreentry
Ventricular isthmus: MV annulus-posterior basilar left ventricular MI scar	VT	Macroreentry or microreentry
Subvalvular right or left ventricular outflow tracts	VT	Reentry/automaticity/triggered activity?
Right or left ventricular dysplasia	VT	Macroreentry or microreentry
Pulmonary veins (ostial regions & muscular "sleeves")	AF, AT, AFL	Automaticity/triggered activity/microreentry?
"Remodeled" atria	AF	Reentry (multiple wavefronts?)
Healed atrial myocardial surgical incision	AT, AFL	Macroreentry or microreentry

AF, atrial fibrillation; AFL, atrial flutter; AT, atrial tachycardia; AV, atrioventricular; AVNRT, atrioventricular node reentrant tachycardia; AVRT, atrioventricular reciprocating tachycardia; IVC, inferior vena cava; IVCD, intraventricular conduction delay; MI, myocardial infarction; MV, mitral valve; PJRT, permanent form of junctional reciprocating tachycardia; SA, sinoatrial; SART, sinoatrial reentrant tachycardia; TV, tricuspid valve; VF, ventricular fibrillation; VT, ventricular tachycardia

ventricle can be excited earlier than would normally be expected. This phenomenon is referred to as *ventricular preexcitation* [51,52]. Based on findings of anatomical and electrophysiological studies, accessory connections can be classified into several forms [51]: (1) accessory AV muscle bundles; (2) accessory nodoventricular muscle bundles; (3) atriofascicular bypass tracts; (4) intranodal bypass tracts; (5) nodal malformations; and (6) fasciculoventricular accessory connections. Some of these accessory connections have been demonstrated to exist only anatomically or electrophysiologically, a few have been demonstrated to exist both anatomically and electrophysiologically, but others are only hypothetical and remain very much debatable. The tachyarrhythmias associated with the ventricular preexcitation syndromes are the best studied examples of reentry (circus movement) and are discussed in detail later in this book (see "Ventricular Preexcitation Syndromes: The Wolff-Parkinson-White Syndrome and Variants" on page 539).

The crista terminalis [53-56] is a ridge of tissue which runs posteriorly from the "tail" of the SA node along the lateral right atrial wall and then medially to merge with the eustachian ridge, which ends near the ostium of the coronary sinus. During its route, the crista and eustachian ridge provide the posterior border of the isthmus of atrial tissue forming the floor of the right atrium lying between the inferior vena cava and tricuspid valve annulus (IVC-TV isthmus). Typical clockwise and counterclockwise atrial flutters traverse this isthmus as part of their macroreentry circuits and this isthmus has become the anatomic target for curative catheter ablation of typical atrial flutters (Figure 1-8). In addition, along its course the crista terminalis appears to provide fertile ground for the origin of atrial tachycardia [53-56] due to automaticity, triggered activity, or reentry. Atrial tachycardia related to a healed atrial scar from a past surgical incision for repair of an atrial septal defect, other congenital heart disease, or valvular heart disease is also been described [57,58]. Most recently, the ostia of the pulmonary veins have been recognized a frequent source of atrial premature depolarizations and rapid atrial tachycardias that can trigger atrial fibrillation and atrial flutter. Ablation of these triggering foci may provide a curative treatment for selected patients with atrial fibrillation and atrial flutter [59,60]. Finally, "remodeling" of the atria due to dilation, enlargement, and stretch resulting from atrial fibrillation may predispose to more atrial fibrillation [61-66]. Atrial tachycardia, atrial flutter, and atrial fibrillation are discussed in more detail later (see "Atrial Tachycardias and Atrial Flutter" on page 609. and "Atrial Fibrillation" on page 657.

Various forms of ventricular tachycardia have been associated with specific anatomical structures. Ventricular tachycardias originating in the right and left ventricular outflow tracts have been identified [67-76]. In each case, the tachycardia focus appears to be located immediately proximal to the pulmonic valve or aortic valve, respectively. The mechanism of these tachycardias are still open to debate and may have characteristics consistent with automaticity, reentry, triggered activity, or possibly all three. Recent data utilizing magnetic resonance imaging suggests that the foci of tachycardia in some of these patients may not be entirely structurally normal [77,78]. Bundle branch reentrant ventricular tachycardia utilizing the main right and left bundle branches along with a poorly-defined trans-septal myocardial pathway for macro-reentry has also been described [79-82]. In addition, fascicular tachycardias that exclusively utilize the His-Purkinje system for macroreentry has also been observed [83-89]. Ventricular tachycar-

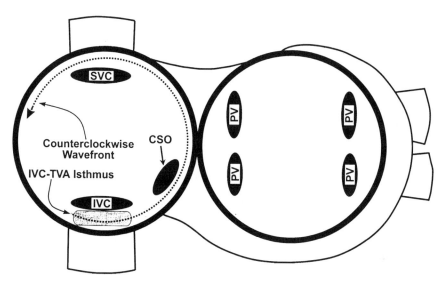

FIGURE 1-8. Cross-section view through the atrioventricular groove at the level of the mitral and tricuspid valve annulae as seen from the cardiac apex. The reentrant wavefront in patients with the typical clockwise and conterclockwise (shown here) forms of atrial flutter conduct through the isthmus bordered by the inferior vena cava (IVC) and the tricuspid valve annulus (TVA). The IVC-TVA isthmus is the anatomic target during ablation of typical atrial flutter. CSO, ostium of the coronary sinus; PV, pulmonary vein; SVC, superior vena cava. See text for additional discussion.

dia related to right and/or left ventricular dysplasia involving replacement of normal myocardium with fat and fibrous tissue has also been reported [90-98]. Clearly the most common and most dangerous cause of ventricular tachycardia is myocardial reentrant ventricular tachycardia related to an old myocardial infarct scar [99-108]. Classically, this form of tachycardia is related to residual viable myocardium, possibly at the border zone of the infarct scar, which contains a zone of slow conduction and unidirectional conduction block. However, recently, the concept of a viable isthmus region lying between two areas of non-conducting tissue has been proposed as a substrate for this form of ventricular tachycardia, in a fashion analogous to atrial flutter in the right atrium. Specifically, in some patients with a posterior basilar and left ventricular myocardial infarct scar, a viable isthmus between the scar and the posterior aspect of the mitral valve annulus may be responsible for macro-reentry in these patients [109,110]. Monomorphic ventricular tachycardia is discussed in detail in on page 687.

CHAPTER 1

References

1. Anderson RH, Janse MJ, van Capelle FJ, et al.: A combined morphological and electrophysiological study of the atrioventricular node of the rabbit heart. *Circ Res* **35**:909-22, 1974.

2. Anderson RH, Becker AE, Tranum-Jensen J, Janse MJ: Anatomico-electrophysiological correlations in the conduction system--a review. *Br Heart J* **45**:67-82, 1981.

3. Becker AE, Anderson RH. Morphology of the human atrioventricular junctional area. In: Wellens HJJ, Lie KI, Janse MJ, eds. *The Conduction System of the Heart: Structure, Function and Clinical Implication.* Leiden, The Netherlands: Sterfest Kroese BV, 263-286: 1976.

4. Becker AE, Anderson RH, Durrer D, Wellens HJ: The anatomical substrates of Wolff-Parkinson-White syndrome. A clinicopathologic correlation in seven patients. *Circulation* **57**:870-9, 1978.

5. Bharati S, Rosen KM, Towne WD, Lev M: The conduction system in the baboon heart. *Chest* **75**:62-6, 1979.

6. Bharati S, Nordenberg A, Bauernfiend R, et al.: The anatomic substrate for the sick sinus syndrome in adolescence. *Am J Cardiol* **46**:163-72, 1980.

7. Janse MJ, Capelle FJV, Anderson RH, et al.: Correlation between electrophysiologic recordings and morphologic findings in the rabbit atrioventricular node. *Arch Int Physiol Biochim* **82**:331-2, 1974.

8. Inoue S, Becker AE: Posterior extensions of the human compact atrioventricular node: a neglected anatomic feature of potential clinical significance. *Circulation* **97**:188-93, 1998.

9. Lev M, Unger PN, Rosen KM, Bharati S: The anatomic substrate of complete left bundle branch block. *Circulation* **50**:479-86, 1974.

10. Lev M, Fox SMD, Bharati S, et al.: Mahaim and James fibers as a basis for a unique variety of ventricular preexcitation. *Am J Cardiol* **36**:880-8, 1975.

11. Lev M, Unger PN, Rosen KM, Bharati S: The anatomic base of the electrocardiographic abnormality left bundle branch block. *Adv Cardiol* **14**:16-24, 1975.

12. McGuire MA, de Bakker JM, Vermeulen JT, et al.: Atrioventricular junctional tissue. Discrepancy between histological and electrophysiological characteristics. *Circulation* **94**:571-7, 1996.

13. Racker DK: Atrioventricular node and input pathways: A correlated gross anatomical and histological study of the canine atrioventricular junctional region. *Anat Rec* **224**:336-354, 1989.

14. Davies MJ, Anderson RH, Becker AE: *The Conduction System of the Heart.* London: Butterworth, 1983.

15. Bharati S, Lev M. The anatomy and pathology of the conduction system. In: Samet P, El-Sherif N, eds. *Cardiac Pacing.* Orlando, FL: Grune & Stratton: 1980.

16. Becker AE: Atrioventricular nodal anatomy revisited. *Learning Center:*17-22, 1994.

17. Fitzgerald D, Lazzara R: Functional anatomy of the conduction system. *Hosp Pract (Off Ed)* **23**:81-90, 92, 1988.

18. Sealy WC, Gallagher JJ, Pritchett EL: The surgical anatomy of Kent bundles based on electrophysiological mapping and surgical exploration. *J Thorac Cardiovasc Surg* **76**:804-15, 1978.

19. Rossi L: Interatrial, internodal and dual reentrant atrioventricular nodal pathways: an anatomical update of arrhythmogenic substrates. *Cardiologia* **41**:129-134, 1996.

20. Keith A, Flack M: The form and nature of the muscular connections between the primary divisions of the vertebrate heart. *J Anat Physiol* **41**:172-189, 1907.

21. James TN: Morphology of the human atrioventricular node, with remarks pertinent to its electrophysiology. *Am Heart J* **62**:756-771, 1961.

22. Hecht HH, Kossmann CE, Childers RW, et al.: Atrioventricular and intraventricular conduction. Revised nomenclature and concepts. *Am J Cardiol* **31**:232-44, 1973.

23. Tawara S: *Das Reizleitungssystem des Saugetierherzens.* Jena: Gustav Fisher, 1906.

24. Truex RC, Smythe MO: Reconstruction of the human atrioventricular node. *Anat Rec* **158**:11-20, 1967.

25. McGuire MA, Johnson DC, Robotin M, et al.: Dimensions of the triangle of Koch in humans. *Am J Cardiol* **70**:829-30, 1992.

26. Widran J, Lev M: The dissection of the atrioventricular node, bundle and bundle branches in the human heart. *Circulation* **4**:863-867, 1951.

27. Racker DK: Sinoventricular transmission in 10 M K+ by canine atrioventricular nodal inputs. Superior atrionodal bundle and proximal atrioventricular bundle. *Circulation* **83**:1738-1753, 1991.

28. Janse MJ, van Capelle FJL, Anderson RH, et al.: Electrophysiology and structure of the atrioventricular node of the isolated rabbit heart. In: Wellens HJJ, Lie KI, Janse MJ, eds. *The Conduction System of the Heart: Structure, Function and Clinical Implication.* Leiden, The Netherlands: Sterfest Kroese BV, 296-315: 1976.

29. Janse MK, Anderson RH, van Capelle FJ, Durrer D: A combined electrophysiological and anatomical study of the human fetal heart. *Am Heart J* **91**:556-62, 1976.

30. Janse MJ: Influence of the direction of the atrial wave front on A-V nodal transmission in isolated hearts of rabbits. *Circ Res* **25**:439-49, 1969.

31. Meijler FL, Janse MJ: Morphology and electrophysiology of the mammalian atrioventricular node. *Physiol Rev* **68**:608-47, 1988.

32. Zipes DP, Mendez C, Moe GK: Evidence for summation and voltage dependency in rabbit atrioventricular nodal fibers. *Circ Res* **32**:170-7, 1973.

33. Sherf L, James TN, Woods WT: Function of the atrioventricular node considered on the basis of observed histology and fine structure. *J Am Coll Cardiol* **5**:770-780, 1985.

34. Oosthoek PW, Viragh S, Lamers WH, Moorman AF: Immunohistochemical delineation of the conduction system. II: The atrioventricular node and Purkinje fibers. *Circ Res* **73**:482-91, 1993.

35. Oosthoek PW, Viragh S, Mayen AE, et al.: Immunohistochemical delineation of the conduction system. I: The sinoatrial node. *Circ Res* **73**:473-81, 1993.

36. Sugi Y, Hirakaw R: Freeze-fracture studies of the sinoatrial and atrioventricular nodes of the caprine heart, with special reference to the nexus. *Cell Tissue Res* **245**:273-279, 1986.

37. Davis LM, Rodefeld ME, Green K, et al.: Gap junction protein phenotypes of the human heart and conduction system. *J Cardiovasc Electrophysiol* **6**:813-22, 1995.

38. Spach MS, Josephson ME: Initiating reentry: the role of nonuniform anisotropy in small circuits. *J Cardiovasc Electrophysiol* **5**:182-209, 1994.

39. Randall WC. Differential autonomic control of SAN and AVN regions of the canine heart: structure and function . In: Mazgalev T, Dreifus LS, Michelson EL, eds. *Progress in Clinical Biological Research: Electrophysiology of the Sinoatrial and Atrioventricular Nodes* . New York: Alan R. Liss, 15-31: 1988.

40. Mines GR: On dynamic equilibrium in the heart. *J Physiol (London)* **46**:349-383, 1913.

41. Lewis T: *The mechanism and graphic registration of the heartbeat.* 3rd ed. London: Shaw & Sons, 1925.

42. Lewis T: Observations upon flutter and fibrillation: IV. Impure flutter: Theory of circus movement. *Heart* **7**:293, 1920.

43. Moe GK, Pastelin G, Mendez R. Circus movement excitation of the atria. In: Little RC, ed. *Physiology of Atrial Pacemakers and Conductive Tissue.* Mt. Kisco, New York: Futura Publishing, 207-220: 1980.

44. Pastelin G, Mendez R, Moe GK: Participation of atrial specialized conduction pathways in atrial flutter. *Circ Res* **42**:386-93, 1978.

45. Allessie MA, Bonke FI, Schopman FJ: Circus movement in rabbit atrial muscle as a mechanism of trachycardia. *Circ Res* **33**:54-62, 1973.

46. Allessie MA, Bonke FI, Schopman FJ: Circus movement in rabbit atrial muscle as a mechanism of tachycardia. II. The role of nonuniform recovery of excitability in the occurrence of unidirectional block, as studied with multiple microelectrodes. *Circ Res* **39**:168-77, 1976.

47. Allessie MA, Bonke FI, Schopman FJ: Circus movement in rabbit atrial muscle as a mechanism of tachycardia. III. The "leading circle" concept: a new model of circus movement in cardiac tissue without the involvement of an anatomical obstacle. *Circ Res* **41**:9-18, 1977.

48. Lev M: Anatomic basis for atrioventricular block. *Am J Med* **37**:742, 1964.

49. Truex RC, Bishof JK, Hoffman EL: Accessory atrioventricular bundles of the developing human heart. *Anat Rec* **135**:45, 1958.

50. Childers R: The AV node: Normal and abnormal physiology. *Prog Cardiovasc Dis* **13**:361, 1977.

51. Anderson RH, Becker AE, Brechenmacher C, et al.: Ventricular preexcitation: A proposed nomenclature for its substrates. *Eur J Cardiol* **3**:27, 1975.

52. Gallagher JJ, Gilbert M, Svenson RH, et al.: Wolff-Parkinson-White syndrome. The problem, evaluation, and surgical correction. *Circulation* **51**:767-85, 1975.

53. Kalman JM, Olgin JE, Saxon LA, et al.: Activation and entrainment mapping defines the tricuspid annulus as the anterior barrier in typical atrial flutter. *Circulation* **94**:398-406, 1996.

54. Olgin JE, Kalman JM, Fitzpatrick AP, Lesh MD: Role of right atrial endocardial structures as barriers to conduction during human type I atrial flutter. Activation and entrainment mapping guided by intracardiac echocardiography. *Circulation* **92**:1839-48, 1995.

55. Olgin JE, Kalman JM, Lesh MD: Conduction barriers in human atrial flutter: correlation of electrophysiology and anatomy. *J Cardiovasc Electrophysiol* **7**:1112-26, 1996.

56. Kalman JM, Olgin JE, Karch MR, et al.: "Cristal tachycardias": origin of right atrial tachycardias from the crista terminalis identified by intracardiac echocardiography. *J Am Coll Cardiol* **31**:451-9, 1998.

57. Kalman JM, VanHare GF, Olgin JE, et al.: Ablation of 'incisional' reentrant atrial tachycardia complicating surgery for congenital heart disease. Use of entrainment to define a critical isthmus of conduction. *Circulation* **93**:502-12, 1996.

58. Lesh MD, Kalman JM, Saxon LA, Dorostkar PC: Electrophysiology of "incisional" reentrant atrial tachycardia complicating surgery for congenital heart disease. *Pacing Clin Electrophysiol* **20**:2107-11, 1997.

59. Haissaguerre M, Jais P, Shah DC, et al.: Spontaneous initiation of atrial fibrillation by ectopic beats originating in the pulmonary veins. *N Engl J Med* **339**:659-66, 1998.

60. Haissaguerre M, Shah DC, Jais P, Clementy J: Role of catheter ablation for atrial fibrillation. *Curr Opin Cardiol* **12**:18-23, 1997.

61. Elvan A, Wylie K, Zipes DP: Pacing-induced chronic atrial fibrillation impairs sinus node function in dogs. Electrophysiological remodeling. *Circulation* **94**:2953-60, 1996.

62. Daoud EG, Knight BP, Weiss R, et al.: Effect of verapamil and procainamide on atrial fibrillation-induced electrical remodeling in humans. *Circulation* **96**:1542-50, 1997.

63. Goette A, Honeycutt C, Langberg JJ: Electrical remodeling in atrial fibrillation. Time course and mechanisms. *Circulation* **94**:2968-2974, 1996.

64. Tieleman RG, Van Gelder IC, Crijns HJ, et al.: Early recurrences of atrial fibrillation after electrical cardioversion: a result of fibrillation-induced electrical remodeling of the atria? *J Am Coll Cardiol* **31**:167-73, 1998.

65. Wijffels MC, Kirchhof CJ, Dorland R, et al.: Electrical remodeling due to atrial fibrillation in chronically instrumented conscious goats: roles of neurohumoral changes, ischemia, atrial stretch, and high rate of electrical activation. *Circulation* **96**:3710-20, 1997.

66. Yue L, Feng J, Gaspo R, et al.: Ionic remodeling underlying action potential changes in a dog model of atrial fibrillation. *Circulation Research* **81**:512-525, 1997.

67. Nibley C, Wharton JM: Ventricular tachycardias with left bundle branch block morphology. *Pacing Clin Electrophysiol* **18**:334-56, 1995.

68. Ng KS, Wen MS, Yeh SJ, et al.: The effects of adenosine on idiopathic ventricular tachycardia. *Am J Cardiol* **74**:195-7, 1994.

69. Lokhandwala YY, Smeets JL, Rodriguez LM, et al.: Idiopathic ventricular tachycardia--characterisation and radiofrequency ablation. *Indian Heart J* **46**:281-5, 1994.

70. Merliss AD, Seifert MJ, Collins RF, et al.: Catheter ablation of idiopathic left ventricular tachycardia associated with a false tendon. *Pacing Clin Electrophysiol* **19**:2144-6, 1996.

71. Mont L, Seixas T, Brugada P, et al.: The electrocardiographic, clinical, and electrophysiologic spectrum of idiopathic monomorphic ventricular tachycardia. *Am Heart J* **124**:746-53, 1992.

72. Okumura K, Yamabe H, Tsuchiya T, et al.: Characteristics of slow conduction zone demonstrated during entrainment of idiopathic ventricular tachycardia of left ventricular origin. *Am J Cardiol* **77**:379-83, 1996.

73. Nishizaki M, Arita M, Sakurada H, et al.: Demonstration of Purkinje potential during idiopathic left ventricular tachycardia: a marker for ablation site by transient entrainment. *Pacing Clin Electrophysiol* **20**:3004-7, 1997.

74. Vora AM, Tang AS, Green MS: Idiopathic left ventricular tachycardia: what is the mechanism? *Pacing Clin Electrophysiol* **20**:2855-6, 1997.

75. Wen MS, Yeh SJ, Wang CC, et al.: Radiofrequency ablation therapy in idiopathic left ventricular tachycardia with no obvious structural heart disease. *Circulation* **89**:1690-6, 1994.

76. Zardini M, Thakur RK, Klein GJ, Yee R: Catheter ablation of idiopathic left ventricular tachycardia. *Pacing Clin Electrophysiol* **18**:1255-65, 1995.

77. Markowitz SM, Litvak BL, Ramirez de Arellano EA, et al.: Adenosine-sensitive ventricular tachycardia: right ventricular abnormalities delineated by magnetic resonance imaging. *Circulation* **96**:1192-200, 1997.

78. Carlson MD, White RD, Trohman RG, et al.: Right ventricular outflow tract ventricular tachycardia: detection of previously unrecognized anatomic abnormalities using cine magnetic resonance imaging. *J Am Coll Cardiol* **24**:720-7, 1994.

79. Blanck Z, Dhala A, Deshpande S, et al.: Bundle branch reentrant ventricular tachycardia: cumulative experience in 48 patients. *J Cardiovasc Electrophysiol* **4**:253-62, 1993.

80. Blanck Z, Deshpande S, Jazayeri MR, Akhtar M: Catheter ablation of the left bundle branch for the treatment of sustained bundle branch reentrant ventricular tachycardia. *J Cardiovasc Electrophysiol* **6**:40-3, 1995.

81. Cohen TJ, Chien WW, Lurie KG, et al.: Radiofrequency catheter ablation for treatment of bundle branch reentrant ventricular tachycardia: results and long-term follow-up. *J Am Coll Cardiol* **18**:1767-73, 1991.

82. De Lima GG, Dubuc M, Roy D, Talajic M: Radiofrequency ablation of bundle branch reentrant tachycardia in a patient with atrial septal defect. *Can J Cardiol* **13**:403-5, 1997.

83. Bogun F, El-Atassi R, Daoud E, et al.: Radiofrequency ablation of idiopathic left anterior fascicular tachycardia. *J Cardiovasc Electrophysiol* **6**:1113-6, 1995.

84. Gonzalez RP, Scheinman MM, Lesh MD, et al.: Clinical and electrophysiologic spectrum of fascicular tachycardias. *Am Heart J* **128**:147-56, 1994.

85. Katritsis D, Heald S, Ahsan A, et al.: Catheter ablation for successful management of left posterior fascicular tachycardia: an approach guided by recording of fascicular potentials. *Heart* **75**:384-8, 1996.

86. Wieland JM, Marchlinski FE: Electrocardiographic response of digoxin-toxic fascicular tachycardia to Fab fragments: implications for tachycardia mechanism. *Pacing Clin Electrophysiol* **9**:727-38, 1986.

87. Vergara I, Wharton JM: Ventricular tachycardia and fibrillation in normal hearts. *Curr Opin Cardiol* **13**:9-19, 1998.

88. Kim SS, Gallastegui J, Welch WJ, Bauernfeind RA: Paroxysmal fascicular tachycardia and ventricular tachycardia due to mechanical stimulation by a mitral valve prosthesis. *J Am Coll Cardiol* **7**:176-9, 1986.

89. Crijns HJ, Smeets JL, Rodriguez LM, et al.: Cure of interfascicular reentrant ventricular tachycardia by ablation of the anterior fascicle of the left bundle branch. *J Cardiovasc Electrophysiol* **6**:486-92, 1995.

90. Berder V, Vauthier M, Mabo P, et al.: Characteristics and outcome in arrhythmogenic right ventricular dysplasia. *Am J Cardiol* **75**:411-4, 1995.

91. Blake LM, Scheinman MM, Higgins CB: MR features of arrhythmogenic right ventricular dysplasia. *AJR Am J Roentgenol* **162**:809-12, 1994.

92. Leclercq JF, Coumel P: Characteristics, prognosis and treatment of the ventricular arrhythmias of right ventricular dysplasia. *Eur Heart J* **10 Suppl D**:61-7, 1989.

93. Leclercq JF, Coumel P: Late potentials in arrhythmogenic right ventricular dysplasia. Prevalence, diagnostic and prognostic values. *Eur Heart J* **14 Suppl E**:80-3, 1993.

94. Leclercq JF, Potenza S, Maison-Blanche P, et al.: Determinants of spontaneous occurrence of sustained monomorphic ventricular tachycardia in right ventricular dysplasia. *J Am Coll Cardiol* **28**:720-4, 1996.

95. Manyari DE, Klein GJ, Gulamhusein S, et al.: Arrhythmogenic right ventricular dysplasia: a generalized cardiomyopathy? *Circulation* **68**:251-7, 1983.

96. Furlanello F, Bertoldi A, Dallago M, et al.: Cardiac arrest and sudden death in competitive athletes with arrhythmogenic right ventricular dysplasia. *Pacing Clin Electrophysiol* **21**:331-5, 1998.

97. Peters S: Right ventricular cardiomyopathy: diffuse dilatation, focal dysplasia or biventricular disease. *Int J Cardiol* **62**:63-7, 1997.

98. Proclemer A, Crani R, Feruglio GA: Right ventricular tachycardia with ventricular dysplasia: clinical features, diagnostic techniques and current management. *Am Heart J* **103**:415-420, 1989.

99. Horowitz LN, Vetter VL, Harken AH, Josephson ME: Electrophysiologic characteristics of sustained ventricular tachycardia occurring after repair of tetralogy of fallot. *Am J Cardiol* **46**:446-52, 1980.

100.   Horowitz LN, Josephson ME, Farshidi A, et al.: Recurrent sustained ventricular tachycardia. 3. Role of the electrophysiologic study in selection of antiarrhythmic regimens. *Circulation* **58**:986-97, 1978.

101.   Horowitz LN, Josephson ME, Harken AH: Epicardial and endocardial activation during sustained ventricular tachycardia in man. *Circulation* **61**:1227-38, 1980.

102.   Horowitz LN, Spielman SR, Greenspan AM, Josephson ME: Mechanisms in the genesis of recurrent ventricular tachyarrhythmias as revealed by clinical electrophysiologic studies. *Ann N Y Acad Sci* **382**:116-35, 1982.

103.   Horowitz LN, Spielman SR, Greenspan AM, Josephson ME: Role of programmed stimulation in assessing vulnerability to ventricular arrhythmias. *Am Heart J* **103**:604-10, 1982.

104.   Josephson ME, Horowitz LN: Recurrent ventricular tachycardia: an electrophysiologic approach. *Med Clin North Am* **63**:53-71, 1979.

105.   Josephson ME, Horowitz LN, Spielman SR, Greenspan AM: Electrophysiologic and hemodynamic studies in patients resuscitated from cardiac arrest. *Am J Cardiol* **46**:948-55, 1980.

106.   Josephson ME: Treatment of ventricular arrhythmias after myocardial infarction. *Circulation* **74**:653-8, 1986.

107.   Josephson ME, Wit AL: Fractionated electrical activity and continuous electrical activity: fact or artifact? *Circulation* **70**:529-32, 1984.

108.   Josephson ME, Almendral JM, Buxton AE, Marchlinski FE: Mechanisms of ventricular tachycardia. *Circulation* **75**:III41-7, 1987.

109.   Wilber DJ, Kopp DE, Glascock DN, et al.: Catheter ablation of the mitral isthmus for ventricular tachycardia associated with inferior infarction. *Circulation* **92**:3481-9, 1995.

110.   Hadjis TA, Stevenson WG, Harada T, et al.: Preferential locations for critical reentry circuit sites causing ventricular tachycardia after inferior wall myocardial infarction. *J Cardiovasc Electrophysiol* **8**:363-70, 1997.

111.   Allessie MA, Lammers WJEP, Rensma PL, et al.: Determinants of re-entry in cardiac muscle. . Philadelphia: Lea & Febiger, 3-15: 1988.

CHAPTER 2

BASIC PRINCIPLES OF CLINICAL CARDIAC ELECTROPHYSIOLOGY

A thorough understanding of basic electrophysiological principles is essential to the proper diagnosis and management of patients with cardiac arrhythmias. Included in this introductory chapter is a discussion of the indications for electrophysiology testing, the equipment and techniques used in a diagnostic electrophysiology study, and the electrophysiological properties of the cardiac conduction system

2.1 Electrophysiology Procedures: Preparation and Performance

The performance of a diagnostic or therapeutic electrophysiological procedure begins well before the patient enters the electrophysiology laboratory. Proper pre-procedure evaluation and selection of patients is, of course, crucial. But so also is the proper organization of the laboratory and its equipment as well as the assembly and training of the requisite personnel, be they medical, nursing, technical, radiological or from the field of biomedical engineering. It cannot be stressed enough that the safe and successful electrophysiological diagnosis and treatment of cardiac arrhythmias requires a dedicated team of specially-trained professionals from a variety of disciplines. These procedures should not be performed unless all these elements are in place.

2.1.1 GENERAL INDICATIONS FOR ELECTROPHYSIOLOGICAL PROCEDURES

In general, electrophysiology testing is indicated in patients with a documented arrhythmia, or symptoms likely due to an arrhythmia, when: 1) a precise electrophysiological diagnosis will effect, direct, or guide the choice of treatment; 2) a therapeutic intervention such as radiofrequency catheter ablation would offer a cure or alleviation of symptoms; or 3) useful prognostic information may be obtained, such as the risk of developing life-threatening brady- or tachyarrhythmias. The American College of Cardiology, American Heart Association, and North American Society of Pacing and Electrophysiology have jointly prepared and published consensus guidelines and indications for diagnostic electrophysiology testing under a variety of clinical situations for both brady-arrhythmias and tachyarrhythmias (Table 2-1. and Table 2-2.)

TABLE 2-1. Summary of indications for intracardiac electrophysiology testing in patients with documented or suspected bradyarrhythmias

Condition	Definitely Indicated	Uncertain or Possible Indication	Not Indicated
Sinoatrial (SA) Node Dysfunction	Symptomatic patients with suspected SA node dysfunction in the absence of documented correlation of symptoms with a bradyarrhythmia.	Patients with documented SA node dysfunction in whom evaluation of atrioventricular or ventriculoatrial conduction or susceptibility to arrhythmias may aid in selection of the best pacing modality.	Symptomatic patients with established association between symptoms and a documented bradyarrhythmia and choice of therapy would not be altered by electrophysiology testing
		To determine the mechanism of sinus bradyarrhythmias, i.e., intrinsic SA node disease, autonomic nervous system dysfunction, medication-induced	Asymptomatic patients with sinus bradyarrhythmias or sinus pauses noted only during sleep, including patients with sleep apnea.
		To evaluate the potential for other arrhythmias to explain the symptoms in symptomatic patients with sinus bradyarrhythmias.	
Acquired Atrioventricular (AV) Block	Symptomatic patients in whom His-Purkinje block, suspected as a cause of symptoms, has not been established.	Patients with 2nd or 3rd degree AV block in whom knowledge of the site of block or its mechanism or response to pharmacological or other temporary intervention may help direct therapy or assess prognosis	Symptomatic patients in whom the symptoms and presence of AV block are correlated with ECG findings.
	Patients with 2nd or 3rd degree AV block treated with a pacemaker who remain symptomatic and in whom another arrhythmia is suspected as a cause of the symptoms.	Patients with premature, concealed junctional depolarizations suspected as a cause of 2nd or 3rd degree AV block (i.e., pseudo AV block).	Asymptomatic patients with transient AV block associated with sinus slowing, e.g., nocturnal AV block, hypervagotonia, etc.
Chronic Intraventricular Conduction Delay	Symptomatic patients in whom the cause of symptoms is unknown.	Asymptomatic patients with bundle branch block in whom pharmacological therapy that could increase conduction delay or produce heart block is contemplated.	Asymptomatic patients with intraventricular conduction delay.
			Symptomatic patients whose symptoms can be correlated with or excluded by ECG events.

Adapted from ACC/AHA Task Force Report [1].

TABLE 2-2. Summary of indications for diagnostic intracardiac electrophysiology studies in patients with documented or suspected tachyarrhythmias

Condition	Indicated	Uncertain or possible indication	Not indicated
Narrow QRS Complex Tachycardia	Patients with frequent or poorly tolerated episodes of tachycardia that do not adequately respond to drug therapy and for whom information about site of origin, mechanism, and electrophysiological properties of the pathways of the tachycardia is essential for choosing appropriate therapy (e.g., drugs, catheter ablation, pacing, or surgery). Patients who prefer ablative therapy to pharmacological treatment.	Patients with frequent episodes of tachycardia requiring drug treatment for whom there is concern about proarrhythmia or the effects of the antiarrhythmic drug on the sinus node or AV conduction.	Patients with tachycardias easily controlled by vagal maneuvers and/or well-tolerated drug therapy who are not candidates for non-pharmacological therapy.
Wide QRS Complex Tachycardia	Patients with wide QRS complex tachycardia in whom correct diagnosis is unclear after analysis of available ECG recordings and for whom knowledge of the correct diagnosis is necessary for patient care.	None	Patients with ventricular tachycardia, supraventricular tachycardia with aberrancy, or preexcited tachycardias diagnosed with certainty by ECG criteria and in whom invasive electrophysiology testing would not influence therapy.
Prolongation of QT Interval	None	Identification of a proarrhythmic effect of a drug in patients experiencing sustained VT or cardiac arrest while receiving the drug. Patients who have equivocal abnormalities of QT interval duration or TU wave configuration, with syncope or symptomatic arrhythmias, in whom catecholamine effects may unmask a distinct QT abnormality.	Patients with clinically manifest congenital QT prolongation, with or without symptomatic arrhythmias. Patients with acquired prolonged QT syndrome with symptoms closely related to an identifiable cause or mechanism.

TABLE 2-2. Summary of indications for diagnostic intracardiac electrophysiology studies in patients with documented or suspected tachyarrhythmias

Condition	Indicated	Uncertain or possible indication	Not indicated
Wolff-Parkinson-White Syndrome	Patients being evaluated for catheter ablation or surgical ablation of an accessory pathway.	Asymptomatic patients with a family history of sudden cardiac death or with ventricular preexcitation but no spontaneous arrhythmia who engage in high-risk occupations or activities and in whom knowledge of the electrophysiological properties of the accessory pathway or inducible tachycardia may help determine recommendations for further activities of therapy.	Asymptomatic patients with ventricular preexcitation, except those in Class II.
	Patients with ventricular preexcitation who have survived a cardiac arrest or have unexplained syncope.	Patients with ventricular preexcitation who are undergoing cardiac surgery for other reasons.	
Wolff-Parkinson-White Syndrome	Symptomatic patients in whom determination of the mechanism of arrhythmia or knowledge of the electrophysiological properties of the accessory pathway and normal conduction system would aid in determining appropriate therapy.		
Non-sustained Ventricular Tachycardia or Frequent Ventricular Ectopy	None	Patients with other risk factors for future arrhythmic events, such as low ejection fraction, positive signal-averaged ECG, and sustained VT on ambulatory ECG recordings in whom electrophysiological studies will be used for further risk assessment and for guiding therapy in patients with inducible VT.	Asymptomatic or mildly symptomatic patients with premature ventricular complexes, couplets, and non-sustained VT without other risk factors for sustained arrhythmias.
		Patients with highly symptomatic, uniform morphology premature ventricular complexes, couplets, and non-sustained VT who are considered potential candidates for catheter ablation.	
Unexplained Syncope	Patients with suspected heart disease & syncope that remains unexplained after appropriate evaluation.	Patients with recurrent unexplained syncope without structural heart disease and with a negative head-up tilt table test	Patients with a known cause of syncope for whom treatment will not be guided by electrophysiological testing.

TABLE 2-2. Summary of indications for diagnostic intracardiac electrophysiology studies in patients with documented or suspected tachyarrhythmias

Condition	Indicated	Uncertain or possible indication	Not indicated
Survivors of Cardiac Arrest	Patients surviving cardiac arrest without evidence of an acute Q wave myocardial infarction (MI).	Patients surviving a cardiac arrest caused by bradyarrhythmia	Patients surviving cardiac arrest occurring within 48 hr of an acute MI.
	Patients surviving cardiac arrest occurring more than 48 hours after the acute phase of a myocardial infarction in the absence of a recurrent ischemic event.	Patients surviving cardiac arrest thought to be associated with congenital long QT syndrome in whom the results of noninvasive diagnostic testing are equivocal	Patients with a cardiac arrest resulting from clearly definable specific causes such as reversible ischemia, severe valvular aortic stenosis, or noninvasively defined congenital or acquired long QT syndrome.
Unexplained Palpitations	Patients with palpitations documented by medical personnel to have inappropriately rapid heart rates but in whom ECG recordings have failed to document the cause of palpitations.	Patients with clinically significant, undocumented, sporadic palpitations, believed to have a cardiac cause.	Patients with palpitations documented to be due to extra-cardiac causes.
	Patients with palpitations preceding syncope.		

Adapted from ACC/AHA Task Force Report [1].

2.1.2 CONTRAINDICATIONS, COMPLICATIONS, AND INFORMED CONSENT

Electrophysiology testing should be performed only on patients who are medically stable and have no acute medical condition that could compromise safety during the study. Contraindications to invasive electrophysiology testing include: critical aortic stenosis, severe hypertrophic obstructive cardiomyopathy, acute respiratory conditions, acute metabolic or electrolyte disturbances, acute exacerbations of congestive heart failure, severe left main coronary artery disease, unstable angina, recent transient ischemic attack or cerebrovascular accident, systemic infections, sepsis, or shock from any cause. Patients with these or other serious acute medical conditions should be stabilized and treated before proceeding with the electrophysiology procedure.

Because electrophysiology procedures may result in depression of, or complete loss of consciousness, elective studies should be performed in the fasting state to prevent any complications resulting from possible aspiration. For baseline studies, antiarrhythmic drugs should be discontinued for at least five half-lives before the study. Normalization, or near-normalization of blood clotting parameters should be attained, especially in the case of catheter ablation procedures, by halting administration of heparin, warfarin, or similar agents for an appropriate period prior to the study. Discontinuation of aspirin prior to the study is generally unnecessary.

The electrophysiologist must discuss the procedure with the patient in detail using clear understandable language. Details of the procedure that should be discussed include the reasons for performing the study, the technical aspects, benefits and risks, and any alternative tests or treatments available in lieu of undergoing this invasive procedure. Ideally, the discussion of the procedure should allow the inclusion of close family members and be undertaken in a non-coercive environment outside of the procedure room. While nurses, support staff, and prepared literature or audiovisual materials can assist in providing information about the procedure, it is critical that the electrophysiologist provide detailed information regarding the benefits, and especially the risks, of the procedure (Table 2-3.) Patients and family members must have an opportunity to ask questions. In the case of language differences, the use of an independent (non-family member) interpreter is recommended. Most commonly, the complications resulting from electrophysiology testing result from the catheterization processes, *per se*, and not from any arrhythmia induced by programmed electrical stimulation. Previous studies have reported a complication rate of electrophysiology testing of less than 2% [2,3] with a death rate less than 0.02% [2].

2.1.3 ELECTROPHYSIOLOGY LABORATORY, EQUIPMENT, AND PERSONNEL

The safe and successful performance of diagnostic and therapeutic intracardiac electrophysiology procedures requires the coordinated effort of well-trained individuals working with well-maintained equipment in a well-designed physical space within a facility offering a core of essential support services. While a variety of commercial vendors are delivering an ever-widening collection of specialized equipment including computer recording systems, fluoroscopy equipment, catheters, and an increasingly exotic array of computerized mapping and ablation system, even the best designed and engineered equipment is useless if not placed in the hands of trained professionals.

TABLE 2-3. Potential complications of diagnostic and therapeutic invasive electrophysiology procedures

Adverse drug reaction or complications of over-sedation including respiratory arrest
Inadvertent induction of non-clinical arrhythmia (e.g., atrial fibrillation, ventricular tachycardia/fibrillation)
Catheter lodgement in cardiac chamber or vascular structure requiring surgical removal
Coronary artery thrombosis or dissection
Death
Deep vein thrombosis and thrombophlebitis
Excessive bleeding, hematoma formation
Hemorrhage requiring transfusion
Hemopericardium and cardiac tamponade
Infection, abscess formation, or sepsis
Myocardial infarction
Perforation of cardiac chambers or major cardiac veins
Pericarditis
Peripheral arterial (including aorta) damage or dissection
Pulmonary embolism
Systemic thromboembolism with infarction
Transient ischemic attack/cerebrovascular accident
Unintentional production of complete atrioventricular block or bundle branch block
Valve or valve apparatus damage with new valvular insufficiency

Laboratory and support personnel
The performance of electrophysiology studies depends upon a group of individuals trained in the different aspects of these highly specialized procedures. It is essential to emphasize that safe and successful performance of electrophysiology procedures requires a team consisting of physicians, nurses, technicians, and support staff including biomedical and radiological engineers. The most productive, safe, and successful electrophysiology laboratories are those that develop a strong collegial and cooperative atmosphere among its team members with a strong sense of mutual respect.

Physicians. The discipline of cardiac electrophysiology has evolved dramatically over the past 30 years since the introduction of the His bundle recording technique in humans. Particularly with the development of therapeutic electrophysiologic techniques such as radiofrequency catheter ablation for supraventricular and ventricular tachycardias and the introduction of tiered-therapy transvenous defibrillator systems, clinical cardiac electrophysiology further defined itself has a full-fledged separate subspecialty of cardiology. Consistent with this evolution, the American Board of Internal Medicine offers certification in Clinical Cardiac Electrophysiology to individuals already certified in Cardiovascular Medicine and who have received additional formal fellowship training in diagnostic and therapeutic electrophysiology. Given the complexity of the field and its techniques, physicians engaged in the practice of cardiac electrophysiology should be expected to have undergone this additional training in an approved clinical training program. Ideally they should demonstrate a minimal level of competence by passing the certifying examination offered by the American Board of Internal Medicine. For most procedures performed in the electrophysiology laboratory, at least one such physician specially trained in cardiac electrophysiology should be responsible for performance of the study. In some complicated cases or difficult ablation procedures, successful and safe performance of the study may be best accomplished with two physicians trained in cardiac electrophysiology.

The assistance of other physicians may be needed from time-to-time, including anesthesiologists, interventional cardiologists, and cardiovascular surgeons. Anesthesiologists are often helpful in providing anesthetic services for pediatric patients and during implantation of cardioverter-defibrillators. Very rarely interventional cardiologists may be needed to assist in the management of complications involving the coronary arteries stemming from electrophysiological procedures. Likewise, the services of cardiovascular surgeons may rarely be necessary to assist in the management of specific complications such as cardiac perforation, tamponade, pneumothorax, or catheter-induced vascular or valvular damage. In addition, cardiac surgeons trained in the techniques of arrhythmia surgery are occasionally necessary in cases where a percutaneous transvenous catheter ablation procedure is unsuccessful at curing an arrhythmia.

Nurses and electrophysiology technicians. Ideally, two specially-trained nurses or one nurse and a electrophysiologically-trained cardiovascular technician should be present during these studies. Their duties are to assure the patient's comfort and safety during the study. They should be familiar with the operation of all the equipment in the laboratory including the recording and fluoroscopic equipment. They should be certified in advanced cardiac life-support and they are responsible for the appropriate and timely operation of safety equipment such as the external cardioverter-defibrillator. They should be familiar with the location and use of other safety and resuscitation equipment. Under the order of the physician, they are responsible for administering intravenous agents such as antiarrhythmic drugs and other medications including benzodiazepines and narcotics. In this regard they must be familiar with local protocols for conscious sedation and monitor the patient's vital signs during the entire course of the study. Depending upon their level of training and expertise, they may also assist in the operation of computerized recording and mapping systems used to collect, display, analyze and store the cardiac rhythms provoked during the study. In many electrophysiology laboratories in which transvenous cardioverter-defibrillator systems are implanted, these individuals must also be trained to prepare for and assist in surgical procedures requiring rigorous sterile technique. Because of the wide variety of skills required and the unique procedures performed in electrophysiology laboratories, it is generally preferable that the nursing or cardiovascular technicians assisting in these procedures be dedicated to the electrophysiology laboratory and not split their time between the electrophysiology labo-

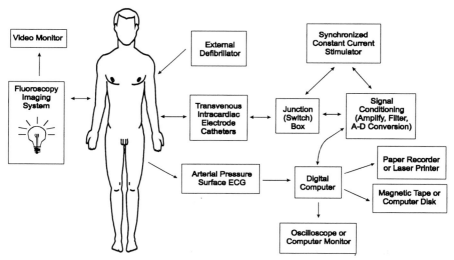

FIGURE 2-1. Schematic diagram illustrating the organization and components of the electrophysiology laboratory. See text for details.

ratory and duties in other settings, such as angiography suites or cardiac catheterization laboratories.

Support staff. The assistance of a well-trained biomedical engineer is essential to assist in the set-up, maintenance, and operation of the myriad of electronic and computer equipment utilized in the modern electrophysiology laboratory. In addition, they often assist in the training of the medical personnel working with this equipment. Most importantly, from the standpoint of patient safety, they must ensure the electrical safety of all the equipment used in the laboratory. Likewise, a radiological technician or engineer is essential in monitoring the fluoroscopy equipment for radiation safety in order to limit radiation exposure to patients and laboratory personnel.

Electrophysiology laboratory organization and equipment
In most cases, a laboratory dedicated to the performance of electrophysiology studies is preferred over a laboratory designed for shared use as a cardiac catheterization/angiography suite. Figure 2-1 schematically displays the components of the electrophysiology laboratory.

Patients are positioned in the supine position on the electrophysiology procedure table. External adhesive defibrillator pads and surface ECG leads (preferably radiolucent) are positioned on the patient's chest (Figure 2-2). At a minimum, recording of ECG leads I, aVF, and V_1 is recommended since they approximate the orthogonal X, Y and Z lead system, although the capability to sample and record an entire 12-lead surface ECG is often useful. During catheter ablation procedures, arterial pressure using an arterial cannula should be continuously recorded. During other types of studies, invasive arterial pressure may be recorded or intermittent pressure recordings obtained with an automatic blood pressure cuff. Low-flow supplemental oxygen administered using a nasal cannula is often used, especially if conscious sedation is employed. Oxygen saturation should also be recorded using an electronic pulse oximeter. Antiseptic preparation of venipuncture sites is accomplished using a surgical iodinated soap or other commercially available preparation. Commercially available sterile drapes should be used to create a sterile field over the patient with strategically-located "cut-outs" for access to the skin around the venipuncture and catheter insertion sites.

The fluoroscopy video system allows visualization of the intracardiac catheters and the outlines of the dense cardiac structures contrasting with the air-filled lungs. In general, a permanent fluoroscopic imaging system is preferred, although a portable C-arm system can be used. In either case, the fluoroscopic system must allow variable positioning of the x-ray tube and image intensifier from far right to far left anterior oblique views. Biplane fluoroscopy which can provide simultaneous right and left anterior oblique views is often very helpful during mapping and catheter ablation procedures.

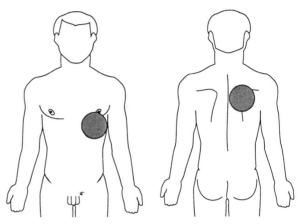

FIGURE 2-2. Commonly used position of adhesive defibrillator pads for patients undergoing electrophysiology procedures. Some electrophysiologists may use an anterior right parasternal position and left anterolateral position (lateral to PMI). See text for details.

At a minimum, the analog signals from the electrode catheters and orthogonal surface ECG leads I, aVF and V_1 must be amplified, filtered and then recorded using a strip chart recorder capable of paper transit speeds of at least 200 mm/sec. In newer multichannel digital recording systems, the analog signals are digitally converted and are displayed using a high resolution computer monitor and stored on magnetic or optical disks for later analysis. Hard-copy records can be made using a laser printer. Whether analog or digital data is collected, a notch filter of 0.1 – 100 Hz should be utilized to record ECG signals. Recording and filtering of intracardiac signals are discussed below (see "Bipolar and unipolar electrode systems" on page 31)

The digital or analog recording system is interfaced with a constant current electronic stimulator (Figure 2-1) allowing synchronous and asynchronous electrical stimulation of cardiac tissues through the electrode catheters. The stimulator must be electrically isolated from the patient and should have the capability to deliver paced cycle lengths between 100 – 2000 msec using increments of 5 – 10 msec. It should allow variable pulse widths from 0.5 – 10 msec and output currents up to 10 mA. The stimulator must be able to perform fixed cycle length pacing as well as deliver up to four independently variable extrastimuli either during the patient's native rhythm or after a variable fixed cycle length pacing train.

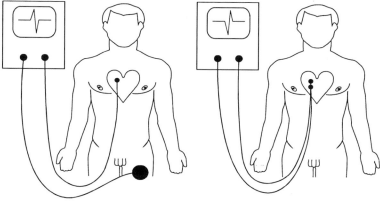

Unipolar Electrogram Recording   Bipolar Electrogram Recording

FIGURE 2-3. Unipolar electrograms are recorded between an indifferent electrode patch on the skin and an intracardiac electrode. A bipolar electrogram is recorded between two closely-spaced electrodes positioned inside the heart.

A junction (or switch) box is the central hardware component between the patient and the recording/stimulation system (Figure 2-1). The metallic pins leading from the electrode catheters positioned in the patient's heart are plugged into the connectors of the junction box (see "Diagnostic and ablation catheters" on page 33) In turn, these connections are "mapped" via software and hardware to the recording system so that each desired cardiac signal is amplified, filtered, recorded, labeled, and stored appropriately. In other words, a His bundle signal should be amplified, filtered, recorded and labeled differently than a signal from the right ventricular apex.

2.1.4 ELECTRODE CATHETERS, INTRACARDIAC ELECTROGRAMS, & ELECTRICAL PACING

Bipolar and unipolar electrode systems
Performance of a diagnostic and therapeutic electrophysiology procedure involves electrical stimulation of various cardiac chambers and recording of local cardiac electrical activity, termed *electrograms*, using temporary *electrode catheters* placed percutaneously in central veins and then maneuvered, under fluoroscopic guidance, into the atria, ventricles, or the lumen of epicardial vessels. Two types of electrode recording systems are available for electrogram recording, *unipolar* and *bipolar* (Figure 2-3).

An electrogram represents a recording of a *voltage* or *electrical potential difference*. A *unipolar electrogram* is the potential difference recorded between an intracardiac electrode in close association with cardiac tissue and a distant *indifferent electrode* patch applied to the body surface (Figure 2-4). By convention, a wavefront of depolarization approaching an electrode results in a *positive* (upward) deflection, while a wavefront receding from an electrode yields a *negative* (downward) deflection. Therefore, a wavefront of depolarization traveling past a unipolar electrode in the heart will produce an electrogram that has a positive and negative deflection representing the approach and recession of the activation wavefront (Figure 2-4, left panel). The rapid transition from

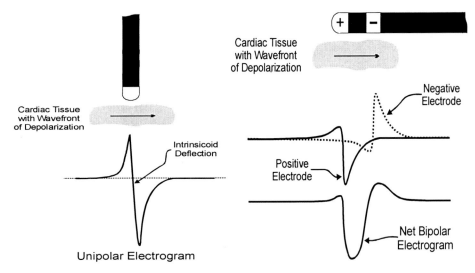

FIGURE 2-4. Schematic illustration of genesis of unipolar (left panel) and bipolar (right panel) electrograms. See text for further discussion.

the positive to negative deflection is termed the *intrinsicoid deflection*. Because a unipolar electrode records a potential difference between widely-spaced electrodes, it will record both local and far-field voltage changes. The exact time of local activation beneath the unipolar electrode, however, can be identified as the point of maximum negative slope (maximum -dV/dt) as the positive deflection changes to negative. This is usually very close to the point where the intrinsicoid deflection crosses the zero baseline. (Strictly speaking this is only true when the positive deflection is the same amplitude as the subsequent negative deflection, but it is a good approximation in almost all cases). In general, a unipolar electrogram is *directionally insensitive* because a local depolarization wavefront approaching the intracardiac unipolar electrode will, regardless of its orientation or direction, result in an initial positive deflection.

Recording of *bipolar electrograms* involves recording a potential difference between a pair of closely-spaced electrodes. One of the electrodes is defined as positive while the other electrode is denoted as negative. Each electrode will record a separate signal, with the resultant bipolar electrogram produced by electronically summing the signals from the positive and negative electrodes (Figure 2-4, right panel). The signal from second electrode will be delayed in time relative to that from the first electrode and the second signal will be inverted compared to the first. Unlike unipolar recordings, bipolar recordings are *directionally sensitive*. If a wavefront of depolarization approaches the electrode pair from a direction opposite to that seen in Figure 2-4, the negative electrode will "see" the depolarization wavefront before, the positive electrode, resulting in an inverted electrode (compare Figure 2-4 and Figure 2-5). The peak negative deflection or positive deflection in a bipolar recording is the time of local activation when the depolarization wavefront passes immediately beneath the midpoint of the bipolar pair. If a bipolar signal has a net negative deflection, then the wavefront of depolarization is reaching the positive electrode first (Figure 2-4), Conversely, if the signal exhibits a net positive deflection, the wavefront reaches the negative electrode first (Figure 2-5). If the wavefront approaches from a direction perpendicular to the bipolar pair, both electrodes will record the same amplitude signal but with reverse polarity resulting in a net zero bipolar signal (Figure 2-5).

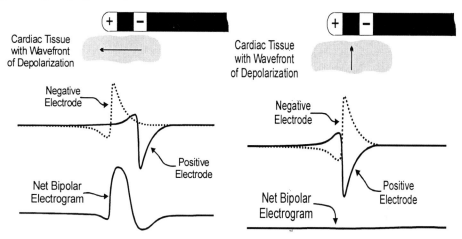

FIGURE 2-5. Bipolar electrogram recorded during reverse direction of the depolarization wavefront (compare left panel with Figure 2-4) results in a net positive bipolar electrogram (left panel). With a perpendicular wavefront (right panel) the resultant net bipolar electrogram is zero.

Bipolar electrodes primarily record local voltage signals and limit the recording of far-field signals and noise. Consequently, the *signal-to-noise ratio* of a bipolar recording is generally greater than that with unipolar recording, making bipolar recording the preferred method of electrogram recording in clinical cardiac electrophysiology. Clinically useful electrode pairs are generally 1 – 5 mm apart. Bipolar signals are normally filtered below 30 – 40 Hz and above 400 – 500 Hz. The eliminated low-frequency signals generally represent far-field voltages, while the high frequency signals are generally noise.

Differences are also observed during electrical pacing with bipolar and unipolar electrode systems. Bipolar pacing produces a small electrical artifact, while unipolar pacing between two distant electrodes produces a large electrical artifact which can significantly distort the local electrograms recorded by nearby bipolar or unipolar recording electrodes.

Diagnostic and ablation catheters

In general, two types of electrode catheters are available from commercial vendors – diagnostic and ablation catheters. *Diagnostic electrode catheters* are the simplest type of catheters (Figure 2-6). They have a pre-formed curve at the distal end which incorporates two or more metal ring electrodes constructed from an inert metal such as platinum. The electrode width varies, but for diagnostic catheters is generally 0.5 – 2-mm. The interelectrode distance likewise varies, but is generally 2 – 10-mm. The smaller the electrode width and interelectrode distance, the smaller the recorded signal amplitude but greater the accuracy of the recorded bipolar signal at representing true local activation.

The commonly used quadripolar (four metal electrodes) diagnostic catheters are typically used for pacing and local recording from the atria and ventricles or recording from the low septal right atrium at the His bundle region. These catheters are constructed with four electrodes (two bipole pairs) near the tip with variable interelectrode spacing generally ranging from 2 – 10-mm. With this catheter arrangement, bipolar pacing can be performed from

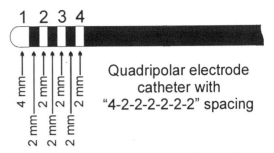

FIGURE 2-6. Schematic diagram of standard quadripolar electrode catheter used for bipolar pacing and recording. For recording, 2 mm to 5 mm interelectrode distance is the most common.

the distal bipole pair while bipolar recording can simultaneously occur using the proximal bipole pair (Figure 2-7). Catheters with 5, 10, 12, 20 or even more electrode pairs are commonly used for mapping the location of accessory connections along the atrioventricular groove within the coronary sinus and great cardiac vein or for localizing the origin of other arrhythmogenic foci within the atria or ventricles. Manipulation of and maneuvering these catheters within the vascularity and cardiac chambers results from the operator torquing the catheter shaft and bending the distal flexible tip, either using a proximal control *steering* mechanism or by pushing gently against the walls of the vessels or cardiac chambers. While diagnostic electrode catheters traditionally have not incorporated a steering mechanism within the catheter shaft, commercial vendors now offer steerable multi-polar electrode catheters which may assist the operator during positioning these catheters.

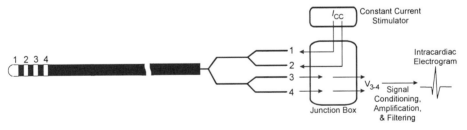

FIGURE 2-7. Simultaneous pacing and recording from a quadripolar electrode catheter. Bipolar electrical pacing is performed using a constant current pulse generator using the distal electrode pair (1 and 2). Bipolar recording of an adjacent patch of cardiac tissue is performed using the proximal electrode pair (3 and 4). The junction box acts as the "traffic cop" directing the stimulation current back to the patient through bipoles 1 and 2, while the recorded potential difference between bipoles 3 and 4 is directed to the signal conditioning equipment, amplifier, and filter before it is displayed on a cathode ray tube or recording paper, or digitally stored on a computer disk or tape.

Ablation catheters are always steerable, allowing the operator to variably bend (and sometimes rotate) the catheter tip using a control mechanism incorporated into a handheld device connected to the proximal end of the catheter that remains outside the patient's body to be manipulated and controlled by the operator. While the precise construction details of the steering mechanism varies, the critical component responsible for the variable bending or rotation of the tip involves thin wires which run along the length of the inner core of the catheter shaft and insert into the distal segments of the flexible tip. Bending or rotating the tip in one direction is accomplished by selectively shortening some wires relative to others running within the catheter shaft. With the explosion of the transvenous techniques to perform endocardial arrhythmia mapping and radiofrequency catheter ablation, many vendors now supply a variety of steerable catheter models designed to work best in different chambers and regions of the heart.

Electrode catheter insertion and positioning
For basic diagnostic electrophysiology studies percutaneous vascular access is most commonly achieved using the right or left femoral veins (Figure 2-8). For diagnostic or

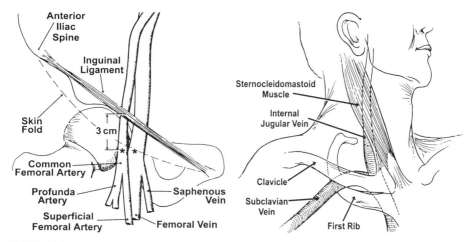

FIGURE 2-8. Regional anatomy of the right femoral region (left panel) and the right neck and clavicular area (right panel). Common insertion sites for diagnostic electrophysiology studies include the right femoral vein and right internal jugular vein. Some electrophysiologists also utilize the right or left subclavian veins. For ablation of left side accessory connections or left ventricular tachyarrhythmias utilizing the retrograde transaortic approach, catheters must be inserted in the right or left femoral artery. See text for further discussion.

therapeutic studies requiring catheter positioning in the coronary sinus/great cardiac vein, vascular access is usually also achieved from central veins cephalad to the heart, including the right or left subclavian veins or right internal jugular vein. Catheters are not inserted directly into the vein. Instead, for convenience, ease of catheter exchange and manipulation, and to reduce the risk of vascular injury, insertion of electrode catheters into central veins is through a *vascular sheath* or *vascular cannula*. Most sheaths used clinically are short, less than 16 cm in length. However, for radiofrequency catheter ablation procedures requiring special catheter stability, unusual catheter positioning, or trans-septal access to the left atrium long specially-designed and shaped sheaths are available from commercial vendors and can be inserted through a femoral vein entry site. Insertion of vascular sheaths is performed using the modified Seldinger technique (Figure 2-9).

Although each patient and electrophysiology study should be viewed as unique and approached as such, in general, patients undergoing diagnostic electrophysiology studies

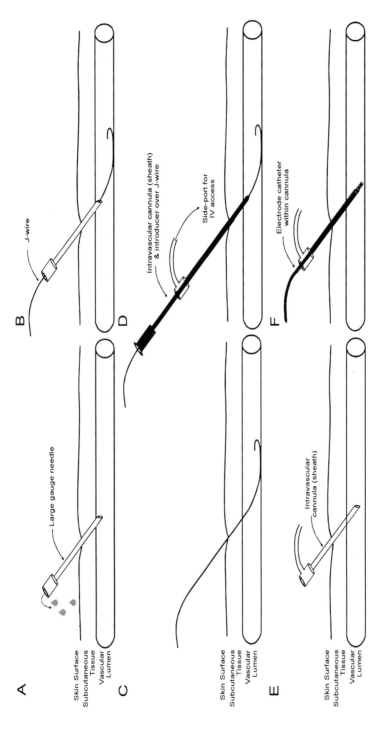

FIGURE 2-9. Percutaneous vascular access using modified Seldinger technique. Panel A, after skin infiltration with local anesthetic, a large gauge needle is used for venipuncture entry into the vein or artery; Panel B, a J-guide wire is passed through the needle lumen into the vessel; Panel C, the needle is removed, leaving the J-wire behind within the vessel lumen; Panel D, a stiff plastic introducer and overlying intravascular cannula (sheath) is passed over the J-guide wire into the vascular lumen; Panel E, the J-wire and intravascular introducer is removed from the vessel and overlying sheath, leaving behind the soft-plastic vascular sheath within the vessel lumen; Panel F, for the duration of the electrophysiologic study the non-thrombotic sheath remains within the vessel lumen allowing easy introduction and removal of electrode catheters.   The vascular sheath contains a diaphragm, to prevent bleed-back, and a side-port for pressure recording or administration of intravenous fluids and drugs.

for documented wide QRS complex tachycardia, assessment of risk of sudden death, or evaluation of a possible arrhythmia cause of syncope require insertion of three diagnostic catheters. Normally, quadripolar electrode catheters are placed at the right ventricular apex and the high right atrium near the sinoatrial node for electrical pacing and electrogram recording. A third quadripolar catheter is placed across the anteroseptal border of the tricuspid annulus in the region of the His bundle in the low septal right atrium (Figure 2-10). Patients undergoing diagnostic studies for narrow QRS complex tachycardias or catheter ablation procedures requiring accurate localization of an accessory connection or origin of an arrhythmia focus usually benefit by inserting a fourth multipolar catheter in the coronary sinus and great cardiac vein using a subclavian or internal jugular vein entry port (Figure 2-10).

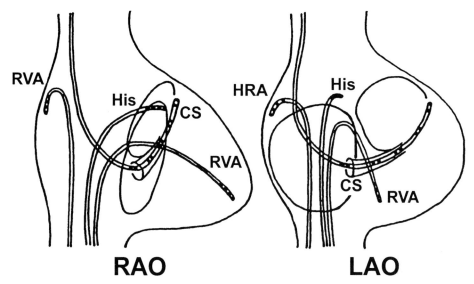

FIGURE 2-10. Schematic diagram illustrating the intracardiac positions of multi-polar electrode catheters used for electrical stimulation and recording. Under x-ray fluoroscopic guidance, transvenous catheter insertion into the cardiac chambers is performed using a percutaneous technique. Illustrated here is the appearance of the catheters using the standard fluoroscopy views of right anterior oblique (RAO) and left anterior oblique (LAO). During a basic electrophysiology study catheters are positioned in the high right atrium (HRA), right ventricular apex (RVA), and at the His bundle position (anterior low septal right atrium straddling the tricuspid valve annulus). For specialized studies in some patients with supraventricular tachycardia, a multi-polar catheter is inserted in the coronary sinus (CS) and advanced into the great cardiac vein traversing the left atrioventricular groove around the mitral valve annulus.

Intracardiac electrograms

Figure 2-11 shows intracardiac bipolar electrograms recorded from the high right atrium near the SA node, His bundle region, and right ventricular apex using quadripolar catheters. Not unexpectedly, during sinus rhythm, the electrogram recorded from the high right atrium precedes the inscription of the atrial electrogram recorded from the electrode catheter in the low septal right atrium. Because the catheter positioned near the His bundle is located at the junction of the right atrium and right ventricle, it records both a local atrial electrogram as well as a right ventricular electrogram resulting from local activa-

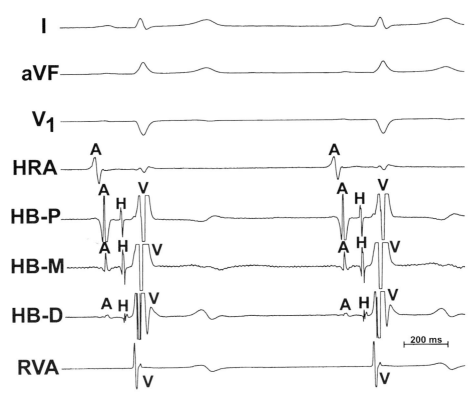

FIGURE 2-11. Intracardiac bipolar recordings from high right atrium (HRA), proximal (HB-P), middle (HB-M), and distal (HB-D) His bundle region, and right ventricular apex (RVA) using quadripolar catheters. Surface ECG leads I, aVF, and V$_1$ are also displayed. This is the standard set-up used in many laboratories for a basic diagnostic study in a patient without supraventricular tachycardia. See text for additional discussion.

tion of the right ventricular septum. Between these two signals is inscribed the His bundle electrogram. This deflection represents electrical activation of the His bundle as the wavefront passes the pair of electrodes on the His bundle catheter.

In patients with presumed or documented supraventricular tachycardia, the set-up is similar except that (usually) five additional bipolar electrograms are recorded from the proximal to distal coronary sinus/great cardiac vein (Figure 2-12).

Pacing protocols and programmed electrical stimulation
Atrial or ventricular muscle tissue consists of single cells with a negative resting potential of about -80 to -90-mV. Activation of single heart cells requires application of an electrical current that moves the cell's resting potential to the *threshold potential*. Once the cell reaches its threshold potential, ion channels open and a self-regenerating all-or-none action potential conducts to adjacent cells spreading throughout the conduction system. The minimum amount of electrical current that must be applied to heart tissue to produce a regenerating wavefront of depolarization is termed the *threshold current* (or simply *threshold*).

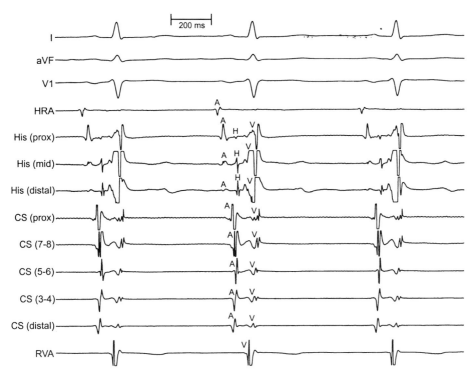

FIGURE 2-12. Basic 13 channel recording during a cardiac electrophysiology study in a patient with documented or presumed supraventricular tachycardia. From top to bottom, recordings taken from surface ECG leads I, aVF, and V_1 along with intracardiac electrograms recorded from high right atrium (HRA), proximal (prox). middle (mid), and distal (dist) electrode pairs of a quadripolar electrode catheter positioned at His bundle region, coronary sinus (CS) catheter positioned within the great cardiac vein along the posterior and lateral AV groove between the left atrium and left ventricle, and right ventricular apex (RVA). Arterial blood pressure (not shown) is often also recorded. For patients undergoing electrophysiology testing for presumed ventricular tachycardia, the coronary sinus catheter is generally not used. Some electrophysiologists only record from two, or rarely one, bipolar electrode pairs in the His bundle region. A, atrial electrogram, H, His bundle electrogram, V, ventricular electrogram.

The electrical conduction properties of cardiac tissues, including the atria, ventricles, and specialized conducting system, are investigated using *programmed electrical stimulation (PES)*. PES involves electrical stimulation of heart tissue using one of a number of pacing protocols. Either the atria or ventricles can be stimulated during electrical pacing. During pacing protocols, electrical stimulation is performed at a particular cycle length. The cycle length represents the time between any two successive stimuli. The relationship between pacing rate (PR) and cycle length (CL) is easily described, i.e., PR = 60,000/CL, with pacing rate expressed as pulses or stimuli per min with cycle length measured in msec. Pacing at a cycle length of 600 msec corresponds to a pacing rate of 100 pulses per minute.

The first type of pacing used in electrophysiological studies is termed *fixed rate* or *fixed cycle length pacing* (Figure 2-13). In this type of pacing, the cycle length (pacing rate) of all the stimuli in the *pacing train* is the same and fixed. For example, fixed cycle length pacing of the right atrium may be performed at a cycle length of 600 msec, which means that the time interval between any two stimuli in the pacing train is 600 msec. The length of the pacing train may range from only a few stimuli to many stimuli. A common length for a pacing train is eight or ten stimuli. Pacing for this duration allows stabilization of the refractory period (see rate-related refractoriness below). Each of the pacing events in a pacing train is referred to as S_1. If the pacing is performed in the atrium, capture and conduction of the S_1 stimulus through the atria results in an atrial depolarization, termed A_1. If the ventricle is being paced, capture and conduction of the S_1 in the ventricle results in a ventricular depolarization, termed V_1.

The second common

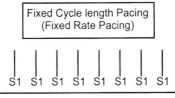

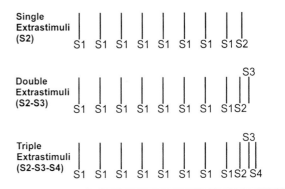

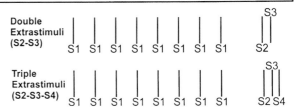

FIGURE 2-13. Schematic representation of two pacing protocols commonly used in electrophysiology studies. During fixed cycle length (fixed rate) pacing, a train of electrical stimuli (S_1) is delivered in which the time between successive stimuli in the train is a fixed time interval (cycle length). During fixed cycle length pacing with premature extrastimuli, the cardiac tissue is stimulated as above, but at the end of the fixed pacing train one or more premature stimuli are delivered earlier than the previous fixed cycle length. In practice, this premature extrastimulus is delivered earlier and earlier during subsequent pacing trains until it fails to depolarize the tissue. This type of pacing is used to determine the refractory periods of the atrium, ventricle, and specialized conduction system and to induce reentrant arrhythmias. The long-short extrastimuli pacing protocol is often used to induce reentrant ventricular tachycardia, especially bundle branch reentrant ventricular tachycardia.

type of pacing protocol performed involves *fixed cycle length (fixed rate) pacing with extrastimuli*. In this type of pacing, a fixed pacing train is followed by the introduction of one or more *premature extrastimuli* at the end of a fixed pacing train (Figure 2-13). For example, if the cycle length of the eight stimuli in the drive train is 600 msec, a ninth stimulus may be added with the time between the last drive stimulus and the premature stimulus being 350 msec instead of 600 msec. This ninth premature stimulus is termed S_2, which can cause premature atrial (A_2) or ventricular (V_2) depolarization. In this example, the S_1-S_2 *coupling interval* or *coupling cycle length* is 350 msec. The reason for introducing premature stimuli is to determine a refractory period (see below) or attempt to induce an arrhythmia. It is common to introduce multiple premature stimuli at the end of a fixed cycle pacing train; often up to three extra stimuli are used. The first extrastimulus is S_2, the second is termed S_3, and the third is referred to as S_4, etc. (with A_2, A_3, A_4, or V_2, V_3, or V_4, corresponding to the resultant atrial or ventricular depolarizations, respectively).

A variant of this second type of pacing is *fixed cycle length pacing with long-short extrastimuli* (Figure 2-13). This type of pacing is often useful for inducing some types of ventricular tachycardia, especially bundle branch reentrant ventricular tachycardia.

2.2   The Basic Diagnostic Electrophysiological Evaluation

Unlike many other specialized procedures which have rigid standardized protocols, to a large degree the electrophysiologist must decide from moment-to-moment what to do next during an invasive electrophysiology study based upon what he or she has just observed in response to a pacing protocol, induced rhythm, or infused drug.

While a complete diagnostic electrophysiological evaluation may entail the use of a variety of pacing protocols in different cardiac chambers before and after the administration of a variety of pharmacological agents, at a minimum the basic diagnostic study has the following main goals: 1) an analysis of baseline rhythm, 2) evaluation of baseline conduction properties, 3) assessment of pacemaker function, 4) programmed electrical stimulation of the atria and ventricles to quantify the refractoriness of the anterograde and retrograde conduction pathways and to assess atrioventricular and ventriculoatrial conduction patterns, 5) attempts to provoke a clinical arrhythmia and, 6) determination of the mechanism of any induced tachy- or bradyarrhythmias (Table 2-4.)

In the remainder of this chapter, we discuss the parameters evaluated and measured during an electrophysiology study, along with some common electrophysiology phenomenon observed during the course of the intracardiac evaluation of the cardiac conduction system.

2.2.1 BASELINE CARDIAC RHYTHM

By analyzing the surface 12-lead ECG, an assessment of the patient's baseline rhythm can be made even before the patient enters the electrophysiology laboratory and preliminary planning for the study can be undertaken. For example, if the patient is in atrial fibrillation or flutter, but the purpose of the study is to evaluate AV node function, the His Purkinje system, or study and ablate an accessory connection that is the source of a recurrent clinical arrhythmia, then plans must be made (and appropriate anticoagulation administered) to perform cardioversion prior to, or at the time of, the study. If the 12-

TABLE 2-4. Standard components of basic diagnostic electrophysiology study

Component	Items/Phenomenon Evaluated	Parameters Measured/Examples
Baseline Rhythm	Surface ECG & intracardiac electrograms	Sinus, AFL, AF, etc.
Baseline Conduction Intervals	Surface ECG intervals	V-V, P-R, Q-T intervals, QRS duration
	Intracardiac intervals	A-H, H-V intervals
Pacemaker Function	SA node function	SNRT, corrected SNRT, SACT, CSM
Anterograde Refractoriness & Conduction Patterns	Atrial and AV refractory periods	AERP, AVN ERP/FRP, WBCL, HP ERP/FRP, anterograde AP ERP/BCL
	AV conduction patterns	NP or AP; AVN FP or AVN SP
	Arrhythmia induction	Mode of induction, QRS axis & morphology, arrhythmia CL
Retrograde Refractoriness & Conduction Patterns	Ventricular and VA refractory periods	VERP, retrograde NP ERP/BCL, retrograde AP ERP/BCL
	VA conduction patterns	NP or AP; AVN FP or AVN SP
	Arrhythmia induction	Mode of induction, QRS axis & morphology, arrhythmia CL
Arrhythmia Induction & Mechanism	Various pacing techniques and procedures; IV drugs	SART, AVNRT, AFL, AT, VT, AVRT, etc.

A, atrial electrogram; AERP, atrial effective refractory period; AF, atrial fibrillation; AFL, atrial flutter; AP, accessory pathway; AV, atrioventricular; AT, atrial tachycardia; AVN, atrioventricular node; AVNRT, atrioventricular node reentrant tachycardia; AVRT, atrioventricular reciprocating tachycardia; BCL, block cycle; CSM, carotid sinus massage; ERP, effective refractory period; FP, fast conduction pathway of the atrioventricular node; FRP, functional refractory period; H, His bundle electrogram; HP, His-Purkinje; IV, intravenous; NP, normal pathway (atrioventricular node and His-Purkinje system); PES, programmed electrical stimulation; SA, sinoatrial; SACT, sinoatrial conduction time; SART, sinoatrial reentrant tachycardia; SNRT, sinus node recovery time; SP, slow conduction pathway of the atrioventricular node; V, ventricular electrogram; VERP, ventricular effective refractory period; VA, ventriculoatrial; VT, ventricular tachycardia; WBCL, Wenckebach block cycle length

lead ECG shows evidence of an old inferior myocardial infarction in a patient with syncope, the electrophysiology study should be specifically directed at finding evidence of inducible monomorphic ventricular tachycardia. The presence of preexcitation should alert the clinician that the patient has an accessory connection and will probably have inducible supraventricular tachycardia. The electrophysiologist should routinely plan each study based upon all the clinical and ECG data available from the patient's clinical record.

2.2.2 BASELINE CONDUCTION INTERVALS

Baseline conduction intervals are measured both from the surface ECG and the intracardiac electrograms (Figure 2-14). The PR, QRS, QT, P-P (A-A), and R-R (V-V) intervals are measured in the usual fashion. The time between the onset of the atrial spike in the

His bundle recording and the onset of the His bundle electrogram is termed the *A-H interval* (Figure 2-14). The A-H interval represents the conduction time from the low septal right atrium through the AV node to the His bundle. Because a major component of the A-H interval is AV node conduction, and since AV node conduction is significantly effected by autonomic tone, the A-H interval can be widely variable. In general, the normal range is from 50 to 150 msec [4-14]. Prolongation of the A-H interval can merely indicate high vagal tone, but may also signify AV node disease or the effect of drugs. With enhanced sympathetic tone, or the administration of catecholamines, the A-H interval shortens. The AV node exhibits decremental conduction properties, meaning that with rapid atrial pacing rates, or with premature atrial stimuli, the AV node conduction time increases and the A-H interval prolongs (see below).

The time between the onset of the His spike and the earliest activation of the ventricle, as measured from either the surface ECG or the ventricular electrogram in the His bundle recording, is termed the *H-V interval* (Figure 2-14). The H-V interval represents the time required for the electrical impulse to conduct from the proximal His bundle until it first activates any portion of the ventricle. This is normally much less than the A-H interval and the normal range for the H-V interval is from 30 to 55 msec [4-14]. An apparent H-V interval of less than 30 msec may result from mistakenly recording the right bundle branch depolarization instead of the His bundle depolarization. Alternatively, a short H-V interval is also observed with ventricular preexcitation caused by anterograde conduction within accessory AV connection. Significant prolongation of the H-V inter-

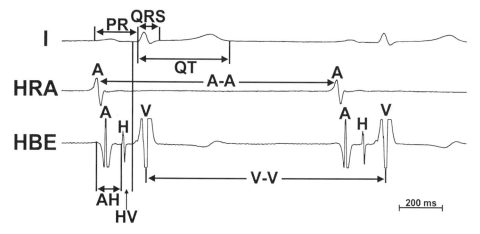

FIGURE 2-14. Measurement of baseline conduction intervals using surface ECG and intracardiac electrograms. Surface ECG lead I is shown. Surface intervals (PR, QRS, QT are measured in the usual ways. The A-A (P-P) interval is the cycle length of atrial depolarization recorded from the surface ECG or intracardiac electrograms. The V-V (R-R) interval is the cycle length of ventricular depolarization recorded from the surface ECG or intracardiac electrograms. During sinus rhythm, the high right atrial (HRA) electrogram occurs earliest. The atrial electrogram (A) recorded at the low septal right atrium by the His bundle (HBE) catheter occurs later. The A-H interval represents the conduction time between the low septal right atrium and the proximal His bundle region (measured in the HBE recording). The His bundle (H) deflection represents the depolarization wavefront traveling through the His bundle as it conducts to the bundle branches and ventricles. The H-V interval represents the time required for the wavefront to conduct from the proximal His bundle to earliest ventricular activation as measured from HBE recording or any surface ECG lead. In this case the earliest ventricular activation is recorded in the His bundle region.

val can occur with drugs, or it may indicate disease within the His-Purkinje system. Unlike the AV node, the His-Purkinje system is not normally significantly affected by levels of autonomic tone and does not exhibit decremental conduction. The His-Purkinje system, however, may exhibit decremental conduction properties when it is exposed to antiarrhythmic drugs, becomes ischemic, or otherwise is diseased.

2.2.3 EVALUATION OF SINOATRIAL NODE PACEMAKER FUNCTION

Evaluation of the native pacemaker function – the SA node – is often the first component of the invasive study performed during the basic diagnostic electrophysiology study (although in diagnostic studies for supraventricular tachycardia, the study generally begins in the ventricle with an analysis of ventriculoatrial conduction). The *sinoatrial conduction time (SACT)* is occasionally evaluated. *Carotid sinus massage* is an easy method to test for the presence of *carotid sinus hypersensitivity* in patients with syncope. However, the most common invasive assessment of sinus node function involves measurement of the *sinus node recovery time (SNRT)* which is normally corrected for sinus rate (the *corrected sinus node recovery time (SNRT_C)*). A detailed discussion of SNRT, $SNRT_C$, and SACT (along with normal and abnormal values) and other means of invasive and non-invasive assessment of SA node function is discussed in "Assessment of Sinoatrial Node Function" on page 458.

Measurement of the SNRT involves fixed cycle length pacing of the high right atrium near the SA node at progressively shorter cycle lengths, beginning with a cycle length just below the sinus cycle length. Each drive train lasts for 60 sec. One minute is allowed for full SA node recovery between drive trains. The interval between the last atrial-paced event and the appearance of the first sinus-derived atrial depolarization is the uncorrected SNRT (Figure 2-15). Care must be taken to ensure that the escape depolarizations at the termination of overdrive pacing originate from the SA node. This can be done by comparing the P-wave morphology of these beats to P-waves generated during sinus rhythm or by having a second electrode catheter in the low right atrium to

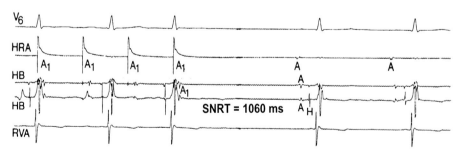

FIGURE 2-15. Surface ECG and intracardiac recording during determination of sinus node recovery time (SNRT). Shown are the surface ECG lead V_6 and intracardiac electrograms from the high right atrium (HRA), His bundle region (HB), and right ventricular apex (RVA). Fixed cycle length pacing of the HRA is performed for one minute (A_1-A_1 = 400 msec) (last four atrial stimuli shown here). The interval between the last atrial-paced event (A_1) and the appearance of the first sinus-derived atrial depolarization (A) is the uncorrected SNRT (1060 msec). H, His bundle electrogram. See text for details.

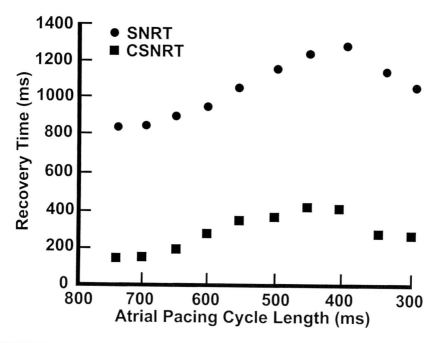

FIGURE 2-16. Family of SNRT and SNRT$_C$ values obtained from a patient with sinus cycle length of 800 msec as a function of atrial pacing cycle length. SNRT, sinus node recovery time; CSNRT, corrected sinus node recovery time.

record the morphology, origin, and timing of electrograms during sinus rhythm and at the termination of the rapid pacing.

In normal persons, the longest SNRT is generally obtained in response to overdrive pacing at a cycle length of 400 – 450 msec. In patients in which abnormal SA node function is highly suspected, overdrive pacing can be performed at various cycle lengths ($\leq$ the sinus cycle length) down to 300 –350 msec, generating a SNRT (and SNRT$_c$) value at each cycle length (Figure 2-16). Since patients with significant SA node dysfunction may have *SA node entrance block*, especially at short pacing cycle lengths, not all atrial pacing will necessarily be effective at overdrive suppression of the SA node pacemaker activity. Therefore, one may find the longest SNRT or SNRT$_c$ is measured in response to overdrive pacing at 500-600 msec rather than at 400 – 500 msec. In general, a SNRT$_c$ $\leq 500 – 550$ msec is considered normal.

2.2.4 ASSESSMENT OF ANTEROGRADE REFRACTORINESS & PATTERNS OF CONDUCTION

Refractory periods and rate-related refractoriness
Refractory periods are the "fundamental currency" of intracardiac electrophysiology and the means by which the electrical properties of cardiac tissues are described and compared (Table 2-5.)

TABLE 2-5. Definition of anterograde periods

Conduction System Component	Effective Refractory Period	Relative Refractory Period	Functional Refractory Period
Atrium	Longest S_1-S_2 that fails to produce an atrial depolarization	Longest S_1-S_2 at which S_2-A_2 is > S_1-A_1	Shortest A_1-A_2 resulting from any S_1-S_2
AV node	Longest A_1-A_2 (measured at the His bundle region) that fails to produce a His bundle depolarization	Longest A_1-A_2 at which A_2-H_2 is > A_1-H_1	Shortest H_1-H_2 resulting from any A_1-A_2
Accessory AV connection	Longest A_1-A_2 interval that fails to depolarize any portion of the ventricles through the accessory connection	Not normally measured	Shortest preexcited V_1-V_2 resulting from any A_1-A_2
His-Purkinje system	Longest H_1-H_2 that fails to result in ventricular depolarization[+]	Longest H_1-H_2 at which H_2-V_2 is > H_1-V_1 or generates an aberrant QRS complex	Shortest V_1-V_2 resulting from any H_1-H_2

S_1, A_1, H_1, V_1: stimulus artifact, atrial, His bundle, and ventricular electrograms during fixed cycle-length pacing train; S_2, A_2, H_2, V_2: stimulus artifact, atrial, His bundle, and ventricular electrograms of premature depolarization; [+]normally not measurable because effective refractory period of AV node is generally > His bundle or His Purkinje system

In general, when a premature stimulus, S_2, is introduced at the end of a fixed pacing train, S_1, the S_2 may or may not generate a self-sustaining depolarizing wavefront in the cardiac tissue depending upon the degree of prematurity of S_2. The S_1-S_2, A_1-A_2, H_1-H_2 or V_1-V_2 coupling intervals are used to determine the refractory periods of cardiac tissues. For example, as the S_1-S_2 coupling interval is made shorter, eventually an S_1-S_2 interval will be reached where S_2 fails to capture the heart tissue.

The *relative refractory period* of a cardiac tissue is defined as the longest premature coupling interval that results in prolonged conduction of the premature impulse compared to the conduction of

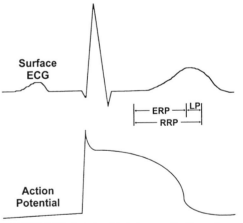

FIGURE 2-17. Relationship between effective refractory period (ERP), relative refractory period (RRP), latency period (LP) and the surface ECG and the ventricular muscle cell action potential. See text for further discussion.

the stimulus delivered during the basic drive train (Figures 2-17 & 2-18). For example, if atrial pacing is being performed, the atrial relative refractory period is the longest S_1-S_2 that results in an S_2-A_2 interval longer than the S_1-A_1 interval.

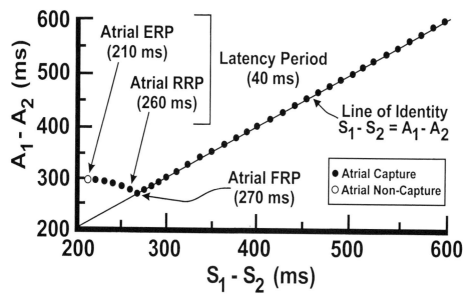

FIGURE 2-18. Determination of atrial functional, relative, and effective refractory periods as well as latency period by plotting A_1-A_2 versus S_1-S_2. A line of identity corresponds to the condition where S_1-S_2 = A_1-A_2. As S_1-S_2 shortens to 270 ms, the atrial functional refractory period (FRP) is reached. As S_1-S_2 shortens below 270 ms the resultant A_1-A_2 deviates from the line of identity as the relative refractory period (RRP) is reached and the latency period is entered. During this period, the A_1-A_2 interval actually increases despite further decreases in S_1-S_2. Eventually, with further shortening of S_1-S_2, the atrial effective refractory period (ERP) is reached. Pacing stimulus intensity at twice diastolic threshold.

The *effective refractory period* of a cardiac tissue is defined as the longest premature coupling interval that fails to conduct through a tissue (Figures 2-17 & 2-18). The atrial effective refractory period is the longest S_1-S_2 coupling interval which fails to depolarize the atria (S_2 without A_2), while the AV node effective refractory period is the longest A_1-A_2 interval which fails to conduct through the AV node to the His bundle.

The relative refractory period is generally slightly longer than the effective refractory period by an amount called the *latency period* (Figures 2-17 & 2-18). While the tissue remains excitable during the latency period, conduction may be slower or even decremental if activation occurs during this period. As seen in (Figure 2-19), when the S_2 stimulus is delivered sufficiently close to the preceding S_1 (i.e., S_1-S_2 interval between atrial relative refractory period and atrial effective refractory period) in the high right atrium, a relatively isoelectric period of delay is noted in the high right atrial recording and the A_1-A_2 interval recorded at the low septal right atrium near the His bundle is much longer than the S_1-S_2 interval recorded by the high right atrial catheter, i.e., the atrial activation (A_2) resulting from S_2 conducts slowly from the high right atrium to the His bundle region.

The *functional refractory period* is the shortest interval between two consecutively conducted impulses out of a cardiac tissue resulting from any two consecutive input impulses into that tissue (Figures 2-18, & 2-20). Note that the functional refractory period is a measure of *output* of a tissue and, unlike the relative refractory period or effective re-

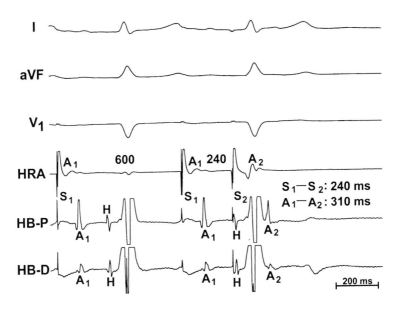

FIGURE 2-19. Demonstration of slow intra-atrial conduction during the atrial latency period. An extrastimulus is delivered to the high right atrium (HRA) at progressively shorter coupling intervals (S_1-S_2) until eventually S_2-A_2 is > S_1-A_1 (atrial relative refractory period). With continued decrease in S_1-S_2, the atrial effective refractory period is eventually reached (not shown). Between these two refractory periods lies the atrial latency period. As shown in this figure, S_2 delivered during the latency period conducts slowly making A_1-A_2 much > than S_1-S_2. HB-P, proximal His bundle recording; HB-D, distal His bundle recording.

fractory period, is a "shortest" interval as opposed to a "longest" interval. In a sense, it is the shortest output interval that can occur in response to *any* input interval in a particular tissue. For example, the atrial functional refractory period is the shortest A_1-A_2 interval in response to any S_1-S_2 interval (Figure 2-18), while the functional refractory period of the AV node is the shortest H_1-H_2 interval resulting from any A_1-A_2 interval (Figure 2-20).

The effective refractory period is not an absolute value but varies depending upon the stimulus intensity of the extrastimulus (Figure 2-21) as well as the cycle length between the fixed stimuli making up the pacing train. The effective refractory period of atrium, ventricle and His-Purkinje systems decreases with decreasing cycle length of the pacing train (*rate-related refractoriness*), while

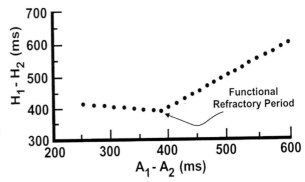

FIGURE 2-20. Plot of H_1-H_2 versus A_1-A_2 to determine functional refractory period of the AV node. See text for details

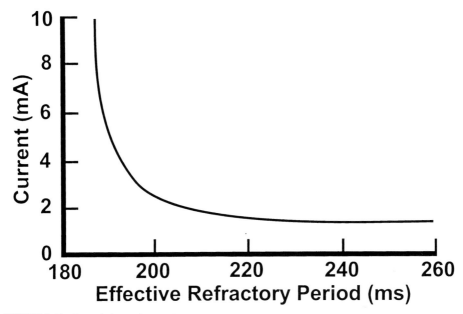

FIGURE 2-21. Strength-interval curve depicting relationship between effective refractory period of ventricular myocardium and stimulating current. The effective refractory period declines as the stimulating current is increased, until eventually an absolute minimum refractory period is reached. Refractory period of atrial or ventricular myocardium is a function of the amplitude of the premature stimuli used to determine the refractory period. Adapted from [69].

the AV nodal effective refractory period increases with decreasing cycle length [15-17]. In the case of atrial, ventricular and His-Purkinje tissues, the shortening of effective refractory period with increased pacing rate is termed "pealing back of refractoriness". It results from the fact that rapid pacing in these tissues causes shortening of the action potential duration. Under normal physiological conditions, the effective refractory period in these tissues is regulated by and usually less than the action potential duration. Therefore, shortening the action potential duration with rapid pacing will decrease the effective refractory period. This rate-related shortening of action potential duration appears to result from a pacing-induced increase of one component of the delayed rectifier K+ current [18-20].

The AV node, on the other hand, displays post-repolarization refractoriness. AV node cells exhibiting slow, Ca++-dependent action potentials may not become re-excitable until after repolarization is complete, even though they exhibit very short action potential duration [21-24]. The ionic mechanisms responsible for these differences are in dispute.

Intra-atrial conduction & atrial activation
Endocardial mapping indicates that normal atrial activation begins in either the high or mid-lateral right atrium, with the former more likely to occur at sinus rates >100/min and the latter more likely at rates < 60/min. These different activation patterns may reflect different exit routes from a single SA node or a SA node consisting of multiple pacemak-

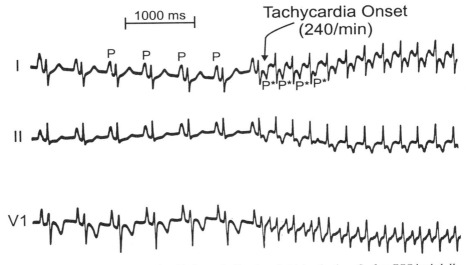

FIGURE 2-22. Change in P-wave axis with change in direction of atrial activation. Surface ECG leads I, II, and V$_1$ were simultaneously recorded immediately before and after the onset of AV reciprocating tachycardia. Prominent positive P-waves are seen in each of these leads during sinus rhythm, indicative of atrial activation proceeding from the high right atrium to the low right atrium. After the onset of tachycardia, the P-waves become negative (P*) in leads I and II and biphasic in lead V$_1$. This tachycardia involves retrograde conduction from the ventricles to the atria through an accessory AV connection and the retrograde atrial depolarization wavefront is proceeding away from the positive poles of leads I, and II and is perpendicular to lead V$_1$. The high right atrium is activated after the lower portions of the atria.

er regions [25]. Spread of the atrial impulse to the right AV junction requires about one-half the time required to reach the left atrial free wall. Whether specific inter-atrial tracts exist between the SA and AV nodes is the subject of debate [26] (see "Functional Anatomy of the Conduction System" on page 1)

When normal atrial activation spreads from the high right atrium to the low right atrium, the surface ECG will display upright P-waves in the inferior leads II, III, aVF (because the depolarization wavefront is moving toward the positive poles of these leads). If, however, atrial activation proceeds in the opposite direction, as occurs with the usual form of atrial flutter or low right atrial tachycardias, the P-wave will be inverted in these leads, because the depolarization wavefront is moving toward the negative poles of the inferior leads (Figure 2-22). The morphology of a P-wave produced by a premature atrial depolarization depends on the location of its origin. Hence, its morphology is usually different from the P-wave produced by the normal SA node depolarization.

Atrial vulnerability

The period of atrial vulnerability roughly corresponds to the interval between the atrial relative refractory period and effective refractory period (latency period). The normal atrial effective refractory period ranges from 150 to 260 msec [17,27-30], while the atrial relative refractory period is normally 10 - 30 msec greater than the atrial effective refractory period. Atrial extrastimuli delivered during the period of atrial vulnerability are often followed by repetitive atrial activity which can become sustained resulting in atrial flutter or fibrillation (Figure 2-23) [31-39]. Atrial extrastimuli with progressively shorter coupling intervals less than the relative refractory period and ever closer to the effective refractory period increase the incidence of repetitive responses and the risk of atrial flutter or fibrillation. In normal atria, the atrial vulnerable period is very brief (usually 10 to 30 msec). However, the vulnerable interval increases as the fixed drive cycle length is made shorter due to a drive cycle length-dependent decrease in the effective refractory period without any reduction in the relative refractory period [40]. The repetitive atrial responses result from reentry of a premature atrial extrastimulus conducting through tissues that are relatively refractory. The conduction velocity is reduced, and in the presence of regions of unidirectional block, sustained reentrant atrial arrhythmias can result.

Anterograde AV conduction pathways
When the high right atrium is electrically stimulated with a suprathreshold stimulus, capture occurs with spread of the wavefront of depolarization throughout both atria. Normally, the wavefront conducts from the atria to the ventricles through the AV node-His-Purkinje system, termed the *normal pathway*. In patients with a normal conduction system this results in a normal PR, A-H and H-V intervals with a short QRS duration due to rapid conduction within the His-Purkinje system.

In the fully developed human heart, fibrous AV rings (annulus fibrosus) almost completely electrically insulates the atrial and ventricular myocardia from each other. In most people, the normal pathway is the only conduction pathway from the atria to the ventricles because only at the AV node/His bundle region is the annulus fibrosus breached and electrical continuity established, permitting cardiac impulse conduction from the atria to the ventricles. As long as the insulation of the annulus fibrosus is not

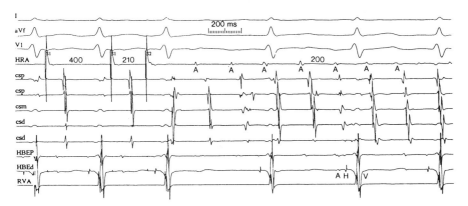

FIGURE 2-23. Atrial extrastimulus delivered during the period of atrial vulnerability results in repetitive atrial responses and sustained atrial flutter. From top to bottom, recordings from surface ECG leads I, aVF and V_1 along with intracardiac electrograms from high right atrium (HRA), five coronary sinus leads (proximal (csp), middle (csm) and distal (csd)), proximal His bundle (HBEP), distal His bundle (HBEd), and right ventricular apex (RVA). After fixed atrial pacing at a cycle length (S_1-S_1) of 400 msec, introduction of an atrial premature stimulus (S_1-S_2 = 210 msec) results in repetitive atrial depolarizations (A-A = 220 msec) and sustained atrial flutter with 3:1 atrioventricular conduction. A, atrial electrogram. H, His bundle electrogram. V, ventricular electrogram.

disrupted anywhere else, atrial impulses are conducted to the ventricle only by way of the AV node-His-Purkinje system. Because of its decremental conduction properties, the AV node functions as a protective barrier delaying AV conduction and preventing rapid one-to-one impulse conduction from the atria to the ventricles. AV nodal conduction is discussed in more detail below (see "Atrial pacing and decremental AV nodal conduction" on page 52) Some patients exhibit dual (fast and slow) AV conduction pathways. Although in many patients this has no functional significance, in some individuals these dual conduction pathways provide the substrate for AV nodal reentrant tachycardia (see "Atrioventricular Nodal Reentrant Tachycardia" on page 487)

In rare patients, AV conduction can occur by both the normal pathway (AV nodal/His-Purkinje system) as well as one or more abnormal conduction pathways, termed *accessory connections* or *accessory pathways*. In some cases, these accessory connections may permit rapid anterograde AV conduction during atrial fibrillation or flutter, possibly resulting in life-threatening consequences if the resultant rapid ventricular response degenerates into ventricular fibrillation. These accessory connections are also critical anatomical components necessary for the development of orthodromic AV reciprocating tachycardia. Accessory connections, ventricular preexcitation, and the Wolff-parkinson-White syndrome are discussed in more detail below (see "Accessory AV connections & the concept of preexcitation" on page 56 and "Ventricular Preexcitation Syndromes: The Wolff-Parkinson-White Syndrome and Variants" on page 539).

Atrial pacing and decremental AV nodal conduction

The AV node exhibits decremental conduction properties, meaning that with rapid atrial pacing, or with premature atrial stimuli, the AV node conduction time (A-H interval) increases (Figure 2-24). If one plots the A_2-H_2 interval versus the A_1-A_2 interval (Figure 2-25) a gradual increase in the A_2-H_2 interval is noted with reductions in A_1-A_2 coupling interval until either the AV node or atrial effective refractory period is reached (Figure 2-24). Similarly, pacing at a critical A_1-A_1 interval results in progressive prolongation of the A-H interval until eventually there is atrial capture without conduction to the His bundle or ventricles (Figure 2-26). In normal hearts, the conduction block almost always occurs within the A-V node, and not the His bundle. The *AV node Wenckebach cycle length* is the longest A_1-A_1 interval which fails to result in one-to-one conduction through the AV node to the His bundle.

Certain individuals may have AV nodes exhibiting multiple trans-nodal conduction pathways. In these patients, the curve relating A_2-H_2 to A_1-A_2 often fails to show a smooth increase in A_2-H_2 with reductions in A_1-A_2, and instead exhibits an abrupt discontinuity at a critical A_1-A_2 coupling interval (Figure 2-27). The explanation for this finding is that many normal AV nodes contain a fast conducting pathway and a slow conducting pathway (Figure 2-28). Normally, conduction occurs preferentially down the fast pathway to activate the His bundle and ventricle. However, because the effective refractory period of the fast pathway is, in general, longer than that of the slow pathway, as the A_1-A_2 coupling interval is decreased, the effective refractory period of the fast pathway is reached and conduction blocks in that pathway. Conduction, however, continues down the non-refractory slow pathway even as the A_1-A_2 coupling interval is shortened

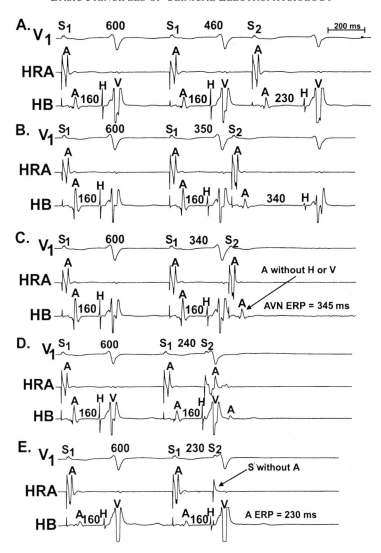

FIGURE 2-24. Demonstration of anterograde AV nodal decremental conduction, AV node effective refractory period, and atrial effective refractory period. In each panel, ECG lead V_1 shown along with intracardiac electrograms from the high right atrium and His bundle region. An eight pulse fixed rate drive train (S_1-S_1) (only last two stimuli shown) is delivered in the HRA followed by increasingly premature extrastimulus (S_2) at coupling intervals (S_1-S_2) of 460 ms (panel A), 350 ms (panel B), 340 ms (panel C), 240 ms (panel D) and 230 ms (panel E). Note that the A-H interval during the drive train is significantly shorter than that seen with an extrastimulus and A-H prolongs as the coupling interval of the extrastimulus decreases (decremental conduction). The AV node effective refractory is reached at the longest A_1-A_2 which fails to conduct to the His bundle (panel C), while the atrial effective refractory period is the longest S_1-S_2 which fails to capture the atria (panel E). A, atrial electrogram; A ERP, atrial effective refractory period; AVN ERP, atrioventricular node effective refractory period; H, His bundle electrogram; V, ventricular electrogram; S, stimulus artifact.

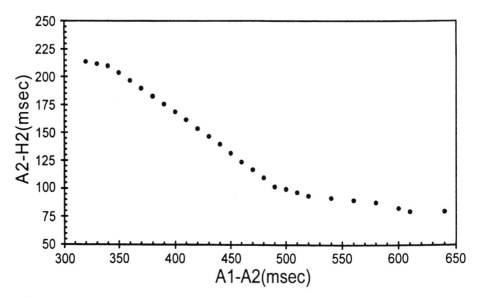

FIGURE 2-25. Plot of A_2-H_2 interval versus A_1-A_2 interval, illustrating normal decremental conduction properties of the AV node. Fixed cycle length pacing of the high right atrium (A_1-A_1 = 650 msec) is followed by the introduction of a premature atrial extrastimulus (A_2). As the duration of the premature coupling interval (A_1-A_2) is reduced, the conduction through the AV node is prolonged (increase in the duration of the A_2-H_2 interval). This increase in AV node conduction time is gradual without any abrupt changes or discontinuities.

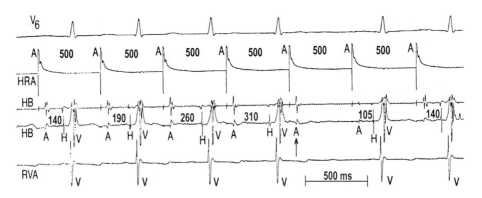

FIGURE 2-26. Normal AV node decremental conduction during fixed cycle length atrial pacing. Intracardiac recording shows AV node Wenckebach phenomenon. Fixed cycle length pacing of the HRA (A-A = 500 msec) results in progressive prolongation of the A-H interval recorded by the His bundle electrographic (HB) lead. With continued pacing, conduction eventually blocks (upward arrow) in the AV node. Note that in the first paced complex following the block the A-H interval is much shorter than in the complex occurring just before the development of block. Recording paper speed 100 mm/sec. A, atrial electrogram. H, His bundle electrogram. RVA, right ventricular apex. V, ventricular electrogram. See text for details.

FIGURE 2-27. Plot of A_2-H_2 interval versus A_1-A_2 interval in a patient with dual AV node pathway physiology. Fixed cycle length pacing of the high right atrium (HRA) (A_1-A_1 = 650 msec) is followed by the introduction of a premature atrial depolarization (A_2). As the premature coupling interval (A_1-A_2) is reduced from 540 msec to 530 msec, there is an abrupt increase in the duration of the A_2-H_2 interval (compare to Figure 2-25). This abrupt increase in AV node conduction time at a discrete premature coupling interval indicates the presence of sudden block in the fast AV nodal pathway with anterograde conduction continuing via the slow AV nodal pathway.

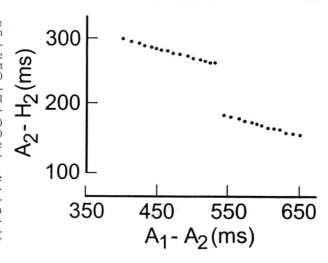

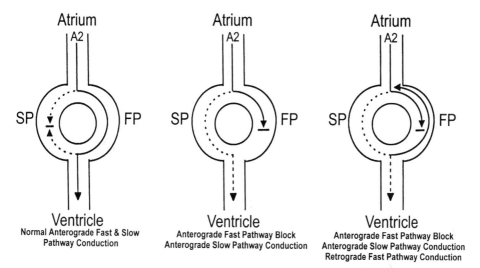

FIGURE 2-28. Schematic diagram of the AV node with fast and slow pathways. See text for details.

further. When the impulse conduction changes from fast pathway to slow pathway, the A-H interval dramatically prolongs because conduction through this AV node pathway is now much slower. This change from fast pathway to slow pathway conduction is marked by an A-H interval "jump" (Figure 2-29). An A-H interval jump is defined as a 50 msec or greater increase in the A-H interval in response to a 10 ms reduction in the A_1-A_2 coupling interval. Because of the prolonged conduction time in the anterograde slow pathway, by the time the impulse reaches the lower junction of the slow and fast pathways, the retrograde fast pathway may no longer be refractory and may conduct the impulse retrograde to re-excite the atria. Meanwhile, if the anterograde slow pathway has recovered, the wavefront of depolarization may reenter this anterograde pathway possibly leading to a sustained circus movement tachyarrhythmia termed the slow-fast form of AV node reentrant tachycardia (Figure 2-28) (see "Atrioventricular Nodal Reentrant Tachycardia" on page 487). However, many individuals with dual AV node pathway physiology will never have a clinical tachycardia. As an interesting, but predictable side-note, if the difference in conduction time between the anterograde slow and fast conduction pathways is longer than the effective refractory period of the His-Purkinje system and ventricle, than a double response can occur, with the ventricles activated twice by a single atrial depolarization, once using the anterograde fast pathway and a second depolarization via the anterograde slow pathway (Figure 2-30).

Accessory AV connections & the concept of preexcitation
As mentioned above, most people only have AV conduction within the normal AV conduction pathway (AV node-His-Purkinje system). Rare patients also exhibit AV conduction occurring within an accessory pathway. Functionally, there are three distinct varieties of accessory connections: those that conduct only in the anterograde direction (from atrium to ventricle), termed *manifest accessory AV connections*; those that conduct

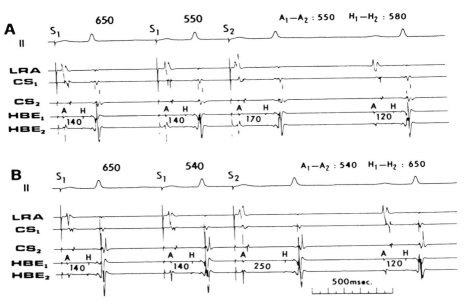

FIGURE 2-29. Intracardiac recording showing jump in A-H interval. From top to bottom in each panel are the surface ECG recording from lead II and endocardial recordings from the low right atrium (LRA), proximal and distal epicardial recordings from the coronary sinus catheter (CS_1 and CS_2, respectively), and proximal and distal endocardial His bundle recordings (HBE_1 and HBE_2, respectively). Panel A: Fixed cycle length pacing of right atrium is performed at a (S_1-S_1) cycle length of 650 msec followed by the introduction of a premature stimulus at a coupling interval (S_1-S_2) of 550 msec (A_1-A_2 = 550 msec). The resultant A-H interval increases from 140 to 170 msec (normal decremental AV node conduction). Panel B: After reducing the S_1-S_2 coupling interval to 540 msec (A_1-A_2 = 540), the A-H interval dramatically increases to 250 msec, indicating conduction block in the fast AV nodal pathway, but with continued anterograde conduction in the slow AV nodal pathway S, stimulus artifact. A, atrial electrogram. H, His bundle electrogram.

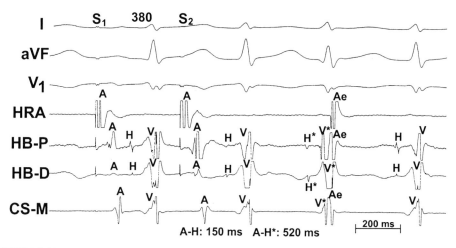

FIGURE 2-30. Double ventricular response in patient with dual AV nodal conduction pathways. Displayed are ECG leads I, aVF, and V_1 and intracardiac electrograms recorded from the high right atrium (HRA), proximal (HB-P) and distal (HP-D) His bundle region, middle coronary sinus (CS-M). After a fixed drive train (S_1-S_1 = 600 ms, not shown), a premature extrastimulus is introduced in the high right atrium coupling interval of (S_1-S_2) of 380 ms. The resultant atrial depolarization conducts within anterograde fast (A-H interval = 150 ms) and slow (A-H* interval = 520 ms) conduction pathways to the ventricle. The His bundle and ventricle are activated twice (H and H*, V and V*, respectively) from the single atrial depolarization. An atrial echo depolarization (Ae) conducts retrograde within the fast AV nodal pathway after anterograde conduction is complete over the slow pathway. Double ventricular activation from a single atrial depolarization can occur if the difference in conduction time between the anterograde slow and fast conduction pathways (in this case, 370 ms) is longer than the effective refractory period of the His-Purkinje system and ventricle. A, atrial electrogram; H His bundle electrogram, V, ventricular electrogram.

only in the retrograde direction (from ventricle to atrium), termed *concealed accessory AV connections*; and those that conduct in both directions (also termed manifest pathways). In addition, within each of theses types, accessory pathways exhibit either rapid all-or-none conduction (i.e., similar to atrial or ventricular muscle) or decremental conduction (i.e., similar to the AV node), with the former much more common than the latter.

When the annulus fibrosus insulation is disrupted by a rapidly conducting *manifest* accessory AV connection, the AV node-His-Purkinje system is short-circuited and the ventricle may be excited earlier than would have otherwise normally occurred (*ventricular preexcitation*). Some areas of ventricular myocardium will be activated via the accessory pathway, while other regions will continue to be activated through the normal pathway. When viewed with surface ECG mapping, this multi-pathway activation of the ventricle manifests characteristic ECG changes (hence the term "manifest" accessory connection) including a shortened P-R interval, slurring of the QRS complex upstroke (*delta (δ) wave*), increased duration of the QRS complex, and often, an atypical QRS complex axis (Figure 2-31). Fast conduction over the AV connection bypassing the AV node accounts for the short P-R (P-δ) interval duration. This abnormal, multi-pathway activation of the ventricle, results in *ventricular fusion*, generating a hybrid QRS complex which is different from that resulting from exclusive conduction over either the normal or accessory pathway. Varying degrees of ventricular preexcitation with dynamic

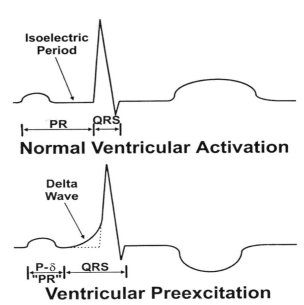

Normal Ventricular Activation

Ventricular Preexcitation

FIGURE 2-31. The delta wave represents anterograde activation of the ventricles through an accessory connection in advance of normal anterograde activation through the AV nodal – His – Purkinje system. See text for further discussion.

variations in the QRS complex configuration can be observed in the same patient at different times. The greater the contribution of ventricular activation through the normal pathway (relative to the accessory connection), the less ventricular preexcitation that will be evident. On the other hand, the greater the contribution to ventricular depolarization through the accessory connection (relative to the normal pathway), the greater the degree of ventricular preexcitation that will occur (Figure 2-32).

Ventricular preexcitation during sinus rhythm is often more pronounced with right-sided than with left-sided accessory AV connections, because right-sided accessory connections are relatively closer to the sinus node. As a result more ventricular activation has already occurred by way of the nearby accessory pathway (more ventricular preexcitation) before the impulse has had a chance to activate the ventricle through the slower conducting and more distant normal pathway. A shift in location of the atrial pacemaker or atrial pacing site can also change the degree of ventricular preexcitation. The closer the site of the ectopic pacemaker to the accessory AV connection, the greater will be the degree of preexcitation. A change in the cardiac cycle length may also cause variation in the degree of ventricular preexcitation. Before reaching the anterograde effective refractory period of an accessory AV connection, atrial pacing at faster rates and atrial premature stimulation with progressively shorter coupling intervals increases the degree of ventricular preexcitation (Figure 2-32). This is because progressive lengthening of AV nodal conduction time associated with shortening of the cardiac cycle length (decremental conduction) permits more ventricular excitation to occur through the accessory connection. Despite the increasing degree of ventricular preexcitation, the atrial stimulus artifact-to-delta wave (P-δ interval) remains constant in non-decrementally conducting accessory connections. Finally vagal stimulation may also be expected to increase the

FIGURE 2-32. Differential contributions to ventricular depolarization through the normal AV conduction pathway and an accessory AV connection result in different degrees of preexcitation (fusion). If all the ventricular activation is through the normal AV nodal (AVN) pathway, normal ventricular activation occurs through the bundle branches and there is no preexcitation. If all the ventricular activation occurs through the accessory connection (AC), *maximal preexcitation* is present. In between these two extremes, ventricular depolarization is the result of variable contributions to ventricular activation (*ventricular fusion*) through both the normal and accessory connections. HB, His bundle; LBB, left bundle branch; RBB, right bundle branch.

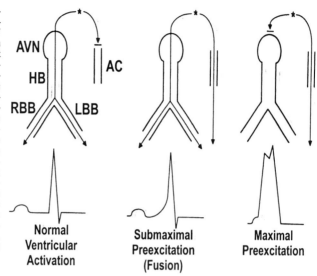

Normal Ventricular Activation

Submaximal Preexcitation (Fusion)

Maximal Preexcitation

degree of preexcitation by prolonging AV nodal conduction time, thereby promoting the contribution of accessory connection conduction to ventricular excitation.

Normalization of the QRS complex morphology with disappearance of ventricular preexcitation may also occur under a variety of situations (Figure 2-33). For example, a reduction in vagal tone during exercise, or by blocking vagal effects with atropine, facil-

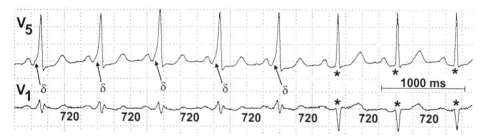

FIGURE 2-33. Short rhythm strip recorded from a patient with a left lateral accessory connection and orthodromic AV reciprocating tachycardia with intermittent preexcitation. ECG leads V_1 and V_5 are shown. On this rhythm strip, the first five QRS complexes exhibit a positive delta (δ) wave (see upward arrows), while the last three QRS complexes (marked by *) lack a delta wave and show no evidence of ventricular preexcitation. The loss of preexcitation occurs despite any change in sinus rate and without evidence of an increase in sympathetic tone or decrease in parasympathetic tone (sinus cycle length remains unchanged at 720 ms) or change in the pacemaker site. Part of the explanation for this finding is that the accessory connection has a long effective refractory period and is located a long distance from the SA node pacemaker. Because of the close proximity of the SA and AV nodes to each other, even very small (?undetectable) changes in the AV nodal conduction time may effect the degree of preexcitation generated by an anatomically distant accessory connection with a long effective refractory period. While strictly speaking, this connection is *manifest* (δ wave evident), if a 12 lead ECG was recorded at the "right time" the accessory connection would appear to be *concealed* (no δ wave seen). Patients with these accessory connections are often said to exhibit *latent preexcitation* because the preexcitation is not always evident and may, in fact, only declare itself under certain conditions such as blockade of AV nodal conduction (adenosine), rapid atrial pacing, or changes in autonomic tone, etc.

itates normal pathway conduction, thereby lessening, or possibly eliminating preexcitation with normalization of the QRS complex. Other situations associated with disappearance of preexcitation and normalization of ventricular activation include: late activation of the accessory AV connection relative to the normal AV conduction pathway; ineffective atrial conduction at the entrance of the accessory AV connection; enhanced AV nodal conduction; and rate-dependent conduction block within the accessory connection at critical cardiac cycle lengths.

Rarely, an atrial impulse conducted simultaneously over the normal and accessory pathways may produce a double ventricular response (1:2 AV conduction) (Figure 2-34). As mentioned above (Figure 2-30), this phenomenon may also occur in patients with dual AV nodal pathways. This can occur because of the marked difference in conduction time between the two AV conduction pathways, with an atrial impulse first activating the ventricle through an accessory pathway and then reactivating the ventricle through the normal pathway. The difference in conduction time between the two AV conduction pathways must be, therefore, longer than the effective refractory period of the His-Purkinje system and ventricle. Slow conduction in the AV node (i.e., presence of dual AV nodal conduction pathways), a minimal degree of retrograde concealed conduction within the His-Purkinje system, and a short effective refractory period of the ventricle fa-

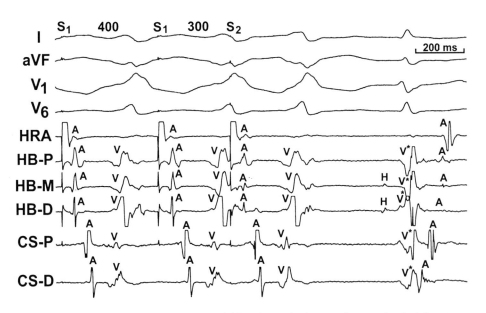

FIGURE 2-34. Demonstration of simultaneous atrial impulse conduction over the normal and a left postero-lateral accessory AV pathways resulting in the production of a double ventricular response (1:2 AV conduction). After a drive train (S₁-S₁ = 400-msec) an atrial extrastimulus is introduced (S₂). The premature atrial impulse activates the ventricle (V) using the accessory connection (preexcitation on surface ECG without His bundle activation) as well as a slow AV nodal pathway (V*) (note His bundle activation (H) and absence of preexcitation on surface ECG). Following this, a single ventriculoatrial echo beat occurs via the accessory connection. Abbreviations: high right atrium (HRA), proximal (HB-P), mid (HB-M) and distal (HB-D) His bundle (HB) region; proximal (CS-P) and distal (CS-D) coronary sinus; A, atrium; H, His bundle; S, stimulus.

vor the development of this phenomenon. Repetition of double ventricular responses during sinus rhythm or an atrial arrhythmia may theoretically generate a non-reentrant form of supraventricular tachycardia.

In patients with the common variety of manifest accessory connection (Kent bundle), fixed atrial pacing at slow rates (just slightly faster than the patient's sinus rate) will result in conduction over both the anterograde normal and accessory pathways. With increasing pacing rate, the anterograde block cycle length of both the normal pathway and the accessory pathway will be reached. In each case, this is defined as the slowest fixed rate of atrial pacing (longest fixed cycle length) at which 1:1 AV conduction over the accessory pathway or normal pathway cannot be maintained. Which block cycle length is reached first is dependent upon which pathway – normal or accessory – has the longest effective refractory period (with the longest effective refractory period within the normal pathway usually residing within the AV node). If the block cycle length of the normal pathway is reached first (i.e. block cycle length of normal pathway > accessory pathway), all AV conduction at faster rates will be within the accessory connection and maximal preexcitation will be present (with no ventricular fusion). If the block cycle length of the accessory pathway is reached first (i.e. block cycle length of accessory pathway > normal pathway), all AV conduction at faster rates will be within the normal pathway and no preexcitation will be evident (also with no ventricular fusion). When pacing at cycle lengths longer than both the accessory and normal pathway block cycle lengths, anterograde conduction will proceed over both the accessory and normal pathways resulting in varying degrees of ventricular fusion and submaximal preexcitation evident. With continued more rapid atrial pacing eventually a cycle length will be reached where either anterograde block is present in both pathways, or the refractory period of the atrial tissue is reached with loss of atrial capture.

Most accessory connections exhibit all-or-none conduction, meaning over a wide range of premature coupling intervals the conduction time of atrial extrastimuli within the accessory connection remains unchanged (*Kent fibers*). However, as alluded to above, in response to atrial extrastimulation, some accessory connections with anterograde conduction exhibit decremental conduction properties, similar to that seen in the AV node. Included in this group are classic *Mahaim fibers* (nodoventricular), as well as some right atriofascicular and rare right and left atrioventricular fibers. From a functional standpoint, the main distinguishing characteristic between these two types of accessory connections during atrial extrastimulation is that the P-to-δ wave interval (or stimulus artifact-to-δ wave interval) remains constant in the case of the Kent fiber (because the conduction time of an extrastimulus within the accessory connection does not change), while the P-to-δ wave interval increases in the case of the Mahaim fiber (because the conduction time of an extrastimulus within the accessory connection increases) (Figure 2-35).

2.2.5 ASSESSMENT OF RETROGRADE REFRACTORINESS & PATTERNS OF CONDUCTION

In general, anterograde AV conduction is better maintained than retrograde (ventriculoatrial) conduction, with AV conduction block occurring in normal individuals at very short A_1-A_1 or A_1-A_2 coupling intervals that are usually (but not always) shorter than the corresponding V_1-V_1 and V_1-V_2 intervals at which ventriculoatrial conduction is blocked. As in the case of anterograde conduction, retrograde conduction may occur within: 1) the normal pathway, i.e., the His-Purkinje-AV nodal pathway; 2) an accessory pathway, i.e., an accessory ventriculoatrial connection; 3) both the normal and accessory pathways.

Retrograde refractory periods
        As with anterograde AV conduction, there are a number of retrograde refractory periods which are routinely measured during the ventricular pacing portion of an electrophysiology study (Table 2-6.)

Normal ventriculoatrial conduction
Fixed rate pacing in the ventricles with or without extrastimuli result in characteristic conduction patterns in a manner analogous to atrial pacing. Conduction may proceed unimpeded from its ventricular origin all the way to the atria. On the other hand, retrograde conduction block may develop anywhere along the ventriculoatrial conduction pathway (Figures 2-36 & 2-37). However, evaluating retrograde conduction, particularly the site

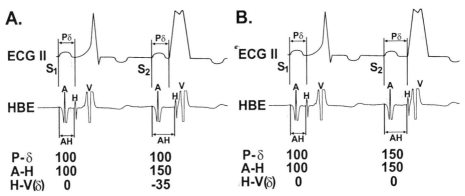

FIGURE 2-35. Schematic diagram illustrating the differences between anterograde conduction patterns in accessory connections exhibiting all-or-none conduction (panel A) and decremental conduction (panel B) in response to an atrial extrastimulus. In the basal state with fixed rate pacing (S_1) there is minimal preexcitation. In both cases the P-δ interval is 100 ms. With the introduction of an extrastimulus (S_2) in the atria the conduction time from the atria to the His bundle through the AV node prolongs from 100 ms to 150 ms. In the case of the accessory connection with non-decremental conduction (panel A), this increased conduction time allows a greater degree of preexcitation (greater proportion of the ventricles activated via the accessory connection) as seen in QRS complex of the surface ECG and the H-V interval changing from zero to -35 ms (i.e., anterograde His bundle activation occurs 35 ms after the earliest ventricular activation through the accessory connection). However, because the conduction time within the accessory connection does not change in response to the extrastimulus, the *P-δ interval does not change* and is still measured at 100 ms. In the case of the accessory connection with decremental conduction properties (Panel B), the extrastimulus is associated with an increase of conduction time in both the AV node and the accessory connection. Because conduction time increases in the accessory connection, the *P-δ interval must increase* (in this case from 100 to 150 ms). Even with this increase in anterograde conduction time within the accessory connection, preexcitation can still increase (as evidence by the increased QRS duration) so long as conduction time within the normal AV nodal pathway increases even more. Many accessory connections exhibiting decremental conduction are atriofascicular (running from the right atrium to a branch of the right bundle branch). In this case the H-V interval may be largely unchanged because His bundle activation actually results from an impulse traveling in the retrograde direction within right bundle branch back to the proximal His bundle. This retrograde His bundle activation can also occur in cases of accessory connections lacking decremental conduction, especially if anterograde conduction of the AV node is prolonged, such as in the case of conduction within a slow AV nodal pathway. Whether His bundle activation is the result of anterograde AV nodal conduction or retrograde right bundle branch conduction can often only be made if right bundle and His bundle electrograms are simultaneously recorded.

TABLE 2-6. Definition of retrograde refractory periods

Conduction System Component	Effective Refractory Period	Relative Refractory Period	Functional Refractory Period
Ventricle	Longest S_1-S_2 that fails to produce a ventricular depolarization	Longest S_1-S_2 at which S_2-V_2 is $> S_1$-V_1*	Shortest V_1-V_2* resulting from any S_1-S_2
AV node	Longest H_1-H_2 (or S_1-H_2) that fails to produce an atrial depolarization near the His bundle region**	Not normally measurable	Shortest A_1-A_2 resulting from any H_1-H_2**
Accessory AV connection	Longest V_1-V_2 interval that fails to depolarize any portion of the atria through the accessory connection	Not normally measurable	Shortest A_1-A_2 resulting from any V_1-V_2++
His-Purkinje system	Longest V_1-V_2 (or S_1-S_2) interval that fails to produce His bundle depolarization**	Not normally measurable	Shortest H_1-H_2 (or S_1-H_2) resulting from any V_1-V_2**

S_1, A_1, H_1, V_1: stimulus artifact, atrial, His bundle, and ventricular electrograms during fixed cycle-length pacing train; S_2, A_2, H_2, V_2: stimulus artifact, atrial, His bundle, and ventricular electrograms of premature depolarization; * earliest V measured on surface ECG or intracardiac recordings; ** assumes that one can clearly record retrograde His bundle activation resulting from premature stimulation; ++ measured near the site of the atrial input of accessory connection assuming all retrograde normal pathway conduction is blocked

of ventriculoatrial block, is more difficult than evaluating conduction in the anterograde direction (Figure 2-37). The reason for this is that during anterograde AV conduction, His bundle activation reliably occurs well before ventricular activation (except in the case of preexcitation) and the His bundle electrogram is predictably found and clearly delineated 30-55 ms before local ventricular activation. On the other hand, during retrograde conduction, the ventricular myocardium near the His bundle or proximal bundle branches may be activated before, or nearly simultaneous with, the His bundle or proximal right and left bundle branches (Figures 2-38 & 2-39). Consequently, the retrograde His bundle, right bundle, or left bundle electrograms may not be recorded because: 1) they are hidden within the much larger local ventricular depolarization recorded by the electrode catheter positioned to record those electrograms or, 2) conduction block has occurred below the level of the His bundle or proximal bundle branches. However, because conduction is rapid within the bundle branches (relative to ventricular muscle), rapid retrograde conduction within the right bundle branch block often results in the retrograde His bundle inscription before local activation of the ventricle in the His bundle region (Figure 2-38). Only by recording *immediately proximal and distal* to a particular site (and *verifying* correct catheter position) can conduction block be said to occur at that particular site.

Conduction in the His-Purkinje system following right apical endocardial activation may proceed within either right or left bundle branch (Figures 2-38 & 2-39). Not uncommonly, conduction proceeds via the right bundle branch at long coupling intervals. At shorter coupling intervals, retrograde conduction block may develop in the right bundle branch. Retrograde conduction, however, may continue within the left bundle branch after a delay resulting from right-to-left transseptal intramyocardial conduction [41,42] (Figures 2-39 & 2-40).

The most common site of retrograde conduction delay or block during ventriculoatrial conduction is in the His-

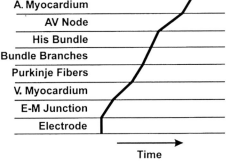

Sites of Potential Retrograde Block (Normal Conduction Pathway)

| A. Myocardium |
| AV Node |
| His Bundle |
| Bundle Branches |
| Purkinje Fibers |
| V. Myocardium |
| E-M Junction |
| Electrode |

Time

FIGURE 2-36. Ladder diagram showing potential sites of retrograde conduction block within the normal pathway. E-M, electrode-myocardial junction; A, atrial; V., ventricular

Purkinje system or at the junction between the Purkinje fibers and ventricular myocardium [42-44]. Retrograde conduction block at this junction may occur because Purkinje fibers normally have a longer action potential duration than ventricular myocardial fibers (see Figure 16-8 on page 738); therefore, Purkinje tissue exhibits a longer period of refractoriness compared to ventricular myocardium. Pacing from the ventricular myocardium may thus encounter relatively refractory Purkinje fibers, which may be manifested as decremental conduction properties and even conduction block below the His bundle (Figures 2-37 & 2-39 through 2-43). Because of the disparate action potential durations in Purkinje fibers and ventricular myocardial fibers, anterograde AV conduction is more easily maintained than retrograde (ventriculoatrial) conduction.

Right ventricular stimulation using fixed cycle ventricular pacing with a single ventricular extrastimulus (V_1-V_2) can be used to study the behavior of the His-Purkinje system/ventricular myocardium as long as a retrograde His bundle deflection can be recorded. Progressive prolongation of His-Purkinje conduction (V_2-H_2) occurs with increasing prematurity of the ventricular extrastimulus (V_1-V_2) in a relatively constant fashion (Figure 2-42). Furthermore, at any given V_1-V_2 interval, the V_2-H_2 interval is shorter at shorter drive cycle lengths (V_1-V_1). Eventually with increasing prematurity, the ventricular effective refractory period is reached (Figures 2-43 & 2-44).

Prior to reaching the ventricular effective refractory period, the introduction of a ventricular extrastimulus may result in repetitive ventricular responses even in individuals with normal hearts. The most common type of response is *bundle branch reentry* [45-49] (Figures 2-43, 2-45, & 2-46). In a significant percentage of patients, fixed right ventricular pacing with ventricular extrastimulation results in retrograde conduction of V_2 via the right bundle branch. This can be proven by observing a retrograde right bundle or His bundle deflection before the ventricular electrogram in the His bundle recording. As the premature coupling interval (V_1-V_2) is reduced, progressive retrograde conduction delay (prolongation of V_2-H_2 or S_2-H_2) occurs in the right bundle branch until block occurs. At this point, the retrograde conduction continues via the left bundle branch after transseptal activation and the retrograde His potential is then observed following the local ventricular electrogram at the His bundle recording site. As the V_1-V_2 interval is further decreased, the V_2-H_2 (or S_2-H_2) further prolongs. When a critical degree of retrograde conduction delay has occurred, excitability can recover in the previously refractory right bundle branch. This allows V_2 to reenter the right bundle branch and conduct anterograde re-exciting the ventricle as V_3 with a left bundle branch block QRS morphology pattern (similar to the QRS complex resulting from right ventricular apex stimulation) [45-49]. In the case of bundle branch reentry, the retrograde His bun-

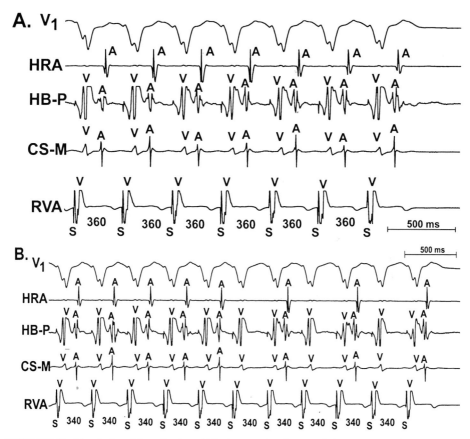

FIGURE 2-37. Ventriculoatrial conduction within the normal pathway and demonstration of the retrograde normal pathway block cycle length. Displayed from top to bottom is ECG lead V_1, along with intracardiac recordings from the high right atrium (HRA), proximal (HB-P) and distal (HB-D) His bundle (HB) region, middle coronary sinus (CS-M), and right ventricular apex (RVA). Panel A: Fixed rate right ventricular pacing is performed at a cycle length of 360 ms results in 1:1 ventriculoatrial conduction with retrograde earliest atrial activation in the His bundle region consistent with retrograde conduction through the normal His bundle-AV nodal pathway. Panel B: The pacing cycle length is reduced to 340 ms and 1:1 ventriculoatrial conduction changes to 2:1 conduction (right half of panel). The exact level of conduction block cannot be determined because the retrograde His bundle electrogram cannot be seen.

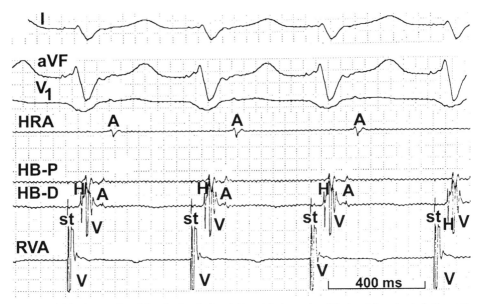

FIGURE 2-38. Retrograde atrial activation during right ventricular pacing. Displayed from top to bottom are surface ECG leads I, aVF, V$_1$, along with intracardiac recordings from the high right atrium (HRA), proximal (HB-P) and distal (HB-D) His bundle (HB) region, and right ventricular apex (RVA). Panel A: During RVA pacing at a cycle length of 500 msec, there is 1:1 ventriculoatrial conduction through the His bundle-AV node axis with each ventricular depolarization (V) followed by an atrial depolarization (A). In this case, retrograde conduction proceeds rapidly up the right bundle branch from the RVA, resulting in activation of the His bundle (H), which can be clearly identified as a discrete sharp deflection (retrograde H). st, stimulus artifact.

dle potential (H$_2$) precedes the anterograde right bundle deflection (RB$_2$) and the H-V interval preceding the extra-beat (H$_2$-V$_3$) is equal to or greater than the H-V interval in sinus rhythm. For patients with normal hearts without a fixed bundle branch conduction delay, bundle branch reentry is rarely sustained and self-terminates after one or two beats.

Retrograde conduction utilizing accessory ventriculoatrial connections
Despite the fact that it is often difficult to record the retrograde His bundle activation, the hallmark of retrograde normal pathway (ventricular myocardium/His-Purkinje-AV node) conduction is that it is decremental (Figure 2-47) and the earliest retrograde atrial activation occurs at the anterior right atrial septum at the site where the maximal His bundle electrogram is recorded during sinus rhythm (Figure 2-47) (unless retrograde AV nodal conduction occurs within the slow pathway, in which case the earliest retrograde atrial activation will be recorded more posteriorly, near to the ostium of the coronary sinus [50]).

If ventriculoatrial conduction occurs within an accessory connection, the retrograde pattern of conduction will be different than that seen in Figure 2-47 (unless the accessory connection lies immediately adjacent to the normal AV node-His bundle and also exhibits decremental conduction properties). For example, in a patient with a concealed left-sided accessory AV connection (which only conducts from the ventricle to atrium), fixed

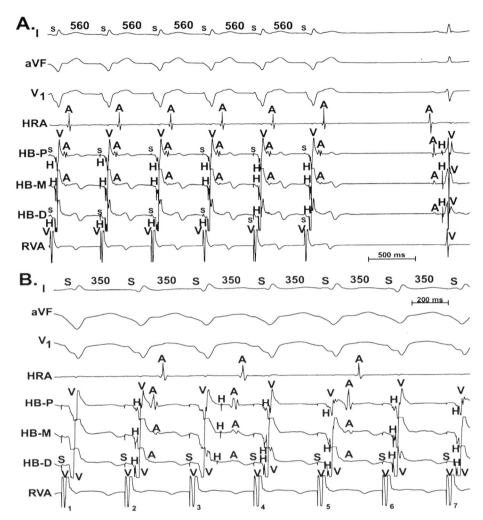

FIGURE 2-39. Fixed cycle length pacing at the right ventricular apex at two different drive cycle lengths shows 1:1 ventriculoatrial conduction (panel A) and conduction block at various levels within the retrograde normal pathway (panel B). Displayed in each panel are ECG lead I, aVF, V$_1$ and intracardiac electrograms recorded from the high right atrium (HRA), proximal (HB-P), middle (HB-M), and distal (HB-D) His bundle regions, and right ventricular apex (RVA). In panel A, S$_1$-S$_1$ drive of 560 ms results in 1:1 ventriculoatrial conduction with the retrograde His bundle electrogram (H) inscribed as the sharp deflection recorded in the early portion of the local ventricular electrogram in each of the HB leads. In panel B, the S$_1$-S$_1$ drive interval is reduced to 350 ms. At this pacing rate there is no longer 1:1 ventriculoatrial conduction. Ventricular depolarization #1 (see numbers at bottom of panel B) captures the ventricle, but there is conduction block in the His-Purkinje system because no retrograde His bundle electrogram is recorded. Ventricular depolarizations #2 and 5 conduct to the atrium with inscription of the His bundle electrogram in the early portion of the local ventricular electrogram after rapid retrograde conduction within the right bundle branch. Ventricular depolarization #3 blocks retrograde in the right bundle branch, conducts transseptal, and then proceeds up the left bundle branch to activate the His bundle which is now inscribed well after the local ventricular electrogram in the His bundle region. Retrograde conduction thereafter continues through the AV node to depolarize the atrium. Ventricular depolarizations #4, 6, and 7 all conduct retrograde via the right bundle branch to activate the His bundle, without continuing onward through the AV node to activate the atrium (i.e., conduction block within the AV node). A, atrial electrogram; H, His bundle electrogram; V, ventricular electrogram; S, stimulus artifact.

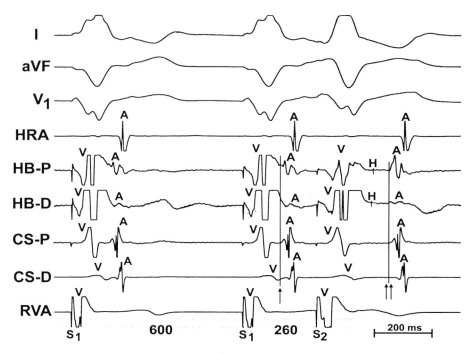

FIGURE 2-40. Ventricular extrastimulation with ventriculoatrial conduction illustrating the normal sequence of retrograde atrial activation and decremental conduction properties of the normal retrograde pathway. Displayed from top to bottom is ECG lead I, aVF, V_1 and intracardiac electrograms recorded from the high right atrium (HRA), proximal (HB-P), and distal (HB-D) His bundle regions, proximal (CS-P) and distal (CS-D) coronary sinus regions, and right ventricular apex (RVA). Ventricular pacing is performed at a fixed cycle length (S_1-S_1) of 600 ms (eight pulses) and then a premature extrastimulus (S_2) is introduced at the RV apex. During the fixed drive train, there is 1:1 ventriculoatrial conduction (although the His bundle electrogram is not seen because it is hidden within the local ventricular depolarization) with the earliest retrograde atrial activation recorded at the His bundle recording site (HB-P and HB-D) (see line with single upward arrow). Also note that the inscription of the atrial electrogram at the proximal coronary sinus (CS-P) recording site is also early and atrial activation at CS-P and the His bundle region clearly precede left atrial activation in the distal coronary sinus (CS-D). Finally notice that the retrograde atrial activation sequence remains the same after the premature stimulus (S_1-S_2 = 260 ms) (see line with double upward arrow), although there has been a marked increase in the ventriculoatrial interval due a prolonged conduction time from the right ventricular apex to the His bundle region (and the retrograde His bundle deflection is now clearly visualized). This conduction delay results from retrograde block of the ventricular extrastimulus in the right bundle branch with trans-septal conduction and resumption of retrograde conduction to the His bundle region via the left bundle branch. A, atrial electrogram; H, His bundle electrogram; V, ventricular electrogram; S, stimulus artifact.

cycle length ventricular pacing will demonstrate ventriculoatrial conduction proceeding exclusively within the accessory connection. In this case, the earliest retrograde atrial activation will be recorded by one of the electrode pairs positioned within the coronary sinus adjacent to the location of the accessory connection (Figure 2-48).

If fixed rate ventricular pacing is performed in a patient with both normal and accessory connections capable of retrograde conduction, various patterns of conduction may occur. Pacing at slow rates (just slightly faster than the patient's sinus rate) may result in conduction over both the retrograde normal and accessory pathways. At these cycle lengths there will be fusion activation of the atria, with some portions of the atria

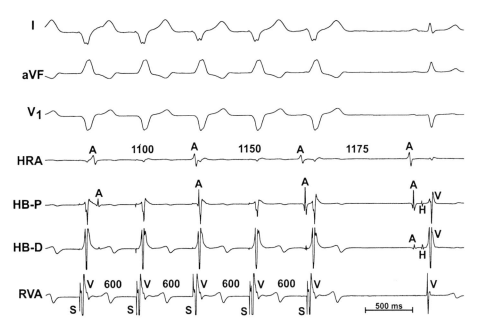

FIGURE 2-41. Fixed rate ventricular pacing with no ventriculoatrial conduction and presumed retrograde conduction block within the His-Purkinje system/ventricular myocardium (below His bundle). Displayed from top to bottom is ECG lead I, aVF, V_1 and intracardiac electrograms recorded from the high right atrium (HRA), proximal (HB-P), middle (HB-M), and distal (HB-D) His bundle regions, and right ventricular apex (RVA). Ventricular pacing is performed at a fixed cycle length (S_1-S_1) of 600 ms. The atrial activation is by the normal sinus mechanism with a "high to low" intra-atrial activation sequence (i.e., high right atrium is activated before the low septal right atrium at the His bundle recording site). Atrial activation is dissociated from the retrograde ventricular depolarizations which block below the His bundle (no retrograde His bundle activation) in the His-Purkinje system/ventricular myocardium. A, atrial electrogram; H, His bundle electrogram; V, ventricular electrogram; S, stimulus artifact.

being activated using the accessory connection while other portions are activated via the normal pathway (see Figure 12-9 on page 549). With increasing pacing rate, the retrograde block cycle lengths of the accessory pathway and the normal pathway, respectively, will be reached. In each case, this is defined as the slowest fixed rate of ventricular pacing (longest fixed cycle length) at which 1:1 ventriculoatrial conduction over the accessory pathway or normal pathway, respectively, cannot be maintained. Which block cycle length is reached first is dependent upon which pathway – normal or accessory – has the longest effective refractory period. If the retrograde block cycle length of the normal pathway is reached first (i.e. block cycle length of normal pathway > accessory pathway), all ventriculoatrial conduction at faster rates will be within the accessory connection (with no atrial fusion). If the block cycle length of the accessory pathway is reached first (i.e. block cycle length of accessory pathway > normal pathway), all ventriculoatrial conduction at faster rates will be within the normal pathway (also with no atrial fusion). A more in-depth discussion of accessory connections, anterograde and retrograde conduction patterns, and their role in AV reciprocating tachycardia is discussed in "Arrhythmia Localization" on page 136, "The Physiology of Ventricular Preexcita-

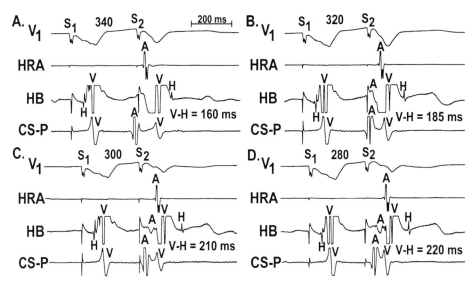

FIGURE 2-42. Decremental retrograde conduction within the ventriculoatrial conduction system below the His bundle. Displayed are ECG lead V_1 and intracardiac electrograms recorded from the high right atrium (HRA), His bundle (HB) region, and proximal coronary sinus (CS-P) region. After a fixed drive train (S_1-S_1 = 600 ms), a premature ventricular extrastimulus is introduced at the right ventricular apex at a coupling interval (S_1-S_2) of 340 ms (panel A), 320 ms (panel B), 300 ms (panel C), or 280 ms (panel D). A, atrial electrogram; H, His bundle electrogram; V, ventricular electrogram; S, stimulus artifact.

tion" on page 539, "Electrophysiology Study" on page 541 and "Radiofrequency Catheter Ablation" on page 586.

2.2.6 CONCEALED CONDUCTION

Concealed conduction refers to incompletely penetrating electrical (non-propagated) impulses in the heart that are themselves electrically silent on the surface ECG but which alter the conduction of subsequent propagated impulses. For example, incomplete penetration of the AV node by premature atrial or ventricular depolarizations can result in the unexpected prolongation of conduction or unexpected failure of propagation of an impulse [51-54]. Figures 2-23, 2-49, 2-50 & 2-51 illustrate examples of concealed conduction involving slowing or blocking of AV nodal or intra-atrial conduction by premature impulses or during atrial flutter. In the situation depicted in Figure 2-49, right atrial premature depolarizations which fail to conduct to the His bundle or ventricles, nevertheless delay subsequent conduction of impulses in the AV node. In Figure 2-50, non-propagated atrial stimuli increase the intra-atrial conduction time of subsequent propagated atrial stimuli.

During atrial flutter (Figure 2-51), many of the rapid atrial depolarizations penetrate into, but do not conduct through the AV node to the His bundle (note atrial depolarizations not followed by His depolarizations in Figure 2-23). Under normal conditions, this concealed conduction functions to prevent rapid 1:1 AV conduction during atrial

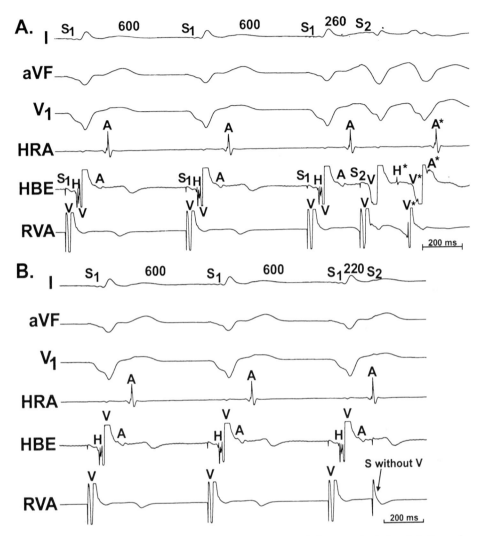

FIGURE 2-43. Retrograde conduction patterns resulting from ventricular extrastimulation. In both panels A and B, ECG leads I, aVF, V_1 and intracardiac electrograms from the high right atrium (HRA), His bundle region (HBE), and right ventricular apex (RVA) are displayed. Fixed drive pacing (S_1-S_1) at the right ventricular apex at a cycle length of 600 ms is followed by a premature extrastimulus with a coupling interval (S_1-S_2) of 260 ms (panel A) and 220 ms (panel B). In panel A, there is 1:1 retrograde ventriculoatrial conduction during the fixed drive with the retrograde His bundle electrogram (H) inscribed as the sharp deflection recorded in the early portion of the local ventricular electrogram in the HBE lead. The premature ventricular depolarization blocks in the retrograde right bundle, conducts transeptal, and then proceeds up the left bundle to activate the His bundle (H*) which is now plainly visible after the large ventricular electrogram recorded by the HBE lead. In addition, retrograde conduction continues through the AV node to activate the atrium (A*). After activating the His bundle (H*), the wavefront conducts anterograde within the previously refractory right bundle branch (bundle branch reentry) to re-excite the ventricle (V*). The S_1-S_2 coupling intervals are further reduced (not shown) until ventricular capture fails at a coupling interval S_1-S_2 of 220 ms (panel B). This is the ventricular effective refractory period. A, atrial electrogram; V, ventricular electrogram.

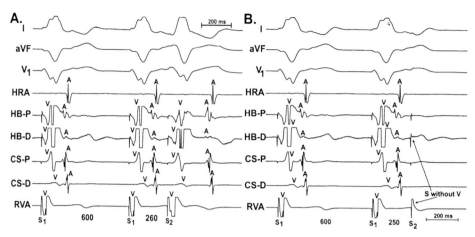

FIGURE 2-44. Retrograde decremental conduction and ventricular effective refractory period. Displayed are ECG leads I, aVF, and V_1 and intracardiac electrograms recorded from the high right atrium (HRA), proximal (HB-P) and distal (HP-D) His bundle region, proximal (CS-P) and distal (CS-D) coronary sinus regions, and right ventricular apex (RVA). After a fixed drive train of eight pulses (S_1-S_1 = 600 ms) delivered at the RVA, a premature ventricular extrastimulus is introduced at the RVA at a coupling interval (S_1-S_2) of 260 ms (panel A) or 250 ms (panel B). In panel A, there is 1:1 ventriculoatrial conduction during the fixed drive train and decremental conduction somewhere within the normal ventriculoatrial pathway during the extrastimulus. Note that the retrograde atrial activation sequence remains unchanged with the earliest atrial activation occurring in the proximal His bundle (HB-P) region and the latest activation in the distal coronary sinus (CS-D). As the ventricular extrastimulus coupling interval is further decreased to 250 ms, there is failure to capture the ventricle. This defines the ventricular effective refractory period. A, atrial electrogram; H, His bundle electrogram; V, ventricular electrogram; S, stimulus artifact.

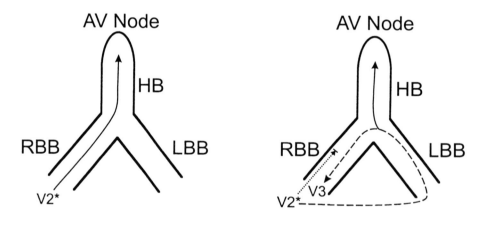

FIGURE 2-45. Schematic illustration showing circuit of bundle branch reentry. A premature right ventricular depolarization (V_2*) normally conducts retrograde in the right bundle branch (RBB), through the His bundle (HB), to the AV node. With greater prematurity, retrograde V_2* conduction is blocked in the RBB but proceeds transseptally and conducts retrograde via the left bundle branch (LBB) to the HB. At the junction of the HB, RBB and LBB, conduction can continue retrograde to the AV node, but also may proceed anterograde within the RBB to re-excite the ventricle (V_3). Reentrant anterograde conduction in the RBB occurs because the delay resulting from transeptal & LBB conduction allows recovery of RBB excitability.

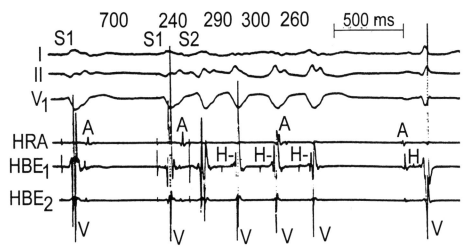

FIGURE 2-46. Surface ECG and intracardiac recording of bundle branch reentry. Recordings top to bottom are from ECG leads I, II, and V_1, along with intracardiac recordings from high right atrium (HRA) and proximal (HBE$_1$) and distal (HBE$_2$) His bundle regions. Right ventricular pacing is performed at a cycle length (S_1-S_1) of 700 msec followed by the introduction of an extrastimulus at a premature coupling interval (S_1-S_2) of 240 msec. During the S_1-S_1 drive train, there is 1:1 ventriculoatrial conduction with the retrograde His bundle depolarization resulting from conduction in the right bundle branch (RBB) buried in the much larger ventricular electrogram recorded at the His bundle region. The premature ventricular depolarization is followed by a series of three spontaneous ventricular depolarizations with left bundle branch block (LBBB) morphology. As schematically illustrated in Figure 2-45, the extrastimulus fails to conduct retrograde in the RBB, and instead proceeds trans-septal and travels retrograde in the left bundle branch (LBB). Once this depolarization reaches the junction of the RBB and His bundle, the RBB is no longer refractory allowing anterograde conduction again to proceed within the RBB. The ventricles are again activated from this reentrant depolarization wavefront with LBBB morphology. The long V-H- interval results because, with the RBB refractory, the His bundle is activated only after the impulse travels the long path from the right ventricle to the left ventricle and then retrograde in the LBB. A, atrial depolarization. H, anterograde His bundle depolarization. H-, retrograde His bundle depolarization. From [66] with permission.

flutter (Figure 2-51, upper panel). However, exercise, with its reduction in parasympathetic and increase in sympathetic tone, can alter the effects of concealed conduction and enhance AV conduction during atrial flutter (Figure 2-51, lower panel). The concealed AV nodal conduction is markedly diminished by the high adrenergic tone of exercise resulting in a increase in the ventricular rate to the atrial flutter rate of 215 beats/min.

2.2.7 GAP PHENOMENON

The *gap phenomenon* refers to an unusual situation whereby atrial premature depolarizations of greater prematurity are more likely to conduct to the ventricles than less premature atrial depolarizations. The resumption of conduction at shorter coupling intervals was originally interpreted as a manifestation of supernormal conduction; however, it is now clear that this phenomenon has a simple physiologic basis.

In general, the gap phenomenon requires a distal region of the conduction system to have an effective refractory period longer than the functional refractory period of a more proximal region. In this case, premature atrial depolarizations block first in the distal location, but with continued prematurity, delay develops in the proximal site permitting

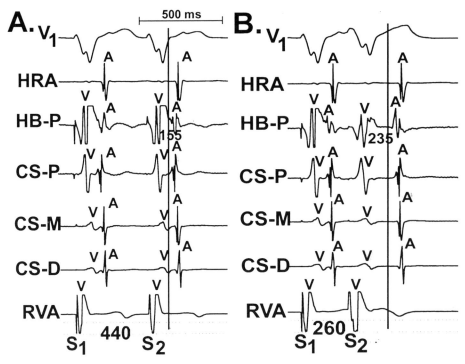

FIGURE 2-47. Decremental conduction properties of the retrograde normal pathway. Displayed are ECG leads V_1 and intracardiac electrograms recorded from the high right atrium (HRA), proximal His bundle region (HB-P), proximal (CS-P), middle (CS-M), and distal (CS-D) coronary sinus regions, and right ventricular apex (RVA). After a fixed drive train (S_1-S_1 = 600 ms, not shown), a premature ventricular extrastimulus is introduced at the right ventricular apex. Note that as the extrastimulus coupling interval (S_1-S_2) decreases from 440 ms (panel A) to 260 ms (panel B), the ventriculoatrial conduction interval (measured as the local ventriculoatrial conduction time in the His bundle recording) increases from 155 ms to 235 ms. Also note that the retrograde atrial activation sequence remains unchanged with the earliest atrial activation occurring in the proximal His bundle (HB-P) region and the latest activation in the distal coronary sinus (CS-D). While the prolongation of conduction time is obvious, the site(s) of conduction delay cannot be identified because the His bundle electrogram is hidden within the ventricular depolarization recorded by the His bundle leads. A, atrial electrogram; H, His bundle electrogram; V, ventricular electrogram; S, stimulus artifact.

time for the distal tissue to recover excitability allowing resumption of distal conduction (Figure 2-52) [42-44,55-60]. While numerous types of gap phenomenon have been demonstrated in human hearts, the most common gaps involve the AV node as the proximal region and various components of the His-Purkinje system as the distal site [42-44,55-60] (Table 2-7.)

Figure 2-53 illustrates an unusual example of the gap phenomenon involving a patient with a right-sided accessory AV connection. Anterograde conduction through the accessory connection results in a wide QRS complex morphology on the surface ECG due to the depolarization wavefront proceeding independent of the His-Purkinje system. In this case, ventricular depolarization must conduct from myocardial cell to myocardial cell without the benefit of the arborizing specialized conduction system. On the other hand, activation of the ventricle through the AV node/His-Purkinje axis results in a rapid, almost simultaneous depolarization of all regions of the ventricles eliciting a narrow

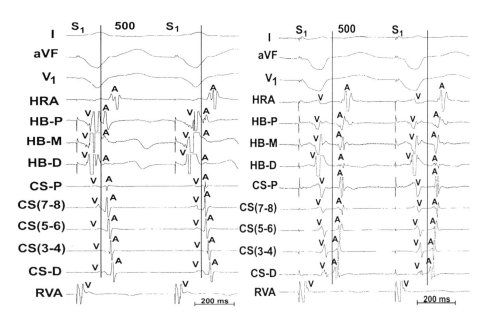

FIGURE 2-48. Fixed rate ventricular pacing with ventriculoatrial conduction using the normal pathway (left A) and a left lateral accessory connection (right B). From top to bottom are displayed surface ECG leads I, aVF, V_1 and intracardiac electrograms from high right atrium (HRA), proximal (HB-P), middle (HB-M), & distal (HB-D) His bundle regions, proximal (CS-P), middle (CS(3-4), CS(5-6), CS(7-8)), & distal (CS-D) coronary sinus/great cardiac vein, and right ventricular apex (RVA). The tip of the coronary sinus catheter (CS-D) is located at the far left lateral mitral annulus within the great cardiac vein, far from the interatrial septum and the His bundle region. Left panel: Fixed rate pacing (S_1-S_1) at 500 ms at the RVA results in ventriculoatrial conduction with the earliest retrograde atrial activation recorded in the His bundle region and progressively later atrial activations recorded as one proceeds from right anterior interatrial septum to the lateral coronary sinus region (CS-D). Right panel: Fixed rate pacing (S_1-S_1) at 500 ms at the RVA results in ventriculoatrial conduction with the earliest retrograde atrial activation recorded in the distal coronary sinus and progressively later atrial activations recorded as one proceeds from the lateral coronary sinus region to the ostium of the coronary sinus (CS-P) and finally the anterior interatrial septum (HB-P). A, atrial electrogram; V, ventricular electrogram.

QRS complex morphology. In the example illustrated in this figure, the patient exhibits exclusive AV conduction through an accessory AV connection and not the AV node/His-Purkinje system, during fixed right atrial pacing at a rate of 150 beats/min. However, a gap exists allowing atrial premature depolarizations delivered at a specific coupling interval to conduct through the AV node/His-Purkinje system, while earlier or later premature atrial depolarizations conduct through the accessory connection. In this case, the accessory AV connection (distal tissue) has an effective refractory period (300 msec) longer than the functional refractory period (295 msec) of the atrium (proximal tissue).

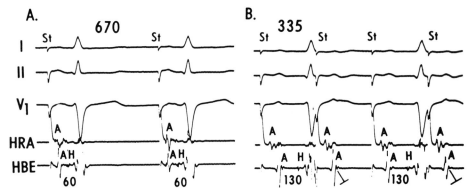

FIGURE 2-49. Demonstration of concealed conduction into the AV node with prolongation of AV nodal conduction time. In both panels, recordings from top to bottom are surface ECG leads I, II, V$_1$ and endocardial electrograms from high right atrium (HRA) and His bundle region (HBE). *Panel A*. Electrical stimulation (St) of the HRA at a St-St cycle length of 670 msec results in 1:1 intra-atrial and AV conduction with an A-H interval of 60 msec. *Panel B*. The rate of atrial stimulation is increased (St-St = 335) resulting in 2:1 AV conduction (A-A cycle length = 335 msec, V-V cycle length = 670 msec) with a A-H interval of 130 msec. Despite the fact that the ventricular rate is identical in *panels A* and *B*, the A-H interval during AV conduction increases from 60 msec to 130 msec when the atrial depolarization rate is doubled. This indicates that the atrial depolarization not conducted to the His bundle or ventricles nevertheless incompletely penetrates the AV node thereby prolonging AV nodal conduction (A-H interval) during the subsequent AV conducted impulse (concealed conduction). St, stimulus artifact. A, electrogram. H, His bundle electrogram.

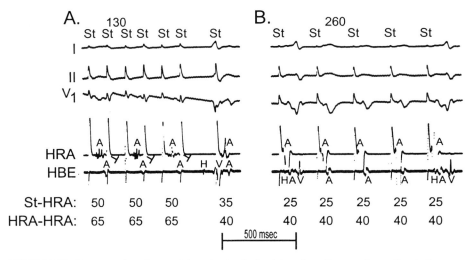

FIGURE 2-50. Demonstration of concealed conduction in the right atrium. Format of recordings is the same as in Figure 2-49. In addition, the conduction times from the stimulus (St) to the HRA and from the HRA to the low right atrium (LRA) is indicated at the bottom of each panel. *Panel A* shows intra-atrial conduction during 2:1 stimulus to atrium conduction at a St-St interval of 130 msec resulting in an atrial depolarization cycle length (A-A) of 260 msec. *Panel B* illustrates intra-atrial conduction during 1:1 stimulus to atrium conduction with both the St-St and A-A intervals equal to 260 msec. Note that with rapid stimulation (St-St = 130 msec), and 2:1 stimulus to atrial conduction, that the intra-atrial conduction time (HRA - LRA) during conducted stimuli is prolonged compared to that seen during 1:1 stimulation, even though the atrial depolarization rate is identical in both instances (260 msec). This indicates that the non-propagated stimulus during rapid pacing partially penetrates the atrium and delays conduction of the subsequent propagated impulse (concealed intra-atrial conduction). St, stimulus artifact,. A, atrial electrogram. H, His bundle electrogram. V, ventricular electrogram. From [67] with permission.

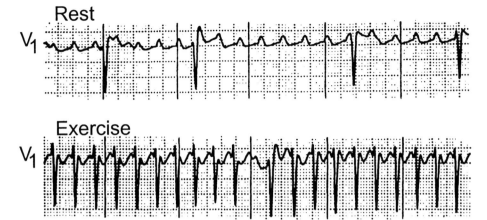

FIGURE 2-51. Effect of exercise on concealed AV nodal conduction during atrial flutter. ECG lead V_1 is recorded in both the upper and lower panels. At rest *(upper panel)* the patient exhibits atrial flutter at a rate of 215/min. The cycle length of the ventricular response varies from 1200 to 2200 msec. The ventricular response is much less than the atrial rate because the rapid atrial input into the decremental-conducting AV node prevents the AV conduction of subsequent atrial inputs (concealed conduction into AV node). An intra-cardiac His bundle recording (not shown) would reveal that non-conducted atrial depolarizations would not be followed by a His bundle depolarization, indicating that conduction block occurs at the level of the AV node (proximal to the His bundle). During exercise *(lower panel)*, the high catecholamine state allows 1:1 AV conduction with the atrial and ventricular rates equal to 215/min. The high adrenergic tone markedly diminishes the effect of concealed AV nodal conduction permitting each atrial input to be conducted through the AV node to the His bundle and ventricles. Paper speed 25 mm/sec.

TABLE 2-7. Classification of gap phenomenon

Type	Distal (initial) site of block	Proximal (delayed) site of block
	Anterograde Conduction	
1	HPS	AV node
2	HPS (distal)	HPS (proximal)
3	HPS	His bundle
4	HPS or AV node	Atrium
5	AV node (distal)	AV node (proximal)
6	HPS	Supernormal conduction
	Retrograde Conduction	
1	AV node	HPS
2	HPS (proximal)	HPS (distal)

AV, atrioventricular; HPS, His-Purkinje system. Adapted from [58].

2.2.8 SUPERNORMAL AND PSEUDO-SUPERNORMAL CONDUCTION

In clinical electrophysiology, supernormal conduction has been classically used to describe situations in which conduction is either better than anticipated or occurs when

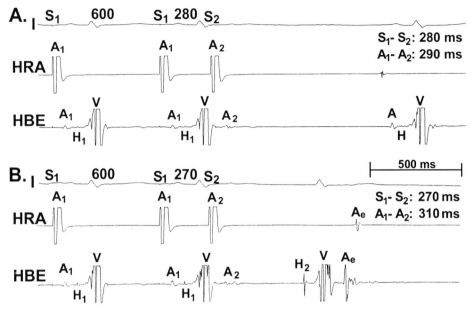

FIGURE 2-52. Intracardiac recordings of type 4 gap phenomenon. Surface ECG lead I is shown at the top of each panel. Fixed rate pacing (S_1-S_1) at 600 ms is performed in the high right atrium (HRA) followed by the introduction of an extrastimulus at a coupling interval (S_1-S_2) of 280 ms (panel A) or 270 ms (panel B). Panel A: The extrastimulus results in an A_1-A_2 interval of 290 ms recorded in the His bundle region (HBE) with the atrial premature depolarization (A_2) failing to conduct through the AV node (A_2 not followed by H_2). Panel B: With a further reduction in S_1-S_2 to 270 ms, the intra-atrial conduction interval (A_1-A_2) recorded at the His bundle region increases to 310 ms. This intra-atrial conduction delay of 20 ms between the HRA and the AV junction (A_1-A_2 increases from 290 ms to 310 ms) occurs despite a 10 ms decline in the extrastimulus coupling interval (S_1-S_2) from 280 to 270 ms. Because of this intra-atrial conduction delay, the AV node has time to recover excitability allowing the atrial extrastimulus (A_2) to conduct to the His bundle (H_2) and ventricle. This phenomenon, whereby AV nodal conduction occurs at long extrastimulus coupling intervals (not shown), is blocked at shorter coupling intervals (panel A), but resumes despite a further reduction in the extrastimulus coupling interval (panel B) is called the gap phenomenon. In general a conduction gap can occur when conduction delay in a proximal tissue (in this case the right atrium) allows previously blocked conduction to resume through a distal tissue (in this case the AV node). The atrial electrogram, A_e, is an atrial echo beat resulting from retrograde activation of the atrium using the retrograde fast AV nodal pathway following anterograde conduction of A_2 within the slow AV nodal pathway. A, atrial electrogram; H, His bundle electrogram, V, ventricular electrogram, S, stimulus artifact.

block was expected [61,62]. It is in dispute whether true supernormal conduction occurs in human hearts and many phenomena that have been attributed to "supernormal conduction" can be explained by concealed conduction, the gap phenomenon, facilitation, rate-related changes in refractoriness, summation and reflection, and dual AV node physiology [63-65]. As such, these examples of "supernormal" phenomena have been more correctly classified as pseudo-supernormal conduction [51,63-65].

However, Figure 2-54 illustrates a series of intracardiac recordings that are difficult to explain without invoking supernormal conduction. In this case, AV conduction and ventricular activation occurs such that the 12-lead ECG exhibits a right bundle branch block pattern. Premature atrial depolarizations delivered after the fixed drive train are conducted without right bundle branch block. With increasing prematurity, the input

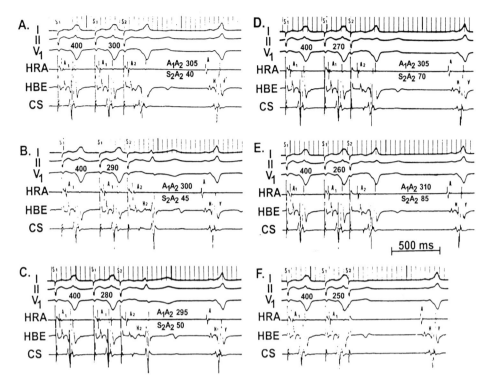

FIGURE 2-53. Unusual demonstration of gap phenomenon in a patient with manifest right-sided accessory connection. In all panels, recordings from top to bottom are surface ECG leads I, II, V_1 and endocardial electrograms from high right atrium (HRA), His bundle region (HBE), and an epicardial recording from the left side of the heart using a coronary sinus catheter (CS). A fixed pacing train is delivered (S_1-S_1 = 400 msec) in the HRA followed by the introduction of a premature stimulus (S_2). In each panel, during the fixed pacing train, conduction proceeds anterograde exclusively via the accessory connection, resulting in ventricular pre-excitation and a wide QRS complex. Panel A: A premature stimulus at a coupling interval (S_1-S_2) of 300 msec results in a premature atrial depolarization with a coupling interval (A_1-A_2) of 305 msec, due to atrial latency associated with the extrastimulus (S_2-A_2 = 40 msec). The resultant ventricular activation is via the accessory pathway (preexcitation with a wide QRS complex). Panel B: With a decrease in S_1-S_2 to 290 msec (resultant A_1-A_2 of 300 msec), premature atrial latency (S_2-A_2) increases even further to 45 msec. However, this input coupling interval (A_1-A_2 = 300 msec) exceeds the accessory pathway's effective refractory period resulting in conduction block in the pathway. Anterograde conduction, nevertheless, continues through the AV node/His-Purkinje system resulting in ventricular activation with a narrow QRS complex. Panel C: Further reductions in S_1-S_2 to 280 msec results only in a small decrease in A_1-A_2 to 295 msec because of an additional increase in atrial latency to 50 msec. Anterograde conduction in the accessory connection is blocked, but continues via the AV node/His-Purkinje system (narrow QRS complex). Panels D-E: With increased extrastimulus prematurity to 270 msec (panel D) and 260 msec (panel E), the atrial latency (S_2-A_2) markedly increases to 70 msec and 85 msec, respectively, resulting in available atrial inputs for AV conduction (A_1-A_2) of 305 msec and 310 msec, respectively. Since these input coupling intervals now exceed the effective refractory period of the accessory connection, anterograde conduction resumes in the accessory pathway as evidenced by ventricular activation with a wide QRS complex morphology. Consequently, there is an approximately 20 msec gap in the S_1-S_2 interval during which conduction proceeds via the AV node/His-Purkinje system. The gap in conduction in the accessory connection is due to the cycle length of the atrial input (A_1-A_2) initially decreasing and then subsequently increasing, because of a progressive increase in atrial latency (S_2-A_2) to a greater degree than the shortening of the S_1-S_2 coupling interval. Panel F: With continued prematurity of S_2 (S_1-S_2 = 250 msec), the atrial effective refractory period is reached. From [68] with permission.

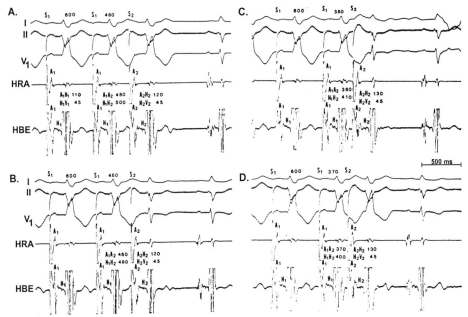

FIGURE 2-54. Evidence of supernormal conduction in the right bundle branch. Recordings from top to bottom in each panel include surface ECG leads I, II, and V_1 and intracardiac electrograms from the high right atrium (HRA) and His bundle region (HBE). Fixed cycle length pacing (S_1-S_1 = 600 msec) is performed in the HRA followed by the introduction of increasingly premature extrastimulus (S_2). During the fixed pacing train, AV conduction occurs with a right bundle branch block (RBBB) QRS complex morphology (see surface leads). Panels A-C: With reductions in the S_1-S_2 (and A_1-A_2) coupling interval from 480 msec to 380 msec, the QRS complex morphology of the premature beat (V_2) changes from the RBBB pattern to a normal pattern. Associated with this change is the finding that the input coupling interval into the RBB (H_1-H_2) actually decreases from 500 msec to 480 msec, with only slight or no changes in the AV nodal (A_1-A_2) and His-Purkinje (H_2-V_2) conduction times. Therefore, despite the increase in prematurity of the input impulse to the RBB (and the absence of any delay in conduction in other portions of the conduction system), conduction within the RBB actually improves, contrary to expectations (supernormal conduction). Panel D: With continued prematurity of S_2, and further reductions of the H_1-H_2 interval to 400 msec, conduction finally blocks in the RBB, resulting again in the RBBB QRS morphology. Consequently, there is a 90-msec window of H_1-H_2 intervals ranging from 500 msec to 410 msec within which conduction is enhanced in the RBB.

coupling interval into the right bundle branch (H_1-H_2) actually decreases, with only a minor or no change in AV nodal and His-Purkinje conduction times. Contrary to expectations, despite the increase in prematurity of the input impulse to the right bundle branch (and the absence of any delay in conduction in other portions of the conduction system), conduction within the right bundle branch actually recovers and results in normal His-Purkinje conduction (narrow QRS complex). This phenomenon can also be seen in the left bundle branch and accessory AV connections.

2.2.9 PROGRAMMED INDUCTION OF CLINICAL ARRHYTHMIAS

In general, most clinical arrhythmias are due to reentry and are inducible using programmed electrical stimulation (fixed cycle length pacing with extrastimuli) (see "Pacing protocols and programmed electrical stimulation" on page 38). In patients undergoing studies for documented or presumed supraventricular tachycardia, the pacing study begins in the ventricle. This would allow early determination of the potential retrograde limb of a reentrant supraventricular tachycardia. For patients with syncope or documented or presumed ventricular tachycardia, the pacing begins in the atrium. This early assessment of sinus node function and anterograde AV conduction properties before induction of any ventricular tachyarrhythmias. Typically during programmed stimulation a pacing train consisting of eight or 10 pulses at a fixed cycle length (faster than the sinus rate) is delivered to stabilize the effective refractory period of the tissue before introducing the extrastimulus (Figures 2-55 & 2-56). It is standard to alternate fixed cycle length trains of 600 or 400 ms with up to three extrastimuli at each drive cycle length. In addition, some electrophysiologists also introduce extrastimuli after sensing eight or 10 sinus beats. During a typical study, a single extrastimulus is introduced following the chosen drive train (e.g., 600 ms) with the S_1-S_2 interval sequentially decremented by 10 ms until the effective refractory period is reached. This is repeated using a drive train at the other cycle length (e.g. 400 ms). This process is repeated at each of the two drive cycle lengths using two extrastimuli. Starting S_1-S_2 and S_2-S_3 at 30 -50 ms above the effective refractory period, the S_2-S_3 interval is reduced in 10 ms increments until capture is again lost. The S_1-S_2 interval is then decremented until the effective refractory period is again reached. During a study designed to induce monomorphic ventricular tachycardia, programmed electrical stimulation is usually initially performed at the right ventricular apex. If no ventricular tachycardia is induced after testing with two extrastimuli, the protocol can be repeated at a second pacing site in the right ventricle, usually the right ventricular outflow tract. Should this fail to induce a clinical arrhythmia, the protocol can be repeated with each of the two drive trains at each of the two sites with three extrastimuli (Figure 2-57).

The likelihood of introducing a non-clinical arrhythmia, or even a totally non-specific tachyarrhythmia, such as ventricular fibrillation, is increased when three extrastimuli are introduced. Because only the induction of monomorphic ventricular tachycardia is considered a specific and clinically-relevant finding, the use of three extrastimuli is delayed until two extrastimuli are tested at each of the two right ventricular sites. Although less common today, in the past, patients with clearly documented monomorphic ventricular tachycardia that were non-inducible using right ventricular pacing would often receive programmed electrical stimulation through a catheter placed in the left ventricle. The rationale for this was that because most circuits responsible for reentrant monomorphic ventricular tachycardia are related to an old left ventricular infarct scar, and since inducing reentry is easier the closer the pacing catheter is to the circuit, it may be possible to induce clinical monomorphic ventricular tachycardia in some patients only by pacing in the left chamber. Because of the increased risk of risks and potential complications associated with left heart catheterization, programmed ventricular stimulation in the left ventricular is not generally performed.

The long-short protocol may be especially useful in patients with suspected bundle branch reentrant ventricular tachycardia. Fixed-rate pacing without extrastimuli (without or with isoproterenol (1 - 5 μg/min) is sometimes effective at inducing some forms of

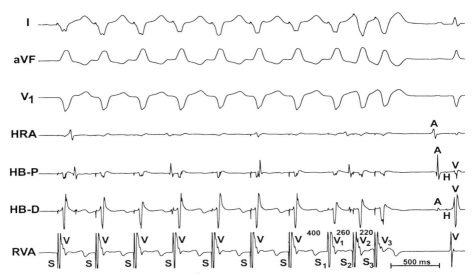

FIGURE 2-55. The most common means to induce reentrant arrhythmias is through programmed electrical stimulation (PES). In this example, PES is performed using an electrode catheter placed at the right ventricular apex (RVA). After a fixed cycle drive train (eight beats at 400 ms), two extrastimuli are introduced (S_1-S_2 = 260 ms and S_2-S_3 = 220 ms). Following the extrastimuli, sinus rhythm resumes (i.e., no arrhythmia is induced). A, atrial electrogram; H, His bundle electrogram; HRA, high right atrium; HB-P, proximal His bundle recording lead; HB-D, distal His bundle recording lead, V, ventricular electrogram.

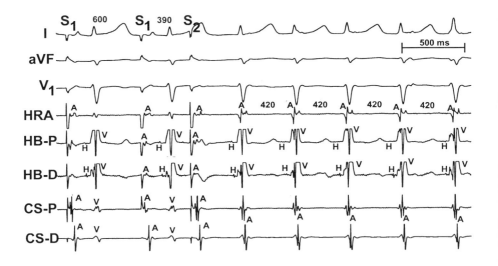

FIGURE 2-56. One of the most common forms of supraventricular tachycardia induced during an electrophysiology study is the typical (slow-fast) form of AV nodal reentrant tachycardia. As shown above, the high right atrium (HRA) is driven at a cycle length of 600 msec. A premature atrial depolarization with a coupling interval (S_1-S_2) of 390 ms blocks anterograde in the fast AV nodal pathway but does conduct in the anterograde slow AV nodal pathway. Retrograde conduction then continues in the retrograde fast AV nodal pathway and a circuit movement tachycardia results with anterograde conduction again within the slow AV nodal pathway. CS-P, proximal coronary sinus; CS-D, distal coronary sinus. Other abbreviations as in Figure 2-55.

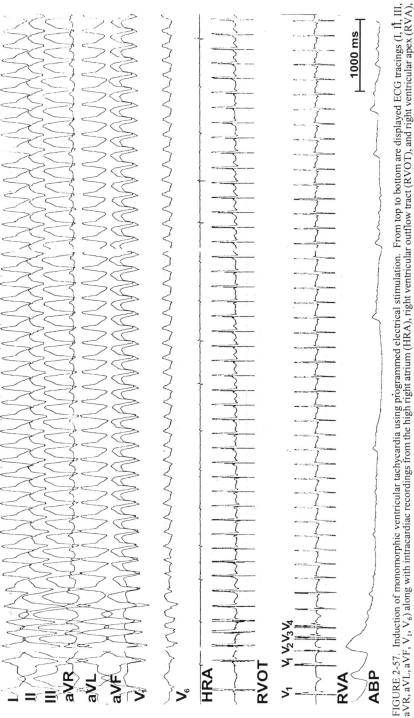

FIGURE 2-57. Induction of monomorphic ventricular tachycardia using programmed electrical stimulation. From top to bottom are displayed ECG tracings (I, II, III, aVR, aVL, aVF, V$_1$, V$_6$) along with intracardiac recordings from the high right atrium (HRA), right ventricular outflow tract (RVOT), and right ventricular apex (RVA), and arterial blood pressure (ABP). In response to a fixed cycle length drive train (eight pulses, V$_1$-V$_1$ = 400 ms) and three premature extrastimuli (V$_2$, V$_3$, V$_4$) delivered to the RVA, sustained monomorphic ventricular tachycardia (cycle length 210 ms) is induced.

supraventricular and monomorphic ventricular tachycardia, especially AV nodal reentrant tachycardia, AV reciprocating tachycardia utilizing an accessory connection, or idiopathic forms of monomorphic ventricular tachycardia occurring in patients with structurally normal hearts which may not result from a reentrant mechanism.

Be prepared to terminate any organized, hemodynamically stable, ventricular or supraventricular tachycardia with overdrive fixed-rate burst pacing and any unorganized or hemodynamically unstable tachyarrhythmia with external electrical countershock. It is also prudent to have readily available in the laboratory a system which allows internal cardioversion-defibrillation in those very rare patients in which ventricular fibrillation cannot be terminated with external shock.

2.2.10 ELECTROPHYSIOLOGICAL EVALUATION OF ARRHYTHMIA MECHANISMS

The final phase of an electrophysiology study involves defining the mechanism of any induced arrhythmia. The electrophysiologist must not only establish whether the arrhythmia is supraventricular or ventricular in origin, but she/he must also strive to determine the precise type of supraventricular or ventricular tachyarrhythmia (Table 2-8.) In addition, the clinical and cellular mechanism should be defined, if possible (see Table 1-1. on page 13 and Table 3-10. on page 115 as well as discussion "Mechanisms of Cardiac Arrhythmias" on page 7).

While much of this remaining book is devoted to defining the mechanisms of various types of clinical arrhythmias using intracardiac recordings, much can be learned regarding the clinical mechanism from a simple analysis of a surface 12-lead ECG recorded during the clinical arrhythmia. Clinical and ECG criteria which aids the clinician in deciding whether a wide QRS complex tachycardia is ventricular tachycardia or, for example, supraventricular tachycardia with aberrant AV conduction is widely available (Table 8-1. on page 442). The two most powerful discriminators between ventricular tachycardia and supraventricular tachycardia is the presence of ventricular fusion beats and AV dissociation recorded on the surface 12-lead ECG (Figure 2-58).

Visibility and analysis of the P-wave morphology on the 12-lead ECG may also assist in discriminating between the various types of supraventricular tachycardias (Figure 2-59). During normal sinus rhythm or sinus tachycardia, the P-wave precedes the QRS complex with a normal PR interval. In addition, the P-wave has a normal upright axis in ECG leads II, III, and aVF. The P-wave morphology and axis during sinoatrial reentrant tachycardia (high cristal focal tachycardia, see "Classification of Atrial Tachycardias" on page 609 & see "Focal Atrial Tachycardia" on page 610) should be identical to that recorded during sinus rhythm. However, unlike sinus tachycardia, sinoatrial reentrant tachycardia has an abrupt onset and termination. Atrial tachycardia is also a paroxysmal tachycardia with P-waves preceding the QRS complex and exhibiting an abnormal P-wave morphology and axis. The P-wave axis during atrial tachycardia is usually markedly different than the P-wave axis seen during sinus rhythm. In the case of the typical slow-fast form of AV nodal reentrant tachycardia, the P-wave is most often undetectable because it is buried in the QRS complex (Figure 2-59). In some patients, however, it can be detected partially buried just at the beginning or just at the end of the QRS complex. These same P-wave relationships may be observed in patients with junctional tachycar-

TABLE 2-8.   Classification of narrow and wide QRS complex tachyarrhythmias

Narrow QRS Complex Tachyarrhythmias
Supraventricular tachyarrhythmias
Sinus tachycardia
Sinoatrial reentrant tachycardia (high cristal focal tachycardia)
Junctional tachycardia
AV nodal reentrant tachycardia
Orthodromic AV reciprocating tachycardia
Atrial tachycardia
Atrial flutter
Atrial fibrillation
Ventricular tachyarrhythmias
Monomorphic ventricular tachycardia
Wide QRS Complex Tachyarrhythmias
Ventricular tachyarrhythmias
Monomorphic ventricular tachycardia
Polymorphic ventricular tachycardia
Torsade de pointes
Ventricular fibrillation
Preexcited tachyarrhythmias
Antidromic AV reciprocating tachycardia (accessory connection is intrinsic part of circuit)
AV nodal reentrant tachycardia (with a bystander accessory connection)
Atrial tachycardia (with a bystander accessory connection)
Atrial flutter (with a bystander accessory connection)
Atrial fibrillation (with a bystander accessory connection)
Supraventricular tachyarrhythmias with pre-existing or functional (rate-related) bundle branch block

dia, but in general, junctional tachycardia exhibits a slower rate (70-130/min) than typical AV nodal reentrant tachycardia. Depending upon the location of the accessory connection and its conduction properties, orthodromic AVRT may have P-waves either partially buried in the QRS complex (septal AV connections) or readily identified as inverted (retrograde) P-waves in the ST segment. The atypical fast-slow form of AV nodal reentrant tachycardia is a form of long RP′ tachycardia with the P-wave inverted in ECG leads II, III, and aVF. Patients with an accessory AV connection with decremental conduction properties can also have an orthodromic AV reciprocating tachycardia that exhibits a long RP′ interval. This form of tachycardia is often referred to as the *permanent form of junctional reciprocating tachycardia (PJRT)* and is discussed in "Ventricular Preexcitation Syndromes: The Wolff-Parkinson-White Syndrome and Variants" on page 539. An electrophysiology study is often required to differentiate PJRT from the atypical form of AV nodal reentrant tachycardia.

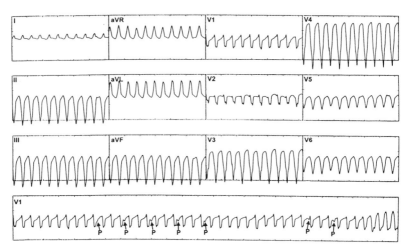

FIGURE 2-58. Surface 12-lead ECG recording obtained from a 45-year old man with a history of a previous anterior myocardial infarction during an episode of his clinical wide QRS complex tachycardia. While electrophysiology testing confirmed that this arrhythmia was ventricular tachycardia, careful analysis of the ECG alone, especially the lead V₁ rhythm strip, would have revealed evidence of P-wave activity (arrows) dissociated from the ventricular rhythm, strongly suggesting the diagnosis of ventricular tachycardia. Also note the axis change of the last three QRS complexes at the far right of the rhythm strip. Paper speed 25 mm/sec.

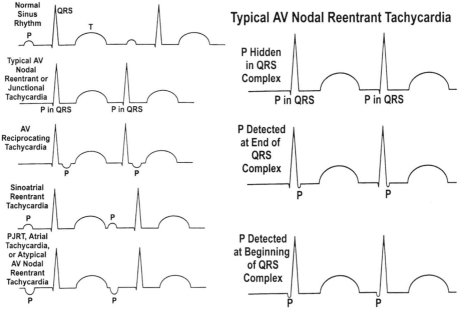

FIGURE 2-59. Schematic diagram illustrating the most common P-wave relationships observed during various forms of supraventricular tachycardia. Schematic ECG lead II shown. Left panel: Comparison of typical P-wave visibility, morphology, and axis during sinus rhythm and various common forms of supraventricular tachycardia. Right panel: During the typical slow-fast form of AV nodal reentrant tachycardia P-waves are usually undetectable (hidden within the QRS complex), rarely remnant P-waves can be detected at the very beginning or end of the QRS complex. Lead V₁ is often best lead to examine in case of AV nodal reentry. PJRT, permanent form of junctional reciprocating tachycardia.

References

1. Zipes DP, DiMarco JP, Gillette PC, et al.: Guidelines for clinical intracardiac electrophysiological and catheter ablation procedures. *J Am Coll Cardiol* **26**:555-73, 1995.
2. Horowitz LN: Safety of electrophysiologic studies. *Circulation* **73**:11-28, 1986.
3. Dimarco JP, Garan H, Ruskin JN: Complications in patients undergoing cardiac electrophysiologic procedures. *Ann Intern Med* **97**:490-3, 1982.
4. Bekheit S, Murtagh JG, Morton P, Fletcher E: Measurements of sinus impulse conduction from electrogram of bundle of His. *Br Heart J* **33**:719, 1971.
5. Castellanos A, Castillo C, Agha A: Contribution of the His bundle recording to the understanding of clinical arrhythmias. *Am J Cardiol* **28**:499, 1971.
6. Castellanos A, Jr., Castillo CA, Agha AS, Tessler M: His bundle electrograms in patients with short P-R intervals, narrow QRS complexes, and paroxysmal tachycardias. *Circulation* **43**:667-78, 1971.
7. Damato AN, Lau SH, et al.: Recording of specialized conducting fibers (A-V nodal, His bundle, and right bundle branch) in man using an electrode catheter technic. *Circulation* **39**:435-47, 1969.
8. Damato AN, Lau SH, Helfant RH, et al.: Study of atrioventricular conduction in man using electrode catheter recordings of His bundle activity. *Circulation* **39**:287-96, 1969.
9. Damato AN, Lau SH: Clinical value of the electrogram of the conduction system. *Prog Cardiovasc Dis* **13**:119-40, 1970.
10. Narula OS, Cohen LS, Samet P, et al.: Localization of A-V conduction defects in man by recording of the His bundle electrogram. *Am J Cardiol* **25**:288, 1970.
11. Narula OS, Scherlag BJ, Samet P, Javier RP: Atrioventricular block: Localization and classification by His bundle recordings. *Am J Med* **50**:146, 1971.
12. Rosen KM: Evaluation of cardiac conduction in the cardiac catheterization laboratory. *Am J Cardiol* **30**:701-3, 1972.
13. Rosen KM, Scherlag BJ, Samet P, Helfant RH: His bundle electrogram. *Circulation* **46**:831-2, 1972.
14. Bekheit S, Murtagh JG, Morton P, Fletcher E: Studies of heart block with His bundle recordings. *Br Heart* **34**:717, 1972.
15. Batsford WP, Akhtar M, Caracta AR, et al.: Effect of atrial stimulation site on the electrophysiological properties of the atrioventricular node in man. *Circulation* **50**:283-92, 1974.
16. Cagin NA, Kunstadt D, Wolfish P, Levitt B: The influence of heart rate on the refractory period of the atrium and the A-V conducting system. *Am Heart J* **85**:358, 1973.
17. Denes P, Wu D, Dhingra R, et al.: The effects of cycle length on cardiac refractory periods in man. *Circulation* **49**:32-41, 1974.
18. Jurkiewicz NK, Sanguinetti MC: Rate-dependent prolongation of cardiac action potentials by a methanesulfonalide class III antiarrhythmic agent: specific block of rapidly activating delayed rectifier K+ current by dofetilide. *Circ Res* **72**:75-83, 1993.
19. Sanguinetti MC, Jurkiewicz NK: Two components of cardiac delayed rectifier K+ current: Differential sensitivity to block by class III antiarrhythmic agents. *J Gen Physiol* **96**:194, 1990.
20. Sanguinetti MC, Jurkiewicz NK: Delayed rectifier outward K+ current is composed of two currents in guinea pig atrial cells. *Am J Physiol* **260**:H393, 1991.
21. Hoffman BF, Paes de Carvalho A, De Mello WC: Transmembrane potentials of single fibres of the atrio-ventricular node. *Nature* **181**:66-67, 1958.
22. Hoffman BF, Paes de Carvalho A, De Mello WC, et al.: Electrical activity of single fibers of the atrio-ventricular node. *Circ Res* **7**:11-18, 1959.
23. Jalife J: The sucrose gap preparation as a model of AV nodal transmission: Are dual pathways necessary for reciprocation or AV nodal echoes. *PACE* **6**:1106, 1983.
24. Simson MB, Spear JF, Moore EN: Electrophysiologic studies on atrioventricular nodal Wenckebach cycles. *Am J Cardiol* **41**:244, 1978.
25. Josephson ME. Electrophysiologic investigation: General concepts. *Clinical Cardiac Electrophysiology: Techniques and Interpretations*. Philadelphia: Lea & Febiger, 28-70: 1993.
26. Sherf L: The atrial conduction system: clinical implications. *Am J Cardiol* **37**:814, 1976.

27. Schuilenburg RM, Durrer D: Conduction disturbances located within the His bundle. *Circulation* **45**:612, 1972.

28. Josephson ME. Atrial flutter and fibrillation. *Clinical Cardiac Electrophysiology: Techniques and Interpretations*. Philadelphia: Lea & Febiger: 1993.

29. Akhtar M, Caracta AR, Lau SH, et al.: Demonstration of intra-atrial conduction delay, block, gap and reentry: a report of two cases. *Circulation* **58**:947-55, 1978.

30. Akhtar M, Damato AN, Batsford WP, et al.: A comparative analysis of antegrade and retrograde conduction patterns in man. *Circulation* **52**:766-78, 1975.

31. Allessie MA, Bonke FI, Schopman FJ: Circus movement in rabbit atrial muscle as a mechanism of trachycardia. *Circ Res* **33**:54-62, 1973.

32. Allessie MA, Bonke FI, Schopman FJ: Circus movement in rabbit atrial muscle as a mechanism of tachycardia. II. The role of nonuniform recovery of excitability in the occurrence of unidirectional block, as studied with multiple microelectrodes. *Circ Res* **39**:168-77, 1976.

33. Allessie MA, Bonke FI, Schopman FJ: Circus movement in rabbit atrial muscle as a mechanism of tachycardia. III. The "leading circle" concept: a new model of circus movement in cardiac tissue without the involvement of an anatomical obstacle. *Circ Res* **41**:9-18, 1977.

34. Allessie MA, Lammers WJ, Bonke IM, Hollen J: Intra-atrial reentry as a mechanism for atrial flutter induced by acetylcholine and rapid pacing in the dog. *Circulation* **70**:123-35, 1984.

35. Boineau JP, Schuessler RB, Mooney CR, et al.: Natural and evoked atrial flutter due to circus movement in dogs. *Am J Cardiol* **45**:1167, 1980.

36. Bennett MA, Pentecost BL: The pattern of onset and spontaneous cessation of atrial fibrillation in man. *Circulation* **41**:981, 1970.

37. Frame LH, Page RL, Hoffman BF: Atrial reentry around an anatomic barrier with a partially refractory excitable gap: A canine model of atrial flutter. *Circ Res* **58**:495, 1986.

38. Haft JI, Lau SH, et al.: Atrial fibrillation produced by atrial stimulation. *Circulation* **37**:70-4, 1968.

39. Killip T, Gault JH: Mode of onset of atrial fibrillation in man. *Am Heart J* **70**:172, 1965.

40. Buxton AE, Marchlinski FE, Miller JM, et al.: The human atrial strength-interval relationship: Influence of cycle length and procainamide. *Circulation* **79**:271, 1989.

41. Akhtar M, Gilbert CJ, Wolf FG, Schmidt DH: Retrograde conduction in the His-Purkinje system. Analysis of the routes of impulse propagation using His and right bundle branch recordings. *Circulation* **59**:1252-65, 1979.

42. Akhtar M: Retrograde conduction in man. *Pacing Clin Electrophysiol* **4**:548-62, 1981.

43. Akhtar M, Damato AN, Caracta AR, et al.: The gap phenomena during retrograde conduction in man. *Circulation* **49**:811-7, 1974.

44. Akhtar M, Damato AN, Caracta AR, et al.: The gap phenomenon during retrograde conduction in man. *Circulation* **49**:811, 1974.

45. Akhtar M, Damato AN, Ruskin JN, et al.: Characteristics and coexistence of two forms of ventricular echo phenomena. *Am Heart J* **92**:174-82, 1976.

46. Akhtar M, Denker S, et al.: Macro-reentry within the His-Purkinje system. *PACE* **6**:1010, 1983.

47. Akhtar M, Damato AN, Batsford WP, et al.: Demonstration of re-entry within the His-Purkinje system in man. *Circulation* **50**:1150-62, 1974.

48. Farshidi A, Michelson EL, Greenspan AM, et al.: Repetitive responses to ventricular extrastimuli: incidence, mechanism, and significance. *Am Heart J* **100**:59-68, 1980.

49. Roy D, Brugada P, Bar FWHM, Wellens HJJ: Repetitive responses to ventricular extrastimuli: Incidence and significance in patients without organic heart disease. *Eur Heart J* **4**:79, 1983.

50. Sung RJ, Waxman HL, Saksena S, Juma Z: Sequence of retrograde atrial activation in patients with dual atrioventricular nodal pathways. *Circulation* **64**:1059-67, 1981.

51. Josephson ME. Miscellaneous phenomena related to atrioventricular conduction. *Clinical Cardiac Electrophysiology: Techniques and Interpretations*. Philadelphia: Lea & Febiger: 1993.

52. Knoebel SB, Fisch C: Concealed conduction. *Cardiovasc Clin* **5**:21, 1973.

53. Moore EN, Knoebel SB, Spear JF: Concealed conduction. *Am J Cardiol* **28**:406, 1971.

54. Zipes DP, Mendez C, Moe GK: Evidence for summation and voltage dependency in rabbit atrioventricular nodal fibers. *Circ Res* **32**:170-7, 1973.

55. Agha AS, Castellanos A, et al.: Type II & type III gaps in bundle branch conduction. *Circ* **47**:325, 1973.

56. Agha AS, Castellanos A, Jr., Wells D, et al.: Type I, type II, and type 3 gaps in bundle-branch conduction. *Circulation* **47**:325-30, 1973.

57. Akhtar M, Damato AN, Batsford WP, et al.: Unmasking and conversion of gap phenomenon in the human heart. *Circulation* **49**:624-30, 1974.

58. Damato AN, Akhtar M, Ruskin J, et al.: Gap phenomena: Antegrade and retrograde. In: Wellens HJJ, Lie KI, Janse MJ, eds. *The Conduction System of the Heart: Structure, Function and Clinical Implications*. Philadelphia: Lea & Febiger: 1976.

59. Moe GK, Mendez C, Han J: Aberrant A-V impulse propagation in the dog heart: A study of functional bundle branch block. *Circ Res* **16**:261, 1965.

60. Wu D, Denes P, Dhingra R, et al.: Nature of the gap phenomenon in man. *Circ Res* **34**:682-92, 1974.

61. Childers RW: Supernormality. *Cardiovasc Clin* **5**:135, 1973.

62. Pick A, Langendorf R, Katz LN: The supernormal phase of atrioventricular conduction. *Circulation* **26**:322, 1962.

63. Gallagher JJ, Damato AN, Caracta AR, et al.: Gap in A-V conduction in man; types I and II. *Am Heart J* **85**:78-82, 1973.

64. Gallagher JJ, Damato AN, Varghese PJ, et al.: Alternative mechanisms of apparent supernormal atrioventricular conduction. *Am J Cardiol* **31**:362-71, 1973.

65. Moe GK, Childers RW, et al,: An appraisal of "supernormal" A-V conduction. *Circulation* **38**:5, 1968.

66. Sung RJ, Juma Z, Saksena S: Electrophysiologic properties and antiarrhythmic mechanisms of intravenous N-acetylprocainamide in patients with ventricular dysrhythmias. *Am Heart J* **105**:811-9, 1983.

67. Sung RJ, Myerburg RJ, Castellanos A: Electrophysiological demonstration of concealed conduction in the human atrium. *Circulation* **58**:940-6, 1978.

68. Nguyen NX, Yang PT, et al.: Effects of beta-adrenergic stimulation on atrial latency and atrial vulnerability in patients with paroxysmal supraventricular tachycardia. *Am J Cardiol* **61**:1031-6, 1988.

69. Greenspan AM, Camardo JS, Horowitz LN, et al.: Human ventricular refractoriness: effects of increasing current. *Am J Cardiol* **47**:244-50, 1981.

CHAPTER 3

PRINCIPLES OF PHARMACOTHERAPY AND ANTIARRHYTHMIC DRUGS

It is at the level of antiarrhythmic drugs and mechanisms of cardiac arrhythmias that cellular cardiac electrophysiology (ionic currents, channels, receptors, etc.) interacts most closely with clinical cardiac electrophysiology. For this reason, we devote a chapter to a review of: 1) the clinical pharmacology and pharmacotherapy of antiarrhythmic drugs; 2) basic cellular electrophysiology of cardiac cells; 3) the regulators and modulators of ionic currents; 4) the targets of antiarrhythmic drugs; 5) cellular mechanisms of action of antiarrhythmic drugs; and 6) mechanisms of cardiac proarrhythmia. This chapter provides much of the basic science material that a clinical electrophysiologist may find useful in understanding the mechanisms of arrhythmias, drug antiarrhythmia and proarrhythmia, and genetic conditions such as the long QT syndromes.

3.1 Principles of Pharmacokinetics and Pharmacodynamics

A knowledge of basic pharmacokinetics and pharmacodynamics is useful to clinicians, in general, and particularly to cardiac electrophysiologists who treat their patients with powerful antiarrhythmic drugs with proarrhythmic potential. This section outlines some of the basic principles of pharmacology [1], especially as it relates to antiarrhythmic drugs.

3.1.1 BASICS OF PHARMACOKINETICS

In general, the processes involved in drug disposition, such as absorption or hepatic metabolism, either usually occur at rates that are *directly proportional* to the concentration of the drug (*first-order or linear kinetics*) or at a constant rate (*zero-order, non-linear, or saturable kinetics*). For example, the rate of drug absorption from the intestine decreases as the concentration of the drug in the intestinal lumen decreases (first-order kinetics). On the other hand, some processes such as hepatic metabolism generally occurs at the maximum (constant) rate and cannot increase further even with additional increases in drug concentration (zero-order kinetics). In general, processes exhibit linear kinetics at low concentrations and saturable kinetics at high concentrations.

A process such as drug elimination often exhibits first-order kinetics
and has an easy mathematical description. The rate of loss of drug from the
body, dC/dt, is proportional to the concentration of the drug (C):

$$\frac{dC}{dt} = -kC$$

where k is a constant, called the first-
order elimination rate constant, and t is
time. Integration yields:

$$C = C°e^{-kt}$$

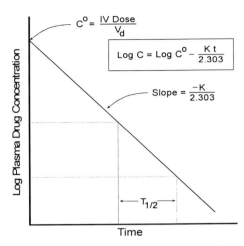

where e is the base of the natural loga-
rithm, $C°$ is the initial concentration of
the drug in the body at time $t = 0$. Taking logarithms yields:

FIGURE 3-1. Plasma concentration as a function of time
for a drug eliminated using first-order kinetics. $T_{1/2}$, elimination half-life. See text for details.

$$\log C = \log \mathcal{C}° - \frac{kt}{2.303}$$

When plasma concentration is plotted on a logarithmic scale, the relationship results in a
straight line (Figure 3-1).

3.1.2 DRUG DISPOSITION

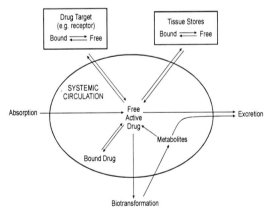

FIGURE 3-2. Schematic representation of factors important in
affecting free active drug concentration and drug disposition. See
text for discussion.

When a drug is administered to a
patient, the disposition of the drug
and the concentration in the serum
and at the cellular or subcellular
target site of action is the net result of a number of processes, including the amount of drug
administered, the absorption into
the systemic circulation, distribution to and binding within tissues,
metabolism and biotransforma-
tion in the liver and other organs,
and excretion by the kidneys, gas-
trointestinal tract, and lungs (Figure 3-2). An understanding of
these factors may assist in pre-
scribing, administering, and evaluating drug efficacy and toxicity in patients under normal and pathological conditions.

Absorption

Following oral administration of a drug a number of factors affect the transfer of active drug from the intestinal lumen to the systemic circulation including but not limited to: 1) dissolution rates of the oral preparation; 2) the physiochemical properties of the preparation (e.g., slow release preparations; 3) rates of transport and/or diffusion of drug across intestinal cell membranes which can be affected by many factors including malabsorption and motility disorders; 4) drug interactions with and binding to other drugs or chemicals within the intestinal lumen; 5) degree of "first pass" drug metabolism in the liver; 6) portal blood flow.

The fraction of drug dose absorbed into the systemic circulation is termed the systemic *bioavailability*. The fraction (F) of drug absorbed is:

$$F = \frac{AUC_{oral}}{AUC_{IV}}$$

where AUC is the total area under the plasma concentration versus time curve from the time the drug is administered until it is completely eliminated from the body and assuming that the clearance of both the oral and intravenous forms of the drug are identical.

Distribution

After absorption into the systemic circulation, the drug is distributed to tissues and organs. In general, a drug distributes rapidly to certain tissues and organs, such as those with the highest blood flow such as the heart, kidneys, lung, liver, etc., termed the *central compartment*. In addition, drug may also distribute more slowly from the systemic circulation or the central compartment to one or more *secondary* or *peripheral compartments* (Figure 3-3).

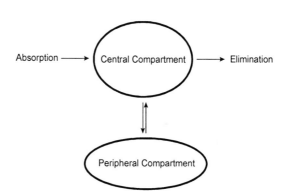

FIGURE 3-3. Two compartment model of drug distribution. See text for discussion.

These compartments are not distinct anatomical entities, but instead represent cross-tissue and cross-organ reservoirs of drug with different "fill" and "empty" according to different kinetic rate constants. Depending upon the drug, the target site of the drug may be within the central or peripheral compartment.

If one considers a drug with one central compartment and one peripheral compartment, the serum concentration (C) versus time (t) is described by a multiexponential equation:

$$C = Ae^{-\alpha t} + Be^{-\beta t}$$

where A and B are coefficients and α and β are first-order rate constants. In essence, this equation says that the serum concentration of a drug at any point in time is the net of the rate of drug distribution to the tissues and the rate of drug elimination from the tissues. α is related to half-life of drug distribution, while β is related to the *half-life of elimination* ($t_{1/2}$):

$$\beta = \frac{0.693}{t_{1/2}}$$

In most cases, drug distribution to its peripheral compartment(s) is rapid, meaning that any subsequent change in serum concentration of the drug with time is dependent upon the rate of elimination ($t_{1/2}$).

Not only is the rate of distribution and elimination important, but the extent of distribution, or *volume of distribution* (V_d), is also a useful concept:

$$V_d = \frac{Cl_S}{\beta}$$

where Cl_S is the systemic clearance of the drug and β is the elimination rate constant. Analogous to the above-mentioned "compartments", the "volume" of distribution does not refer to a identifiable anatomical or physiological volume. Instead, V_d is a "functional volume" and represents nothing more than a proportionality constant relating the serum concentration to the overall amount of drug in the body. Drugs that extensively bind to tissues or are concentrated within cells will have a large V_d while drugs having little tissue binding or remain largely trapped within the vascular compartment by binding to plasma proteins will have a small V_d.

Metabolism
Metabolism, primarily in the liver, can have important effects on the serum concentration of active drug. Most commonly hepatic enzyme systems convert an active drug to an inactive form or, in some cases, convert a less active or inactive pro-drug to more active drug metabolite. The efficiency of hepatic enzymes to metabolize drugs depends on a number of factors including genetics, underlying diseases, or previous exposure to other drugs, chemicals, or toxins. For example, procainamide, with predominantly class IA antiarrhythmic effects is acetylated a greater or lesser degree to N-acetyl-procainamide which has class III effects. Propafenone, which itself is an active drug with a short half life, is variably metabolized to other active metabolites which are even more potent than the parent pro-drug.

Elimination
In general, drug elimination is accomplished by hepatic metabolism and renal excretion of unchanged drug or drug metabolites. Therefore, total systemic *clearance* (Cl_S) of a drug is the sum of hepatic and renal clearances:

$$Cl_S = Cl_H + Cl_R$$

where Cl_H and Cl_R are the hepatic and renal clearances, respectively, of that drug. Clearance is an important concept because, in the steady state, the dosing regimen of a drug will depend directly upon Cl_S. The elimination half-life $(t_{1/2})$ is related to clearance (Cl_S) and volume of distribution (V_d) by the following equation.

$$t_{1/2} = \frac{0.693 \cdot V_d}{Cl_S}$$

Analysis of this equation reveals that elimination half-life is affected by altering either a drug's volume of distribution or its clearance. An increase in tissue binding of drug (increase in V_d) or a decrease in hepatic or renal clearance (increase in Cl_S) will increase the half-time of elimination. Changes in these parameters due to age, disease states, or interaction with other drugs concomitantly administered can dramatically affect drug elimination and consequently may significantly alter the dosing regimen. For example, renal insufficiency may increase $t_{1/2}$ of sotalol, which is cleared by the kidneys, necessitating a reduction in dosage to avoid potential proarrhythmia (torsade de pointes).

3.1.3 STEADY-STATE DRUG DOSING

The processes discussed above – *absorption, distribution, metabolism, elimination* – determine the rate of drug accumulation in the body and the time-dependent serum drug concentration. Figure 3-4 schematically illustrates the accumulation of an orally administered drug with successive doses until a steady-state is achieved. The following equation can be used to calculate the average serum concentration at steady-state $(\overline{C}_{SS})$.

$$\overline{C}_{SS} = \frac{F \cdot Dose_m}{Cl_S \cdot \tau} = \frac{F \cdot Dose_m \cdot t_{1/2}}{0.693 \cdot V_d \cdot \tau}$$

where F is the fraction of the maintenance dose $(Dose_m)$ absorbed, Cl_S is systemic clearance, τ is the time between doses, V_d is the volume of distribution, and $t_{1/2}$ is the elimination half-life. As seen from this equation, the final *average* steady state concentration is directly dependent upon the bioavailability, dose, elimination half-life and inversely dependent upon the clearance, volume of distribution and time between doses.

During continuous intravenous infusion, the peak and trough fluctuations in drug concentration are eliminated allowing the clinician to maintain stable steady state concentrations (Figure 3-4). Assuming a one-compartment model, the desired steady state drug concentration during a constant intravenous infusion (C_{SS}) can be calculated using the above equation and the infusion rate (IR):

$$C_{SS} = \frac{IR}{Cl_S} = \frac{IR \cdot t_{1/2}}{0.693 \cdot V_d}$$

where

$$IR = \frac{F \cdot Dose_m}{\tau}$$

The time required to achieve steady-state is the same regardless of intravenous or oral administration or the dose of the drug, i.e., approximately four times the elimination half-life (Figure 3-4). Therefore one can infuse the maintenance dose and the steady state concentration will be approximately achieved in a four elimination half-lives. However, in some cases it may be beneficial to quickly reach a therapeutic concentration

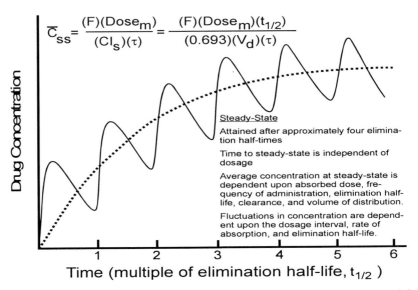

$$\overline{C}_{ss} = \frac{(F)(Dose_m)}{(Cl_s)(\tau)} = \frac{(F)(Dose_m)(t_{1/2})}{(0.693)(V_d)(\tau)}$$

Steady-State

Attained after approximately four elimination half-times

Time to steady-state is independent of dosage

Average concentration at steady-state is dependent upon absorbed dose, frequency of administration, elimination half-life, clearance, and volume of distribution.

Fluctuations in concentration are dependent upon the dosage interval, rate of absorption, and elimination half-life.

Time (multiple of elimination half-life, $t_{1/2}$)

FIGURE 3-4. Serum drug concentration during repetitive administration or continuous intravenous infusion based upon a one-compartment model. Solid line represents time course of drug concentration resulting from repeated administration at intervals equal to the elimination half-life of a rapidly absorbed drug. The dotted line illustrates the accumulation pattern during administration of an equivalent dosage by continuous intravenous infusion. See text for discussion and definition of terms and abbreviations.

near the final steady-state concentration. In this case, a loading dose can be administered just prior to initiating the maintenance dose. The intravenous loading dose is the product of the desired steady-state concentration in the central compartment (C_{ss}) and the volume of the central compartment (V_C).

$$LoadingDose_{IV} = C_{SS} \cdot V_C$$

The oral loading dose depends upon the oral maintenance dose ($Dose_m$), the elimination half-life ($t_{1/2}$), and the dosing interval (τ).

$$LoadingDose_{Oral} = \frac{Dose_m}{1 - e^{(-0.693\tau)/(t_{1/2})}}$$

The therapeutic plasma drug concentration is generally quoted as a concentration range. The actual therapeutic (as well as toxic) level can vary considerably from patient-to-patient; therefore, the published therapeutic ranges for various cardiac drugs should be used only as guidelines (Table 3-1.) Despite administration of a reasonable maintenance dose, measurement of plasma drug concentrations may be useful either when the desired therapeutic effects are not being achieved or toxic side-effects are noted. In order to achieve therapeutic effects and avoid toxic effects, larger or smaller than expected maintenance doses may be required in individual patients depending upon their unique rates of drug clearance. In addition, age, the presence of other interacting drugs, and disease states effecting renal and hepatic function may significantly alter the plasma concentration. A variety of pharmacokinetic data for commonly used antiarrhythmic drugs are summarized in Tables 3-1., 3-2., 3-3., 3-4., 3-5., and 3-6.

TABLE 3-1. Pharmacokinetic data of commonly used antiarrhythmic drugs*

Drug	Oral Availability (%)	Urinary Excretion (%)	Plasma Protein Bound (%)	Clearance (ml/min/kg)	Volume of Distribution (l/kg)	Half-life (hrs)	Effective Concentrations (μg/ml)
Quinidine	80 (sulfate) 71 (gluconate)	18	87	4.7	2.7	6.2	2-6
Procainamide	83	67	16	N/A	1.9	3-4	3-14
Disopyramide	83	55	65-90	1.2	0.59	6.0	>1.5
Phenytoin	90	2	89	N/A	0.64	6-24	>10
Lidocaine	35	2	70	9.2	1.1	1.8	1.5-6
Tocainide	89	38	10	2.6	3.0	13.5	6-15
Mexiletine	87	4-15	63	6.3	4.9	9.2	0.7-2.0
Propafenone	40-50	NS	90	11.2	3.6	2.5-7.5	0.2-3.0
Flecainide	70	48	61	5.6	4.9	11	0.4-0.8
Moricizine	35-40	35	95	N/A	4	2-6	0.1
Sotalol	90-100	80-90	NS	N/A	1.2-2.4	7-18	N/A
Amiodarone	46	0	99.98	1.9	66	25-53 days	0.5-2.5
Bretylium	23	77	0-8	10.2	5.9	8.9	0.5-1.5
N-acetyl-procainamide	83	81	10	3.1	1.4	6.0	21
Ibutilide	N/A	82	40	29	11	2-12	N/A
Dofetilide	>90	50		4.7-5.8	2.8-6.3	7-10	N/A

*References [2-45].
N/A, not available; NS, not significant.

TABLE 3-2. Clinical pharmacologic profile of class I antiarrhythmic drugs

Vaughan-Williams Drug Class	Name of Drug	Elimination Half-Life	Route of Excretion	Dosage* and Interval	Effect on Resting ECG	Therapeutic Serum Level
Class IA Na$^+$ Channel Blockers	Quinidine	4 - 17 hr	Primarily hepatic	PO: 200-400 mg q4-6hr (sulfate); 324-648 mg q8hr (gluconate)	Prolongs QRS, QT, and PR (±)	2 - 5 µg/ml
	Procainamide	3 - 6 r	Variable renal & hepatic	PO: 50-100 mg/kg/day in divided doses, q3-4hr or q6hr (long-acting); IV loading: no more than 100 mg q5 min to 1 gm or 12-15 mg/kg	Prolongs QRS, QT, and PR (±)	4 - 10 µg/ml (NAPA active metabolite = 10 -20 µg/ml)
	Disopyramide	4 - 10 hr	Variable renal & hepatic	PO: 100-200 mg q6-8hr (long-acting)	Prolongs QRS, QT, and PR (±)	2 - 5 µg/ml
CLASS IB Na$^+$ Channel Blockers	Lidocaine	2 - 4 hr	Hepatic	IV loading: 1 mg/kg bolus, then 0.5 mg/kg bolus after 20 min, then 30 mg/kg/min continuous infusion	No significant effect	1.5 - 5 µg/ml
	Phenytoin	18 - 24 hr	Hepatic	PO loading: 14 mg/kg; IV loading: 50 mg q 5min up to total dose 12 mg/kg; PO 0r IV maintenance: 200 - 400 mg/day	No significant effect	5 - 20 µg/ml
	Mexiletine	12 - 24 hr	Hepatic	PO: 100 - 300 mg q 8hr	No significant effect	0.5 - 2 µg/ml
	Tocainide	12 - 15 hr	Hepatic & renal	PO: 200 - 600 mg q 8hr	No significant effect	3 - 10 µg/ml
CLASS IC Na$^+$ Channel Blockers	Flecainide	15 - 30 hr	Primarily hepatic	PO: 100 - 200 mg q 12hr	Prolongs PR and QRS	0.2 - 1 µg/ml
	Propafenone	2 - 24 hr (extensive metabolites)	Hepatic	PO: 150 - 300 mg q 8hr	Prolongs PR and QRS	Active metabolites preclude establishment
	Moricizine	N/A	N/A	PO: 200 - 300 mg q 8hr	Prolongs PR and QRS	Not established

* Patients with decreased hepatic or renal function may require lower dosage. Always consult manufacturers package insert for latest dosing information.

TABLE 3-3. Clinical pharmacologic profile of class II, III, IV antiarrhythmic drugs

Vaughan-Williams Drug Class	Name of Drug	Elimination Half-Life	Route of Elimination	Dosage* and Interval	Effect on Resting ECG	Therapeutic Serum Level
CLASS II β-Adrenergic Blockers	Propranolol	3 - 4 hours	Hepatic	PO: 10 - 80 mg q 6hr (or equivalent long-acting formulation)	Prolongs PR (±); shortens QT; sinus bradycardia	50 - 100 ng/ml
	Metoprolol	6 - 12 hours	Hepatic	PO: 50 - 200 mg q 12hr	Prolongs PR (±); shortens QT; sinus bradycardia	Not established
	Esmolol	9 minutes	Red blood cell esterases	IV loading: 500 mg/kg over 1 min. IV maintenance: 25 mg/kg/min initially; increase by 25 - 50 mg/kg/min q 5min until desired effect or until maximum of 300 mg/kg/min	Prolongs PR (±); shortens QT; sinus bradycardia	0.15 - 2 µg/ml
CLASS III K$^+$ Channel Blockers	d,l-Sotalol	8 - 10 hours	Renal	PO: 80 - 320 mg q 12h	Prolongs PR, QT; sinus bradycardia	Not established
	Amiodarone	13 - 103 days	Hepatic	PO loading: 800 - 1600 mg/day (divided) for 1 - 3 weeks, then 600 - 800 mg/day for 4 weeks. PO maintenance: 100 - 400 mg/day	Prolongs PR, QRS, QT; sinus bradycardia	Not established (1 - 2 mg/ml?)
	Bretylium	4 - 16 hours	Primarily renal	IV loading: 5 mg/kg with additional doses of 10 mg/kg (effect may be delayed). IV maintenance: 5 - 10 mg/kg g6 h or infusion 1 - 2 mg/min	Prolongs QT; sinus bradycardia	Not established
	Ibutilide	2 - 12 hours	Renal/Hepatic	IV: 1.0 mg infused over 10-min; may repeat 2nd dose of 0.5 - 1.0 mg.	Prolongs QT	Not established
	Dofetilide	7 - 10 hours	Renal/Hepatic	PO: N/A	Prolongs QT	1.4 - 6.4 ng/ml
CLASS IV Ca^{++} Channel Blockers	Verapamil	3 - 7 hours	Hepatic	IV initial: 2.5 - 10 mg over 2 - 3 min; repeat in 30 min if necessary. IV maintenance: 0.125 mg/min. PO: 120 - 480 mg/day divided q 6 - q 8 h or long-acting formulation	Prolongs PR	15 - 100 ng/ml
	Diltiazem	2 - 5 hours	Hepatic	PO: 30 - 120 mg q 8hr or equivalent long-acting formulation	Prolongs PR (±)	30 - 130 ng/ml

* Patients with decreased hepatic or renal function may require lower dosage. Always consult manufacturers package insert for latest dosing information.

TABLE 3-4. Clinical pharmacologic profile of unclassified antiarrhythmic drugs

Vaughan-Williams Drug Class	Name of Drug	Drug Half-Life	Route of Elimination	Dosage* and Interval	Effect on Resting ECG	Therapeutic Serum Level
OTHERS Purinergic Blockers	Adenosine	< 10 seconds	Red blood cell adenosine deaminase	IV: 3 -12 mg rapid bolus	Prolongs PR	Not established
Na$^+$/K$^+$ Pump Blockers	Digoxin	36 hours	Primarily renal	PO or IV loading: 1 - 1.5 mg divided over 24 hr, then 0.125 - 0.375 mg daily for maintenance	Prolongs PR; depresses ST segment; flattens T wave	1 - 2 ng/ml
	Digitoxin	4 - 6 days	Primarily hepatic	PO or IV loading: 1 - 1.2 mg divided over 24 hr, then 0.1 - 0.2 mg daily for maintenance	Prolongs PR; depresses ST segment; flattens T wave	10 - 20 ng/ml

* Patients with decreased hepatic or renal function may require lower dosage. Always consult manufacturers package insert for latest dosing information.

TABLE 3-5. Potential adverse side effects of class I antiarrhythmic drugs

Vaughan-Williams Drug Class	Name of Drug	Potential Adverse and Toxic Effects
Class IA Na$^+$ Channel Blockers	Quinidine	Diarrhea & other GI symptoms, cinchonism, hepatic granuloma & necrosis, thrombocytopenia, rashes, hypotension, heart block, tachyarrhythmias, torsade de pointes, fever, lupus-like syndrome
	Procainamide	Lupus-like syndrome, confusion, disorientation, GI symptoms, rash, hypotension, arrhythmias, torsade de pointes, blood dyscrasias, fever
	Disopyramide	Anticholinergic effects, hypotension, heart failure, tachyarrhythmias, torsade de pointes, heart block, nausea, vomiting, diarrhea, hepatic toxicity, acute psychosis, agranulocytosis, constipation, hypoglycemia
CLASS IB Na$^+$ Channel Blockers	Lidocaine	Drowsiness or agitation, slurred speech, tinnitus, disorientation, coma, seizures, paresthesias, cardiac depression, especially with excessive accumulation in heart failure or liver failure or infusions for more than 24 hours
	Phenytoin	Ataxia, nystagmus, drowsiness, coma, blood dyscrasias, cardiac toxicity with rapid IV injection, fever, rash, hepatic granulomas and necrosis
	Mexiletine	GI upset, fatigue, nervousness, dizziness, tremor, sleep upset, convulsions, visual disturbances, psychosis, fever, hepatic toxicity, blood dyscrasias
	Tocainide	GI upset, paresthesias, dizziness, tremor, confusion, nightmares, psychotic reactions, coma, seizures, rash, fever, arthralgia, agranulocytosis, aplastic anemia, thrombocytopenia, hepatic granulomas, interstitial pneumonitis
CLASS IC Na$^+$ Channel Blockers	Flecainide	Bradycardia, heart block, ventricular fibrillation, sustained ventricular tachycardia, heart failure, dizziness, blurred vision, nervousness, headache, GI upset, neutropenia
	Propafenone	Bradycardia, heart block, ventricular fibrillation, sustained tachycardia, heart failure, dizziness, lightheadedness, metallic taste, dysgeusia, GI upset, bronchospasm
	Moricizine	Bradycardia, heart block, ventricular fibrillation, sustained tachycardia, heart failure, dizziness, nausea, GI upset

TABLE 3-6. Potential adverse side effects of class II, III, IV and unclassified antiarrhythmic drugs

Vaughan-Williams Drug Class	Name of Drug	Potential Major Adverse and Toxic Effects
CLASS II β-Adrenergic Blockers	Propranolol, Metoprolol, Esmolol, etc.	Heart block, hypotension, heart failure, bronchospasm
CLASS III K⁺ Channel Blockers	d,l-Sotalol	Heart block, hypotension, heart failure, bronchospasm, ventricular tachyarrhythmias
	Amiodarone	Acute pulmonary toxicity, pulmonary fibrosis, bradycardia, heart block, ventricular tachyarrhythmias, GI upset, hepatitis, phospholipidosis, ataxia, tremor, dizziness, photo-sensitivity, blue-grey skin, corneal deposits, hyper- or hypothyroidism, increased serum cholesterol
	Bretylium	Orthostatic hypotension, nausea & vomiting, ventricular arrhythmias, increased response to catecholamines
	Ibutilide	Torsade de pointes (more likely in patients with bradycardia and significant left ventricular dysfunction).
	Dofetilide	Torsade de pointes.
CLASS IV Ca⁺⁺ Channel Blockers	Verapamil, Diltiazem	Heart block, hypotension, bradycardia, dizziness, headache, fatigue, peripheral edema, nausea, constipation, Stevens-Johnson syndrome
OTHERS Purinergic Blockers	Adenosine	Transient dyspnea, chest discomfort (non-myocardial), hypotension
Na⁺/K⁺ Pump Blockers	Digoxin, Digitoxin	Anorexia, nausea, vomiting, diarrhea, abdominal pain, headache, confusion, abnormal vision, bradycardia, AV block, arrhythmias

3.2   Molecular and Biophysical Targets for Antiarrhythmic Drugs

Before undertaking a discussion of the cellular mechanism of action of antiarrhythmic drugs it is helpful to review the basic cellular electrophysiology of cardiac cells, including ion channels, transmembrane currents, membrane receptors, and second messenger systems.

3.2.1 NATURE OF THE CELLULAR RESTING POTENTIAL

To understand the origin of the resting potential in cardiac cells, the concept of *diffusion potentials* must be appreciated. Consider the situation depicted in Figure 3-5. In panel A, a membrane impermeable to water and ions separates two halves of a water-filled container. If NaCl and KCl are added to side 1, there is no ionic movement across the membrane to side 2 because the membrane is impermeable to ion movement. In panel B is depicted an identical system in all respects except that this membrane is *semipermeable*, allowing transmembrane movement only of K^+ ions. In this case, after the addition of NaCl and KCl to side 1, there will be a net diffusion of K^+ ions from side 1 (the region of high K^+ concentration) to side 2 (the region of low K^+ concentration). This net diffusion results because the force represented by the concentration gradient tends to draw K^+ ions from the region of high concentration to a region of low concentration. It is important to note, however, that as K^+ diffuses from side 1 to side 2, another counterbalancing force starts to develop, namely an electrical force tending to push K^+ from side 2 back into side 1. This force develops because with the transmembrane movement of each K^+ ion, the sum of all charges in side 2 is a net positive, while the sum of all charges in side 1 is net negative. Therefore, with continued diffusion of K^+ from side 1 to side 2, an *electric potential difference* (*diffusion potential*, measured in millivolts (mV)) begins to develop across this semipermeable membrane. The diffusion of K^+ from side 1 to 2 will continue until an *equilibrium* condition is reached. At equilibrium (panel C), the concentration force tending to draw K^+ ions into side 2 is equal to and opposite the electrical force tending to push K^+ ions back into side 1. When the opposing concentration

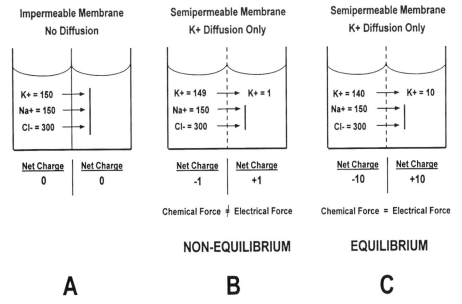

FIGURE 3-5. Role of semipermeable membrane in the genesis of the cardiac cellular resting potential. See text for details.

and electrical forces are equal in this equilibrium condition, the stable diffusion potential across the semipermeable membrane is termed an *equilibrium potential.* In this case, it would be a *K+ equilibrium potential (E_K),* because the membrane is only permeable to K+. The K+ equilibrium potential is the membrane potential at which there is no net movement of K+ ions. If side 1 represents the intracellular space, and side 2 the extracellular space, then this stable transmembrane potential would be the resting potential, i.e., the K+ equilibrium potential and the resting potential would be identical. Similarly, there is also a membrane potential at which there is no net movement of Na+, Cl-, and Ca++ ions (E_{Na}, E_{Cl}, and E_{Ca}, respectively). However, it is essential to emphasize that these ions and equilibrium potentials will *only* contribute to the membrane potential if the membrane is permeable to them. At rest, the normal ventricular or atrial muscle cell has a membrane permeability for potassium, P_K, which is much greater than that for Na+ (P_{Na}), Ca2+ (P_{Ca}), or Cl- (P_{Cl}). Since, at the normal resting potential the cell is largely impermable to these other ions, they contribute little to the resting potential. Consequently, in most cardiac cells, the resting or maximum diastolic potential will be very close to E_K, because P_K >>P_{Na}, P_{Cl}, or P_{Ca} at this level of membrane potential.

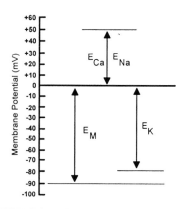

In cardiac cells, the intracellular K+ concentration $[K^+]_i$, is normally 30 to 40 times as large as the extracellular K+ concentration, $[K^+]_o$, whereas the extracellular Na+ concentration, $[Na^+]_o$, is 10 to 20 times as large as the intracellular Na+ concentration, $[Na^+]_i$. An equation (*Nernst equation*) has been derived enabling the calculation of equilibrium potentials. For the K+ equilibrium potential, E_K:

$$E_K = \frac{RT}{zF}\ln\frac{[K_{out}]}{[K_{in}]}$$

FIGURE 3-6. The resting potential approximates the potassium equilibrium potential, E_K, because the permeability to potassium ions, P_K, is much greater than P_{Na} or P_{Ca}. See text for details.

where R is the universal gas constant, T is the absolute temperature, F is the Faraday constant, and z is the ionic charge. (Strictly speaking, the Nernst equation requires the use of ionic activities rather than concentrations as used here). It is important to emphasize that E_K is the transmembrane potential at which net diffusion-dependent K+ currents, are equal to zero. From another standpoint, E_K represents the energy stored in the K+ electrochemical gradient and in that sense E_K is the electromotive force (EMF) of the "K+ battery".

As alluded to above, in addition to the K+ battery, the Na+ battery (E_{Na}), the Ca++ battery (E_{Ca}), and the Cl- battery (E_{Cl}) are also important in cardiac cells. An equation analogous to the Nernst equation for the E_K can be written for each of the equilibrium potentials (batteries) due to these ions. The transmembrane potential at any particular time is the result of the interaction of these various ionic batteries. In cardiac cells at their normal resting potential, P_K >> P_{Na} and P_{Ca}, and the membrane potential very closely approximates E_K (-80 to -90 mV). During the upstroke of a normal action potential, P_{Na} and $P_{Ca} >> P_K$, therefore, the membrane potential approaches E_{Na} and E_{Ca} (>+50 mV). The changing transmembrane voltage during the action potential (see below) merely reflects changes in the relative contributions of these various "ionic batteries" to the net transmembrane potential difference.

3.2.2 IONIC CHANNELS AND TRANSMEMBRANE CURRENTS

Transmembrane ionic currents are of two basic types. Most currents are *diffusion-dependent*, with ions traversing the membrane through pores or channels down their electrochemical gradient, by way of a non-carrier-mediated passive diffusion process as outlined in the above section. Evidence also suggests that some transmembrane ionic currents are generated by an energy-requiring pump which moves ions across the membrane against their electrochemical gradient apparently by way of a membrane-bound carrier. Such an ionic current is said to be an *electrogenic pump current*. Regardless of the mechanism, by convention an outward current is defined as the net movement of positive charge out of the cell, while an inward current is defined as the net movement of positive charge into the cell. Outward currents, are denoted with a positive sign, whereas inward currents are denoted with a negative sign.

Diffusion-dependent ionic currents traverse the membrane lipid bilayer through channels. Channels are large glycoproteins that span the membrane bilayer and which can form a transmembrane pore when subjected to an appropriate stimulus (Figure 3-7). The formation of the channel pore appears to result from a conformational change in the channel protein. Pioneering experimental and theoretical work suggests that ion channels can exist in three states (Figure 3-8): *rested* (R); *inactivated* (I); and *activated* (A). For example, Na⁺ channels exist in the R-state at negative levels of membrane potential near the resting potential. In the R-state, the channels are closed but can be opened by an appropriate stimulus, in this case a depolarizing voltage pulse. At more positive membrane potentials, Na⁺ channels are in the I-state, which is also a closed state; however, unlike channels in the R-state that are poised to be activated, channels in the I-state must

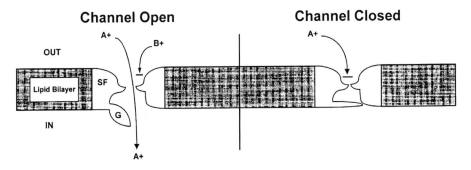

FIGURE 3-7. Schematic diagram of transmembrane ion channels. Channels are transmembrane proteins that span the lipid bilayer. When open, the channels form a hydrophilic pore that allows passage of ions that can meet the size requirements of the selectivity filter (SF). Some form of gating (G) structure is present which obstructs the pore and prevents passages of even the correct-sized ions when the channel is closed. See text for details.

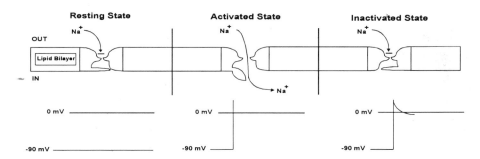

FIGURE 3-8. Three states of ion channels. Ion channels can exist in the resting (closed), activated (open), and inactivated (closed) states. While both the resting and inactivated states are "closed" states, they differ in that the resting channel can be activated (opened) by membrane depolarization, whereas the inactivated channel cannot. See text for details.

be returned to the negative level of membrane potential before they can be reactivated, i.e., the channel cannot go from the I-state to the A-state without going through the R-state (Figure 3-8). Between these two levels of membrane potentials, Na^+ channels are in the A-state, or open state, and are able to conduct Na^+ ions. Gating is the process whereby the appropriate stimulus induces a conformational change in the protein allowing pore formation and channel opening. Channels that are opened may stay open until the stimulus is removed, or may close after a period of time even if the stimulus continues.

A variety of stimuli are known to open channels. Some channels are *voltage-gated*, meaning that they open (form a transmembrane pore) when the transmembrane potential is within a particular range. Strictly speaking, opening of voltage-gated ion channels is a statistical event; at certain membrane potentials the channel is statistically more likely to be in the A-state than the R-state, while at other membrane potentials the R-state is more likely than the A-state or I-state. Other channels are *ligand-gated,* and open when a chemical mediator binds to the channel protein or an associated structure. Other channels, termed *mechanically-gated*, open in response to mechanical deformation of the membrane such as occurs during stretch. A variety of neurohumoral mediators may modulate the opening and closing behavior of ion channels (see "Neurohumoral Regulators of Ionic Currents" on page 109).

It is important to appreciate that even if a channel is open, conduction of ions is not assured unless other conditions are met. Firstly, the channel pore must have a larger diameter than the diameter of the ion in question. In fact, because ions are generally associated with water molecules, the diameter of the pore may have to be greater than the hydrated ionic diameter. Therefore, ion channels generally exhibit *selectivity* for certain ions or groups of ions. Secondly, even if the ionic diameter is sufficiently small, a net ionic current will only flow if there is a net driving force for the ion in question. Thirdly, the resistance or conductance of ions through the channel pore may vary with levels of the membrane potential, even though the channel remains open.

In cardiac cells, voltage-dependent currents play the greatest role in generation of the resting and action potential, although "background leak currents" which result from ion passage through channels that appear to be open all the time also play a role, particularly in sinus and AV node cells. A large number of normal and abnormal ionic currents have been identified in cardiac cells (Table 3-7.) Not all of these currents are operative in all cardiac tissues at all times. Inward currents are by convention defined as the net movement of positive charges into the cell; outward currents are defined as the net movement of positive charges out of the cell. Outward currents are arbitrarily defined as positive currents, while inward currents are denoted as negative currents.

TABLE 3-7. Transmembrane ionic currents in cardiac cells

	Current	Description
Inward Currents	i_{Na}	Inward Na^+ current during action potential upstroke
	i_{Ca-L}	Inward Ca^{++} current during action potential upstroke and plateau
	i_{Ca-T}	Inward Ca^{++} current at negative diastolic potentials
	i_{TI}	Non-selective transient inward current carried by Na^+ activated when myoplasmic Ca^{++} rises above normal levels during diastole
	i_{SA}	Inward current carried by channels activated by stretch
	i_{NaCa}	Inward Na^+ current carried by electrogenic Na^+/Ca^{++} exchange system
	i_f	Non-selective inward current carried by Na^+ activated at negative potentials; contributes to the generation of pacemaker depolarization during diastole
	i_{Na-B}	Background inward Na^+ current
Outward Currents	i_K	Outward delayed-rectifier K^+ current; contributes to repolarization. Composed of rapidly inactivating component, i_{KR}, and slowly inactivating component, i_{KS}.
	i_{Ks}	Slowly inactivating component of delayed rectifier.
	i_{Kr}	Rapidly inactivating component of delayed rectifier.
	i_{K1}	Outward inwardly-rectifying K^+ current; contributes to repolarization and resting potential
	i_{TO}	Outward K^+ current activated briefly during depolarization
	$i_{K(Ach)}$	Outward K^+ current activated by acetylcholine or adenosine
	$i_{K(ATP)}$	Outward K^+ current inhibited by high levels of ATP
	$i_{K(Ca)}$	Outward K^+ current activated by high myoplasmic $[Ca^{++}]$
	i_{Cl}	Outward Cl^- current; may contribute to repolarization
	i_{NaK}	Outward Na^+ current carried by electrogenic Na^+/K^+ exchange system
	i_{NaCa}	Outward Na^+ current carried by electrogenic Na^+/Ca^{++} exchange system; may contribute to Ca^{++} entry during the plateau and aid repolarization

3.2.3 ACTION POTENTIAL GENERATION IN CARDIAC CELLS

In general, cardiac cells exhibit two types of action potentials (Figure 3-9). Fast-response action potentials are generated in cells which possess i_{K1} and fast i_{Na} channels and have very negative resting potentials. Slow-response action potentials are generated in cells which lack i_{K1} and i_{Na} channels and exhibit a more positive resting potential near -50 to -40 mV. Fast action potentials occur normally in atrial, ventricular, His-Purkinje, and some AV nodal cells, although their contour varies slightly. Slow action potentials are normally confined to SA and many AV nodal cells, particularly those in the compact AV node. Under experimental or pathological conditions, many cells which normally only generate fast action potentials, can exhibit both these levels of resting potential and therefore generate both slow and fast action potentials. If i_{K1} is blocked, the cell will depolarize to -40 to -50 mV; at this membrane potential fast Na+ channels are inactivated and if the cell is excited only slow action potentials will be generated.

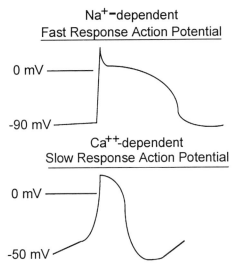

FIGURE 3-9. Fast and slow response action potentials. Na+-dependent fast response action potentials are generated from a low resting potential near -90 mV in atrial, ventricular and His-Purkinje cells. Ca++-dependent slow response action potentials are generated from a less negative resting potential near -40 to -50 mV in sinoatrial and some atrioventricular nodal cells. See text for details.

Sinoatrial and atrioventricular node cells
Figure 3-10 (panel A) graphically displays the ionic currents involved in the generation of the slow action potentials in nodal cells. Note that the upstroke of the action potential results from i_{Ca-L} and i_{Ca-T}, with repolarization resulting primarily from i_K. i_{Na} and i_{K1} channels are largely absent in these cells. Diastolic depolarization results from a combination of a slow increase in the decay of i_K in association with the constant background Na+ current, i_{Na-B}, and increasing magnitude of if and, possibly, i_{Ca-T}. Activation of $i_{K(Ach)}$ and the Na+/K+ pump current may shorten the action potential, hyperpolarize the cell, and may decrease the rate of diastolic depolarization.

Atrial, ventricular and His-Purkinje cells
Figure 3-10 (panel B) graphically displays the ionic currents responsible for generation of the fast action potential in atrial, ventricular and His-Purkinje cells. The action potentials in all these cells are basically the same, except the plateau phase varies. The plateau is generally longest in His-Purkinje cells and shortest in atrial cells, with ventricular cells

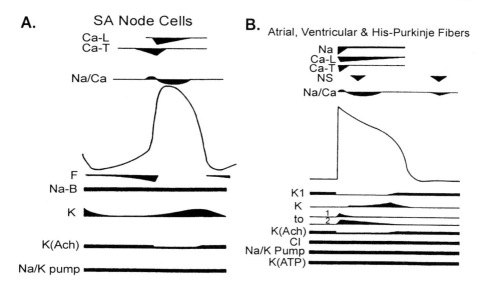

FIGURE 3-10. Schematic illustration of currents involved in the generation of slow action potentials in SA (and some AV) nodal cells (panel A) and fast action potentials in atrial, ventricular, and His-Purkinje cells (panel B). Adapted from [51]. See text for details.

having a plateau phase of intermediate duration. The upstroke of the action potential in these cells results from i_{Na}, i_{Ca-L}, i_{Ca-T}, with the plateau resulting from a balance between the inward currents, primarily i_{Ca-L}, and the outward currents i_K and i_{TO}, with i_{NaCa} having a variable effect. Repolarization results as the outward currents overwhelm the decaying inward currents. In atrial cells, activation of $i_{K(Ach)}$, and possibly i_{Cl}, i_{NaK}, and outward component of i_{NaCa}, may also contribute to repolarization and shortening of the action potential duration.

3.2.4 NEUROHUMORAL REGULATORS OF IONIC CURRENTS

General principles
A variety of neurohumoral mediators modulate cardiac ionic currents and action potential conduction (Table 3-8.). In general, this process involves a number of stereotyped processes including: 1) agonist binding to specific membrane-bound receptor; 2) activation of receptor-coupled GTP-binding proteins (G proteins); 3) the activated G proteins either directly alter specific ion channel conductances, or indirectly modulate ionic conductances by modulating a variety of intracellular enzyme systems or the production of a number of intracellular mediators. The agonists and receptors involved include α- and β-adrenergic agents, M$_2$-cholinergic agents, A$_1$-purinergic agents, and angiotensin. The intracellular enzymes/mediators include: 1) adenylyl cyclase and the cyclic adenosine monophosphate (cAMP)–dependent protein kinase (protein kinase A, PKA); 2) phospholipase C (PLC), inositol triphosphate (IP$_3$), diacylglycerol (DAG), and protein kinase C (PKC); 3) phospholipase A$_2$ and arachidonic acid (AA). The ionic currents effected include i_f, i_K,

TABLE 3-8. Overview of cardiac cell receptor-effector coupling systems

Receptor	G-Protein	Possible Intracellular Mediators	Effected Channels
β_1-Adrenergic	G_S	Activation of AC/cAMP/PKA system Direct coupling of G-protein to ion channels	Increased i_f, i_K, i_{Cl}, i_{NaK}, i_{TO}, i_{Ca-L} Decreased i_{Na}
α_1-Adrenergic	?G_i, ?G_o	Activation of PLC/IP$_3$ system Activation of PLC/DAG/PKC system Direct coupling of G-protein to ion channels	Increased i_{NaK}, ?i_{TI}, i_K Decreased i_{K1}, i_{TO}
M_2-Cholinergic	?G_i, ?G_o	Inhibition of AC/cAMP/PKA system Activation of PLC/DAG/PKC system Activation of PLA$_2$/AA system Direct coupling of G-protein to ion channels	Increased $i_{K(Ach)}$, ?i_K Decreased i_f Reversal of β_1-adrenergic increase in i_{Ca-L}, ?i_K, i_f
AII-Angiotensin	?G_i, ?G_o	Activation of PLC/DAG/PKC system	Increased i_{Na}
A_1-Purinergic	?G_i, ?G_o	Direct coupling of G-protein to ion channels	Increased $i_{K(Ach)}$ Reversal of β_1-adrenergic increase in i_{Ca-L}, i_f

AA, arachidonic acid; AC, adenylate cyclase; cAMP, cyclic adenosine monophosphate; DAG, diacylglycerol; IP$_3$, inositol triphosphate; PKA, protein kinase A (cAMP-dependent protein kinase); PKC, protein kinase C; PLA$_2$, phospholipase A$_2$; PLC, phospholipase C

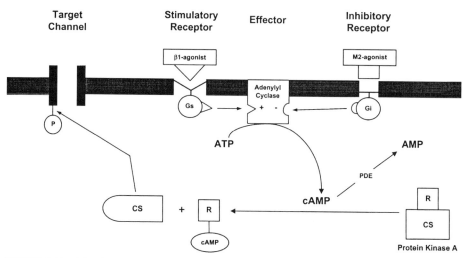

FIGURE 3-11. Adenylyl cyclase/protein kinase A receptor-effector coupling system. Abbreviations: AMP, adenosine monophosphate; ATP, adenosine triphosphate; cAMP, cyclic adenosine monophosphate; CS, catalytic subunit of protein kinase A; Gi, inhibitory GTP-binding protein; Gs, stimulatory GTP-binding protein; P, phosphorylation of protein; PDE, phosphodiesterase; R, regulatory subunit of protein kinase A.

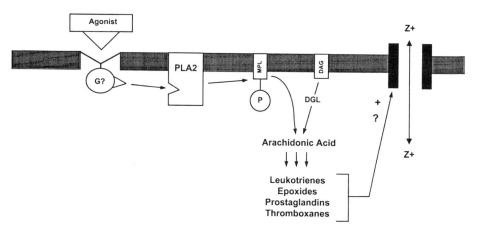

FIGURE 3-12. Phospholipase A2/arachidonic acid receptor-effector coupling system. Abbreviations: DAG, diacyglycerol; DGL, diacyglycerol lipase; G?, uncharacterized stimulatory GTP-binding protein; MPL, membrane phospholipids; P, phosphorylated protein; PLA2, phospholipase A2; Z+, generic ion.

i_{Cl}, i_{NaK}, i_{TO}, i_{Ca-L}, i_{Na}, i_{TI}, i_{K1}, and $i_{K(Ach)}$. These receptor-effector coupling systems are summarized in Figures 3-11 through 3-13 and Table 3-8..

Adrenergic receptors
Activation of β_1-adrenergic receptors (Figure 3-11) by agonists such as epinephrine, norepinephrine, or isoproterenol results in activation of a specific G protein (G_s) which

stimulates adenylyl cyclase to catalyze the formation of cAMP. cAMP, in turn, releases the regulatory subunit from the catalytic subunit of PKA allowing the phosphorylation of the target ionic channel. G_s also appears to directly activate some ionic channels, independent of channel phosphorylation. Presumably, it is this channel phosphorylation, or direct G protein activation, which increases i_F, i_K, i_{Cl}, i_{NaK}, i_{TO} and i_{Ca-L}, and decreases i_{Na}.

Activation of α_1-adrenergic receptors also appears to modulate some ionic currents, increasing i_K, i_{NaK}, i_{TI}, and decreasing i_{TO}, i_{K1}. These effects appear to be mediated either by direct interaction of the G protein with the ion channel, or effector-receptor coupling to the PLC/IP$_3$ (Figure 3-12) or PLC/DAG/PKC enzyme systems (Figure 3-13).

Cholinergic receptors

Cholinergic agents which bind to muscarinic (M$_2$) receptors increase $i_{K(Ach)}$ and possibly i_K, decrease i_F, and reverse the β_1-adrenergic activation of i_{Ca-L}. The reversal of the β_1-adrenergic activation of i_{Ca-L} or i_F is mediated through an inhibitory G protein, G_i, which inhibits the adenylyl cyclase-induced increase in cAMP (Figure 3-11). The increase in $i_{K(Ach)}$, and possibly i_K, and the decrease in if may also be mediated by activation of the PLC/DAG/PKC (Figure 3-12)and PLA2/AA systems (Figure 3-13).

Purinergic receptors

The purinergic agents adenosine and adenosine triphosphate also can activate the K$^+$ current $i_{K(Ach)}$ and reverse the β_1-adrenergic enhancement of i_{Ca-L} and i_F. The latter effect is mediated through the inhibitory G protein, G_i, while the activation of $i_{K(Ach)}$ may be due to direct coupling of the G protein to the channel, although the precise mechanism is unclear.

Angiotensin receptors

There is evidence that angiotensin II can increase i_{Na}. This effect appears to be mediated by the PLC/DAG/PKC system.

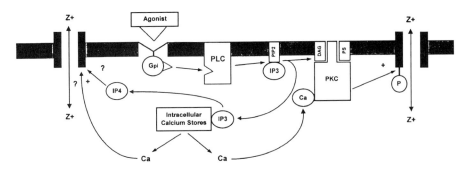

FIGURE 3-13. Phosphatidylinositide receptor-effector coupling system. Abbreviations: Ca, calcium ion; DAG, diacylglycerol; Gpi, stimulatory GTP-binding protein for phosphatidylinositide system; IP3, inositol triphosphate; IP4, inositol tetraphosphate; P, phosphorylation of protein; PIP2, phosphatidylinositol biphosphate; PKC, protein kinase C, PLC, phospholipase C; PS, phosphatidylserine; Z+, generic ion.

3.3 Classification of Antiarrhythmic Drugs

3.3.1 MODIFIED VAUGHAN WILLIAMS CLASSIFICATION

The most widely-used antiarrhythmic drug classification was proposed by Vaughan Williams [46,47] and later modified [48-50] (Table 3-9.). While this classification has severe limitations, its virtual universal usage makes an understanding of it essential. By the Vaughan Williams classification, class I drugs are those that primarily block Na^+ channels and decrease the rate of depolarization in cells exhibiting Na^+-dependent action potentials, while class III drugs primarily block K^+ channels and therefore prolong repolarization. Class II includes agents that block adrenergic receptors, while class IV are Ca^{++}-channel blocking drugs and decrease the upstroke velocity of Ca^{++}-dependent action potentials.

TABLE 3-9. Modified Vaughan Williams classification of antiarrhythmic drugs

Class	Pharmacological Effect	Antiarrhythmic Drugs
IA	Depress rapid action potential upstroke and decrease conduction velocity (Na^+ channel blockade) and significantly prolong repolarization (K^+ channel blockade)	Quinidine, Procainamide, Disopyramide, Diphenylhydantoin
IB	Depress rapid action potential upstroke in abnormal tissue (little effect in normal tissue) and enhance repolarization	Mexiletine, Lidocaine, Tocainide, Moricizine
IC	Markedly depress rapid action potential upstroke and decrease conduction velocity (Na^+ channel blockade) but exert little effect on repolarization (K^+ channel blockade)	Propafenone, Encainide, Flecainide, Moricizine
II	Drugs which block adrenergic receptors	Propranolol, Metoprolol, Atenolol, etc.
III	Drugs which primarily block K^+ channels and slow repolarization (little or no Na^+ channel blockade)	Sotalol, Amiodarone, Bretylium, Ibutilide, N-acetylprocainamide
IV	Drugs which block Ca^{++} channels	Verapamil, Diltiazem, etc.

3.3.2 SICILIAN GAMBIT CLASSIFICATION

In 1991, a new more comprehensive and physiologically-based classification system was proposed by the Task Force of the Working Group on Arrhythmias of the European Society of Cardiology [51-53]. This system focuses on the *targets* of antiarrhythmic drugs, whether they are ion channels, pumps, or effector-receptor coupling systems (Figure 3-14). These targets are also effected by the autonomic nervous system and circulating neurohumors. Competing or complementary alterations in ionic currents by antiarrhyth-

mic drugs and neuromediators can modulate cardiac conduction and refractoriness via
intracellular second messenger systems.

The Sicilian Gambit investigators further focused on the mechanisms of clinical cardiac arrhythmias and identified the vulnerable parameter to be targeted for the best antiarrhythmic effect (Table 3-10.). Finally, they further narrow the focus by suggesting which ionic currents will modulate the vulnerable parameter (Figure 3-10.). Using this analysis they come up with a classification of antiarrhythmic drugs based more upon cellular electrophysiological effects than surface ECG changes (Figure 3-15).

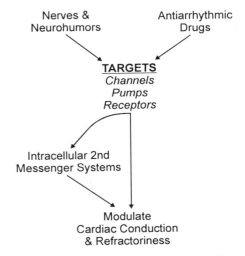

FIGURE 3-14. Rationale for Sicilian Gambit classification of antiarrhythmic drugs based upon molecular targets of the drugs. See text for details.

3.4   Modulated Receptor Theory of Antiarrhythmic Drug Action

3.4.1 THREE STATES OF ION CHANNELS

According to the Hodgkin-Huxley theory of ion channels, Na^+ channels can exist in three states (Figure 3-8). As previously touched on above, the resting (R) state is a closed state present at cells the resting potential. A resting channel can be opened with depolarization. The inactivated (I) state is a closed state present at low levels of membrane potential. An inactivated channel cannot be opened even, with depolarization, unless it is first returned to the resting state. The activated (A) state is the open state of the channel allowing the transmembrane conduction of ions. The channel briefly passes through the activated state enroute from the R-state to I-state.

According to the modulated receptor theory of antiarrhythmic drugs action [55-60], antiarrhythmic drugs can interact with the open, closed, and inactivated states (Figure 3-16). According to this theory, drug-free channels can exhibit voltage-dependent transitions between R-, A-, and I-states. The affinity of drug for channels in each of these states varies and each state has a characteristic association (k) and dissociation (I) rate constants. As with drug-free channels, drug-bound channels exhibit voltage-dependent transitions between RD-, AD-, and ID-states. Drug-bound channels do not conduct ions, even when in the A-state.

TABLE 3-10. Cellular mechanisms possibly responsible clinical cardiac arrhythmias

Mechanism of arrhythmia	Vulnerable parameter (antiarrhythmic effect)	Ionic currents which may modulate vulnerable parameter
Automaticity		
Enhanced normal automaticity	Phase 4 depolarization (decrease)	I_f, I_{Ca-T} (block); $I_{K(Ach)}$ (activate)
Abnormal automaticity	Maximum diastolic potential (hyperpolarize)	I_K, $I_{K(Ach)}$ (activate)
	Phase 4 depolarization (decrease)	I_{Ca-L}, I_{Na} (block)
Triggered Activity		
Early afterdepolarizations	Action potential duration (shorten) or early afterdepolarizations (suppress)	I_K (activate); I_{Ca-L}, I_{Na} (block)
Delayed afterdepolarizations	Calcium overload (unload) or delayed afterdepolarizations (suppress)	I_{Ca-L} (block); I_{Ca-L}, I_{Na} (block)
Reentry		
Primary impaired conduction (long excitable gap) due to depressed Na$^+$ channels	Excitability and conduction (decrease)	I_{Na} (block)
Primary impaired conduction (long excitable gap) due to slow Ca^{2+} current	Excitability and conduction (decrease)	I_{Ca-L} (block)
Primary impaired conduction (long excitable gap) due to anisotropy	Excitability and conduction (decrease)	Gap junction (block)
Conduction impaired by encroaching on refractoriness (short excitable gap)	Effective refractory period (prolong)	I_K (block); I_{Ca-L}, I_{Na} (activate)
Other mechanisms		
Reflection	Excitability (decrease)	I_{Na}, I_{Ca-L} (block)
Parasystole	Phase 4 depolarization (decrease)	I_f (block) (if maximum diastolic potential is high)

Modified and adapted from [51,52,54]

Drug	Channels						Receptors				Pumps	ECG Effects			
	Na			K	Ca	f	α	β	M_2	A_1	Na-K ATPase	PP	PR	QRS	QT
	Fast	Med	Slow												
Lidocaine	Low											→			↓
Mexiletine	Low											→			↓
Tocainide	Low											→			↓
Moricizine	High (I)											→		↑	
Disopyramide		High (A)		Moderate								→	↑↓	↑	↑
Procainamide		High (A)		Moderate					Low			→	↑	↑	↑
Quinidine		High (A)		Moderate			Low		Low			↓	↑↓	↑	↑
Propafenone		High (A)						Moderate				↑	↑	↑	
Flecainide			High (A)	Low								→	↑	↑	
Encainide			High (A)									→	↑	↑	
Verapamil	Low				High		Moderate					↑	↑		
Diltiazem					Moderate							↑	↑		
Bretylium				High			Agonist/Antagonist	Agonist/Antagonist				↑			↑
Sotalol				High				High				↑	↑		↑
Amiodarone	Low			High	Low		Moderate	Moderate				↑	↑		↑
Nadolol								High				↑	↑		
Propranolol	Low							High				↑	↑		
Atropine									High			↓	↓		
Adenosine										Agonist		↑	↑		
Digoxin									Agonist		High	↑	↑		↓

Relative potency of block: ○ Low ◍ Moderate ● High

□ Agonist ⬟ Agonist/Antagonist

A = Activated state blocker

I = Inactivated state blocker

FIGURE 3-15. Sicilian Gambit classification of antiarrhythmic drugs. Adapted from [51,52]. See text for details.

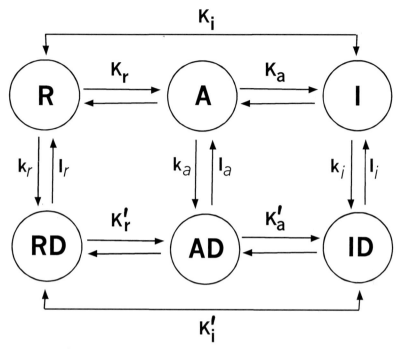

FIGURE 3-16. Schematic diagram summarizing the modulated receptor theory of antiarrhythmic drug action. Adapted from [60,95]. See text for details and abbreviations.

Clinically useful antiarrhythmic drugs exhibit a low affinity for the rested state and a high affinity for activated or inactivated states. During diastole antiarrhythmic drugs unbind from the channel (RD —> R + D). Tetrodotoxin, from the Japanese Puffer fish, has a high affinity for rested state and is a highly toxic drug. A-state blockers show a marked increase in block during the action potential upstroke. I-state blockers exhibit a marked increase in channel block during the plateau phase of action potential, not during the upstroke. Mixed I- and A state blockers show an abrupt increase in block during upstroke of action potential, followed by slow increase during the plateau until a steady-state of block is achieved.

Access to and from the membrane-bound A-state and I-state channels can be achieved using either the hydrophilic or lipophilic pathways (Figure 3-17). Because some antiarrhythmic drugs are ionized at physiological pH, or even more strongly under acidic conditions (which may exist during ischemia), these drugs will vary in their ability to traverse the hydrophilic and lipophilic pathways. Non-ionized drugs easily traverse the lipophilic pathway and therefore can bind to and unbind from channels in either their I- or A-state (Figure 3-17). On the other hand, ionized antiarrhythmic drugs can only access the channel using the hydrophilic pathway and, therefore, can bind to, or leave the channel, only when the channel is in the A-state. Acidosis, increases the proportion of the ionized fraction of ionizable drugs, such as lidocaine. Thus, these ionized drugs cannot readily unbind from inactivated channels because they cannot traverse the lipophilic

CHAPTER 3

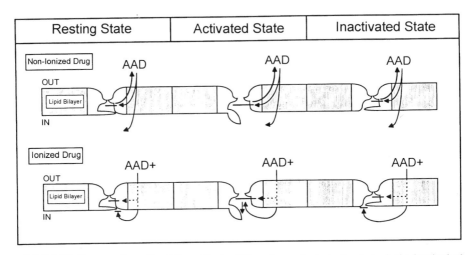

FIGURE 3-17. Transmembrane lipophilic and hydrophilic pathways for ionized and non-ionized antiarrhythmic drugs. Non-ionized drugs have ready access to its channel binding site through the lipophilic pathway regardless of the state of the channel. Ionized drugs, in general cannot traverse the lipophilic pathway, but can easily use the hydrophilic pathway to access the channel only during the activated (open) state. See text for details.

pathway. Therefore, during diastole, recovery from block is slowed in ischemic tissues enhancing the antiarrhythmic effect of these drugs in these tissues.

3.4.2 CLASSIFICATION OF BLOCK

Tonic block
Tonic block is defined as the steady-state level of channel block in the baseline state. It represents the sum total of non-stimulated block of all channels, i.e., RD + AD + ID. Very little tonic block is R-state block because rested channels have a very low affinity for antiarrhythmic drugs. Most tonic block is due to the level of non-stimulated block present in the tissue resulting from drug binding to activated or inactivated channels, not rested channels.

Use-dependent block
Use-dependent block is block that develops during the A- and I-states which does not dissipate (unblock) during diastole (R-state). Figure 3-18 schematically displays the effect of use-dependent block using a potent Na^+ channel blocking agent, such as one of the class IC drugs. Use-dependent block can only be observed if the rate of unblocking during the R-state (rate of drug dissociation from the channel) is slower than the rate of blocking during the A- and I-states (rate of association of drug with channel). If an open or inactivated channel has a higher affinity for the drug then the rested channel, and the rate of dissociation of the drug from the rested channel is sufficiently slow compared to the rate of channel activation, use-dependent block will be seen to occur. Agents which exhibit fast recovery from block (dissociation time constant short), such as lidocaine

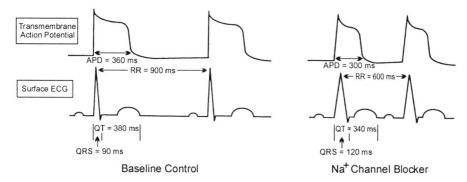

FIGURE 3-18. Sodium channel blockade and use-dependent block. Na^+ channel blockers decrease phase 0 (rapid upstroke) of the Na^+-dependent action potential that is more marked at faster heart rates (use-dependent block). This decrease in the velocity of phase 0 is manifested as an increase in the duration of the QRS complex at shorter R-R intervals. Na^+ channel blockers have no significant effect on the rate-related shortening of the action potential duration and QT interval, both of which are primarily K^+ channel-dependent processes. See text for additional details.

($T_{0.67}$ = 230 msec) will exhibit use-dependent block only if the stimulation rate (rate of channel opening) is fast (<700 msec, or three times $T_{0.67}$). Quinidine, with a $T_{0.67}$ = 4.7 sec, will exhibit use-dependent block at much longer pacing cycle lengths.

A number of factors can enhance use-dependent block (Table 3-12.) Firstly, any increase in heart rate resulting in increased number of action potential upstrokes and plateaus per unit time will increase the amount of use-dependent block caused by A- or I-state blockers, especially those with long time constants for dissociation of drug from receptor. In the case of Na^+ channel blockers with long time constants for unbinding (flecainide), use-dependent block can be marked. Because of this, these drugs are theoretically the most potent in treating tachyarrhythmias, i.e., they block more channels the faster the heart rate.

An increase in action potential duration will likewise increase use-dependent block because this increases the time for drugs to bind to inactivated channels (in the case of I-state blockers), as well as decreasing the duration of diastole, thereby decreasing the time for recovery from block. The net effect is to increase the degree of use-dependent block. Clinically, drugs that exert little I-state blocking will have little effect on arrhythmias occurring in tissues with short plateau phases, i.e., lidocaine has virtually no effect on atrial arrhythmias. Drugs that prolong the action potential duration, such as amiodarone, can also increase the degree of their own, or other, I-state blocking. Amiodarone may increase antiarrhythmic effectiveness of procainamide, propafenone, flecainide, or quinidine.

Heart cells that are depolarized, such as seen in diseased tissues have a greater proportion of their channels in the A- or I-states. Consequently, antiarrhythmic drugs that have an affinity for these states, will have a greater potency in these tissues. This is possible explanation for relative safety of antiarrhythmic drugs in patients with normal hearts (low proarrhythmia).

Increasing the drug concentration will also increase use-dependence. Also, as mentioned above, acidosis which results in an increase fraction of ionized drug which cannot

TABLE 3-11. Time constant of recovery from Na$^+$ channel block

Drug	Vaughan Williams Class	Unbinding Time Constant* (sec)
Lidocaine	IB	0.23
Mexiletine	IB	0.47
Tocainide	IB	1.1
Moricizine	IB	1.3
Quinidine	IA	4.7
Procainamide	IA	6.3
Disopyramide	IA	12.2
Lorcainide	IC	13.2
Propafenone	IC	15.5
Flecainide	IC	15.5
Encainide	IC	20.3
Nicainoprol	IC	47.1
Prajmaline	IC	184.3

Adapted from [61,62].

diffuse through the lipid phase during diastole and therefore remains on the channel longer compared with an equivalent unionized drug, increasing use-dependent block. Finally, assuming everything else is held constant, increasing the antiarrhythmic drug molecular weight decreases the rate of unbinding during diastole which increases use-dependent block.

Reverse use-dependence

In the case of reverse use-dependence there is less block of ion channels with increased use of channels. In other words, even though more time is spent in the A- or I-state, there is less channel block, i.e., there is less drug effect despite an increased use of the channels (Figure 3-19). In the case of K$^+$ channel blockers, this would mean less action potential duration prolongation (QT prolongation) despite increased stimulation rate or heart rate. Because drugs exhibiting reverse use-dependence are less effective at higher heart rates, this property should limit the effectiveness of these agents at terminating tachyarrhythmias. Na$^+$ channel blockers do not appear to exhibit reverse use-dependence.

The cellular electrophysiologic basis for reverse use-dependence is not clearly established but may involve the failure of K$^+$ channel blockers to block the slow component of the delayed rectifier K$^+$ current. Recall that the inward depolarizing currents primarily responsible for prolonging the action potential duration include the L-type Ca^{++} current, i_{Ca-L}, and possibly the electrogenic Na$^+$/Ca^{++} exchange current, $i_{Na/Ca}$. The outward currents which promote repolarization and shorten the action potential duration in-

TABLE 3-12.   Factors that enhance use-dependent block

Factor	Mechanism of enhancement of use-dependent block
Increased Heart Rate	Increased proportion of time channel is in I- and A-state results in more channels being blocked by I- and A-state blockers
Increased Action Potential Duration	Increased proportion of time channel is in I-state results in more channels being blocked by I-state blockers
Membrane Depolarization	Greater proportion of channels are in I- or A-state in depolarized cells than in cells with a normal resting potential
Increased Drug Concentration	More channels are blocked because more drug is available
Acidosis	Ionized antiarrhythmic drug cannot diffuse through lipid phase during diastole and therefore remains on the channel longer compared with an equivalent unionized drug
Increased Drug Molecular Weight	Everything else being constant, as the molecular weight of the drug increases, the rate of unbinding during diastole decreases

clude the inward rectifying K$^+$ current, i_{K1}, the transient outward K$^+$ current, i_{TO} and the delayed rectifier K$^+$ current, i_K. In reality, however, the delayed rectifier K$^+$ current i_K consists of two components, i_{Kr} and i_{Ks}. i_{Kr} is blocked by most class III K$^+$ channel blockers, but not i_{Ks}. i_{Ks} has a very slow decay after activation. Therefore, rapid pacing of the heart results in shortening of the action potential duration because with each subsequent action potential the residual i_{Ks} results in earlier repolarization, i.e., the net outward repolarizing K$^+$ current is increased hastening repolarization. Consequently, rapid pacing or heart rates will tend to decrease the action potential duration prolongation due to class III antiarrhythmic drugs. With increased stimulation rate, the residual i_{Ks} overwhelms the antiarrhythmic drug-induced block of i_{Kr}, shortening action potential duration and decreasing effective refractory period. The apparent observation of reverse use-dependence is not due to less block at higher stimulation rates, but instead is due to slow decay of another outward current which overwhelms and counters the presumed normal use-dependence which is ongoing.

3.4.3 TERMINATION OF REENTRY BY ANTIARRHYTHMIC DRUGS

Concept of excitable gap

Reentrant tachyarrhythmias result when a wavefront of depolarization travels around a circumscribed path of cardiac tissue, each time reentering a previously unexcitable region. For reentry to occur, at least two conditions must exist including 1) an area of slow conduction and, 2) a region of unidirectional block. As seen in Figure 1-6 on page 9, a premature depolarization blocks in one limb of the circuit and proceeds to conduct slowly in the anterograde direction in the other limb. Because conduction is so slow, by the time the wavefront reaches the lower junction of the two limbs it can contin-

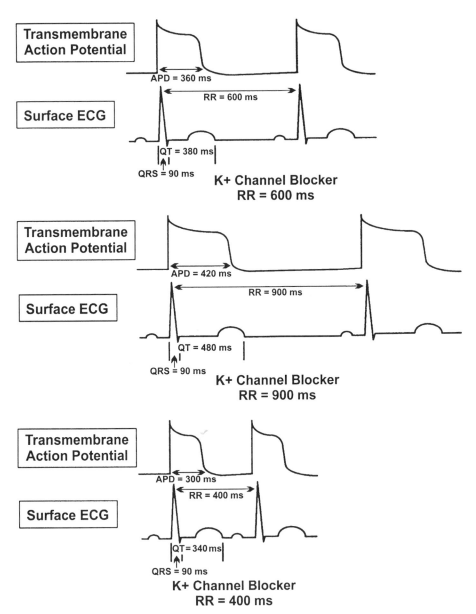

FIGURE 3-19. Potassium channel blockade and reverse use-dependence. K$^+$ channel blockers exert their primary effect on repolarization by prolonging action potential duration and the QT interval. These effects are more marked at long R-R intervals (compare *top panel* to *middle panel*) than at shorter R-R intervals (*bottom panel*). Unlike Na$^+$ channel blockers, pure K$^+$ channel blockers have no significant effect on phase 0 of the Na$^+$-dependent action potential and do not increase the duration of the QRS complex.

ue to conduct in the retrograde direction back to its origin. By the time it reaches its origin, the tissue is no longer refractory and the depolarization wavefront can reenter the integrate limb. If this process continues uninterrupted a circus movement tachycardia can be sustained.

Figure 3-20 depicts an example of a depolarizing wavefront traversing a circular reentry circuit. The depolarization wave leaves in its wake a length of cardiac tissue that is absolutely refractory because the Na$^+$ channels in this region are in the I-state. No matter how much current is applied in this region, this absolutely refractory tissue cannot be excited. Only after a specific period of time elapses, termed the *absolute refractory period*, can this tissue be re-excited. In reality, there is a graded region of variable or *relative refractoriness* in tissue behind the region of absolute refractoriness. This tissue can be excited, but only if an above normal amount of depolarizing current is applied. If the velocity of the depolarization wave is slow enough, or the path of the reentrant circuit is long enough, the leading edge of the depolarization wavefront will return to that refractory region after it again becomes excitable. The length of the excitation wave, or *wavelength*, is the product of the conduction velocity and the refractory period.

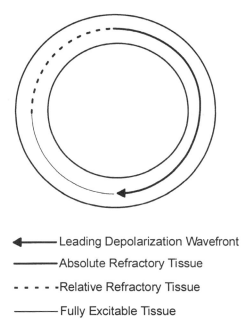

← ——— Leading Depolarization Wavefront

——— Absolute Refractory Tissue

- - - - - Relative Refractory Tissue

——— Fully Excitable Tissue

FIGURE 3-20. Excitable gap model of reentry. The excitable gap is that portion of the reentry circuit that is fully excitable. The wavelength of the depolarization wave is equal to the length of the circuit that is absolutely and relatively refractory and is the product of the conduction velocity of the wavefront (m/sec) and the duration of the refractory period (sec). See text for details.

If the wavelength is greater than the path of the reentrant circuit, then the circus movement tachycardia cannot be sustained because the leading edge of the depolarization wavefront "runs into", or abuts, the tail of the excitation wave and it can no longer propagate in the unexcitable tissue. The *excitable gap* corresponds to the length of tissue in the reentry circuit between the end of the relative refractory period and the leading edge of the depolarizing wavefront.

Role of antiarrhythmic drugs in altering the excitable gap
From the standpoint of the excitable gap model, an "ideal" antiarrhythmic drug would enhance conduction velocity of the depolarization wavefront and increase the absolute refractory period, both of which increase the depolarization wavelength and "narrow the excitable gap" (Figure 3-21). Conversely, a proarrhythmic drug would slow conduction

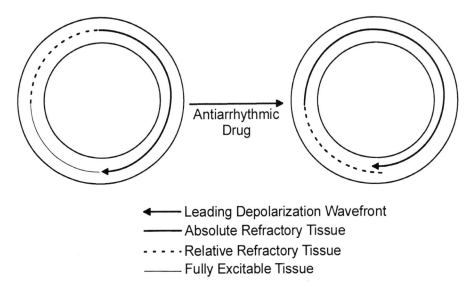

Leading Depolarization Wavefront
Absolute Refractory Tissue
Relative Refractory Tissue
Fully Excitable Tissue

FIGURE 3-21. Effect of antiarrhythmic drugs on the excitable gap. When the depolarization wavelength exceeds the physical path of the reentrant circuit, propagation cannot be sustained because the leading edge of the depolarization "runs into" inexcitable tissue. Ideal antiarrhythmic drugs will narrow the excitable gap by increasing the refractory period and enhancing conduction velocity. If the gap is extinguished, the tachycardia will terminate. While there are many drugs that increase the refractory period, there are no drugs currently available which enhance conduction, particularly in the diseased tissue which is often the substrate for reentrant arrhythmias. See text for details.

velocity of the depolarization wavefront and decrease the absolute refractory period, both of which decrease the depolarization wavelength and "widen the excitable gap". The refractory period will be increased by increases in the action potential duration, decreases in the rate of membrane depolarization, or any factor that enhances use-dependent block (Table 3-12.) The action potential conduction velocity will be decreased by reductions in the rate of membrane depolarization or an alteration in cable properties, such as the diameter of the cells, the internal or external longitudinal resistances, the structure and function of the intercalated disks and gap junctions, or the membrane resistance. In reality, while all clinically-available Na^+ channel blocking drugs may modestly lengthen the refractory period, they fail to enhance conduction velocity (Figure 3-22). In fact, their primary effect is to decrease conduction velocity; therefore, they exert both antiarrhythmic and proarrhythmic effects. Similarly, while the most potent of the K^+ channel blocking drugs may have a dramatic effect on the refractory period, especially at low heart rates (see "Reverse use-dependence" on page 120), they have only a modest effect on conduction velocity, and in no case does any clinically-available K^+ channel blocker enhance conduction velocity

There are undoubtedly many reasons why antiarrhythmic drugs are ineffective in suppressing tachyarrhythmias. One possibility is that the effect of the antiarrhythmic drug to increase the refractory period is balanced by its opposite effect to slow conduction velocity; therefore, the tendency to narrow the excitable gap (increase refractory period) is countered by the tendency to widen the excitable gap (decrease conduction velocity), resulting in no antiarrhythmic effect. Another possibility is that the reentry circuit may have a variable path. Any increase in the path of reentry circuit will counter the effect of the antiarrhythmic drug to narrow the excitable gap.

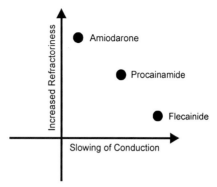

FIGURE 3-22. Graphical comparison of the two critical components of antiarrhythmic drug effectiveness: refractoriness and conduction for three commonly used antiarrhythmic dugs. See text for details.

3.5 Proarrhythmic Effects of Antiarrhythmic Drugs

By their nature as chemical agents which alter the conduction properties and refractoriness of cardiac tissue, one would predict that all antiarrhythmic drugs may potentially have proarrhythmic effects. Proarrhythmia is often difficult to define and even more difficult to diagnose with certainty. Any untoward rhythm disturbance noted while a patient is receiving an antiarrhythmic drug is usually blamed on the drug, even if the drug is guiltless. In these cases, it is often too risky to maintain the patient on the drug and therefore it is discontinued. Establishment of certainty of proarrhythmia by re-challenging the patient with the drug is usually viewed as contraindicated or unethical and therefore the question of cause and effect often remains unanswered. Nevertheless, a number of investigators have attempted to define and classify proarrhythmia (Table 3-13.)

The most feared proarrhythmia is the provocation of fast mono- or polymorphic ventricular tachycardia in a patient who is otherwise at virtually no risk of having these arrhythmias. Consequently, the use of powerful antiarrhythmic drugs in patients with non-life-threatening arrhythmias, particularly if there is an alternative treatment such as radiofrequency catheter ablation, should be approached with extreme caution. On the other hand, some of the patients with the highest risk of proarrhythmia from antiarrhythmic drugs are those with significant heart disease with marked reductions in left ventricular function (Table 3-14.) Unfortunately, these are the exact patients which ordinarily would benefit from the antiarrhythmic effect of these drugs. However, it is this proarrhythmic danger which has resulted in the dramatic decline in the use of these drugs in this population along with the dramatic increase in the popularity of the implantable cardioverter-defibrillator for these patients.

The most common groups of drugs that cause proarrhythmia are the potent Na^+ and K^+ channel blockers. In the former case, the dramatic reductions in conduction velocity can predispose to proarrhythmia using a reentrant mechanism resulting in recurrent, or

TABLE 3-13. Definition and classification of proarrhythmia

Aggravation of pre-existent tachyarrhythmia

  Statistically significant increase in frequency of arrhythmia episodes

  Increase in duration of episodes, e.g. convert non-sustained into sustained arrhythmia

  Increase in rate of a tachyarrhythmia

  Altered response of arrhythmia to non-pharmacologic therapy, typically DC countershock

  Significant increase in the difficulty of termination and/or suppression of a tachyarrhythmia

  Development of incessant tachyarrhythmia that cannot be terminated

  Spontaneous onset of sustained ventricular tachyarrhythmias

  Easier inducibility of sustained tachyarrhythmia (fewer extrastimuli) compared with baseline electro-physiology study

Development of previously unobserved tachyarrhythmia

  Newly inducible sustained or spontaneously-occurring tachyarrhythmia in patient receiving antiar-rhythmic drug

      Torsade de pointes (polymorphic VT) - class IA and Class III antiarrhythmic drugs

      Monomorphic VT - class IC antiarrhythmic drugs

Exacerbation or development of new bradyarrhythmia

  Sinoatrial node dysfunction (sinus node, sinoatrial junction)

  Disturbances of atrioventricular conduction (AV node, His-Purkinje system)

From [63-74].

TABLE 3-14. Predisposing and contributing factors to proarrhythmia

  Reduced left ventricular ejection fraction

  Increased severity of structural heart disease

  Increased risk with increased severity of arrhythmia under treatment

  Myocardial ischemia

  History of ventricular tachycardia or fibrillation

  Worsening congestive heart failure

  Rapid escalation of dose

  High plasma levels of drug

  Alterations in hepatic or renal clearance

  Electrolyte disturbance (hypokalemia, hypomagnesemia)

  Diuretic use

  Individual (genetic) variations in drug metabolism with accumulation of active metabolites

  Bradycardia

  Atrial fibrillation (with variable R-R intervals)

From [64-66,75-94]

even incessant, monomorphic ventricular tachycardia. In the latter case, the dramatic prolongation of repolarization can lead to early afterdepolarizations and torsade de pointes. However, aggravation of a pre-existing arrhythmia is often proarrhythmia and new bradyarrhythmias may result from use of these agents.

References

1. Fenster PE: Clinical pharmacology: Clinical uses of pharmacokinetic principles in prescribing cardiac drugs. *Med Clin North Am* **6**:1281-1293, 1984.
2. Woodings-Scott RA, Smalley J, Visco J, Slaughter RL: The pharmacokinetics and pharmacodynamics of quinidine and 3-hydroxyquinidine. *Br J Clin Pharmacol* **26**:415-421, 1988.
3. Ochs HR, Greenblatt DJ, Woo E: Clinical pharmacokinetics of quinidine. *Clin Pharmacokinet* **5**:150-168, 1980.
4. Follath F, Ganzinger U, Schuetz E: Reliability of antiarrhythmic drug plasma concentration monitoring. *Clin Pharmacokinet* **8**:63-82, 1983.
5. Le Corre P, Gibassier D, Sado P, Le Verge R: Stereoselective metabolism and pharmacokinetics of disopyramide enantiomers in humans. *Drug Metab Dispos* **16**:858-864, 1988.
6. Siddoway LA, Roden DM, Woosley RL: Clinical pharmacology of propafenone: pharmacokinetics, metabolism and concentration-response relations. *Am J Cardiol* **54**:9D-12D, 1984.
7. Siddoway LA, Roden DM, Woosley RL: Clinical pharmacology of old and new antiarrhythmic drugs. *Cardiovasc Clin* **15**:199-248, 1985.
8. Siddoway LA, Woosley RL: Clinical pharmacokinetics of disopyramide. *Clini Pharmacokinet* **11**:214-222, 1986.
9. Siddoway LA, Thompson KA, McAllister CB, et al.: Polymorphism of propafenone metabolism and disposition in man: clinical and pharmacokinetic consequences. *Circulation* **75**:785-91, 1987.
10. Siddoway LA, Schwartz SL, Barbey JT, Woosley RL: Clinical pharmacokinetics of moricizine. *Am J Cardiol* **65**:21D-25D; discussion 68D-71D, 1990.
11. Siddoway LA, McAllister CB, Wilkinson GR, et al.: Amiodarone dosing: a proposal based on its pharmacokinetics. *Am Heart J* **106**:951-6, 1983.
12. Siddoway LA, Barbey JT, Roden DM, Woosley RL: Pharmacologic evaluation of standard and controlled-release disopyramide. *Angiology* **38**:184-7, 1987.
13. Grasela TH, Sheiner LB, Rambeck B, et al.: Steady-state pharmacokinetics of phenytoin from routinely collected patient data. *Clin Pharmacokinet* **8**:355-364, 1983.
14. Crowley JJ, Koup JR, Cusack BJ, et al.: Evaluation of a proposed method for phenytoin maintenance dose prediction following an intravenous loading dose. *Eur J Clin Pharmacol* **32**:141-148, 1987.
15. Cusack B, O'Malley K, Lava J, et al.: Protein binding and disposition of lignocaine in the elderly. *Eur J Clin Pharmacol* **29**:323-329, 1985.
16. Nattel S, Zipes DP: Clinical pharmacology of old and new antiarrhythmic drugs. *Cardiovasc Clin* **11**:221-48, 1980.
17. Nattel S, Rinkenberger RL, Lehrman LL, Zipes DP: Therapeutic blood lidocaine concentrations after local anesthesia for cardiac electrophysiologic studies. *N Engl J Med* **301**:418-20, 1979.
18. Nattel S, Gagne G, Pineau M: The pharmacokinetics of lignocaine and b-adrenoceptor antagonists in patients with acute myocardial infarction. *Clin Pharmacokinet* **13**:293-316, 1987.
19. Nattel S, Feder-Elituv R, Matthews C, et al.: Concentration dependence of class III and beta-adrenergic blocking effects of sotalol in anesthetized dogs. *J Am Coll Cardiol* **13**:1190-4, 1989.
20. Gillis AM, Kates RE: Clinical pharmacokinetics of the newer antiarrhythmic agents. *Clin Pharmacokinet* **9**:375-403, 1984.
21. Brockmeyer NH, Breithaupt H, Ferdinand W, et al.: Kinetics of oral and intravenous mexiletine: lack of effect of cimetidine and ranitidine. *Eur J Clin Pharmacol* **36**:375-378, 1989.
22. Thomson AH, Murdoch G, Pottage A, et al.: The pharmacokinetics of R- and S-tocainide in patients with acute ventricular arrhythmias. *Br J Clin Pharmacol* **21**:149-154, 1986.

23. Tjandra-Maga TB, Verbessent R, Van Hecken A, et al.: Flecainide: single and multiple oral dose kinetics, absolute bioavailability and effect of food and antacid in man. *Br J Clin Pharmacol* **22**:309-316, 1986.

24. McQuinn RL, Pentikainen PJ, Chang SF, Conrad GJ: Pharmacokinetics of flecainide in patients with cirrhosis of the liver. *Clin Pharmacol Ther* **44**:566-72, 1988.

25. Murray KT, Barbey JT, Kopelman HA, et al.: Mexiletine and tocainide: a comparison of antiarrhythmic efficacy, adverse effects, and predictive value of lidocaine testing. *Clin Pharmacol Ther* **45**:553-61, 1989.

26. Murray KT: Ibutilide. *Circulation* **97**:493-7, 1998.

27. Atkinson AJ, Ruo TI, Piergies AA, et al.: Pharmacokinetics of N-acetylprocainamide in patients profiled with stable isotope method. *Clin Pharmacol Ther* **46**:182-189, 1989.

28. Connolly S, Lebsack C, Winkle RA, et al.: Propafenone disposition kinetics in cardiac arrhythmia. *Clin Pharmacol Ther* **36**:163-8, 1984.

29. Connolly SJ, Kates RE: Clinical pharmacokinetics of N-acetylprocainamide. *Clin Pharmacokinet* **7**:206-220, 1982.

30. Rapeport WG: Clinical pharmacokinetics of bretylium. *Clin Pharmacokinet* **10**:248-256, 1985.

31. Somani P: Basic and clinical pharmacology of amiodarone: relationship of antiarrhythmic effects, dose and drug concentrations to intracellular inclusion bodies. *J Clin Pharmacol* **29**:405-412, 1989.

32. Veronese ME, Mclean S, Hendriks R: Plasma protein binding of amiodarone in a patient population: measurement by erythrocyte partitioning and a novel glass-binding method. *Br J Clin Pharmacol* **26**:721-731, 1988.

33. Hollmann M, Brode E, Hotz D, et al.: Investigations on the pharmacokinetics of propafenone in man. *Arzneimittelforschung* **33**:763-70, 1983.

34. Naccarelli GV, Lee KS, Gibson JK, VanderLugt J: Electrophysiology and pharmacology of ibutilide. *Am J Cardiol* **78**:12-6, 1996.

35. Sager PT: New advances in class III antiarrhythmic drug therapy. *Curr Opin Cardiol* **14**:15-23, 1999.

36. Granberry MC: Ibutilide: a new class III antiarrhythmic agent. *Am J Health Syst Pharm* **55**:255-60, 1998.

37. Cropp JS, Antal EG, Talbert RL: Ibutilide: a new class III antiarrhythmic agent. *Pharmacotherapy* **17**:1-9, 1997.

38. Rasmussen HS, Allen MJ, Blackburn KJ, et al.: Dofetilide, a novel class III antiarrhythmic agent. *J Cardiovasc Pharmacol* **20 Suppl** 2:S96-105, 1992.

39. Smith DA, Rasmussen HS, Stopher DA, Walker DK: Pharmacokinetics and metabolism of dofetilide in mouse, rat, dog and man. *Xenobiotica* **22**:709-19, 1992.

40. Tham TC, MacLennan BA, Burke MT, Harron DW: Pharmacodynamics and pharmacokinetics of the class III antiarrhythmic agent dofetilide (UK-68,798) in humans. *J Cardiovasc Pharmacol* **21**:507-12, 1993.

41. Le Coz F, Funck-Brentano C, Morell T, Ghadanfar MM, Jaillon P: Pharmacokinetic and pharmacodynamic modeling of the effects of oral and intravenous administrations of dofetilide on ventricular repolarization. *Clin Pharmacol Ther* **57**:533-42, 1995.

42. Walker DK, Alabaster CT, Congrave GS, et al.: Significance of metabolism in the disposition and action of the antidysrhythmic drug, dofetilide. In vitro studies and correlation with in vivo data. *Drug Metab Dispos* **24**:447-55, 1996.

43. Antonaccio MJ, Gomoll A: Pharmacologic basis of the antiarrhythmic and hemodynamic effects of sotalol. *Am J Cardiol* **72**:27A-37A, 1993.

44. Antonaccio MJ, Gomoll A: Pharmacology, pharmacodynamics, and pharmacokinetics of sotalol. *Am J Cardiol* **65**:12A-21A, 1990.

45. Hanyok JJ: Clinical pharmacokinetics of sotalol. *Am J Cardiol* **72**:19A-26A, 1993.

46. Vaughan Williams EM: Classification of antidysrhythmic drugs. *Pharmacol Ther [B]* **1**:115-38, 1975.

47. Vaughan Williams EM: Classifying antiarrhythmic actions: by facts or speculation. *J Clin Pharmacol* **32**:964-77, 1992.

48. Harrison DC: Future perspectives in antiarrhythmic drugs. *Ann N Y Acad Sci* **432**:314-21, 1984.

49. Harrison DC: Antiarrhythmic drug classification: new science and practical applications. *Am J Cardiol* **56**:185-7, 1985.

50. Harrison DC: Current classification of antiarrhythmic drugs as a guide to their rational clinical use. *Drugs* **31**:93-5, 1986.
51. Task Force of the Working Group on Arrhythmias of the European Society of Cardiology: The Sicilian Gambit: A new approach to the classification of antiarrhythmic drugs based on their actions on arrhythmogenic mechanisms. *Circulation* **84**:1831-1851, 1991.
52. Rosen MR, Chevalier P: The Sicilian Gambit: A pathophysiologic approach to antiarrhythmic therapy. *Primary Cardiology* **21**:18-22, 1995.
53. Schwartz PJ, Zaza A: The Sicilian Gambit revisited--theory and practice. *Eur Heart J* **13 Suppl F**:23-9, 1992.
54. Breithardt G, Camm AJ, Campbell RWF, et al.: *Antiarrhythmic Therapy: A Pathophysiologic Approach.* Armonk, NY: Futura Publishing Company, Inc., 1994.
55. Hille B: Ionic selectivity, saturation, and block in sodium channels. A four- barrier model. *J Gen Physiol* **66**:535-60, 1975.
56. Hille B: Ionic channels of nerve: questions for theoretical chemists. *Biosystems* **8**:195-9, 1977.
57. Hille B: Ionic channels in excitable membranes. Current problems and biophysical approaches. *Biophys J* **22**:283-94, 1978.
58. Hille B: *Ionic Channels of Excitable Membranes.* 2nd ed. Sunderlund, MA: Sinauer Associates, 1992.
59. Hille B: Gating in sodium channels of nerve. *Annu Rev Physiol* **38**:139-52, 1976.
60. Hondeghem LM, Katzung BG: Antiarrhythmic agents: the modulated receptor mechanism of action of sodium and calcium channel-blocking drugs. *Annu Rev Pharmacol Toxicol* **24**:387-423, 1984.
61. Campbell T. Subclassification of class I antiarrhythmic drugs. In: Vaughan Williams EM, Campbell TJ, eds. *Antiarrhythmic Drugs.* Berlin: Springer-Verlag, 135-155: 1989.
62. Vaughan Williams EM: Subgroups of class 1 antiarrhythmic drugs. *Eur Heart J* **5**:96-8, 1984.
63. Rinkenberger RL, Prystowsky EN, Jackman WM, et al.: Drug conversion of nonsustained ventricular tachycardia to sustained ventricular tachycardia during serial electrophysiologic studies: identification of drugs that exacerbate tachycardia and potential mechanisms. *Am Heart J* **103**:177-84, 1982.
64. Horowitz LN, Zipes DP, Bigger JT, Jr., et al.: Proarrhythmia, arrhythmogenesis or aggravation of arrhythmia--a status report, 1987. *Am J Cardiol* **59**:54E-56E, 1987.
65. Horowitz LN, Greenspan AM, Rae AP, et al.: Proarrhythmic responses during electrophysiologic testing. *Am J Cardiol* **59**:45E-48E, 1987.
66. Podrid PJ. Aggravation of arrhythmia by antiarrhythmic drugs. In: Podrid PJ, Kowey PR, eds. *Cardiac Arrhythmia: Mechanisms, Diagnosis, and Management.* 1st ed. Baltimore, MD: Williams & Wilkins, 507-522: 1995.
67. Poser RF, Podrid PJ, Lombardi F, Lown B: Aggravation of arrhythmia induced with antiarrhythmic drugs during electrophysiologic testing. *Am Heart J* **110**:9-16, 1985.
68. Rae AP: Proarrhythmic responses during electrophysiologic testing. *Cardiol Clin* **4**:487-96, 1986.
69. Rae AP, Kay HR, Horowitz LN, Spielman SR, Greenspan AM: Proarrhythmic effects of antiarrhythmic drugs in patients with malignant ventricular arrhythmias evaluated by electrophysiologic testing. *J Am Coll Cardiol* **12**:131-9, 1988.
70. Ruskin JN, McGovern B, Garan H, et al.: Antiarrhythmic drugs: a possible cause of out-of-hospital cardiac arrest. *N Engl J Med* **309**:1302-6, 1983.
71. Torres V, Flowers D, Somberg J: The clinical significance of polymorphic ventricular tachycardia provoked at electrophysiologic testing. *Am Heart J* **110**:17-24, 1985.
72. Torres V, Flowers D, Somberg JC: The arrhythmogenicity of antiarrhythmic agents. *Am Heart J* **109**:1090-7, 1985.
73. Bigger JT, Jr., Sahar DI: Clinical types of proarrhythmic response to antiarrhythmic drugs. *Am J Cardiol* **59**:2E-9E, 1987.
74. Buxton AE, Josephson ME: Role of electrophysiologic studies in identifying arrhythmogenic properties of antiarrhythmic drugs. *Circulation* **73**:II67-72, 1986.
75. Creamer JE, Nathan AW, Camm AJ: The proarrhythmic effects of antiarrhythmic drugs. *Am Heart J* **114**:397-406, 1987.
76. Ben-David J, Zipes DP: Torsades de pointes and proarrhythmia. *Lancet* **341**:1578-82, 1993.

77. Akhtar M, Breithardt G, Camm AJ, et al.: CAST and beyond. Implications of the Cardiac Arrhythmia Suppression Trial. Task Force of the Working Group on Arrhythmias of the European Society of Cardiology. *Circulation* **81**:1123-7, 1990.

78. Nathan AW, Hellestrand KJ, Bexton RS, et al.: Proarrhythmic effects of the new antiarrhythmic agent flecainide acetate. *Am Heart J* **107**:222-8, 1984.

79. Nathan AW, Hellestrand KJ, Bexton RS, et al.: The proarrhythmic effects of flecainide. *Drugs* **29 Suppl 4**:45-53, 1985.

80. Josephson ME: Antiarrhythmic agents and the danger of proarrhythmic events. *Ann Intern Med* **111**:101-3, 1989.

81. Josephson RA, Chahine RA, Morganroth J, et al.: Prediction of cardiac death in patients with a very low ejection fraction after myocardial infarction: a Cardiac Arrhythmia Suppression Trial (CAST) study. *Am Heart J* **130**:685-91, 1995.

82. Zipes DP: Proarrhythmic effects of antiarrhythmic drugs. *Am J Cardiol* **59**:26E-31E, 1987.

83. Zipes DP: Proarrhythmic events. *Am J Cardiol* **61**:70A-76A, 1988.

84. Buxton AE, Rosenthal ME, Marchlinski FE, et al.: Usefulness of the electrophysiology laboratory for evaluation of proarrhythmic drug response in coronary artery disease. *Am J Cardiol* **67**:835-42, 1991.

85. Lazzara R, Szabo B, Patterson E, Scherlag BJ. Mechanisms for proarrhythmia with antiarrhythmic drugs. In: Zipes DP, Jalife J, eds. *Cardiac Electrophysiology: From Cell to Bedside*. Philadelphia, PA: W.B. Saunders, 402-407: 1990.

86. Woosley RL: CAST: implications for drug development. *Clin Pharmacol Ther* **47**:553-6, 1990.

87. Woosley RL: New concepts affecting the use of antiarrhythmic agents. *Cardiovasc Drugs Ther* **4 Suppl 3**:541-4, 1990.

88. Wyse DG, Morganroth J, Ledingham R, et al.: New insights into the definition and meaning of proarrhythmia during initiation of antiarrhythmic drug therapy from the Cardiac Arrhythmia Suppression Trial and its pilot study. The CAST and CAPS Investigators. *J Am Coll Cardiol* **23**:1130-40, 1994.

89. Carlsson L, Almgren O, Duker G: QTU-prolongation and torsades de pointes induced by putative class III antiarrhythmic agents in the rabbit: etiology and interventions. *J Cardiovasc Pharmacol* **16**:276-285, 1990.

90. Camm AJ: Clinical trials of arrhythmia management: methods or madness. *Control Clin Trials* **17**:4S-16S, 1996.

91. Camm AJ, Kautzner J: Assessment of arrhythmias after myocardial infarction in the post-CAST era. *Can J Cardiol* **12 Suppl B**:9B-19B; discussion 27B-28B, 1996.

92. Greene HL, Roden DM, Katz RJ, et al.: The Cardiac Arrhythmia Suppression Trial: first CAST ... then CAST-II. *J Am Coll Cardiol* **19**:894-8, 1992.

93. Starmer CF, Romashko DN, Reddy RS, et al.: Proarrhythmic response to potassium channel blockade. Numerical studies of polymorphic tachyarrhythmias. *Circulation* **92**:595-605, 1995.

94. Velebit V, Podrid P, Lown B, et al.: Aggravation and provocation of ventricular arrhythmias by antiarrhythmic drugs. *Circulation* **65**:886-94, 1982.

95. Hondeghem LM, Snyders DJ: Class III antiarrhythmic agents have a lot of potential but a long way to go. Reduced effectiveness and dangers of reverse use dependence. *Circulation* **81**:696-690, 1990.

CHAPTER 4

PRINCIPLES OF ELECTRODE CATHETER ABLATION

Surgical destruction of critical areas of cardiac tissue as a means to "cure" patients with tachyarrhythmias has been the subject of investigation by cardiologists, cardiac electrophysiologists, and cardiac surgeons for many years. Initially, most efforts were directed at patients with Wolff-Parkinson-White Syndrome [1,2] or ventricular tachycardia [3-7]. Since the development of those highly-invasive surgical techniques, a number of less invasive techniques using a variety of "energy sources" have been under investigation. These have ranged from chemical ablation using ethanol [8,9], to ablation using a direct current shock [10-13] and, most prominently, to the highly successful use of radiofrequency (RF) energy for the low-risk cure of many different cardiac arrhythmias [14-16]. In this chapter we discuss the fundamental principles involved in the performance of electrode catheter ablation. Included in this section is a discussion of the induction of the clinical arrhythmia, localization or "mapping" of the critical tissue that is the target for the ablation procedure, delivery of the destructive energy to the target tissue, and finally, verification of successful elimination of the arrhythmia.

4.1 Indications for Ablation of Cardiac Arrhythmias

Although the indications for catheter ablation procedures is an evolving process, the most recently published consensus guidelines are summarized in Table 4-1. In general, RF electrode catheter ablation is a therapeutic option in any patient with a symptomatic tachyarrhythmia that is refractory to medical therapy or in any symptomatic patient who wishes to avoid antiarrhythmic drug therapy. While RF ablation was initially used to target AV nodal reentrant tachycardia [17,18] and AV reciprocating tachycardia utilizing an accessory connection [19-22], the technique is now used for patients with ventricular tachycardia [23-29], atrial tachycardia [25,30-32], atrial flutter [33-35] and, most recently, even atrial fibrillation [36-38].

4.2 ABCs of Electrode Catheter Ablation

In general, successful catheter ablation involves four steps, *induction*, *localization*, *ablation* and *verification* (Table 4-2.) Reliable and reproducible arrhythmia *induction* has two purposes. Firstly, it provides a firm, clear-cut endpoint of success when the arrhythmia becomes non-inducible following the ablation. Secondly, during the arrhythmia the reentry circuit or arrhythmia focus can be precisely *localized* using standard mapping

TABLE 4-1. Summary of indications for therapeutic intracardiac electrophysiology studies in patients with documented or suspected tachyarrhythmias

Procedure	Indicated	Uncertain or Possible Indication	Not Indicated
RF Catheter Ablation and Modification of AV Junction for Ventricular Rate Control of Atrial Tachyarrhythmias	Patients with symptomatic atrial tachyarrhythmias who have inadequately controlled ventricular rates, unless primary ablation of the atrial tachyarrhythmia is possible	Patients with dual-chamber pacemaker and pacemaker-mediated tachycardia that cannot be treated effectively by drugs or by reprogramming the pacemaker	Patients with atrial tachyarrhythmias responsive to drug therapy acceptable to the patient
	Patients with symptomatic atrial tachyarrhythmias with ventricular rate controlled by drugs but where either the medication is not tolerated or the patient prefers not to take medication		
	Patients with symptomatic non-paroxysmal junctional tachycardia that is drug resistant, drugs are not tolerated, or the patient does not wish to take medication		
	Patients resuscitated from sudden cardiac death due to atrial flutter or atrial fibrillation with rapid ventricular response in the absence of an accessory pathway		
RF Catheter Ablation for AV Node Reentrant Tachycardia (AVNRT	Patients with symptomatic sustained AVNRT that is drug resistant or the patient is intolerant or does not desire long-term drug therapy	Patients with sustained AVNRT identified during electrophysiological study or catheter ablation of another arrhythmia	Patients with AVNRT responsive to drug therapy that is well tolerated and preferred by the patient to catheter ablation
		The finding of dual AV node pathway physiology and atrial echo beats without inducible AVNRT during electrophysiological study in patients suspected to have AVNRT clinically	The finding of dual AV nodal pathway physiology (with or without echo beats) during electrophysiological testing in patients in whom AVNRT is not suspected clinically

Adapted from [39].

TABLE 4-1. Summary of indications for therapeutic intracardiac electrophysiology studies in patients with documented or suspected tachyarrhythmias

Procedure	Indicated	Uncertain or Possible Indication	Not Indicated
RF Catheter Ablation of Atrial Tachycardia, Flutter, and Fibrillation	Patients with atrial tachycardia that is drug resistant or the patient is drug intolerant or does not desire long-term drug therapy Patients with atrial flutter that is drug resistant or the patient is drug intolerant or does not desire long-term drug therapy	Atrial flutter/atrial tachycardia associated with paroxysmal atrial fibrillation when the tachycardia is drug resistant or the patient is drug intolerant or does not desire long-term drug therapy Patients with atrial fibrillation and evidence of a localized site(s) of origin when the tachycardia is drug resistant or the patient is drug intolerant or does not desire long-term drug therapy	Patients with atrial arrhythmia that is responsive to drug therapy, well tolerated, and preferred by the patient to ablation Patients with multiform atrial tachycardia
RF Catheter Ablation of Accessory Pathways	Patients with symptomatic AV reentrant tachycardia that is drug resistant or the patient is drug intolerant or does not desire long-term drug therapy Patients with atrial fibrillation (or other atrial tachyarrhythmia) and a rapid ventricular response via the accessory pathway when the tachycardia is drug resistant or the patient is drug intolerant or does not desire long-term drug therapy	Patients with AV reentrant tachycardia or atrial fibrillation with rapid ventricular rates identified during electrophysiology study for another arrhythmia Asymptomatic patients with ventricular pre-excitation whose livelihood or profession, important activities, insurability, or mental well-being or the public safety would be affected by spontaneous tachyarrhythmias or the presence of the ECG abnormality Patients with atrial fibrillation and controlled ventricular rate via an accessory pathway Patients with a family history of sudden cardiac death	Patients who have accessory pathway-related arrhythmias that are responsive to drug therapy, well tolerated, and preferred by the patient to ablation

Adapted from [39].

TABLE 4-1. Summary of indications for therapeutic intracardiac electrophysiology studies in patients with documented or suspected tachyarrhythmias

Procedure	Indicated	Uncertain or Possible Indication	Not Indicated
RF Catheter Ablation of Ventricular Tachycardia (VT)	Patients with symptomatic sustained monomorphic VT when the tachycardia is drug resistant or the patient is drug intolerant or does not desire long-term drug therapy	Non-sustained VT that is symptomatic when the tachycardia is drug resistant or the patient is drug intolerant or does not desire long-term drug therapy	Patients with VT that is responsive to drug, ICD, or surgical therapy and that therapy is well tolerated and preferred by the patient to catheter ablation
	Patients with bundle branch reentrant ventricular tachycardia		Unstable, rapid, multiple, or polymorphic VT that cannot be adequately localized by current mapping techniques
	Patients with sustained monomorphic VT and an ICD who are receiving multiple shocks not manageable by reprogramming or concomitant drug therapy		Asymptomatic and clinically benign non-sustained VT

Adapted from [39].

techniques. After localization, energy is delivered to the target tissue, thereby *ablating* the critical portion of the arrhythmia circuit or focus. Finally, to *verify* the success of the ablation procedure, non-inducibility should be confirmed to document the elimination of the arrhythmia.

TABLE 4-2. General procedure for ablation of cardiac arrhythmias

---

Induction (*provocation*) of the *clinical* arrhythmia (even one beat), preferably reliably and reproducibly.

Localization (*"mapping"*) of the target tissue, be it a small arrhythmia focus (in the case of automatic or triggered arrhythmia, or microreentrant circuit), or a critical region of a macroreentrant circuit.

Delivery of energy to the target tissue *(ablation)* using available equipment, technologies & energy source.

Verification (*confirmation*) that the arrhythmia focus or circuit is either completely eliminated or damaged sufficiently to prevent recurrence of the arrhythmia.

4.3 Arrhythmia Induction

Induction of the arrhythmia serves several purposes. Firstly, it provides the opportunity to define and study the arrhythmia mechanism (e.g., AV nodal reentrant tachycardia, AV reciprocating tachycardia, atrial tachycardia, etc.). Secondly, it is often crucial to establish that the arrhythmia is *reliably and reproducibly* inducible. Reliable and reproducible inducibility establishes an end-point by which ablation success can be gauged. Thirdly, induction of a sustained arrhythmia is often essential in order to "map" or localize its point of origin, or the critical region of its reentrant circuit, thereby identifying the target for ablation.

Most clinical arrhythmias are due to reentry, and thus, are generally induced using programmed electrical stimulation (see "Pacing protocols and programmed electrical stimulation" on page 38 and "Programmed Induction of Clinical Arrhythmias" on page 80). For most reentrant arrhythmias, including supraventricular and ventricular tachyarrhythmias, pacing protocols using one or more extrastimuli have been found to be most useful. Extrastimuli serve the purpose of "peeling back refractoriness" of cardiac tissues, allowing a premature stimulus to enter the reentry circuit and trigger the arrhythmia. Some reentrant supraventricular tachyarrhythmias, such as AV nodal reentrant tachycardia, atrial tachycardia, or AV reciprocating tachycardia also may be provoked using fixed cycle length pacing without extrastimuli. In some cases, catecholamine infusion (isoproterenol), may assist in the inducibility of supraventricular, and some ventricular, tachyarrhythmias. The forms of monomorphic ventricular tachycardia that occur in patients with structurally normal hearts, may also be inducible with programmed stimulation using extrastimuli. More often, however, they are provoked using decremental fixed cycle length pacing without or with isoproterenol infusion. In some cases, it is not unusual for these forms of ventricular tachycardia to be reliably induced using a catecholamine infusion alone, without any electrical stimulation. This is particularly true in those arrhythmias due to catecholamine-sensitive automaticity or triggered activity related to delayed afterdepolarizations. Rarely, arrhythmias are incessant, or occur spontaneously, and therefore do not require special pacing protocols or pharmacological agents for induction.

4.4   Arrhythmia Localization

The most important, and the most difficult aspect of the ablation procedure is to localize ("*map*") the target for the delivery of the RF energy. The safety and success of ablation procedures is directly related to the accuracy of the mapping procedure. It is essential that the electrophysiologist avoid excessive, unnecessary, and non-therapeutic ablations.

Most of the details of mapping techniques as they pertain to particular arrhythmias are discussed in the chapters that follow. However, it is helpful to have an overview of some of the mapping tools available to the electrophysiologist. It should be stressed that not all of these techniques are useful in all patients or in all arrhythmias. In general, however, each type of tachyarrhythmias is usually *best* mapped using only one or two of these techniques. One of the most active areas of current research involves investigating new mapping techniques.

4.4.1   ELECTROGRAM-GUIDED ANATOMIC MAPPING

The simplest method of mapping to localize the target for catheter ablation involves positioning the catheter tip to a certain anatomic location where the arrhythmia focus (or a critical region of the reentry circuit) is known to reside. In this case, the initial positioning of the catheter is guided by fluoroscopy imaging of the cardiac silhouette using the anteroposterior and right and left anterior oblique views. Fine-tuning of the catheter position is accomplished by real-time analysis of cardiac electrograms. The most common application of electrogram-guided anatomic mapping is for AV node modification in patients with AV nodal reentrant tachycardia (see "Atrioventricular Nodal Reentrant Tachycardia" on page 487). For this arrhythmia, the target tissue is the area of slow AV nodal pathway conduction. Very typically, this tissue is located at the atrial side of the tricuspid annulus slightly anterior and superior to the ostium of the coronary sinus. Using the fluoroscopic right anterior oblique view, the approximate correct position for the tip of the ablation catheter is shown in Figure 4-1 (the coronary sinus can be localized by placement of catheter within the coronary sinus/great cardiac vein). Further optimization of the location is achieved by analyzing the electrograms recorded by the distal mapping/ablation electrodes and the His bundle recording catheter. Successful ablation of the slow conduction pathway is usually achieved when the distal bipolar electrode of the ablation catheter records a small atrial deflection and a large ventricular deflection. Ideally, the ratio of the amplitude of the ventricular and atrial electrograms should be 2:1 or greater. Often, an optimum stable position for the ablation catheter is attained when its curve parallels the sweep of the curve of the His bundle catheter. The recording catheter at the His bundle region defines the location of the proximal His bundle by recording a large His bundle electrogram. The operator must avoid ablating near the site of the His

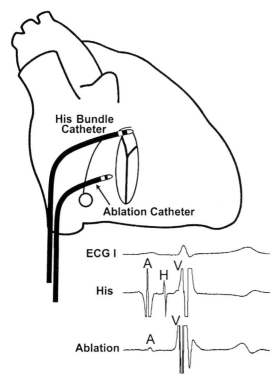

His Bundle
Catheter

Ablation Catheter

ECG I

His

Ablation

FIGURE 4-1. Electrogram-guided anatomic ablation of slow AV node pathway
conduction. Shown here is a schematic diagram illustrating the approximate fluoroscopic appearance (right anterior oblique
view) of the mapping/ablation catheter relative to the His bundle catheter and the
ostium of the coronary sinus. Shown in the
lower portion of the figure are typical
examples of electrograms recorded by the
His bundle catheter and the mapping/abla-
tion catheter when optimally positioned for
ablation of slow pathway conduction. Usually, successful ablation of slow pathway
conduction is achieved when the ventricular
electrogram has at least twice the amplitude
of the atrial electrogram. However, many
electrophysiologists prefer an even larger
ratio, which ensures that the tip of the ablation electrode is very close to the tricuspid
annulus.

bundle and the compact AV node lest complete AV block be produced. While the technique of electrogram-guided anatomic mapping is most commonly used for ablation of
the slow pathway region, some electrophysiologists also may attempt localization of the
retrograde fast and slow conduction pathways by recording the earliest sequence of retrograde atrial activation during ventricular pacing [40]. Rarely, patients with AV nodal
reentrant tachycardia may exhibit retrograde conduction via a posteriorly-located slow
conduction pathway that, in general, has an atrial insertion slightly anterior and superior
to the ostium of the coronary sinus. Under these circumstances, the earliest atrial activity
of the retrograde slow pathway conduction provides the target for the delivery of RF energy during the ablation procedure. Unfortunately, most patients with AV nodal reentrant tachycardia only exhibit retrograde conduction using the fast conduction pathway.
During retrograde conduction via this pathway, the earliest retrograde atrial activation is
generally recorded anteriorly, close to the recording site of the His bundle electrogram.

Electrogram-guided anatomic mapping is also commonly used for the ablation of
typical clockwise and counterclockwise atrial flutter that utilizes the isthmus of tissue
between the tricuspid annulus and the inferior vena cava (Figure 4-2) (also see "Macroreentrant Atrial Tachycardia" on page 626). Optimum ablation technique involves
both anatomic guidance with fluoroscopy imaging and recording of electrograms using
the mapping/ablation catheter. The goal of this ablation is to create a linear RF lesion
across this isthmus, thereby producing bidirectional conduction block within this tissue.

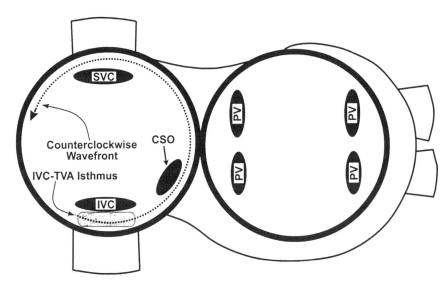

FIGURE 4-2. Cross-section view through the atrioventricular groove at the level of the mitral and tricuspid valve annulae as seen from the cardiac apex. The counterclockwise atrial flutter wavefront conducts through the isthmus bordered by the inferior vena cava (IVC) and the tricuspid valve annulus (TVA). The IVC-TVA isthmus is the anatomic target during ablation of typical atrial flutter. CSO, ostium of the coronary sinus; PV, pulmonary vein; SVC, superior vena cava. See text for additional discussion.

With conduction blocked through this isthmus, the occurrence of typical clockwise or counterclockwise atrial flutter is prevented. In the left anterior oblique view, the correct catheter position for ablation is at the 5 or 6 o'clock position along the tricuspid annulus (middle portion of the lower edge of the tricuspid annulus) (Figure 4-2). Figure 4-3 displays proper catheter position when viewed using a right anterior oblique view. During this ablation procedure, RF application must be delivered at both borders of the isthmus (near the tricuspid annulus, and the edge near the inferior vena cava), as well as the intervening tissue. Analysis of the real-time electrograms recorded from the distal electrodes of the mapping/ablation catheter (in conjunction with the fluoroscopic images) helps define the precise position of the catheter tip along the line from the tricuspid border to the inferior vena cava border (Figure 4-3). The ratio of the amplitude of the atrial and ventricular electrograms can be used to judge if the electrode tip is positioned more toward the tricuspid annulus or inferior vena cava borders, or is located within the middle of the isthmus.

4.4.2 PACE-MAPPING

The technique of pace-mapping is applicable to patients with some forms of ventricular tachycardia and those with Wolff-Parkinson-White Syndrome with anterograde AV conduction in the accessory connection (see "Ventricular Preexcitation Syndromes: The Wolff-Parkinson-White Syndrome and Variants" on page 539 and "The Spectrum of Monomorphic Ventricular Tachycardia" on page 687). In general, pace mapping is use-

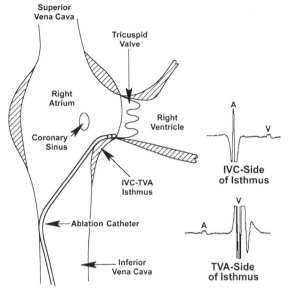

Superior
Vena Cava

Tricuspid
Valve

Right
Atrium

Right
Ventricle

Coronary
Sinus

IVC-TVA
Isthmus

Ablation Catheter

Inferior
Vena Cava

A

V

IVC-Side
of Isthmus

V

A

TVA-Side
of Isthmus

FIGURE 4-3. Electrogram-guided anatomic ablation of typical atrial flutter
circuit. Shown here is a schematic illustration of a right anterior oblique fluoroscopic view. The goal of this ablation is
to create a linear RF lesion across this
isthmus, thereby producing bidirectional
conduction block within this tissue. At
the inferior vena cava (IVC) border, the
amplitude of the atrial electrogram is
much larger than the ventricular electrogram. In fact, it is not unusual to only
record an atrial electrogram at this position. At the tricuspid valve annulus
(TVA) border, the recorded ventricular
electrogram will be much larger than the
atrial electrogram. During this ablation
procedure, a series of RF lesions are created that extend from the TVA side to
the IVC side. The presence of bidirectional conduction block can be established using pacing maneuvers.

ful in ventricular tachycardia due to triggered or automatic activity, but not ventricular
tachycardia due to reentry. The principle of pace-mapping is simple: the electrical activation of the heart resulting from pacing during sinus rhythm at the site of the origin of
an arrhythmia may closely match the pattern of activation generated by the arrhythmia itself. For example, assume that ventricular tachycardia originates from microscopic focus in the right ventricle. Recording a surface 12-lead ECG during ventricular pacing
from the arrhythmia origin should result in a QRS morphology nearly identical to that
generated by the ventricular arrhythmia itself (Figure 4-4). Delivery of RF energy at this
site would be expected to destroy the arrhythmia focus and eliminate the arrhythmia.
This technique is routinely used to successfully ablate the arrhythmia focus responsible
for ventricular tachycardia originating in the right ventricular outflow tract of patients
with structurally normal hearts (Figure 4-5).

Pace-mapping is generally not useful in patients with ventricular tachycardia due to
structural heart disease, especially those individuals with a remote myocardial infarction.
Part of the reason for this is that the reentry circuit responsible for ventricular tachycardia in these patients is situated within or near an infarct scar and my have a complicated
microanatomy. The reentrant tissue may have multiple reentry loops, blind passages,
and alternative exit sites to the working myocardium (see Figure 15-25 on page 722). In
addition, localizing the critical point within the reentry circuit using ventricular-paced
mapping during sinus rhythm is very unlikely. This is because even if ventricular pacing
is performed at a critical site within the reentry circuit, the pattern of ventricular activation resulting from this pacing is very likely to be different than that generated by the
ventricular tachycardia (Figure 4-6, also see "Mapping Using Concealed Entrainment"
on page 147 and Figure 4-18). Conversely, while pacing at the exit site of the reentry
circuit during sinus rhythm may generate a QRS pattern very similar to that inscribed

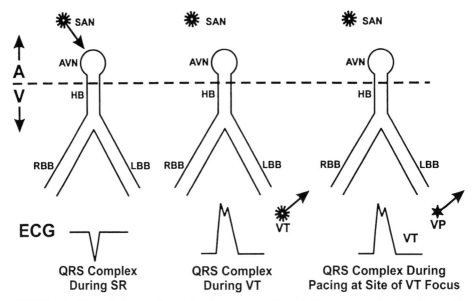

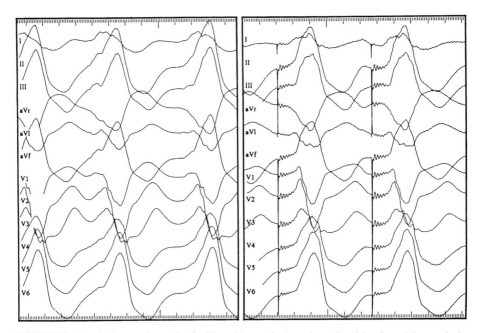

FIGURE 4-4. Schematic diagram illustrating the technique of ventricular-paced mapping in patients with ventricular tachycardia. A, atrium; AVN, atrioventricular node; HB, His bundle; RBB, right bundle branch; LBB, left bundle branch; VT, ventricular tachycardia; VP, ventricular pacing; SR, sinus rhythm; SAN sinoatrial node; V, ventricle. See text for discussion

FIGURE 4-5. Ventricular-paced mapping for idiopathic ventricular tachycardia arising from right ventricular outflow tract. The mapping/ablating electrode is positioned in the right ventricular outflow tract. Note the close similarity of 12-lead QRS morphology of the ventricular tachycardia (left panel) and ventricular-paced rhythm (right panel). Delivery of RF energy at this site eliminated the arrhythmia. Paper speed 200 mm/sec

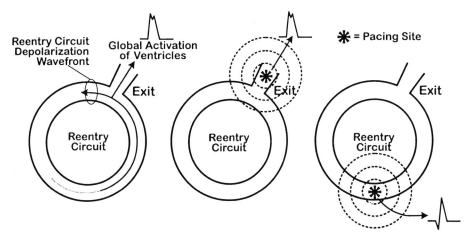

FIGURE 4-6. Schematic illustration of a potential problem associated with ventricular-paced mapping during sinus rhythm using a simplified hypothetical reentrant circuit. During ventricular tachycardia (VT), the reentrant wavefront exits from the reentry circuit to activate the ventricles, generating QRS complexes on the surface ECG (left panel). If ventricular pacing is performed at the exit site of the reentry circuit during sinus rhythm (middle panel), the inscribed QRS complexes will be very similar or identical to those generated during VT. RF ablation at the exit site, however, will not eliminate the VT because a critical area of the reentry circuit remains unaffected. If ventricular pacing is performed at a critical area of the reentry circuit during sinus rhythm (right panel), the QRS complexes on the surface ECG will not be identical to those inscribed during VT. This is because the spread of excitation from the pacing electrode (dashed lines) generates a different activation pattern than that which occurs during VT. Although ablation at this site may be successful, there is no way to know, based upon the ventricular-paced map, that the pacing/ablating electrode is within the reentrant circuit. See below "Mapping Using Concealed Entrainment" on page 147 and Figure 4-18.

during the tachyarrhythmia, because the exit site is not a critical region of the reentry circuit, RF ablation at this site is unlikely to eliminate the arrhythmia. Mapping of ventricular tachycardia in patients with structural heart disease often requires specialized pacing and analysis techniques, including entrainment with concealed fusion (see below "Mapping Using Concealed Entrainment" on page 147 and "Ventricular Tachycardia Associated With Structural Heart Disease" on page 714).

Pace mapping can also assist in the localization of the ventricular insertion site of accessory connections that are capable of anterograde AV conduction. If AV conduction is blocked through the normal AV conduction pathway and instead proceeds exclusively via the accessory AV connection, ventricular activation will originate entirely from the ventricular insertion site of the accessory connection (Figure 4-7). Consequently, 12-lead ECG recordings can be obtained during both maximum preexcitation (exclusive AV conduction through the accessory connection) and during pacing at the putative ventricular insertion site of the accessory connection. The surface activation patterns during maximal preexcitation and with ventricular pacing at the insertion site of the accessory connection should be identical. This technique, of course, can only be performed in patients with manifest Wolff-Parkinson-White syndrome (anterograde conduction in the accessory connection) in whom positioning of the catheter tip electrode at the ventricular insertion site is possible. In general, this latter criterion is met most often in the case of left-sided accessory connections. In this case, the operator must use the retrograde tran-

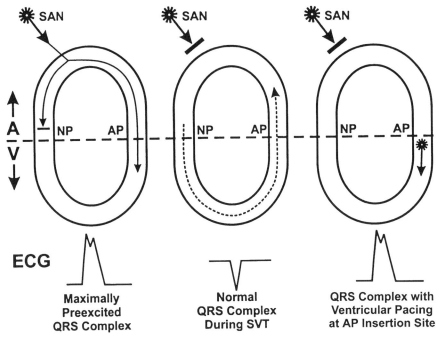

FIGURE 4-7. Schematic diagram illustrating the technique of ventricular pace-mapping in patients with Wolff-Parkinson-White syndrome and a manifest accessory pathway. During sinus rhythm, AV conduction can occur by both the normal AV conduction pathway and the accessory connection. If conduction only proceeds via the accessory pathway (left panel), the ventricles are activated exclusively from a single wavefront emanating from the ventricular insertion of the accessory connection. This results in maximal preexcitation of the ventricle, reflected by the inscription of a wide QRS complex. During orthodromic AV reciprocating tachycardia, all AV conduction occurs through the normal AV conduction system, resulting in a normal QRS complex (middle panel). If pacing is performed at the ventricular insertion site of the accessory pathway, the resultant QRS complex should match the maximally preexcited QRS complex. By matching the ventricular-paced QRS complex with the maximal preexcited QRS complex, the location of the ventricular insertion of the accessory pathway can be identified. A, atrium; AP, accessory pathway; NP, normal AV conduction pathway; SAN sinoatrial node; SVT, supraventricular tachycardia; V, ventricle.

saortic approach (see below "Procedural Approach to Catheter Ablation" on page 162) to reach the ventricular insertion site.

Theoretically, the pace mapping technique should be applicable to *focal* atrial as well as ventricular tachycardias (whether they be due to triggered activity, abnormal automaticity, or microreentry). Pace mapping in the ventricle is possible because detecting differences and similarities in QRS morphology is straightforward. However, attempting to use pace mapping for atrial tachyarrhythmias is problematic due to the necessity to compare P-wave morphologies on the surface 12-lead ECG obtained during atrial pacing and the atrial arrhythmia. Because of the small amplitude of P-waves and the distortion induced by the stimulus artifact, reliable comparison of P-wave morphologies can be difficult.

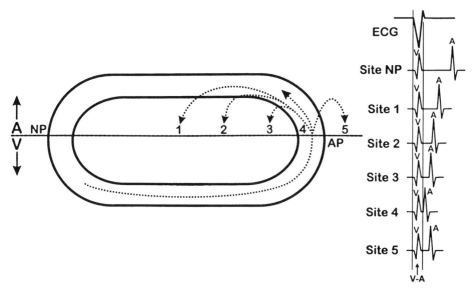

FIGURE 4-8. Schematic diagram illustrating example of activation mapping during supraventricular tachycardia utilizing the normal AV conduction pathway (NP) for anterograde AV conduction and an accessory pathway (AP) for ventriculoatrial (VA) conduction. During tachycardia, the earliest retrograde atrial activation and the shortest VA interval are recorded by a bipolar electrode pair positioned at the site of the accessory connection (site 4). Retrograde atrial activation is progressively later, and VA intervals progressively longer, at recording sites more distant from the location of the accessory pathway.

4.4.3 ACTIVATION MAPPING

Intraoperative mapping of epicardial and endocardial activation using a large number of electrodes allowing simultaneous recording from many myocardial sites has been used to map tachyarrhythmia foci. This technique allows localization of reentrant pathways by computer analysis of activation times, thereby allowing reconstruction of the reentry circuit. However, activation mapping using the percutaneous catheter technique is more difficult, primarily because of the limited number of electrodes that can be applied to restricted areas of endocardium.

Catheter-based activation mapping is most useful in patients with supraventricular tachycardia due to an accessory AV connection, as illustrated in Figure 4-8. Orthodromic AV reciprocating tachycardia utilizes a large reentrant circuit with anterograde AV conduction occurring within the normal AV conduction system, while retrograde (ventriculoatrial) conduction proceeds within the accessory AV connection. Accessory AV connections bridge the atria and ventricles at one or more points along the annulus fibrosus, which electrically insulates the upper chambers from the lower chambers (except at the His bundle region). During supraventricular tachycardia, the earliest site of retrograde atrial activation occurs at the atrial insertion of the accessory connection. If a multipolar electrode catheter is positioned along the right or left AV annulus, the earliest site of retrograde atrial activation can be readily identified, relative to other atrial sites activated later (Figure 4-8). The bipolar electrode pair positioned closest to the accessory AV connection will record the earliest atrial activation during orthodromic AV reciprocating tachycardia. Atrial activation must be measured relative to some constant time point. The ventriculoatrial interval is measured between the onset of the earliest ventricular activation and the earliest retrograde atrial activation recorded in the multipolar mapping or ablation catheter. It is important to measure the earliest ventricular activation, which is usually recorded by the onset of a QRS complex on the surface ECG, and not the local ventriculoatrial interval recorded by a closely spaced bipolar electrode pair. The electrode pair recording the shortest ventriculoatrial interval and the earliest site of retrograde atrial activation marks the presumptive atrial insertion site of the accessory connection and the target site for RF energy delivery. The major problem with activation mapping is that all measurements are *relative* to some presumed fixed time point. Consequently, a "short" ventriculoatrial interval may not be the "shortest". There is no *absolute* measurement of activation that guarantees that the mapping electrode is at *the earliest* site of activation.

Theoretically, activation mapping can also assist in the localization of a reentry circuit in patients with atrial and ventricular tachycardias (Figure 4-9). However, there are problems associated with the use of activation mapping for these arrhythmias. Activation mapping generally does not allow identification of the *critical* segment of a reentrant circuit. Because of the small lesion size produced by RF energy (see "Delivery of Ablation Energy" on page 153), RF ablation should be directed at a small, restricted area

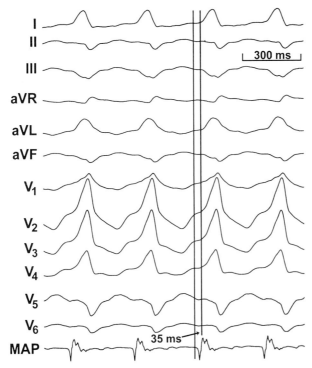

FIGURE 4-9. Use of activation mapping for ablation of left ventricular tachycardia (VT) in a patient without evidence of structural heart disease. The VT was reliably induced by programmed stimulation (not shown). Entrainment with concealed fusion verified that the catheter tip of the ablating catheter (MAP) was within (or very near) the reentry circuit (see Figure 4-18 below). Delivery of RF energy at this site terminated the tachycardia and rendered it non-inducible. As shown here, the onset of the local ventricular electrogram at this site preceded ventricular activation by 35-msec. Although this was the successful ablation site (and was predicted as such by concealed entrainment), activation mapping alone would not necessarily predict this location as the eventual successful site of ablation. There is no *a priori* reason to believe that the recorded ventricular electrogram is really "early enough" or even "early" at all. See text for additional discussion.

of the reentry circuit or a discrete area of slow conduction. In addition, reentrant circuits causing monomorphic ventricular tachycardia may be small. As a result, electrical activation occurring *within* the reentry circuit is electrically silent on the surface ECG. The reentrant depolarization wavefront must exit from the reentrant loop and globally activate the ventricles before the tachycardia can be manifested on the surface ECG. Recording of the actual reentrant impulse within the circuit is only possible if a catheter electrode is positioned at the precise endocardial location of the circuit. If a single electrode catheter could record from the entire reentry circuit, continuous electrical activity would be recorded because some region of the reentry circuit is always subject to activation by the reentrant impulse. However, the ventricles as a whole are only activated when the reentrant impulse exits from the circuit and conducts through the ventricular myocardium (Figure 4-10). Unlike the scenario shown in Figure 4-8 in which an "early" site of retrograde atrial activation (albeit not necessarily the "earliest" site of activation) can be identified at a critical area of the reentrant circuit (i.e., an accessory AV connection at the AV annulus), within the reentry circuit responsible for ventricular tachycardia there are no "early" or "late" electrograms (Figure 4-10). If an electrogram is recorded within the circuit, it may be misinterpreted as being "late" because it is inscribed between two QRS complexes. However, these mid-diastolic potentials are often excellent indicators that the mapping electrode is positioned within the reentry circuit. The ventricular myocardium outside the reentry circuit is a *bystander*, only activated secondarily

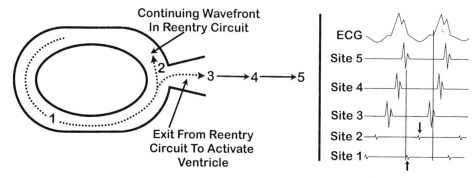

FIGURE 4-10. Schematic diagram illustrating the potential problems with activation mapping of a reentrant arrhythmia (left panel). Conduction within the reentry circuit is not detectable on the surface ECG. After exiting from the reentry circuit, the depolarization wavefront activates the ventricular myocardium as a whole, resulting in the inscription of the QRS complex on the surface ECG. Endocardial electrograms are recorded from sites 1-5. Only sites 1 and 2 are within the reentry circuit. Electrograms recorded from these sites during ventricular tachycardia are shown (right panel). The earliest activation of the ventricle is recorded at site 3 (note electrogram at site 3 precedes the onset of the QRS complex). Activations at sites 4 and 5 succeed activation at site 3, and electrograms recorded at those sites are inscribed later than that at site 3. Within the small reentry circuit, the reentrant impulse continues to circulate and locally activate tissue, even when the ventricle as a whole is in electrical diastole. Therefore, there is no 1:1 association between activation of any particular portion of the reentry circuit and the global ventricular activation as marked by the QRS complex. The ventricles as a whole are merely bystanders to the ongoing continuous electrical activity in the reentry loop. Consequently, the electrograms recorded at sites 1 and 2 are neither "early" or "late" relative to the QRS complex. For example, the electrogram at site 1 (upward arrow) may be misinterpreted as "late" because it occurs well after the onset of a QRS complex; however, it is in reality very "early" because it originates from the reentry circuit. On the other hand, is the electrogram at recorded at site 2 (downward arrow) "early" or "late"? Because it is mid-way between two QRS complexes, these mid-diastolic potentials may be reliable indicators that the electrode recording them is at the site of the reentry circuit.

from the primary reentrant impulse circulating within the reentry loop. Finding an "early" activation site in the bystander ventricular myocardium relative to the QRS onset on the surface ECG may not be helpful in identifying a target site for RF ablation. Even if the exit site is localized, it is generally not a critical area of the circuit; therefore, ablation at this site will not eliminate the tachycardia.

New technologies for activation mapping of cardiac arrhythmias are on the horizon. Specialized mapping systems currently available or under investigation include: 1) epicardial mapping through the coronary sinus venous system using a specially-designed system of micro-electrode catheters, 2) a basket catheter with upwards of 32 pairs of electrodes that is placed in a cardiac chamber for computerized mapping of endocardial activation, and 3) a computer-generated color-coded three-dimensional endocardial activation map created using either electromagnetic or high resolution non-contact imaging

Traditional multielectrode-mapping techniques may be difficult and time consuming, particularly in patients with non-sustained tachycardias or with arrhythmias not easily inducible. A so-called *basket catheter* with multiple splines and electrodes (typically eight splines and eight electrodes on each spline) may facilitate mapping of selected atrial and ventricular tachycardias. In this fashion, multipolar three-dimensional recording of tachycardias has been facilitated in the clinical electrophysiology laboratory. Automated analysis of 64 or more simultaneously-recorded electrograms with computer assisted three-dimensional reconstruction and animation may speed and enhance ease of localization, even in patients exhibiting only sporadic single beats of the tachycardia.

Catheter-based technology allowing high-resolution electromagnetic anatomic mapping of the heart is now available (see Figure 15-24 on page 721) [41,42]. A miniature location sensor is mounted at the tip of a standard, deflectable mapping/ablation catheter. The real-time location and orientation of the sensor inside the heart is determined by rapid analysis of the sensed electromagnetic fields relative to a set of known radiated fields. The system reconstructs a three-dimensional map from endocardial sites that have been sequentially mapped. Furthermore, individual local activation times are determined for every mapped site with respect to a predetermined reference time. The local activation times are provided in a variety of formats, such as a color-coded isochronal map, and the electrophysiologic information is superimposed on the anatomy of the respective mapped areas of the heart chamber.

Recent studies have demonstrated spatial and temporal accuracy and reproducibility and initial clinical utility. The reliable re-navigation of the ablation catheter to a site that had been identified earlier seems to be of advantage in selected cases. After the collection of a number of mapping points, the focus can be identified during mapping of even brief episodes of atrial tachycardia, as the site with the earliest local activation time, relative to a predetermined reference time. Subsequently, accurate re-navigation, according to the three-dimensional map of the chamber, can be attempted during sinus rhythm, followed by radiofrequency application.

The system is capable of not only mapping activation wavefronts of the arrhythmia but also for mapping isopotential (voltage) regions generated by bipolar electrogram amplitudes. Diseased atrial or ventricular tissues, surgical scars, patches and artificial materials such as conduits and baffles can then be identified. The advantages over electrode mapping under fluoroscopy include: 1) multiple electrode catheters do not need to be inserted; 2) three-dimensional visualization of the activation map; 3) identification of diseased areas and conduction barriers by the voltage map and; 4) significant reduction in the time of fluoroscopy exposure.

While electroanatomic mapping may offer an advantage for some patients with tachyarrhythmias, this mapping technique still requires contact of the catheter with the earliest site of endocardial activation. Enhanced speed and the ability to map non-sustained tachycardias would be achieved with a multi-point non-contact electrode. As currently implemented, the non-contact mapping system includes a non-contact multielectrode array incorporated into a balloon-tipped catheter. The catheter can be inserted into cardiac chambers to map a variety of arrhythmias. Real-time mathematical reconstruction of more than 3000 electrograms is performed using a minicomputer, and the electrograms can be superimposed onto a computer model of the endocardium, creating isopotential and isochronal maps.

4.4.4 MAPPING USING SPECIAL POTENTIALS

As discussed above, during activation mapping it may be impossible to decide – based upon timing alone – whether an electrogram definitely originates within a critical region of the reentry circuit. In some cases, the recording of "special potentials" exhibiting characteristic morphologies or unique timing may aid in the localization of the target tissue for RF ablation. As already mentioned, some investigators have suggested that slow pathway potentials may be recorded in the region of the slow conduction pathway in the posterior Triangle of Koch in patients with AV node reentrant tachycardia [18,43]. The significance of these are in dispute and evidence suggests that these potentials may be non-specific findings [44]. Other examples include Mahaim potentials (Figure 4-11) [45,46] and accessory pathway potentials [47,50] that may identify the ablation target in patients with AV reciprocating tachycardia (Figure 4-12). Purkinje potentials have assisted the localization of the ablation site in patients with fascicular tachycardia [51]. Many investigators have used fractionated electrograms to identify the critical site of slow conduction in the reentry circuit in patients with monomorphic ventricular tachycardia [52-56] (Figure 4-13). Finally, mid-diastolic potentials may be recorded within the reentry circuits of patients with atrial and ventricular tachycardias [23,57-60] (Figure 4-10).

4.4.5 MAPPING USING CONCEALED ENTRAINMENT

Many studies have shown that reentry circuits may have a complicated structural and functional organization [61-64]. However, much of the behavior of the dominant loops of many reentrant circuits can be modeled as a simple circular pathway with separate entry and exit sites as shown in (Figure 4-14). Typically, a slow conduction zone will exist somewhere in the reentry circuit. In a small reentry circuit, such as that often associated with monomorphic ventricular tachycardia in a patient with a previous myocardial infarction, the depolarization of tissue within the reentry circuit does not produce electrical activity detectable on the surface ECG; the reentrant wavefront must spread from the cir-

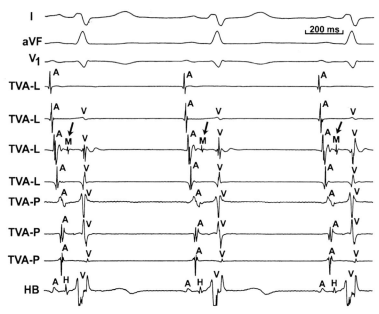

FIGURE 4-11. Recording of so-called "Mahaim pathway potentials" in a patient with a right lateral atriofascicular accessory connection exhibiting anterograde only (decremental) conduction with minimal preexcitation during sinus rhythm. The patient had an inducible wide QRS complex tachycardia resulting from AV nodal reentrant tachycardia with bystander anterograde conduction within the accessory connection. A steerable multipolar electrode catheter was positioned along the tricuspid valve annulus (TVA) from the region of the coronary sinus, extending laterally and then superiorly to the high lateral TVA. This catheter position allowed recording of electrograms at the posterior (P) and lateral (L) aspects of the TVA. Note the prominent Mahaim (M) pathway potential at the lateral TVA (downward arrows). Radiofrequency catheter ablation at this site eliminated the Mahaim potential, preexcitation, and the inducible wide QRS complex tachycardia (not shown). The AV nodal reentrant tachycardia was also subsequently ablated (not shown). A, atrium electrogram; H, His bundle (HB) electrogram; M, Mahaim potential; V, ventricular electrogram.

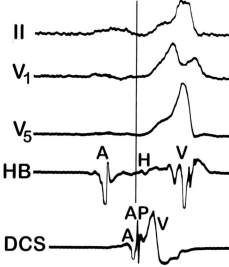

FIGURE 4-12. Recording of possible accessory pathway potential (AP) in a patient with a left free wall accessory connection. Ablation at this site resulted in elimination of accessory pathway conduction. Note the recording of the delta wave on the surface ECG leads. The AP precedes the His bundle electrogram and the onset of the delta wave. Surface ECG leads II, V_1 and V_5 are shown along with intracardiac electrograms from the distal coronary sinus (DCS) and His bundle (HB) region. A, atrial electrogram; H, His bundle electrogram; V, ventricular electrogram.

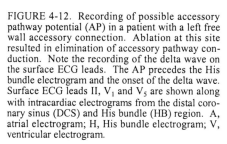

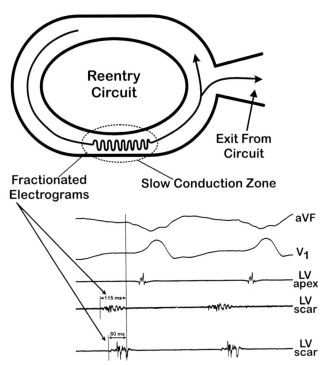

FIGURE 4-13. Fractionated endocardial electrograms recorded from the region of a left ventricular (LV) myocardial scar in a patient with a history of a myocardial infarction. The low amplitude fractionated electrograms may originate from an area of slow conduction within the reentry circuit. The earliest onset of the fractionated electrograms are inscribed during ventricular diastole, well before the activation of the ventricle as whole (as marked by the onset of the QRS complex on the surface ECG). The site of recording of fractionated electrograms is often used by electrophysiologists as a target site for RF ablation.

cuit to activate the heart. For example, in the case of monomorphic ventricular tachycardia, the reentrant depolarization must exit from the reentry circuit in order to activate the entirety of the ventricular myocardium. The entry site to a reentrant circuit is also important. It is generally assumed that in order for a clinical reentrant tachycardia to occur spontaneously, a premature depolarization must enter the reentrant pathway triggering a recurrent circus activation. Within the reentry circuit, the leading edge of the continuously advancing activation wavefront depolarizes tissue, leaving refractory tissue at a variable distance in its wake. A repolarizing wavefront similarly advances behind the depolarization wavefront, reestablishing the excitability of the tissue in the reentrant circuit. Consequently, the wave of activation and recovery has a *wavelength* corresponding to the distance between the leading edge of the depolarization wavefront and the trailing edge just completing the repolarization process. As discussed above (see "Concept of excitable gap" on page 121), the wavelength of the excitation wave is the product of conduction velocity and refractory period. If there is a significant area of slow conduction within the circuit (Figure 4-13), the circus activity can perpetuate because the slow zone allows time for recovery of excitability of adjacent refractory tissue.

The *excitable gap* represents that portion of the reentry circuit lying in the wake of the advancing tachycardia depolarization/repolarization wave that is no longer refractory and can be re-excited by another depolarization wavefront (Figure 4-14). As with the propagating tachycardia wave, the excitable gap is continuously advancing around the reentry circuit. Therefore, the region of the reentrant circuit tissue that is excitable at any

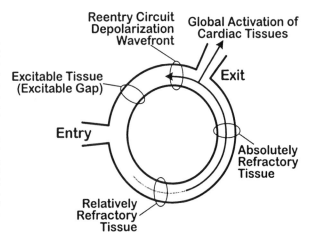

FIGURE 4-14. Simplified hypothetical reentry circuit. The reentrant wavefront circulates within the protected circuit and exits to globally activate working cardiac tissue. The excitable gap consists of non-refractory (excitable) tissue, that can theoretically be accessed via the entry site to the circuit. The most distal portion of the depolarization/repolarization wave may not be absolutely refractory to re-activation. Instead, this recovering area of tissue may be relatively refractory, meaning that it may be capable of conducting an activation impulse, but with a significantly reduced conduction velocity. See text for further discussion.

particular time is continuously changing. An appropriately timed ectopic depolarization will only activate the tissue encompassed by the excitable gap (assuming the ectopic depolarization can otherwise conduct through an intervening tissue and enter the reentry circuit). The excitable gap is defined by the window of time during which a conducted premature stimulus is capable of entering the reentry circuit. An appropriately timed extrastimulus that conducts into the reentry circuit when that region of tissue is excitable (i.e., within the excitable gap) may, therefore, potentially alter the conduction and behavior of the reentrant impulse.

Resetting is a phenomenon whereby an induced premature depolarization interacts with a tachycardia in its reentrant circuit, simultaneously terminating and reinitiating the tachycardia (Figure 4-15) and producing less than a full compensatory pause (Figure 4-16). As seen in Figure 4-15, if the extra-depolarization (S_2) propagates into an excitable portion of the reentry circuit conduction can continue in two directions. Firstly, conduction may proceed in the *antidromic* direction, colliding with and extinguishing the oncoming reentrant wavefront. Secondly, conduction may also proceed in the *orthodromic* direction (i.e., the direction followed by the original tachycardia impulse). Assuming antidromic collision occurs and conduction of the orthodromic wavefront is not blocked by "over-running" the refractory "tail" of the preceding reentrant impulse, the orthodromic impulse will continue to propagate within the reentry circuit, thereby reinitiating the tachycardia. The first beat of this reinitiated tachycardia exits from the reentrant circuit earlier than expected. The tachycardia is thus "advanced" by the extent that the extrastimulus wavefront arrives prematurely at the entrance site to the reentry circuit. The interval between the extrastimulus and the first beat of the reinitiated tachycardia is termed the *return cycle*. In the case of a reentrant arrhythmia, the coupling intervals over which resetting occurs can be considered an estimate of the duration of the excitable gap. The morphology of the return cycle beat should be identical to the morphology of the baseline tachycardia. In the case of a ventricular or atrial tachycardia, the 12-lead ECG morphology of the first QRS complex or P-wave, respectively, following the extrastimulus should be identical to the QRS complex or P-wave recorded during the tachycardia. This

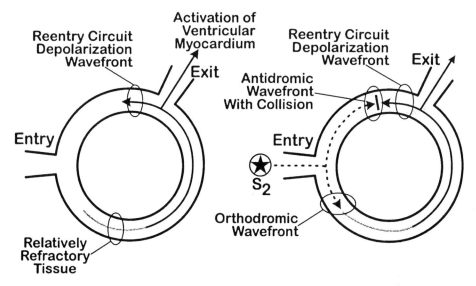

FIGURE 4-15. Schematic diagram illustrating the resetting phenomenon in a hypothetical simple reentry circuit with separate entry and exit sites. Collision of the antidromic wavefront with the oncoming tachycardia impulse terminates the tachycardia, but it is simultaneously reinitiated by the orthodromic wavefront, resulting in a return cycle (see Figure 4-16). If antidromic collision is accompanied by orthodromic conduction block, the tachycardia is terminated. This would occur if the orthodromic wavefront of the conducted extrastimulus (S$_2$) is extinguished by encroaching on the refractory period of the preceding depolarization wavefront. See text for additional discussion.

is because the return cycle depolarization originates within the reentry circuit and should exit from the circuit just as the tachycardia does.

Resetting may also produce *fusion* (Figure 4-16). By definition, fusion represents activation of the myocardium by two separate wavefronts of depolarization. In the case of the resetting phenomenon, fusion can occur because the myocardium is activated by one wavefront generated by the tachycardia and a second wavefront produced by the pacing stimulus. Fusion will be evident if the reentrant tachycardia impulse exits the reentry circuit before it collides with the antidromic wavefront within the reentry circuit. Fusion can be detected by body surface electrocardiography (*ECG fusion*) (Figure 4-16) if the dual depolarization waves separately activate sufficient areas of ventricular (QRS fusion) or atrial (P-wave fusion) myocardium. Fusion can also occur in small areas of reentrant circuits and only be detected locally by recording bipolar intracardiac electrograms (*local fusion*). Fusion that is undetectable by surface electrocardiography has been termed *concealed fusion*. The demonstration of concealed fusion may assist in identifying a critical region of a reentrant circuit and may provide a target for RF catheter ablation.

Classic *manifest entrainment* involves the use of overdrive pacing at a rate slightly faster than the tachycardia to produce continuous resetting with fusion. The classic criteria for recognition of entrainment [65-71] include: 1) fixed fusion at a given paced cycle length without termination of the tachycardia; 2) progressive ECG fusion with tachycardia termination, meaning that the contribution of the pacing-induced wavefront of depo-

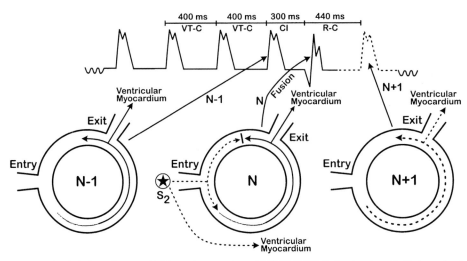

FIGURE 4-16. Schematic example illustrating resetting with ECG (QRS) fusion in a hypothetical reentrant circuit in the ventricle. The extrastimulus (S_2) that enters the reentrant circuit produces antidromic and orthodromic wavefronts. The former collides with the oncoming tachycardia wavefront, while the latter conducts in the non-refractory tissue behind the "tail" of the tachycardia depolarization/repolarization wave. The fusion beat (N) results from ventricular activation by both the exiting tachycardia impulse as well as the propagation of the extrastimulus to other regions of the ventricular myocardium. The first ventricular activation following the fusion depolarization (N+1) results from the exit of the extrastimulus-induced orthodromic wavefront from the reentrant circuit and, therefore, generates a QRS morphology identical to that inscribed during the ventricular tachycardia. In this example, the return cycle (R-C) is measured from the onset of the pacing stimulus to the next QRS complex resulting from of the conduction of the orthodromic wavefront. The duration of R-C is the sum of two time intervals; namely, the conduction time of the depolarization from the stimulating electrode to the entry point of the reentry circuit and the conduction time within the circuit between the entry and exit points. Therefore, the R-C interval may vary depending upon the location of the stimulating electrode relative to the circuit entry and the distance between the entry and exit sites. The R-C can also be measured at the onset of an electrogram recorded at the pacing site, or even an electrogram recorded within the reentry circuit (neither shown here). In this example, the coupling interval (CI) of the extrastimulus is 300 ms, the return cycle (R-C) interval is 440 ms, and the cycle length of the ventricular tachycardia (VT-C) is 400 ms. A full compensatory pause (400 ms + 400 ms = 800 ms) is greater than the measured interval (300 ms + 440 ms = 740 ms).

larization to the fusion QRS morphology increases relative to that contributed by the tachycardia wavefront as the pacing cycle length is shortened; 3) the demonstration of electrogram fusion in which an endocardial site is activated from two different directions (as indicated by relative timing, different electrogram morphologies, or different stimulus artifact-to-electrogram intervals) during pacing at two different rates that do not terminate the tachycardia and; 4) resumption of the tachycardia at the previous cycle length upon cessation of pacing with a non-fused QRS complex.

Resetting with concealed fusion can be demonstrated by delivery of a single extrastimulus within a critical region of the reentry circuit. As seen in Figure 4-17, if an extrastimulus is delivered within the slow conduction zone of a reentry circuit during a ventricular tachycardia, an orthodromic and antidromic wavefronts are generated. The returning wavefront responsible for the preceding tachycardia activation and the antidromic depolarization from the conducted extrastimulus are extinguished when they collide within the reentry circuit. The orthodromic wavefront from the extrastimulus propagates to the exit site, advancing the tachycardia and producing a QRS complex that is identical to that inscribed by the tachycardia. Because fusion activation within the reentry circuit is occurring (*electrogram or local fusion*), but a fusion QRS complex is not detected by the surface ECG, the phenomenon is termed resetting with concealed fusion.

If the pacing/recording electrode is located within the reentrant circuit, the interval between the last stimulus artifact and the next depolarization at the pacing site, termed the *post-pacing interval*, should be identical to the cycle length of the tachycardia (Figure 4-17). However, the post-pacing interval measured between the stimulus artifact and the onset of the return QRS complex recorded on the surface ECG is identical to the coupling interval of the premature stimulus (Figure 4-17). The morphology of the premature QRS complex will be identical to that inscribed during the tachycardia. *Entrainment with concealed fusion*, also commonly known as *concealed entrainment*, represents continuous resetting with concealed fusion. Concealed entrainment can be demonstrated by performing fixed cycle length pacing at a critical region of the circuit at a rate slightly faster than the tachycardia rate (Figure 4-18). Analysis of the post-pacing interval as discussed above and in Figure 4-17 is performed after delivery of the last pacing stimulus of the drive train.

4.5   Delivery of Ablation Energy

Electrode catheter ablation has revolutionized the treatment of cardiac arrhythmias. The use of RF current in medicine was first developed almost 75 years ago by Drs. Harvey Cushing and W. T. Bovie who introduced the electrosurgical unit for cutting of tissue and coagulation during surgical procedure [72]. Today, RF energy is widely used for an ever-increasing number of applications, including the production of lesions in the central and peripheral nervous system and dessication of a variety of malignant tumors. RF electrode catheter ablation was first used to produce lesions in experimental animals [14,15,73] and quickly evolved as a treatment option in patients [16,74-78]. Because RF is clearly the dominant energy source used for ablation procedures, the discussion that follows will only focus on the RF ablation technique. There are a number of other energy sources for cardiac ablation that are under investigation (Table 4-3.)

4.5.1 BIOPHYSICS OF RADIOFREQUENCY ENERGY DELIVERY

RF energy generates tissue injury by conversion of electrical energy into heat. Depending upon the output voltage and the modulation of the current, RF current can cause electrosurgical cutting, fulguration, or dessication. The typical RF generator used for catheter ablation delivers a continuous unmodulated sine wave alternating current at frequencies of 500 to 1000-kHz with a typical root-mean-square voltage of $40 - 70$-V. Using this type of RF current, electrosurgical dessication (low power, heat-induced coagulation necrosis) results and turns out to be very effective for ablation of cardiac arrhythmias. For dessication to occur, the electrode must be in direct contact with the tissue allowing steady current flow from the metal conductor into the tissue.

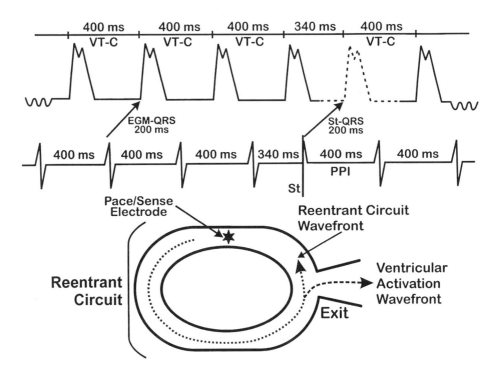

FIGURE 4-17. Schematic diagram illustrating resetting with concealed fusion. The wavefront producing ventricular tachycardia (VT) circulates within the reentry circuit. The surface ECG recording is displayed in the top portion of the diagram. A pacing and recording electrode is positioned within the slow conduction zone of the circuit and the recorded local electrogram is depicted below the ECG tracing. The cycle length of the ventricular tachycardia (VT-C) is 400 ms. The interval from the onset of the local electrogram in the circuit to the onset of the surface QRS complex (EGM-QRS) is 200 ms. An extrastimulus (St) is delivered by the pacing electrode at a coupling interval of 340 ms after the onset of a local electrogram. As previously discussed, the antidromic wavefront is extinguished after colliding with the oncoming VT depolarization (Figure 4-16). The orthodromic wavefront continues to conduct within the excitable tissue of the circuit, eventually exiting to activate the working ventricular myocardium outside the circuit, resetting the tachycardia. The orthodromic wavefront eventually returns to the pacing/recording electrode and another local electrogram is inscribed. As recorded within the circuit by the electrode, the interval from the pacing stimulus to the return local electrogram, also known as the post-pacing interval (PPI), is 400 ms, identical to the cycle length of the ventricular tachycardia. Also the morphology of the premature QRS is identical to the morphology of the QRS complex inscribed during VT. These findings characterize the phenomenon of resetting with concealed fusion and are diagnostic of a reentrant arrhythmia. The demonstration of resetting with concealed fusion means that the pace/sense electrode is positioned within the reentrant circuit. Ablation at this site may result in successful elimination of the arrhythmia. Concealed entrainment (not shown) is merely continuous resetting with concealed fusion that is produced by fixed cycle length pacing at a rate slightly faster than the VT rate.

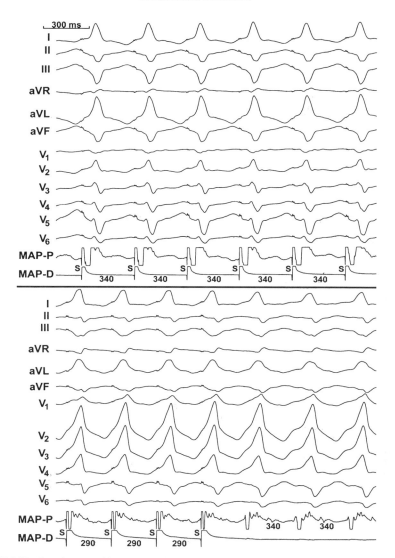

FIGURE 4-18. Entrainment with concealed fusion in a patient with ventricular tachycardia (VT) (same patient as in Figure 4-9). RF ablation at this site eliminated the VT. Prior to ablation, ventricular pacing (cycle length (CL) = 340-msec) at this site during sinus rhythm (SR) (upper panel) generated a QRS morphology distinctly different than that inscribed during the VT (Figure 4-9 and right side of lower panel). This illustrates that ventricular pace mapping during SR is not a reliable way to identify a potential target site for ablation in patients with reentrant VT. During ventricular pacing while in SR, global ventricular activation proceeds differently compared to the pattern of ventricular activation during VT (see Figure 4-6). This is because during the VT the wavefront of depolarization is forced to exit from the circuit at a site that may be far from the site of ventricular pacing during SR. Consequently, a distinctly different QRS morphology is inscribed during VT (lower panel, right side) compared to that inscribed during ventricular pacing at the same site while in SR (upper panel). As seen in the lower panel, pacing at this site during VT at a rate slightly faster than the tachycardia (CL = 290-msec) resulted in *entrainment with concealed fusion* with the inscribed QRS morphology (lower panel, left side) identical to that generated during the VT (lower panel, right side). After cessation of pacing, the VT resumes at its previous rate. MAP-D and MAP-P, distal and proximal bipolar electrode pairs on the mapping/pacing catheter. S, pacing stimulus artifact.

TABLE 4-3. Methods of surgical and catheter ablation of cardiac tachyarrhythmias

Method of Ablation	Mechanism of Tissue Damage	Clinical Examples
Surgical resection/transection	Physical excision or interruption of arrhythmia focus or critical zone	VT, AVNRT, AT, AF, AFL, AVRT, WPW
Low and high energy direct current	Barotrauma, electroporation, radiative heating	VT, AVNRT, AT, AF, AFL, AVRT, WPW
Chemical (ethanol, collagen)	Chemical toxicity; vascular occlusion	VT
Cryothermal ablation	Freezing	VT, AF
Radiofrequency ± modifications (e.g. saline-cooled tip)	Resistive heating	VT, AVNRT, AT, AF, AFL, AVRT, WPW
Microwave	Radiative heating	VT, AT AFL, AVRT
Laser (argon, Nd:YAG)	Heating (photocoagulation), tissue vaporization	VT, AVNRT, WPW, AVRT, AFL
Ultrasound	Mechanical vibration and heat production	AF (PV ostium)

AF, atrial fibrillation; AFL, atrial flutter; AT, atrial tachycardia; AVNRT, atrioventricular nodal reentrant tachycardia; AVRT, atrioventricular reciprocating tachycardia; PV, pulmonary vein; VT, ventricular tachycardia; WPW, Wolff-Parkinson-White Syndrome

In almost all cases, RF energy is delivered in a unipolar fashion between the tip electrode and a dispersive grounding electrode patch applied to the skin (Figure 4-19). The tip electrode is of small size and approximates a point source compared to the large surface area of the skin patch electrode (≥ 10 cm^2). In rare cases, RF current may be delivered in a bipolar fashion between two closely spaced electrodes. Because RF current is alternating, there is no true "cathode" and "anode" meaning the patch and tip electrodes can be connected to either pole of bipolar generator output connector. Because RF energy, unlike DC energy, does not cause cellular depolarization or activation of cardiac, skeletal, or nervous tissue, its application causes minimal pain in most patients, even when conscious, eliminating the need for general anesthesia. In addition, the frequency employed for RF ablation (500 – 1000 kHz) is high enough to avoid the induction of atrial or ventricular fibrillation.

During a cardiac ablation procedure, the alternating RF electrical current travels from the tip electrode through the cardiac myocardium and intervening body tissues to the grounding patch electrode. The passage of current through the tissues results in *resistive* or *ohmic* heating. Resistive heating, *h*, is proportional to the square of the current

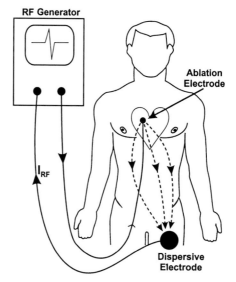

FIGURE 4-19. Schematic diagram of the electrical circuit used during radiofrequency (RF) electrode catheter ablation. RF current flows from the tip electrode positioned at the target tissue in the heart to the dispersive patch electrode on the skin. Current density and resistance are highest at the tip electrode, so essentially all heating is generated at the tip-tissue interface.

density, J, and the current density is inversely proportional to the square of the distance from the tip electrode (radius, r):

$$h \propto J^2$$

$$J \propto \frac{1}{r^2}$$

By combining these two equations it becomes clear that resistive heating decreases with the fourth power of distance from the tip of the ablation electrode:

$$h \propto \frac{1}{r^4}$$

Within an RF current circuit, resistive heating occurs in an area with both a high current density and a high electrical resistance. During RF electrode catheter ablation, the current density and electrical resistance are highest at the electrode tip. Because the current density declines with the square of the distance from the electrode, significant ohmic heating will only occur within the narrow rim immediately surrounding the electrode tip (Figure 4-20). Deeper tissue heating only results from *conductive* spread of heat from the region of resistive heating. *In vitro* and *in vivo* studies have shown that the tissue temperature declines dramatically with distance from the tip electrode, resulting in a steep temperature gradient radiating from the tip electrode [79]. Resistive or conductive heat is dissipated via flowing blood within the cardiac chambers at the endocardial surface or by blood flowing through nearby vascular structures (*convective heat loss*). Little or no heating occurs at the site of the dispersive skin electrode because of the large sur-

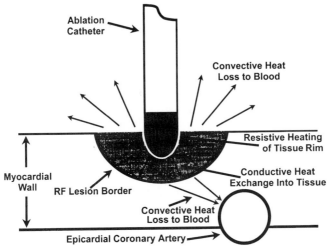

FIGURE 4-20. Schematic diagram illustrating the mechanism of lesion production during RF ablation. A narrow rim (approximately 1 mm) of resistive heating is produced immediately adjacent to the electrode. Heat flow outward from this area extends the size of the RF lesion (conductive heat exchange). Heat is dissipated both endocardially by intracardiac blood flow and epicardially by high velocity blood flow in an adjacent coronary artery.

face area of the patch electrode and the resultant low current density. Consequently, it is rare to observe skin burns except in cases of prolonged applications of RF energy when inadequate conductive gel uniformly covers the patch electrode in contact with the skin.

Any factors that increase resistive or conductive heating at the electrode-tissue interface will also increase the radial temperature gradient and, consequently, lesion size. Factors that affect lesion size are summarized in Table 4-4. Consequently lesion size is directly proportional to RF current output and inversely proportional to impedance between the tip and dispersive electrode. However, the steady-state temperature recorded at the ablation electrode-tissue interface is a more accurate predictor of lesion size (width and depth) than the measured power, current, or energy (Figure 4-21) [79].

An important determinant of tip temperature is the firmness of contact between the electrode tip and the underlying tissue [80]. Because resistive heating only occurs immediately at the electrode-tissue interface (because the high current density required for significant heating), the lesser the surface area contact of the tip with the tissue, the less heating (resistive or conductive) that can occur.

TABLE 4-4. Determinants of lesion size in RF ablation

Delivered power

Duration of energy delivery

Electrode size

Impedance of tissue and catheter system

Electrode contact pressure and tip orientation relative to tissue

Convective heat loss via blood flow

Cooled-tip electrode catheter system

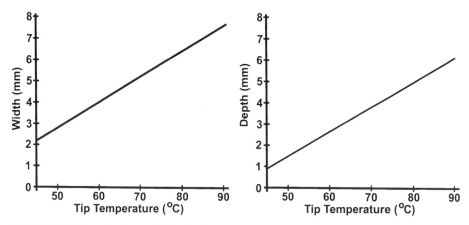

FIGURE 4-21. There is a linear relationship between RF lesion width (left panel) or RF lesion depth (right panel) and RF electrode-tissue interface temperature. Adapted from [79].

Consequently, the lesion size is limited by the development of an impedance rise at excessive tip-tissue interface temperatures. Theoretically, limiting tip temperatures to < 100 °C by continuous cooling of the catheter tip may permit delivery of higher amplitudes of RF current. This may result in higher and deeper resistive heating, thereby extending the radial tissue temperature gradient (due to both resistive and conductive heating) and increasing the lesion size. Data does indeed suggest that lesions created with tip electrodes employing the saline-cooling technology are significantly larger than those created with standard RF technology [81-83]. Lesion size can also be increased by delivery RF current in a bipolar manner [84].

The electrode size is also an important determinant of the lesion size [85]. Theoretically, a larger-sized tip electrode should create a larger lesion and a higher tip-tissue interface temperature, presuming no change in current density. However, to maintain an equivalent current density with the larger tip would require use of a RF generator with higher power, sometimes beyond the standard 50-watts found in commercially available devices. For example the mean steady-state power required to maintain an electrode tip-tissue interface temperature of 80 °C was 16 watts for a 4-mm electrode, 47-watts for an 8-mm electrode, and 61-watts for a 12-mm electrode [86]. Ablation catheters with 4-mm tip electrodes twice the lesion volume as compared with catheters with 2-mm electrodes [87]. However, the effects of tip size are not straightforward. Using a cooled-tip system, recent data indicates that smaller electrodes (2-mm versus 5-mm tips) result in transmission of a greater *fraction* of the RF power to the tissue and produce a higher tissue temperature and larger lesion size [82]. Therefore, small electrode configurations may be more efficient at energy delivery than large electrodes in a saline-cooled system, potentially mitigating the need for high-powered RF generators.

The duration of RF application is also an important determinant of the lesion size. The rate of tissue heating at the tip-tissue interface is rapid (resistive heating) with steady-state temperature reached within a few seconds. Longer time is required for heating deeper tissue layers because of the need for conductive heat exchange. Consequently, the rate of lesion growth is initially rapid (local resistive heating) and then slows as conductive heating occurs. The half-time of lesion growth is 7-10 sec with the maximum lesion size achieved after 30-40 sec of RF delivery [88,89]. There is no evidence that lesion size increases with RF energy applications longer than 50 sec.

The temperature of the electrode tip in close contact with the tissue increases during RF current application due to heat that is reflected from the tissue surface. The temperature of the tip-tissue interface can be monitored by incorporating a thermistor at the tip of the ablation electrode. The ability to monitor and regulate the tip-tissue interface temperature with feedback loop circuitry included in the RF generator allows moment-to-moment control over the ablation process and lesion production. In fact temperature monitoring of the electrode-tissue interface is the preferred manner to deliver of RF current. Temperature monitoring ensures adequate tissue contact and the development of the highest possible current density at the tip-tissue interface; electrode-tissue interface temperature is the best available correlate of lesion size (Figures 4-21 & 4-22). The ability of temperature monitoring to predict lesion size has been shown *in vitro* [79,85,89] and *in vivo* [90,91], probably because it is the best indicator of tissue contact [80].

Temperature monitoring is important not only to assure a successful delivery of sufficient RF energy to the tissue, but also to potentially reduce the risk of adverse conse-

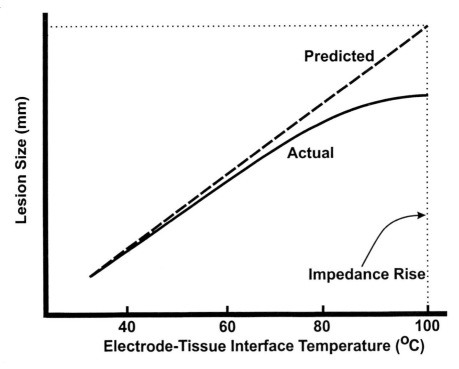

FIGURE 4-22. Lesion size increases with temperature at the electrode-tissue interface. However, the actual lesion size that develops is less than predicted size because of the sudden increase in impedance that occurs at approximately 100 °C and temperature-dependent changes in conductivity. See text for further discussion.

quences secondary to an impedance rise. The lesion size is limited by the fact that the temperature of the tissue immediately apposed to the tip cannot increase above 100 °C (Figure 4-22). Temperatures greater than 100 °C at the electrode-tissue interface usually results in boiling of blood plasma and tissue fluids, denaturation of proteins, and coagulum formation at the tip. The tip coagulum results in a sudden increase in electrical impedance and a subsequent dramatic decline in RF current density at the tip-tissue interface, and consequently, ineffective tissue heating. Sudden increases in impedance are associated with sudden boiling and often audible popping. Effective heating is usually associated with a 5–15 Ω decline in impedance [80]. A large decline in impedance often heralds a sudden increase in impedance due to overheating and coagulum formation. Potential significant complications associated with impedance increases include thrombus formation and the production of superheated gas pockets of gas that may rapidly expand and damage myocardium.

4.5.2 TISSUE EFFECTS OF RADIOFREQUENCY ENERGY

Evidence suggests that irreversible myocardial injury occurs at temperatures greater than 50-52 °C [92]. RF current delivered by an electrode catheter usually produces a well-demarcated coagulation necrosis of the myocardium without destruction of the surrounding normal tissue. Lesion size is usually 5-10 mm in diameter, with the shape usually being spherical or oval [88,93,94]. The acute RF lesion is a well-demarcated area of coagulation necrosis surrounded by a a rim of hemorrhage and inflammatory cells [14,15,73,93,94]. Chronic RF lesions exhibit significant contraction with a reduction of volume. Microscopically the lesions are composed of fibrous scar, fat cells, cartilage, granulation tissue, and infiltration by chronic inflammatory cells [14,15,73]. Interestingly, RF lesions created in the atria and ventricles of infant sheep show a more than a doubling in size over a 9-month period [95], raising a concern about the performance of RF ablation procedures in very young children.

In *in vitro* studies, hyperthermia is associated with: 1) significant depolarization of the resting potential at temperatures > 45 °C; 2) a temperature-dependent increase in the maximum rate of rise of the action potential upstroke and decrease in action potential amplitude and duration; 3) development of abnormal automaticity at temperatures > 45 °C; 4) reversible loss of cellular excitability at an average temperature of 48 °C and; 5) irreversible tissue damage at temperatures ≥ 50 °C [96]. At temperatures > 50 °C, irreversible contracture of the myocardium develops, probably secondary to a non-specific increase in membrane permeability to Ca^{2+} and heat-induced damage to sarcoplasmic reticulum and failure of cytosolic Ca^{2+} re-uptake systems. Experimental studies *in vivo* show that RF ablation results in a marked decrease in microvascular perfusion extending outside the acute RF lesion. Microvascular endothelial injury has been documented by electron microscopy well beyond the demarcated pathological lesion (up to 6-mm) [97]. This reported decrease in myocardial blood flow beyond the acute lesion may explain the clinical observation of delayed success of catheter ablation in some patients with apparent initially unsuccessful procedures [98,99]. Progression of the region of myocardial necrosis may cause delayed loss of conduction in these cases.

4.5.3 PROCEDURAL APPROACH TO CATHETER ABLATION

Catheter ablation of cardiac arrhythmias requires positioning of the tip of an electrode catheter at specific sites in one of the four heart chambers. Access to the right heart is relatively straightforward and direct; the right atrium and right ventricle can be entered through a central vein, most commonly the right or left femoral, subclavian, or right internal jugular. Access to the left ventricle, and especially the left atrium, is more problematic. For ablation of left-sided accessory connections, many electrophysiologists choose the retrograde transaortic approach for patients with native aortic valves. The use of this technique is contraindicated in patients with mechanical aortic valves, and many electrophysiologists do not recommend its use in patients with bioprosthetic aortic valves. With this technique, the ablation catheter is carefully passed retrograde from the right or left femoral artery to the aortic root. Once there, the operator creates a J-shaped bend in the distal catheter segment using the device's steering features. The distal catheter is then prolapsed across the aortic valve in a fashion similar that used to insert a "pigtail" catheter into the left ventricular when performing a left ventricular angiogram. It is crucial that the J-curved tip of the catheter be used to traverse the aortic valve in order to minimize the risk of damage to an aortic valve leaflet. Once in the left ventricle, the curve can be released and catheter tip manipulated to the putative arrhythmia focus. Many electrophysiologists use this approach for ablation of left ventricular tachycardias or the ventricular insertion of accessory connections. In some patients, the ablation of the atrial insertion of a left free wall accessory connection may also be performed using this technique by steering the catheter retrograde across the mitral valve and positioning the tip on the atrial side of the annulus.

For patients with mechanical (or possibly bioprosthetic) aortic valves, aortic stenosis, severe aortic or peripheral arterial disease, or those with arrhythmias originating in the left atrium, the transseptal catheterization technique is often required to gain access to the left heart. The purpose of this technique is to cross from the right atrium to the left atrium through the *fossa ovalis*. Possibly up to 25% of patients have a patent foramen ovale that can be crossed directly by probing the interatrial septum using the tip of the ablation catheter (sometimes inadvertently during a right heart procedure). In the remainder of the patients, the fossa ovalis must be breached by a mechanical puncture using a special needle and catheter combination (Figure 4-23). Some electrophysiologists preferentially use this technique for ablation of the atrial insertion of most left-sided accessory AV connections. In addition, this technique also allows ready access to left atrial arrhythmias originating in the pulmonary veins or along the mitral annulus. Finally, the focus of left ventricular tachycardias in some patients may be more easily approached using the transseptal technique with anterograde passage of the catheter tip across the mitral valve into the left ventricle.

The transseptal catheterization technique should be avoided in patients who cannot lie flat as well as those with distorted anatomy due to congenital heart disease, severe right atrial enlargement, significant deformity of the chest or spine, left atrial thrombus or myxoma, or are fully anticoagulated with warfarin. The potential risk of the transseptal technique is not the puncture of the fossa ovalis, *per se*, but rather the possibility that an adjacent structure, such as the aorta, posterior atrial wall, or coronary sinus will be inadvertently entered. For these reasons, attention to detail and technique is essential for the successful and safe performance of this procedure. In centers that perform the transseptal catheterization regularly the mortality and major complication rate is less than 0.1%.

Performance of the technique of transseptal catheterization requires a thorough understanding of the regional anatomy of the right atrial septum. As viewed from the feet with the patient lying supine, the interatrial septum runs obliquely from 1 o'clock to 7 o'clock (Figure 4-24). The fossa ovalis, with a diameter of approximately 2-cm is located superiorly and posteriorly to the coronary sinus and significantly posterior to the tricuspid valve annulus, right atrial appendage, and His bundle region. Facilitation of the procedure is accomplished by positioning a "pig-tail" catheter in the aortic root and electrode catheters at the His bundle region and within the coronary sinus, allowing easy fluoroscopic identification of these structures. After entry to the left atrium is established, the "pig-tail"

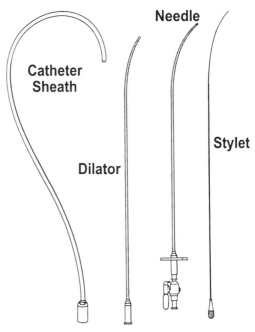

FIGURE 4-23. Equipment used for transseptal catheterization including Mullins sheath, internal dilator, Brockenbrough needle, and needle stylet.

catheter is removed, while the electrode catheters are retained for performance of the subsequent diagnostic and therapeutic electrophysiology study. The area of the fossa ovalis is bounded anteriorly and superiorly by the aortic root and posteriorly by the posterior free wall of the right atrium. In most patients, the fossa has a prominent superior ridge, termed the *limbus*. The transseptal procedure should only be performed from the right femoral vein. The required equipment used in most laboratories includes: 1) Mullins sheath with dilator, 2) Brockenbrough needle, 3) 3-way manifold connected to a pressure transducer, radiographic contrast, and saline, 4) 145 cm J-guide wire (Figure 4-23). To perform the procedure, the Mullins sheath and its internal dilator are positioned in the superior vena cava over the J-guide wire. After flushing the sheath/dilator system with saline, the Brockenbrough needle is advanced through the lumen of the internal dilator to a point just beneath the tip opening of the dilator. Normally, the Brockenbrough needle and paired dilator combination are manufactured such that the needle tip is positioned just beneath the tip of the dilator when there is a "thumb-widths" distance between the directional metal flange near the needle hub and the entry port of the dilator. After flushing the needle and filling its lumen with contrast media, the needle, dilator, and sheath system is firmly grasped using both hands and the system rotated until the di-

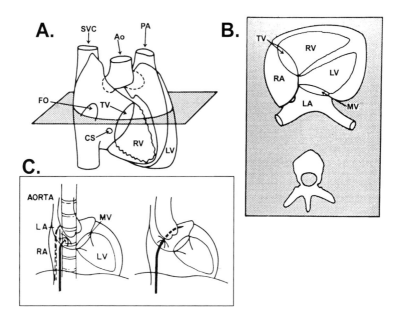

FIGURE 4-24. Cardiac anatomical relationships important for the performance of the transseptal left heart catheterization technique. The position of the fossa ovalis (FO) is shown relative to adjacent structures (panel A). Cross section of the heart through the FO viewed from below (panel B) demonstrating the poster-omedial direction of the interatrial septum and the proximity of the posterior and lateral wall of the right atrium. As the catheter tip slides over the aortic root (panel C, left-side), it appears to move rightward on to the spine. Continued withdrawal of the catheter results in more rightward movement into the FO. Puncture of the FO with advancement of the catheter into the LA is shown (panel C, right-side). Ao, aorta; CS, ostium of coronary sinus; LA, left atrium; LV, left ventricle; MV, mitral valve; PA, pulmonary artery; RA, right atrium; RV, right ventricle; SVC, superior vena cava; TV, tricuspid valve. From [103] with permission.

rectional indicator at the needle hub is pointing at 4:30 o'clock. This maneuver directs the catheter system tip into a posteromedial orientation, approximately perpendicular to the interatrial septum. The entire system is then slowly withdrawn form the patient under fluoroscopic guidance, predominantly using the left anterior oblique view. In so doing, the catheter system exits the superior vena cava and the tip slides over the bulge of the ascending aorta and then moves into the right atrium, but leftward toward atrial septum. With continued withdrawal, the catheter system tip appears to make a sudden leftward "jump" as the catheter traverses the limbus and then "dives" into the fossa ovalis. At this point, the operator may feel the transmitted contractile waves generated by the movement of the atrial septum against the catheter system in contact with the atrial endocardium. When the operator determines that the catheter tip is optimally positioned it is useful to inject contrast media through the needle. Only when the tip is closely opposed to the atrial septum will injected contrast "stain" the septum, confirming the septal location. At this point, in some patients, the catheter tip may spontaneously cross into the left atrium through a patent foramen ovale with little further manipulation. However, before advancing the needle or the tip of the catheter system it is crucial to view catheter positioning using the right anterior oblique view. The tip of the Mullins dilator should be pointing at the atrial septum at a position well posterior to the coronary sinus and His bundle, but not so posterior as to threaten the posterior wall of the right atrium when the catheter tip and/or needle is advanced. In some patients, left atrial entry can be achieved merely by slowly advancing the stiff tip of the catheter system superiorly until it abuts the limbus. A "popping" sensation is often experienced as the tip of the catheter system breeches the fossa ovalis. In most patients, however, this maneuver will fail to breech the septum and the needle will need to be advanced out the tip of the dilator across the septum. Verification of the location of the needle tip can be accomplished by pressure recording, withdrawal of oxygenated blood, or injection of contrast showing streaming into the left atrium. Once accomplished, the entire catheter system should be advanced an additional very short distance and the directional indicator directed more toward 3 o'clock to ensure that the needle and catheter tip are safely directed away from the posterior left atrial wall and toward the anteriorly-positioned the mitral valve. Next, with the needle and sheath held firmly in position, the dilator is slowly advanced over the needle into the left atrium. At this point, the needle is now safely positioned back within the dilator. Finally, holding the dilator and needle in a stable position, the Mullins sheath is slowly advanced over the dilator into the left atrium. Thereafter, the needle is first removed from the dilator lumen and then the dilator is removed from the sheath. The latter should be performed slowly while syringe suction is applied to the side-port of the sheath. This ensures that no air is drawn into the lumen of the Mullins sheath from the "piston-effect" caused by removing the long, lumen-occluding, dilator. The sheath should then be flushed, taking great care to avoid the introduction of air bubbles into the sheath or left atrium.

During the transseptal procedure the operator must be continuously aware of the catheter tip location and orientation as well as the position of the needle. The catheter system should never be manipulated in the superior vena cava, right atrium, or left atrium with the needle extended beyond the tip. The only time the needle should be advanced out the end of the dilator is when proper positioning at the fossa ovalis is confirmed fluoroscopically. As with all catheterization procedures, transseptal catheterization should be performed by, or under the guidance of, an experienced operator.

4.5.4 COMPLICATIONS OF CATHETER ABLATION PROCEDURES

The potential complications of catheter ablation procedures are primarily related to the arterial or venous cannulation or the intracardiac catheter manipulation and are identical to those described for standard diagnostic electrophysiology studies (see "Potential complications of diagnostic and therapeutic invasive electrophysiology procedures" on page 27) [100-102].

4.6   Confirmation of Successful Ablation

In order to reliably determine if an ablation procedure was successful, it is crucial that the arrhythmia be easily and reproducibly inducible. In general, if ablation eliminates inducibility in these patients, an *acute* cure can be assumed. A chronic or durable cure can only be determined during long-term clinical follow-up.

In patients with incessant tachycardia or a manifest accessory connection, successful ablation is generally heralded by sudden termination of the tachycardia or sudden disappearance of the delta wave. However, even when success appears indisputable, additional measures should be taken to ensure that the arrhythmia is eliminated. In the case of patients with accessory connections, even if anterograde conduction is eliminated (marked by disappearance of the delta wave), retrograde conduction may be preserved. In these cases, a manifest accessory connection is converted into a concealed pathway. Unless ventricular pacing is performed to evaluate the retrograde ventriculoatrial conduction pattern, the failure to eliminate the accessory connection will not be recognized. In addition, usually in these cases, orthodromic AV reciprocating tachycardia may still be induced, although, in some patients, induction may require isoproterenol. In some cases, retrograde conduction may be preferentially eliminated by ablation without affecting anterograde conduction. The mapping and ablation procedure should be continued until conduction in both the anterograde and retrograde directions is eliminated.

Ideally, the "hard" ablation endpoint in patients with typical or atypical AV nodal reentrant tachycardia is complete elimination of the slow conduction pathway. However, in patients with easy and reproducibly inducible AV nodal reentrant tachycardia, elimination of inducibility despite the presence of residual slow pathway conduction is often used an endpoint for success. In these cases, a residual "A-H jump" may remain following the ablation, but only single AV nodal echo beats should be allowed. Tachycardia should not be inducible, even during an isoproterenol infusion. This "softer" endpoint for ablation success is used when continued ablation attempts are deemed to put the patient at high risk of ablation-induced AV block. Multiple echo beats or non-sustained AV nodal reentrant tachycardia are not reliable endpoints, even in patients with easily and reproducibly inducible sustained tachycardia.

In patients with paroxysmal atrial or ventricular tachycardias, assessment of acute success is usually established by demonstrating non-inducibility. In these cases, even the presence of inducible non-sustained forms of the arrhythmia indicates that a durable cure is unlikely. Therefore, in these patients a complete pacing and pharmacological evaluation is often indicated, with repeated use of programmed stimulation and decremental pacing, at times along with an infusion of isoproterenol (in absence of contraindications).

In patients with the idiopathic forms of right or left ventricular tachycardia, sustained tachycardia is often not reliably and reproducibly inducible. In many patients with these arrhythmias, only non-sustained salvos may be induced and, in some patients, only frequent ventricular premature depolarizations may occur, even with a high dose isoproterenol infusion. Therefore, verification of an acute cure in these patients may necessitate elimination of all ventricular premature depolarizations with a characteristic morphology and axis.

The inducibility of some arrhythmias may be non-specific. For example, the typical clockwise and counterclockwise forms of atrial flutter may be inducible in patients who have never had these arrhythmias clinically. Conversely, in patients with well documented occurrences of typical clockwise or counterclockwise atrial flutter, the arrhythmias may not be inducible even with aggressive pacing protocols. In those patients with the clinically-evident atrial flutter, the endpoint for acute success is not merely non-inducibility. In addition, bidirectional conduction block should be produced within the atrial isthmus and should be documented by confirming the presence of a line of conduction block within this region (see "Macroreentrant Atrial Tachycardia" on page 626).

Inducibility of atrial fibrillation is a non-specific finding. However, many patients with paroxysmal atrial fibrillation may have their arrhythmia initiated by a triggering arrhythmia, such as atrial premature depolarizations or salvos of rapid atrial tachycardia. In these patients, the triggering arrhythmia may be reliably inducible by pharmacological agents such as isoproterenol, adenosine, or phenylephrine. If this is the case, then mapping and ablating the focus of the triggering arrhythmia may result in acute cure of the paroxysmal atrial fibrillation. Consequently, if the triggering arrhythmia is reliably inducible, confirmation that the triggering focus is eliminated may be possible and can be used as an endpoint for successful acute cure of paroxysmal atrial fibrillation in these patients.

4.7 Future Directions

Rapidly evolving changes in technology are most likely to affect future changes in ablation therapy in the areas of: 1) mapping the precise location of the arrhythmia focus or reentrant circuit; 2) energy sources used for ablation; and 3) catheter systems to deliver the controlled destructive power. In particular, enhanced RF with cooled-tip technology, microwave, cryothermia, laser, or ultrasound may play a niche role in the ablation of atrial and ventricular tachycardias and atrial fibrillation. Further improvements in computerized non-contact and contact mapping systems are also inevitable.

References

1. Sealy WC, Hattler BG, Jr., Blumenschein SD, Cobb FR: Surgical treatment of Wolff-Parkinson-White syndrome. *Ann Thorac Surg* **8**:1-11, 1969.
2. Sealy WC, Gallagher JJ, Wallace AG: The surgical treatment of Wolff-Parkinson-White Syndrome: evolution of improved methods for identification and interruption of the Kent Bundle. *Ann Thorac Surg* **22**:443-57, 1976.
3. Harken AH, Josephson ME, Horowitz LN: Surgical endocardial resection for the treatment of malignant ventricular tachycardia. *Ann Surg* **190**:456-60, 1979.
4. Harken AH, Horowitz LN, Josephson ME: The surgical treatment of ventricular tachycardia. *Ann Thorac Surg* **30**:499-508, 1980.
5. Harken AH, Wetstein L, Josephson ME: Mechanisms and surgical management of ventricular tachyarrhythmias. *Cardiovasc Clin* **15**:287-300, 1985.
6. Harken AH, Josephson ME: Recurrent ventricular tachycardia: how effective is surgical management? *Am J Surg* **145**:718-23, 1983.
7. Josephson ME, Harken AH, Horowitz LN: Endocardial excision: a new surgical technique for the treatment of recurrent ventricular tachycardia. *Circulation* **60**:1430-9, 1979.
8. Kay GN, Bubien RS, Dailey SM, et al.: A prospective evaluation of intracoronary ethanol ablation of the atrioventricular conduction system. *J Am Coll Cardiol* **17**:1634-40, 1991.
9. Kay GN, Epstein AE, Bubien RS, et al.: Intracoronary ethanol ablation for the treatment of recurrent sustained ventricular tachycardia. *J Am Coll Cardiol* **19**:159-68, 1992.

10. Kuck KH, Jackman WM, Pitha J, et al.: Percutaneous catheter ablation at the mitral annulus in canines using a bipolar epicardial-endocardial electrode configuration. *Pacing Clin Electrophysiol* **11**:760-75, 1988.

11. Morady F, Scheinman MM, Griffin JC, et al.: Results of catheter ablation of ventricular tachycardia using direct current shocks. *Pacing Clin Electrophysiol* **12**:252-7, 1989.

12. Fisher JD, Scavin GM, Roth JA, et al.: Direct current shock ablation: quantitative assessment of proarrhythmic effects. *Pacing Clin Electrophysiol* **14**:2154-66, 1991.

13. Rosenquist M, Lee MA, Moulinier L, et al.: Long-term follow-up of patients after transcatheter direct current ablation of the atrioventricular junction. *J Am Coll Cardiol* **16**:1467-74, 1990.

14. Huang SK, Graham AR, Hoyt RH, Odell RC: Transcatheter desiccation of the canine left ventricle using radiofrequency energy: a pilot study. *Am Heart J* **114**:42-8, 1987.

15. Huang SK, Bharati S, Graham AR, et al.: Closed chest catheter desiccation of the atrioventricular junction using radiofrequency energy--a new method of catheter ablation. *J Am Coll Cardiol* **9**:349-58, 1987.

16. Borggrefe M, Budde T, Podczeck A, Breithardt G: High frequency alternating current ablation of an accessory pathway in humans. *J Am Coll Cardiol* **10**:576-582, 1987.

17. Jackman WM, Beckman KJ, McClelland JH, et al.: Treatment of supraventricular tachycardia due to atrioventricular nodal reentry, by radiofrequency catheter ablation of slow-pathway conduction. *N Engl J Med* **327**:313-8, 1992.

18. Moulton K, Miller B, Scott J, Woods WT, Jr.: Radiofrequency catheter ablation for AV nodal reentry: a technique for rapid transection of the slow AV nodal pathway. *Pacing Clin Electrophysiol* **16**:760-8, 1993.

19. Haissaguerre M, Gaita F, Marcus FI, Clementy J: Radiofrequency catheter ablation of accessory pathways: a contemporary review. *J Cardiovasc Electrophysiol* **5**:532-52, 1994.

20. Haissaguerre M, Gaita F, Fischer B, et al.: Radiofrequency catheter ablation of left lateral accessory pathways via the coronary sinus. *Circulation* **86**:1464-8, 1992.

21. Borggrefe M, Hindricks G, Haverkamp W, Breithardt G: Catheter ablation using radiofrequency energy. *Clin Cardiol* **13**:127-31, 1990.

22. Kuck KH, Schluter M: Radiofrequency catheter ablation of accessory pathways. *Pacing Clin Electrophysiol* **15**:1380-6, 1992.

23. Klein LS, Miles WM: Ablative therapy for ventricular arrhythmias. *Prog Cardiovasc Dis* **37**:225-42, 1995.

24. Borggrefe M: Catheter ablation of incessant ventricular tachycardia. *Isr J Med Sci* **32**:868-71, 1996.

25. Strasberg B, Zeevi B, Kusniec J, et al.: Radiofrequency catheter ablation of ectopic atrial tachycardia. *Isr J Med Sci* **33**:112-6, 1997.

26. Stevenson WG, Friedman PL, Kocovic D, et al.: Radiofrequency catheter ablation of ventricular tachycardia after myocardial infarction. *Circulation* **98**:308-14, 1998.

27. Stevenson WG, Friedman PL, Ganz LI: Radiofrequency catheter ablation of ventricular tachycardia late after myocardial infarction. *J Cardiovasc Electrophysiol* **8**:1309-19, 1997.

28. Rodriguez LM, Smeets JL, Timmermans C, et al.: Radiofrequency catheter ablation of sustained monomorphic ventricular tachycardia in hypertrophic cardiomyopathy. *J Cardiovasc Electrophysiol* **8**:803-6, 1997.

29. Morady F, Harvey M, Kalbfleisch SJ, et al.: Radiofrequency catheter ablation of ventricular tachycardia in patients with coronary artery disease. *Circulation* **87**:363-72, 1993.

30. Goldberger J, Kall J, Ehlert F, et al.: Effectiveness of radiofrequency catheter ablation for treatment of atrial tachycardia. *Am J Cardiol* **72**:787-93, 1993.

31. Ivanov MY, Evdokimov VP, Vlasenco VV: Predictors of successful radiofrequency catheter ablation of sinoatrial tachycardia. *Pacing Clin Electrophysiol* **21**:311-5, 1998.

32. Chiladakis JA, Vassilikos VP, Maounis TN, et al.: Successful radiofrequency catheter ablation of automatic atrial tachycardia with regression of the cardiomyopathy picture. *Pacing Clin Electrophysiol* **20**:953-9, 1997.

33. Cosio FG, Lopez Gil M, Arribas F, Goicolea A: Radiofrequency catheter ablation for the treatment of human type 1 atrial flutter. *Circulation* **88**:804-5, 1993.

34. Cosio FG, Arribas F, Lopez-Gil M, Palacios J: Radiofrequency catheter ablation of atrial flutter circuits. *Arch Mal Coeur Vaiss* **89 Spec No 1**:75-81, 1996.

35. Saxon LA, Kalman JM, Olgin JE, et al.: Results of radiofrequency catheter ablation for atrial flutter. *Am J Cardiol* **77**:1014-6, 1996.

36. Haissaguerre M, Shah DC, Jais P, Clementy J: Role of catheter ablation for atrial fibrillation. *Curr Opin Cardiol* **12**:18-23, 1997.

37. Haissaguerre M, Jais P, Shah DC, et al.: Right and left atrial radiofrequency catheter therapy of paroxysmal atrial fibrillation. *J Cardiovasc Electrophysiol* **7**:1132-44, 1996.

38. Haissaguerre M, Jais P, Shah DC, et al.: Spontaneous initiation of atrial fibrillation by ectopic beats originating in the pulmonary veins. *N Engl J Med* **339**:659-66, 1998.

39. Zipes DP, DiMarco JP, Gillette PC, et al.: Guidelines for clinical intracardiac electrophysiological and catheter ablation procedures. A report of the American College of Cardiology/American Heart Association Task Force on Practice Guidelines (Committee on Clinical Intracardiac Electrophysiologic and Catheter Ablation Procedures), developed in collaboration with the North American Society of Pacing and Electrophysiology. *J Am Coll Cardiol* **26**:555-73, 1995.

40. Sung RJ, Waxman HL, Saksena S, Juma Z: Sequence of retrograde atrial activation in patients with dual atrioventricular nodal pathways. *Circulation* **64**:1059-67, 1981.

41. Smeets JLRM, Ben-Haim SA, Rodriguez LM, et al.: New method for non-fluoroscopic endocardial mapping in humans. Accuracy assessment and first clinical results. *Circulation* **97**:2426-2432, 1998.

42. Schilling RJ, Peters NS, Davies W: Simultaneous endocardial mapping in the human left ventricle using a non-contact catheter. Comparison of contact and reconstructed electrograms during sinus rhythm. *Circulation* **98**:887-898, 1998.

43. Haissaguerre M, Gaita F, Fischer B, et al.: Elimination of atrioventricular nodal reentrant tachycardia using discrete slow potentials to guide application of radiofrequency energy. *Circulation* **85**:2162-75, 1992.

44. Kuo CT, Lauer MR, Young C, et al.: Electrophysiologic significance of discrete slow potentials in dual atrioventricular node physiology: implications for selective radiofrequency ablation of slow pathway conduction. *Am Heart J* **131**:490-8, 1996.

45. Heald SC, Davies DW, Ward DE, et al.: Radiofrequency catheter ablation of Mahaim tachycardia by targeting Mahaim potentials at the tricuspid annulus. *Br Heart J* **73**:250-257, 1995.

46. Mounsey JP, Griffith MJ, McComb JM: Radiofrequency ablation of a Mahaim fiber following localization of Mahaim pathway potentials. *J Cardiovasc Electrophysiol* **5**:432-7, 1994.

47. Jackman WM, Friday KJ, Yeung-Lai-Wah JA, et al.: New catheter technique for recording left free-wall accessory atrioventricular pathway activation. Identification of pathway fiber orientation. *Circulation* **78**:598-611, 1988.

48. Niebauer MJ, Daoud E, Goyal R, et al.: Assessment of pacing maneuvers used to validate anterograde accessory pathway potentials. *J Cardiovasc Electrophysiol* **6**:350-6, 1995.

49. Simmers TA, Hauer RN, Wever EF, et al.: Unipolar electrogram models for prediction of outcome in radiofrequency ablation of accessory pathways. *Pacing Clin Electrophysiol* **17**:186-98, 1994.

50. Tai YT, Lee KL, Lau CP: Catheter induced mechanical stunning of accessory pathway conduction: useful guide to successful transcatheter ablation of accessory pathways. *Pacing Clin Electrophysiol* **17**:31-6, 1994.

51. Nogami A, Naito S, Tada H, et al.: Verapamil-sensitive left anterior fascicular ventricular tachycardia: results of radiofrequency ablation in six patients. *J Cardiovasc Electrophysiol* **9**:1269-78, 1998.

52. Stevenson WG, Weiss JN, Wiener I, et al.: Fractionated endocardial electrograms are associated with slow conduction in humans: evidence from pace-mapping. *J Am Coll Cardiol* **13**:369-76, 1989.

53. Josephson ME, Wit AL: Fractionated electrical activity and continuous electrical activity: fact or artifact? *Circulation* **70**:529-32, 1984.

54. Ideker RE, Lofland GK, Bardy GH, et al.: Late fractionated potentials and continuous electrical activity caused by electrode motion. *Pacing Clin Electrophysiol* **6**:908-14, 1983.

55. Kadish AH, Rosenthal ME, Vassallo JA, et al.: Sinus mapping in patients with cardiac arrest and coronary disease-- results and correlation with outcome. *Pacing Clin Electrophysiol* **12**:301-10, 1989.

56. de Bakker JM, van Capelle FJ, Janse MJ, et al.: Fractionated electrograms in dilated cardiomyopathy: origin and relation to abnormal conduction. *J Am Coll Cardiol* **27**:1071-8, 1996.

57.   Fitzgerald DM, Friday KJ, Wah JA, et al.: Electrogram patterns predicting successful catheter ablation of ventricular tachycardia. *Circulation* **77**:806-14, 1988.

58.   Sosa E, Scanavacca M, D'Avila A, et al.: Endocardial and epicardial ablation guided by nonsurgical transthoracic epicardial mapping to treat recurrent ventricular tachycardia. *J Cardiovasc Electrophysiol* **9**:229-39, 1998.

59.   Strickberger SA, Man KC, Daoud EG, et al.: A prospective evaluation of catheter ablation of ventricular tachycardia as adjuvant therapy in patients with coronary artery disease and an implantable cardioverter-defibrillator. *Circulation* **96**:1525-31, 1997.

60.   Jadonath RL, Snow JS, Goldner BG, Cohen TJ: Radiofrequency catheter ablation as primary therapy for symptomatic ventricular tachycardia. *J Invasive Cardiol* **6**:289-95, 1994.

61.   Stevenson WG, Khan H, Sager P, et al.: Identification of reentry circuit sites during catheter mapping and radiofrequency ablation of ventricular tachycardia late after myocardial infarction. *Circulation* **88**:1647-70, 1993.

62.   Stevenson WG: Functional approach to site-by-site catheter mapping of ventricular reentry circuits in chronic infarctions. *J Electrocardiol* **27 Suppl**:130-8, 1994.

63.   Khan HH, Stevenson WG: Activation times in and adjacent to reentry circuits during entrainment: implications for mapping ventricular tachycardia. *Am Heart J* **127**:833-42, 1994.

64.   Stevenson WG, Sager PT, Friedman PL: Entrainment techniques for mapping atrial and ventricular tachycardias. *J Cardiovasc Electrophysiol* **6**:201-16, 1995.

65.   MacLean WA, Plumb VJ, Waldo AL: Transient entrainment and interruption of ventricular tachycardia. *Pacing Clin Electrophysiol* **4**:358-66, 1981.

66.   Kay GN, Epstein AE, Plumb VJ: Incidence of reentry with an excitable gap in ventricular tachycardia: a prospective evaluation utilizing transient entrainment. *J Am Coll Cardiol* **11**:530-8, 1988.

67.   Brugada P, Wellens HJ: Entrainment as an electrophysiologic phenomenon. *J Am Coll Cardiol* **3**:451-4, 1984.

68.   Waldo AL, Plumb VJ, Arciniegas JG, et al.: Transient entrainment and interruption of the atrioventricular bypass pathway type of paroxysmal atrial tachycardia. A model for understanding and identifying reentrant arrhythmias. *Circulation* **67**:73-83, 1983.

69.   Okumura K, Henthorn RW, Epstein AE, et al.: Further observations on transient entrainment: importance of pacing site and properties of the components of the reentry circuit. *Circulation* **72**:1293-307, 1985.

70.   Okumura K, Olshansky B, Henthorn RW, et al.: Demonstration of the presence of slow conduction during sustained ventricular tachycardia in man: use of transient entrainment of the tachycardia. *Circulation* **75**:369-78, 1987.

71.   Henthorn RW, Okumura K, Olshansky B, et al.: A fourth criterion for transient entrainment: the electrogram equivalent of progressive fusion. *Circulation* **77**:1003-12, 1988.

72.   McLean A: The Bovie electrosurgical current generator. *Arch Surg* **18**:1863-73, 1929.

73.   Huang SK, Bharati S, Lev M, Marcus FI: Electrophysiologic and histologic observations of chronic atrioventricular block induced by closed-chest catheter desiccation with radiofrequency energy. *Pacing Clin Electrophysiol* **10**:805-16, 1987.

74.   Langberg JJ, Chin MC, Rosenqvist M, et al.: Catheter ablation of the atrioventricular junction with radiofrequency energy. *Circulation* **80**:1527-35, 1989.

75.   Langberg JJ, Desai J, Dullet N, Scheinman MM: Treatment of macroreentrant ventricular tachycardia with radiofrequency ablation of the right bundle branch. *Am J Cardiol* **63**:1010-3, 1989.

76.   Langberg J, Griffin JC, Herre JM, et al.: Catheter ablation of accessory pathways using radiofrequency energy in the canine coronary sinus. *J Am Coll Cardiol* **13**:491-6, 1989.

77.   Jackman WM, Wang XZ, Friday KJ, et al.: Catheter ablation of atrioventricular junction using radiofrequency current in 17 patients. Comparison of standard and large-tip catheter electrodes. *Circulation* **83**:1562-76, 1991.

78.   Jackman WM, Wang X, Friday KJ, et al.: Catheter ablation of accessory atrioventricular pathways (Wolff-Parkinson-White syndrome) by radiofrequency current. *New Engl J Med* **324**:1605-1611, 1991.

79.   Haines DE, Watson DD: Tissue heating during radiofrequency catheter ablation: a thermodynamic model and observations in isolated perfused and superfused canine right ventricular free wall. *Pacing Clin Electrophysiol* **12**:962-76, 1989.

80. Haines DE: Determinants of lesion size during radiofrequency catheter ablation: the role of electrode-tissue contact pressure and duration of energy delivery. *J Cardiovasc Electrophysiol* **2**:509-15, 1991.

81. Ruffy R, Imran MA, Santel DJ, Wharton JM: Radiofrequency delivery through a cooled catheter tip allows the creation of larger endomyocardial lesions in the ovine heart. *J Cardiovasc Electrophysiol* **6**:1089-96, 1995.

82. Nakagawa H, Wittkampf FH, Yamanashi WS, et al.: Inverse relationship between electrode size and lesion size during radiofrequency ablation with active electrode cooling. *Circulation* **98**:458-65, 1998.

83. Nakagawa H, Yamanashi WS, Pitha JV, et al.: Comparison of in vivo tissue temperature profile and lesion geometry for radiofrequency ablation with a saline-irrigated electrode versus temperature control in a canine thigh muscle preparation. *Circulation* **91**:2264-73, 1995.

84. Chang RJ, Stevenson WG, Saxon LA, Parker J: Increasing catheter ablation lesion size by simultaneous application of radiofrequency current to two adjacent sites. *Am Heart J* **125**:1276-84, 1993.

85. Haines DE, Watson DD, Verow AF: Electrode radius predicts lesion radius during radiofrequency energy heating. Validation of a proposed thermodynamic model. *Circ Res* **67**:124-9, 1990.

86. Langberg JJ, Gallagher M, Strickberger SA, Amirana O: Temperature-guided radiofrequency catheter ablation with very large distal electrodes. *Circulation* **88**:245-9, 1993.

87. Langberg JJ, Lee MA, Chin MC, Rosenqvist M: Radiofrequency catheter ablation: the effect of electrode size on lesion volume in vivo. *Pacing Clin Electrophysiol* **13**:1242-8, 1990.

88. Wittkampf FH, Hauer RN, Robles de Medina EO: Control of radiofrequency lesion size by power regulation. *Circulation* **80**:962-8, 1989.

89. Haines DE, Verow AF: Observations on electrode-tissue interface temperature and effect on electrical impedance during radiofrequency ablation of ventricular myocardium. *Circulation* **82**:1034-8, 1990.

90. Hindricks G, Haverkamp W, Gulker H, et al.: Radiofrequency coagulation of ventricular myocardium: improved prediction of lesion size by monitoring catheter tip temperature. *Eur Heart J* **10**:972-84, 1989.

91. Langberg JJ, Calkins H, el-Atassi R, et al.: Temperature monitoring during radiofrequency catheter ablation of accessory pathways. *Circulation* **86**:1469-74, 1992.

92. Whayne JG, Nath S, Haines DE: Microwave catheter ablation of myocardium in vitro. Assessment of the characteristics of tissue heating and injury. *Circulation* **89**:2390-5, 1994.

93. Huang SK, Graham AR, Wharton K: Radiofrequency catheter ablation of the left and right ventricles: anatomic and electrophysiologic observations. *Pacing Clin Electrophysiol* **11**:449-59, 1988.

94. Huang SK, Graham AR, Bharati S, et al.: Short- and long-term effects of transcatheter ablation of the coronary sinus by radiofrequency energy. *Circulation* **78**:416-27, 1988.

95. Saul JP, Hulse JE, Papagiannis J, et al.: Late enlargement of radiofrequency lesions in infant lambs. Implications for ablation procedures in small children. *Circulation* **90**:492-9, 1994.

96. Nath S, Lynch CD, Whayne JG, Haines DE: Cellular electrophysiological effects of hyperthermia on isolated guinea pig papillary muscle. Implications for catheter ablation. *Circulation* **88**:1826-31, 1993.

97. Nath S, Whayne JG, Kaul S, et al.: Effects of radiofrequency catheter ablation on regional myocardial blood flow. Possible mechanism for late electrophysiological outcome. *Circulation* **89**:2667-72, 1994.

98. Stein KM, Lerman BB: Delayed success following radiofrequency catheter ablation. *Pacing Clin Electrophysiol* **16**:698-701, 1993.

99. Langberg JJ, Borganelli SM, Kalbfleisch SJ, et al.: Delayed effects of radiofrequency energy on accessory atrioventricular connections. *Pacing Clin Electrophysiol* **16**:1001-5, 1993.

100. Horowitz LN: Safety of electrophysiologic studies. *Circulation* **73**:11-28, 1986.

101. Horowitz LN, Kay HR, Kutalek SP, et al.: Risks and complications of clinical cardiac electrophysiologic studies: a prospective analysis of 1,000 consecutive patients. *J Am Coll Cardiol* **9**:1261-8, 1987.

102. Scheinman MM: Catheter ablation for cardiac arrhythmias, personnel, and facilities. North American Society of Pacing and Electrophysiology Ad Hoc Committee on Catheter Ablation. *Pacing Clin Electrophysiol* **15**:715-21, 1992.

103. Ross J: Considerations regarding the technique for transseptal left heart catheterization. *Circulation* **34**:391-399, 1966.

CHAPTER 5

PRINCIPLES OF PACEMAKER THERAPY

The first implantable devices used to treat cardiac arrhythmias were permanent pace-makers. Initially implanted in the late 1950s, they were originally used to treat patients with syncope due to complete AV block. Pacemaker treatment has now significantly expanded to include patients with symptomatic sinoatrial node dysfunction and lesser degrees of AV block, including high degree AV block or Mobitz type II second degree AV block. In addition, permanent pacing is now indicated for selected patients with hyper-trophic and dilated cardiomyopathies, even though they have no symptomatic bradycardia, as well as some patients with the long QT syndrome and torsade de pointes. Even today, there may be rare patients with symptomatic supraventricular tachycardias not amenable to ablation therapy that may be effectively and reliably treated with overdrive atrial pacing delivered from an implanted pacemaker. Finally, there is preliminary evidence that some patients with paroxysmal atrial fibrillation may be more likely to maintain sinus rhythm with multiple-site atrial pacing.

This chapter cannot hope to be exhaustive in its discussion of pacemakers. The focus here will be on principles and not the specifics of any particular device. In addition, one of the most critical components of device therapy is follow-up, particularly trouble-shooting of suspected device or lead malfunction, and analysis of the appropriateness of observed device activity. While we touch on some of this, for the most part these topics are best learned by hands-on experience with the devices and their external programming systems.

5.1 Historical Perspectives

Surprisingly, the development cardiac pacing dates to the late 1920s and the efforts of two physicians working independently, Mark C. Lidwill and Albert S. Hyman [1-3]. However, it was not until the "rediscovery" of this technology in the early 1950s by Paul Zoll [4] that electrical pacing rapidly began to evolve in parallel with the development of hospital-based medicine, especially cardiac catheterization, coronary care units and cardiac surgery. The first fully implantable cardiac pacemakers became available in the late 1950s (Table 5-1.)

Modern pacemaker systems consist of a battery-powered pulse generator that delivers an electrical current impulse to the endocardium through specialized wires (or leads). If suprathreshold, this electrical impulse generates a propagating depolarization wave which spreads throughout the myocardium. Programmable electronic circuitry within the pulse generator can both regulate the amplitude of the delivered current impulse along with sensing spontaneous or paced cardiac activity. Programming is facilitated using external devices that use radiofrequency signals or magnetic fields to instantaneously alter an number of programmable parameters. Digitized data and electrograms stored in the pulse generator can also be retrieved using the external telemetry system. The following discussion covers many of the fundamental concepts of pacemaker therapy. For a more exhaustive presentation the reader is referred to a number of excellent sources devoted to this subject [20-22].

TABLE 5-1. Early historical milestones in the development of cardiac pacing technology

1929	First report of development of an external cardiac stimulator connected to a plunge electrode placed in the ventricle using a transthoracic approach [3]
1932	Development of a mechanically-powered pulse generator and atrial plunge electrode [1,2]
1950	Development of a percutaneous transvenous bipolar electrode catheter used to electrically pace the right atrium of experimental animals [5]
1952	External pacemaker with subcutaneous needle electrodes (subsequently external chest electrodes) [4]
1956	External pacemaker automatically triggered by sensing [6]
1957	Transistorized, battery-powered P-synchronous pacemaker [7]
1957	Myocardial wire with external pulse generator [8]
1958	Myocardial wire with portable, external pulse generator [9]
1958	Percutaneously-inserted transvenous endocardial lead with external pulse generator first used in humans [10,11]
1958	Development of fully-implantable pacemaker with rechargeable battery [12]
1959	Development of radiofrequency pacemaker [13,14]
1959	Bipolar myocardial electrode with portable, external pulse generator [15]
1959	Introduction of P-synchronous pacemaker [16]
1960	Development of inductive-coupled pacemaker [17]
1960	Battery-powered implantable pacemaker [18]
1960	P-synchronous pacemaker with catheter electrodes [19]

5.2   Indications for Pacemaker Therapy

The initial indication for pacemaker therapy was complete AV block with syncope. Over time, the indications for pacemaker use has significantly broadened to include selected patients with a variety of conditions including:

- Acquired AV block in adults
- Chronic bifascicular/trifascicular block
- Post-acute myocardial infarction
- Sinoatrial node dysfunction
- Dilated cardiomyopathy
- Post-cardiac transplantation
- Hypersensitive carotid sinus and neurocardiogenic syndromes
- Overdrive pacing to terminate tachycardias
- Prevention of tachycardia
- Hypertrophic cardiomyopathy

The specific indications for pacemaker therapy are outlined below in Table 5-2.

5.3   Basic Concepts & Biophysical Aspects of Pacing

5.3.1 BASIC ELECTRICAL PRINCIPLES

The fundamental purpose of a permanent pacemaker system is to stimulate the heart chambers to contract using the minimum energy while optimizing pulse generator longevity. An understanding and optimal use of pacemaker systems requires an appreciation for the basic principles of electricity (Table 5-3.)

The fundamental biophysical law which governs electrical pacing is Ohm's law, formulated by the German physicist Georg Simon Ohm (1787–1854):

$$V = I \times R \qquad \text{(Eq 1)}$$

where V is the *electromotive force* or *voltage* that drives current flow (measured in *volts*), I is the magnitude of the *current* which flows (measured in *amperes*), and R is the *resistance* to current flow (measured in *ohms* (Ω)). One ampere is a unit of electrical current produced by one volt acting through a resistance of one ohm.

Other commonly used parameters include *charge* and *energy*. Charge (measured in *amperes-hour* or *Coulombs*) is defined as the product of current (I) and time (t):

$$Charge = I \times t \qquad \text{(Eq 2)}$$

Energy (measured in *joules*) is defined as the product of voltage (V) and charge ($I \times t$):

$$Energy = V \times I \times t \qquad \text{(Eq 3)}$$

TABLE 5-2. Indications for implantation of permanent pacemakers

Condition	Indicated	Uncertain or Possible Indication	Not Indicated
Acquired AV block in adults	Third degree AV block, permanent or intermittent, at any anatomic level, associated with any one of the following conditions: 1) bradycardia with symptoms presumed to be due to AV block; 2) arrhythmias and other medical conditions that require drugs that result in symptomatic bradycardia; 3) documented periods of asystole ≥ 3.0 sec or any escape rate < 40/min in awake, symptom-free patients; 4) after catheter ablation of the AV junction (permanent pacing as a planned part of the treatment); 5) postoperative AV block that is not expected to resolve; 6) neuromuscular diseases with AV block such as myotonic muscular dystrophy, Kearns-Sayre syndrome, Erb's dystrophy (limb-girdle), and peroneal muscular atrophy. Second degree AV block, permanent or intermittent, regardless of the type or site of block, with symptomatic bradycardia.	Asymptomatic third degree AV block, permanent or intermittent, at any anatomic sight, with ventricular rates of 40/min or faster. Asymptomatic type II second degree AV block, permanent or intermittent. Asymptomatic type I second degree AV block at intra-His or infra-His levels found incidentally at EP testing performed for other indications. First degree AV block with symptoms suggestive of pacemaker syndrome and documented alleviation of symptoms with temporary AV pacing. Marked first degree AV block (≥ 300 ms) in patients with LV dysfunction and symptoms of congestive heart failure in whom a shorter AV interval results in hemodynamic improvement, presumably by decreasing left atrial filling pressure	Asymptomatic first degree AV block (see section on bifascicular and trifascicular block). Asymptomatic type I second degree AV block at the supra-His (AV node) level, or not known to be intra- or infra-Hisian. AV block expected to resolve and unlikely to recur (e.g., drug toxicity, Lyme disease).

AV, atrioventricular; EP, electrophysiology; ICD, implantable cardioverter-defibrillator; LV, left ventricular; SA, sinoatrial; SVT, supraventricular tachycardia; VT, ventricular tachycardia. Adapted from [23].

TABLE 5-2. Indications for implantation of permanent pacemakers

Condition	Indicated	Uncertain or Possible Indication	Not Indicated
Chronic bifascicular or trifascicular block	Intermittent third degree AV block. Type II second degree AV block.	Syncope not proved to be due to AV block when other likely causes have been excluded, specifically VT. Incidental finding of prolonged HV interval ($\geq$ 100 ms) during EP testing in asymptomatic patients. Incidental finding of non-physiological, pacing-induced infra-His block during EP testing.	Fascicular block without AV block or symptoms. Fascicular block with first degree AV block without symptoms.
After acute phase of myocardial infarction	Persistent second degree AV block in the His-Purkinje system with bilateral bundle branch block or third degree AV block within or below the His-Purkinje system after acute myocardial infarction. Transient second or third degree infra-nodal AV block and associated bundle branch block. Persistent and symptomatic second or third degree AV block at the level of the AV node.	Persistent second or third degree AV block at the level of the AV node.	Transient AV block in the absence of intraventricular conduction defects. Transient AV block in the presence of isolated left anterior fascicular block. Acquired left anterior fascicular block in the absence of AV block. Persistent first degree AV block in the presence of old (or age indeterminate) bundle branch block.

AV, atrioventricular; EP, electrophysiology; ICD, implantable cardioverter-defibrillator; LV, left ventricular; SA, sinoatrial; SVT, supraventricular tachycardia; VT, ventricular tachycardia. Adapted from [23].

TABLE 5-2. Indications for implantation of permanent pacemakers

Condition	Indicated	Uncertain or Possible Indication	Not Indicated
SA node dysfunction	SA node dysfunction with documented symptomatic bradycardia, including frequent sinus pauses that produce symptoms. In some patients, bradycardia may be a consequence of essential long-term drug therapy for which there is no acceptable alternatives.	SA node dysfunction occurring spontaneously or as a result of necessary drug therapy, with heart rate < 40 beats/min when a clear association between significant symptoms consistent with bradycardia and the actual presence of bradycardia has not been documented.	SA node dysfunction in asymptomatic patients, including those in whom substantial sinus bradycardia (heart rate ≤ 40 beats/min) is a consequence of long-term drug therapy.
	Symptomatic chronotropic incompetence.	In minimally symptomatic patients with chronic heart rate < 30 beats/min while awake.	SA node dysfunction in patients with symptoms suggestive of bradycardia that are clearly documented as not associated with a slow heart rate.
			SA node dysfunction with symptomatic bradycardia due to essential drug therapy.
Dilated cardiomyopathy	Indications as per SA node dysfunction or AV block (see above).	Symptomatic, drug-refractory dilated cardiomyopathy with prolonged P-R interval when acute hemodynamic studies have demonstrated hemodynamic benefit of pacing.	Asymptomatic dilated cardiomyopathy.
			Symptomatic dilated cardiomyopathy when patients are rendered asymptomatic by drug therapy.
			Symptomatic ischemic cardiomyopathy.
Post-cardiac transplantation	Indications as per SA node dysfunction or AV block (see above).	Symptomatic bradyarrhythmias/chronotropic incompetence that, although transient, may persist for months and require intervention.	Asymptomatic bradyarrhythmias following cardiac transplantation.

AV, atrioventricular; EP, electrophysiology; ICD, implantable cardioverter-defibrillator; LV, left ventricular; SA, sinoatrial; SVT, supraventricular tachycardia; VT, ventricular tachycardia. Adapted from [23].

TABLE 5-2. Indications for implantation of permanent pacemakers

Condition	Indicated	Uncertain or Possible Indication	Not Indicated
Hypersensitive carotid sinus and neurovascular syndromes	Recurrent syncope caused by carotid sinus stimulation; minimal carotid sinus pressure induces ventricular asystole of at least 3 sec duration in the absence of any medication that depresses the SA node or AV conduction.	Recurrent syncope without clear, provocative events and with a hypersensitive cardioinhibitory response.	A hyperactive cardioinhibitory response to carotid sinus stimulation in the absence of symptoms.
		Syncope of unexplained origin when major abnormalities of SA node function or AV conduction are discovered or provoked during EP testing.	A hyperactive cardioinhibitory response to carotid sinus stimulation in the presence of vague symptoms of dizziness, light-headedness, or both.
		Neurally-mediated syncope with significant bradycardia reproduced by head-up tilt with or without isoproterenol or other provocative maneuvers.	Recurrent syncope, light-headedness, or dizziness in the absence of a hyperactive cardioinhibitory response
			Situational vasovagal syncope in which avoidance behavior is effective.
Overdrive pacing to terminate tachycardias	Symptomatic recurrent SVT that is reproducibly terminated by pacing after drug therapy and catheter ablation has failed to control the arrhythmia or produce intolerable side effects.	Recurrent SVT or atrial flutter that is reproducibly terminated by pacing as an alternative to drug therapy or ablation.	Tachycardias frequently accelerated or converted to fibrillation by pacing.
	Symptomatic recurrent sustained VT as part of an ICD system.		The presence of accessory pathways with the capacity for rapid anterograde conduction whether or not the pathways participate in the mechanism of the tachycardia.

AV, atrioventricular; EP, electrophysiology; ICD, implantable cardioverter-defibrillator; LV, left ventricular; SA, sinoatrial; SVT, supraventricular tachycardia; VT, ventricular tachycardia. Adapted from [23].

TABLE 5-2. Indications for implantation of permanent pacemakers

Condition	Indicated	Uncertain or Possible Indication	Not Indicated
Prevention of tachycardia	Sustained pause-dependent VT, with or without prolonged QT, in which the efficacy of pacing is thoroughly documented.	High-risk patients with congenital long QT syndrome.	Frequent or complex ventricular ectopic activity without sustained VT in the absence of the long QT syndrome.
		AV reentrant or AV node reentrant SVT not responsive to medical or ablative therapy.	Long QT syndrome due to reversible causes.
		Prevention of symptomatic or drug-refractory recurrent atrial fibrillation.	
Hypertrophic cardiomyopathy	Indications as per SA node dysfunction or AV block (see above).	Medically refractory, symptomatic hypertrophic cardiomyopathy with significant resting or provoked LV outflow obstruction.	Asymptomatic or medically-controlled patients.
			Symptomatic patients without evidence of LV outflow obstruction.

AV, atrioventricular; EP, electrophysiology; ICD, implantable cardioverter-defibrillator; LV, left ventricular; SA, sinoatrial; SVT, supraventricular tachycardia; VT, ventricular tachycardia. Adapted from [23].

TABLE 5-3. Basic electrical parameters and relationships

Parameter	Description
EMF or Voltage (V)	Electromotive force which is the force driving the current to flow. The magnitude of the EMF is a function of the chemicals and electrochemical reaction occurring within the battery. Measured in volts.
Current (I)	The flow of charge in response to a driving voltage or potential difference. Measured in amperes.
Resistance (R) or Impedance	The resistance to flow of current measured in ohms (Ω). According to Ohm's law, current flow is directly proportional to the driving voltage and inversely proportional to the resistance of the pathway through which the current flows ($I = V/R$). The terms resistance and impedance can generally used interchangeably in electrical systems based on direct current.
Charge (Q)	The quantity of electricity that has flowed (or is available to flow) in a unit time (= $I \times t$). Charge is the consumable component, analogous to the quantity of water in a reservoir; after it flows out of the reservoir (battery) and consumed it is no longer available for further use. Measure in ampere-hours (coulombs). A *coulomb* is a unit of charge equal to 6×10^{18} electrons.
Capacitance (C)	The *farad* is the unit of capacitance. The capacitance measures the ability of a capacitor to store charge. Capacitance is defined as the ratio of the charge to voltage ($F = C/V$). A capacitor is essentially two conducting plates separated by an insulator. Given a particular conductor, insulator, and insulator thickness, the capacitance is proportional to the surface area of the plates. To increase the charge stored by a capacitor, one can either increase the surface area (to produce more capacitance) or increase the voltage across the capacitor plates.
Energy (E)	Energy is commonly expressed in joules. A joule is the energy of an electrical pulse with a duration of one second with an amplitude of one volt and one ampere ($E = V \times I \times t$). This formula is exactly accurate for steady voltages and currents, but is only an approximation when they are changing throughout the pulse. It is precise for rectangular waveforms, but not for capacitive discharge waveforms.
Voltage or Current Gradient	The *electric field* (or *voltage gradient*) is defined as voltage difference per distance, expressed in volts/cm. The analogous unit for current is the *current gradient* or *current density,* expressed in units of current per area, e.g., mA/cm^2.

While the words "*impedance*" and "resistance" are often used interchangeably, strictly speaking the term "resistance" is used to describe the impedance of an electrical circuit that has no energy storage capability. Resistance is the property of an electrical conductor by which it opposes flow of electricity and dissipates electrical energy away from the electric circuit, usually as heat. In direct current circuits lacking capacitors or inductors, impedance and resistance are identical. In an alternating current circuit, impedance is not only a function of the resistance (which is a property of the conductor), but also of any inductance and capacitance in the circuit (this is because inductors and

A. Relationship Between Voltage & Current Flow

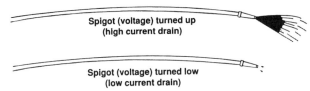

Spigot (voltage) turned up
(high current drain)

Spigot (voltage) turned low
(low current drain)

B. Relationship Between Resistance & Current Flow

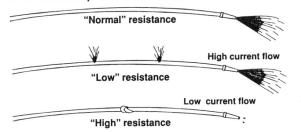

"Normal" resistance

High current flow

"Low" resistance

Low current flow

"High" resistance

FIGURE 5-1. Relationship between voltage, resistance, and current. Panel A: Using the garden hose analogy, the higher the voltage (the greater the pushing force), the greater the current flow (flow of water). The higher the current flow the greater the rate of battery depletion. Panel B: If the garden hose has holes in it, the resistance to flow is reduced and current (water) is lost through the hose at locations other than at the nozzle. This results in high current flow and premature battery drainage. Conversely, if there is a high resistance, such as a conductor break, the current will be very low or absent. In the absence of adequate current, the myocardial threshold for activation will not be reached. Courtesy of Medtronic, Inc.

capacitors build-up voltages that oppose current flow). In a pacemaker or implantable defibrillator system the resistive factors within the circuit include the lead conductor resistance, the resistance between the electrode and the myocardium, and the polarization resistance, which is the resistance to current flow that results from the accumulation of charges of opposite polarity in the myocardium at the electrode-tissue interface. Because of these complex multiple resistive elements (and small capacitive components), the use of the term "impedance" is most appropriate when describing the sum of all resistances to current flow within a pacing or implantable defibrillation system.

The interrelationship of the three components, voltage, current, and the total resistance (impedance), can be likened to the flow of water through a hose (Figure 5-1). Voltage represents the force by which current (water) is delivered through a hose (lead) with total resistance (impedance) represented by the nozzle (the electrode and electrode-tissue interface) and the tubing (the lead conductor). The crucial resistance in any pacemaker system is the series resistance contained within the lead system and lead-tissue interface. In cases of a lead insulation break, a second *parallel* resistance will develop within the system. Because resistance to current flow through the insulation break to biological tissues will be low, usually much lower than the resistance within the lead and lead-tissue interface system itself (usually 300 – 1200 Ω), current flow is shunted from its intended target, the myocardium, to non-cardiac tissues through the insulation break. This may result in failure of the current stimulus to activate the target cardiac tissue because this battery charge is "lost" through the low-resistance shunt of the insulation break. The insulation break may also result in high current drainage from the battery through the parallel low resistance, causing rapid battery depletion. An insulation break can cause the measured impedance to decrease to below 300 Ω. In the case of a conductor break, pacing impedance will be very high. While this decreases the rate of battery drainage, the very low (or non-existent) current flow may prevent activation of the myocardium. With a conductor break the measured impedance may increase to above 2000 Ω or become infinite.

5.3.2 COMPONENTS OF IMPLANTABLE PACING SYSTEMS

Transvenous permanent pacemaker systems consist of a pulse generator, which is designed to be replaceable, and an insulated wire or lead, which is designed to function indefinitely (Figure 5-2). Within the pulse generator case or "can" is the microelectronic circuit board which contains one or more CMOS (complementary metal-oxide semiconductor) chip(s) and other circuit components including resistors and capacitors. The solid-state semiconductor circuitry makes modern pulse generators extremely reliable with a very low incidence of device failures. In addition, the complex logic capabilities of advanced semiconductors permits the extensive programmability of today's pacemakers.

Two kinds of electrical behavior can be exhibited by a pulse generator, *constant current* and *constant voltage* behavior. The pacemaker pulse generator discharges through two resistances in series – an internal resistance within the pulse generator and an external resistance (the pacing electrode and lead), termed the *load*. In the constant current system, the internal resistance is much higher than the external resistance. Therefore, variability in the load has little effect on the overall system resistance and therefore little effect on

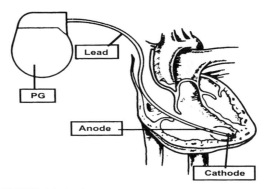

FIGURE 5-2. Basic components of a permanent pacing system include a pulse generator (PG) which contains the battery and a microelectronic circuit board and an insulated pacing lead (bipolar or unipolar) with the electrode(s) at the tip.

the magnitude of current. In other words, current remains fairly constant over a relatively wide range of external resistances (severe increases in lead resistance such as occurs with a lead fracture will, of course, severely reduce current flow). Constant current pulse generators are most commonly used in temporary pacing systems in which the external resistance often varies because of differences in the non-standardized lead systems utilized for temporary pacing. Presently, all available implantable pulse generators are constant voltage sources. These devices have a low internal resistance so that the external load will contribute a much larger percentage to the overall total resistance of the system. In this case, changes in lead resistance will have a much larger effect on current flow with current varying directly with lead resistance in accordance with Ohm's Law.

The critical component of the pacing system is the *pacing wire* or *pacing lead* (Figure 5-3). The essential components of a pacing lead are: 1) *conductor*; 2) *connector pin*; 3) *insulation*; 4) *electrode*; 5) *lead assembly*. The metallic portion of the lead which contacts the heart tissue and through which the stimulating current is delivered is the *electrode* (Figure 5-3). The lead and electrode(s) must function to deliver current efficiently and indefinitely; therefore, they must possess certain properties and characteristics.

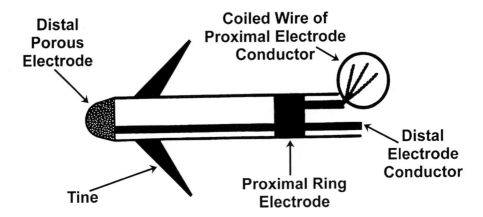

FIGURE 5-3. Anatomy of a bipolar lead. Most modern leads used are bipolar and consist of a porous-tip electrode and a proximal-positioned ring electrode. The coiled-wire co-axial *conductors* for these electrodes run the length of the lead and are each covered by an *insulator*. The dual conductors in the core are then covered by a outer insulator, usually polyurethane or silicone. Unipolar leads generally have a smaller diameter lead body than bipolar leads because they contain only a single conductor coil

The *conductor* is a very thin wire that carries electrical impulses from the pulse generator to the distal tip electrode for pacing and carries intracardiac signals from the tip electrode to the pulse generator for sensing. The conductor is commonly constructed using a metal alloy (often containing combinations of iridium, cobalt, iron, chromium, molybdenum, nickel, silver, or manganese) with a very low resistance to current flow, permitting efficient transfer of current from the pulse generator to the tip electrode. Most commonly, nickel or nickel-silver alloys are used for the conductor, not only because they provide a relatively low resistance pathway, but also because they are durable, flexible, and resistant to corrosion. In general, there are three types of conductors: 1) *unifilar*; 2) *multifilar*; 3) *cable*. A unifilar conductor is a single wire coil that is wound around a central axis in a spiral manner. Coiling the wire helps to facilitate flexibility without breakage. A multifilar conductor consists of two or more wire coils that are wound in parallel together around a central axis in a spiral manner. This construction helps to reduce impedance in the conductor and builds in redundancy if a filar were to fracture. A cable conductor consists of two or more wires that are twisted together as a strand and then bundled with other strands around each other like a rope. Today, most leads use multifilar construction ensuring that if there is a fracture of one or more of the filaments, the remaining intact filaments will permit continued lead function. However, in this situation, intermittent sensing and pacing may occur heralding a potential lead failure.

Leads are constructed as *unipolar*, *bipolar* or *multipolar* depending upon the number of separate conductors included in the lead. Although unipolar leads are not commonly used today, almost all of those manufactured use a multifilar design with a multifilar coil surrounded by insulation. Unipolar leads have the advantage of a small diameter, less rigid lead body. Bipolar leads are generally manufactured using a *co-axial* construction in which an insulated layer is positioned between two concentric multifilar conductor coils. Rarely, some bipolar leads are manufactured using a *co-radial* construction (also called parallel-wound) whereby two insulated coils are wound next to each other. Other uncommon construction designs include parallel coil design in which two separately coiled insulated conductors lie parallel to each other and to the long axis of the lead body. In addition some leads are manufactured with a combination of these various designs. Historically, bipolar leads have had larger diameters than unipolar leads. However, the introduction of coaxial conductor designs, along with advanced insulation technology and smaller conductor coils and cables, there has been a dramatic reduction in the diameter of bipolar leads. Also, the additional conductor coil and added insulation tends to make bipolar leads slightly stiffer than unipolar leads.

Both unipolar and bipolar pacing leads require a tip electrode (*cathode*, negatively-charged) and an indifferent electrode (*anode*, positively-charged) to complete the electrical circuit. In unipolar construction, the single conductor carries the pacing stimulus to the tip electrode that is in contact with the myocardium, while in a bipolar design, one of the two conductors carries the pacing stimulus to the tip electrode. The primary difference between unipolar and bipolar leads is in the location of the indifferent electrode (Figure 5-4). With a unipolar lead, cardiac tissue, body tissue, and body fluid conducts the electrical current from the cathode (tip electrode) to the anode (pacemaker case or "can"). Pacing and sensing is performed between these two distant electrodes. With a bipolar lead, the second conductor conducts the electrical current from the cathode (tip electrode) to adjacent ring electrode (anode) (Figure 5-3). In a bipolar system, both the

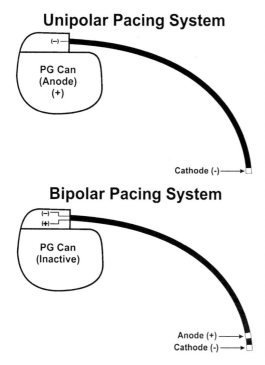

Unipolar Pacing System

Bipolar Pacing System

FIGURE 5-4. Comparison between unipolar and bipolar pacing systems. During unipolar pacing only the cathode is in contact with heart tissue. Current flows from the cathode electrode in the heart to the pulse generator (PG) which functions as the anode. During unipolar pacing the stimulus artifact is large in amplitude. During bipolar pacing both the cathode and the anode are in contact with heart tissue. Current flows from the cathode to the immediately adjacent anode resulting in a stimulus artifact which is of small magnitude. The PG can is electrically inactive in a bipolar pacing system. The unipolar system has lower resistance than the bipolar system because of the larger surface area of the anode in the unipolar system. This results in a slightly higher voltage stimulation threshold in a bipolar system compared with a unipolar system. The amplitude of the atrial and ventricular electrograms measured by a unipolar system is the same as that measured by the bipolar system. However, the unipolar system, because of the wide electrode spacing, is more sensitive to far-field signals, potentially permitting detection of stimulus artifacts from adjacent cardiac chambers.

cathode and anode are closely adjacent and reside intracardiac. In a unipolar system, the cathode and anode are located far apart and only the cathode is positioned endocardially. Sensing by a unipolar lead system may result in detection of far-field voltage signals such as external *electromagnetic interference* (*EMI*) or internal somatic muscle activity (*myopotentials*). This *oversensing* may result in failure to deliver a pacing stimulus. Furthermore, since the current of the pacing stimulus in a unipolar system flows from the cathode (in the heart) to the pulse generator case (usually located in the left subclavian region), skeletal muscle within this pathway may be stimulated to contract, often with uncomfortable consequences for the patient. The main advantage to bipolar leads is the much-reduced risk of oversensing (because of the immediately adjacent paired electrodes). In addition, bipolar leads are associated with a significant decline in the skeletal muscle or phrenic nerve stimulation because of the smaller electrical field (tip-to-ring compared to tip-to-case).

The lead connector functions to provide an attachment point between the lead conductor(s) and the connector block of the pulse generator. A high precision mechanical fit between the connector pin and the connector port in the connector block is crucial for reliable transmission of current from the pulse generator to the cathode without leakage or loss. Fortunately device manufacturers have agreed upon a single standard for the dimensions of lead connector pins, termed *IS-1* (Figure 5-5). The International Organization for Standardization and the International Electrotechnical Commission jointly developed this connector standard in 1992. Leads conforming to this standard will fit the connector port of any device with a connector block manufactured in accordance with this standard. Both bipolar and unipolar IS-1 lead connectors are 3.2 mm in diameter and have sealing rings and a short connector pin. Sealing rings assure reliable insulation of the pacing lead electrical connection from surrounding body tissues and fluids. Unipolar and bipolar leads are labeled IS-1 UNI and IS-1 BI, respectively. For older, chronically implanted leads, special adapters may be required to connect the old leads to a replacement generator, unless the vendor has specifically manufactured a connector block with connector ports to fit those leads.

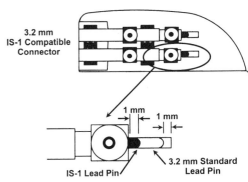

FIGURE 5-5. Schematic diagram illustrating IS-1 lead pin and connector block. See text for details. Courtesy of Guidant/CPI, Inc.

The lead insulator is a non-conducting material that prevents electrical current from escaping into the tissue surrounding the lead. Insulation also protects the conductor from corrosion due to exposure to body fluids and tissues. Insulation materials all possess a number of properties that make them more or less attractive as useful lead insulators: 1) *tensile strength*; 2) *elongation*; 3) *tear strength*; 4) *abrasion*; 5) *compression set*; 6) *crush*; 7) *creep*. Tensile strength refers to the force necessary to cause the material to break. Elongation is the amount of stretch that occurs before a material breaks. Tear strength represents the force necessary to cause a material to tear. In general, once a material is nicked or has a small tear, it is very easy for the tear to progress. Abrasion means the wearing away (scrapping) of material caused by frictional forces created due to adjacent objects sliding against each other. Compression set refers to the permanent deformation of a material after being subjected to compressive forces over time. Compression set is usually manifested by localized areas of thinning of the lead insulation. Crush is the resistance to rupture as a material is compressed between two objects. In the case of the pacing lead, the resistance to crush becomes important when a lead is implanted using a subclavian intravenous access between the clavicle and first rib. Creep, also known as stretch, is the time-dependent dimensional change (usually thinning) due to movement or flow of a polymer under load. Creep most often occurs if there is any excessive stretching of the lead.

Silicone and *polyurethane* are the most commonly used insulation materials for implantable pacing leads. Silicone is a soft, highly flexible material that has been used as a pacing lead insulator for more than 30 years. It is widely used for both the outer and inner insulator in many of the leads manufactured worldwide. Polyurethane is firmer and stiffer than silicone and has been used for more than 20 years. Silicone has the advantages of being inert (chemically inactive), biocompatible (does not induce an inflammatory reaction), and biostable (material remains unchanged *in vivo*). The disadvantages of silicone are that it has a high coefficient of friction (it's "sticky"), making it more prone to abrasion, nicks, tears, and surface wear (although, unlike polyurethane, silicone nicks and tears can be repaired with medical adhesive). Furthermore, silicone leads generally need to be constructed with a slightly larger diameter than equivalent polyurethane leads because it has a lower tear strength (a thicker coat of insulation is required to provide equivalent resistance to tears). Platinum-cured silicone rubber, characterized by improved mechanical strength, has partially alleviated the problems of low tear strength and high friction coefficient. Polyurethane has the advantages of being biocompatible, having a low coefficient of friction, and high tear strength. Consequently, polyurethane leads can generally be manufactured with a smaller cross-sectional diameter. Unique disadvantages of polyurethane include its tendency to develop *environmental stress cracking* and *metal ion oxidation*. Environmental stress cracking refers to cracking of the polyurethane insulation caused by the hostile *in vivo* environment. Metal ion oxidation results from the interaction of macrophage-induced peroxides with metal ions from the conductor, producing a mixture that works to destroy the polyurethane insulation. Historically, polyurethane leads have not performed as well as silicone leads due to environmental stress cracking and metal-induced oxidation.

The purpose of the pacing lead electrode(s) is to both deliver a stimulus to the myocardium as well as detect (*sense*) intracardiac signals. In essence, the electrode(s) act as the long-term interface between the lead and the myocardium. The goal of electrode design is to produce electrodes resulting in low, stable pacing thresholds associated with a high pacing impedance to enhance longevity (minimize current flow). In addition, ideal lead design will ensure optimal sensing of intrinsic cardiac signals, while minimizing interference from non-cardiac electrical signals. Electrode design features that impact electrical characteristics and performance include the: 1) *fixation mechanism*; 2) *polarity*; 3) *surface material*; 4) *size*; 5) *surface structure*; 6) *steroid elution*.

The fixation mechanism provides the means to stabilize the electrode to the moving endocardium. Ideally the electrode should contact the endocardium so as to provide stable contact, with little induced myocardial trauma, and producing minimal local inflammatory and fibrotic reaction. A lead utilizing a *passive fixation* (Figure 5-6) mechanism means that no part of the lead itself is actually embedded in the endocardium. Rather the lead tip is trapped in the trabeculae and/or held in position by its pre-formed shape. The most successful passive mechanism involves *tines* or "fins" to "catch" trabeculi in the heart. In the right atrium, only the appendage is trabeculated. Consequently use of a passive fixation mechanism in the atrium requires the presence of an atrial appendage and the use of a tined pre-formed "J" shaped lead. *Active fixation* (Figure 5-6) means that a part of the lead is actually embedded in the endocardium, providing a secure attachment. The most common active fixation mechanism involves a "corkscrew" shaped screw-in helix electrode. Two types of screw-in mechanisms are available, a *fixed-screw* lead and an *extendible/retractable* screw-in lead. With the fixed-screw type, the screw is always protruding and the lead body must be rotated in a clockwise fashion to advance the fixed screw into the myocardium. To minimize problems associated with advancing a lead

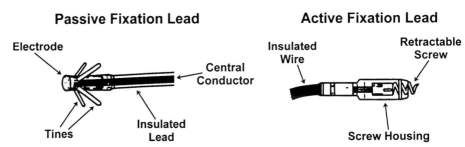

FIGURE 5-6. Two types of transvenous permanent pacemaker leads are available. Passive fixation leads have tines which provide a structural framework to which can attach fibrous tissue to provide a long-lasting firm attachment of the lead to the endocardial surface. In actuality passive leads delay the lead fixation process until fibrous ingrowth has occurred. With active fixation leads, a corkscrew-shaped device is used to "screw" the lead-tip into the endocardium. Some manufacturers have a screw which can retract into a housing, while other manufacturers have a non-retractable screw which is covered by a soluble material (usually a rapidly dissolving sugar such as mannitol) which encapsulates and protects the screw until it is uncovered a few minutes after the lead has been positioned in the heart. The screw may also function as the electrode, although more commonly the actual electrode (usually a porous tip electrode) is positioned proximal to the screw and contacts the endocardium after the screw is advanced into the tissue.

with a protruding screw through the vascular structures and the tricuspid valve apparatus, a sugar (usually mannitol) "shroud" initially covers the screw. After introduction of the lead into the vascular system, the sugar begins to dissolve, eventually exposing the screw. The time required for dissolution of the sugar coating is usually sufficient to provide adequate time to pass the lead into the right atrium or ventricle. With the extendible/retractable screw-in lead, on the other hand, the screw is initially retracted within a housing. Therefore, the screw is "hidden" as the lead is advanced into the heart. After the lead tip is positioned, the screw can be extended using a special tool that comes with the lead. Active fixation leads are usually required for patients lacking a right atrial appendage (secondary to cardiac surgery) or well developed trabeculae in the appendage or right ventricle. In addition, if the operator desires to position the electrode at an atypical position outside the atrial appendage or the right ventricular apex, an active fixation lead is generally recommended.

The choice of polarity can have a significant effect on electrical performance characteristics. As already discussed (see above), the lead size, the amplitude of the stimulus artifact, and the risk of inappropriate stimulation of skeletal muscle or nerves are different in unipolar lead systems compared with bipolar systems. While stimulation threshold is not significantly affected by polarity, sensing is superior in bipolar systems compared with unipolar systems. Bipolar leads can sense cardiac depolarization with greater accuracy and bipolar systems are less likely to sense electrical signals from outside the heart, such as from skeletal muscle or from electromagnetic interference. In addition, bipolar atrial leads are much less susceptible to far-field R-wave sensing from ventricular depolarization. Finally, bipolar lead systems have built in redundancy and provide programming flexibility. If a conductor fractures in a bipolar lead system, programming to a unipolar configuration provides an option to preserve lead function. A unipolar system can only be programmed to the unipolar mode and lacks conductor redundancy.

Surface material also is an important design feature in pacemaker electrodes. Many electrically conductive materials have been used for the surface material of electrodes. Platinum and activated carbon are used extensively in modern lead electrodes because they are corrosion resistant, biocompatible, and exhibit low polarization properties. Surface corrosion and inflammatory reactions directed against the electrode can compromise the stability of electrode performance. Polarization is the build-up of opposite charges on the electrode surface that opposes current flow through the electrode into the surrounding myocardial tissues (see below). Some electrode materials exhibit more polarization at the electrode surface than other materials.

Electrode size can have important implications for electrode performance and pacing system longevity. Reducing the geometric electrode surface area is associated with an increase of the pacing impedance (Figure 5-7). Pacing impedance is the resistance to current flow from the pulse generator to the myocardial tissue and is inversely proportional to current drain. Increased impedance at the tip electrode delivers energy more efficiently, thus allowing lower output voltage settings to ensure myocardial capture (Figure 5-8). The higher the impedance during pacing, the lower the rate of current drain from the battery; a reduced rate of current drainage translates into a longer battery life. The average geometric surface area of electrodes has decreased significantly over the past few years. In the past, it was common

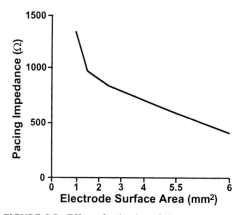

FIGURE 5-7. Effect of reduction of electrode size on pacing impedance. See text for details. Courtesy of Medtronic, Inc.

for pacing electrodes to have a geometric surface area of approximately 50 mm². Current electrodes have a geometric surface area of 1.2 – 8 mm².

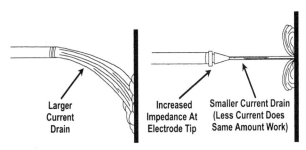

FIGURE 5-8. Schematic diagram illustrating the relationship between impedance of the pacing electrode and current flow. See text for details. Courtesy of Medtronic, Inc.

While reducing electrode size increases pacing impedance, it also increases polarization at the electrode surface (Figure 5-9), mitigating the advantages of size reduction on pacing impedance. When an electrical current flows, the electrode (cathode) attracts positively charged ions. Initially, the movements of these positive charges result in the flow of current from the electrode to the myocardium. As the current pulse continues, a layer of charge surrounds the tip electrode and produces a capacitative effect. This polarization impedes current flow from the electrode into the tissue. If polarization is excessive, a substantial amount of lead current is required merely tó overcome the resistance to current flow, meaning less current is available for activation of the myocardium. Consequently, the output voltage must be increased to deliver an adequate stimulation current, a maneuver that may shorten battery life. Figure 5-10 summarizes the advantages of optimizing electrode size and surface structure.

Changing the surface structure of the electrode can counter a high electrode polarization. Commonly, the electrode surface is made more porous (Figure 5-3), which also increases the geometric surface area of the electrode and reduces polarization. The collective spaces within a platinized porous electrode make up the larger functional surface area, which minimizes the polar-

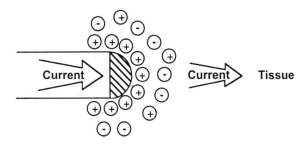

FIGURE 5-9. Schematic diagram illustrating mechanism of electrode polarization. Polarization increases as electrode surface area decreases. See text for details. Courtesy of Medtronic, Inc.

ization potential of the geometrically smaller electrode (more of the output voltage appears at the stimulating electrode). Porous electrodes also enhance sensing because the larger functional surface area provides more electrode area for sensing. Finally, tissue in-growth within the porous structure stabilizes electrode position, ensuring reliable electrode-myocardial contact.

The final feature that can dramatically effect acute and chronic lead performance is the incorporation of steroid elution in the lead design (Figure 5-11). Steroid-eluting electrodes provide a continuous elution of tiny doses of dexamethasone from a silicone rubber binder. Steroid elution limits the inflammatory process at the electrode-tissue interface. As a result of the decreased inflammatory response, there is less fibrous reaction around the tip electrode. Some manufacturers coat the electrode with a steroid mixture rather than providing a steroid matrix for constant elution. While the benefits of the latter approach are well established, it is not clear if the former approach is equally beneficial on pacing thresholds. Steroid elution has been shown to prevent the typical post-implant increase in pacing threshold and reduce the level

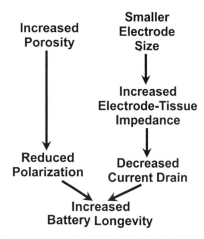

FIGURE 5-10. Battery longevity is enhanced by reducing the size and increasing the porosity of pacing electrodes. See text for further discussion. Courtesy of Medtronic, Inc.

of chronic pacing thresholds compared to conventional smooth metal electrodes (Figure 5-12). Steroid eluting leads may also improve chronic sensing by minimizing development of a fibrous cap around the electrode tip. Steroid elution, particularly when used in conjunction with porous electrodes, can significantly improve long-term sensing, especially in low signal environments such as the atrium.

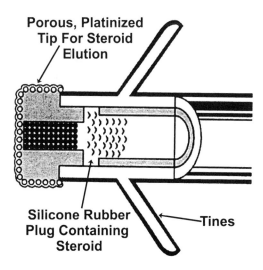

FIGURE 5-11. Steroid eluting leads are constructed with a dexamethasone-containing plug at the tip. Slow elution of the steroid inhibits inflammatory reaction at the tip limiting the post-implant acute increase in pacing threshold. Courtesy of Medtronic, Inc.

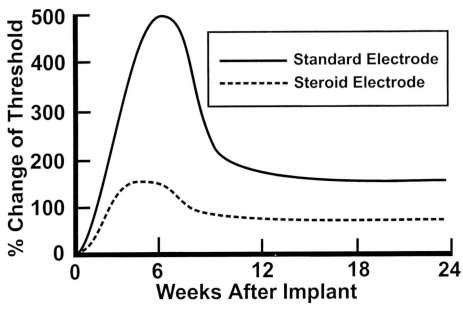

FIGURE 5-12. Acute and chronic rise in stimulation threshold following implantation of standard leads and steroid-eluting leads. Pacemaker leads manufactured with steroid-eluting electrodes result in a reduction in acute and chronic stimulation thresholds. See text for details.

5.3.3 CARDIAC ELECTRICAL STIMULATION

Cardiac stimulation by a pulse generator involves the passage of an electric current between the cathode (negative electrode) and anode (positive electrode) of the pacemaker system. The amplitude and duration of the current pulse (Figure 5-13) must be great enough to initiate a regenerative depolarization in the surrounding myocardium. If this results, "capture" of the chamber paced (atrium or ventricle) is said to have occurred. The "failure to capture" results if the duration and amplitude of the current pulse is not sufficient to reach the myocardial *threshold* for activation (Figure 5-14). In pacemaker systems the electromotive force for current flow resides within the *cell* or *battery*. Currently,

Programmable stimulation parameters:

☛ **Pulse Width**
☛ **Pulse amplitude**

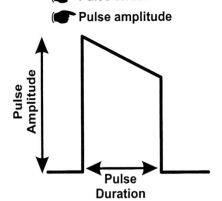

FIGURE 5-13. The stimulating "square-wave" current pulse from a pacemaker generator has a leading edge pulse amplitude and a pulse duration. Both parameters are programmable. See text for details.

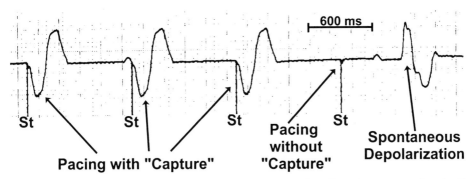

FIGURE 5-14. Pacing stimuli may or may not result in cardiac activation. Shown here, some pacing stimuli (St) result in capture of the ventricle, while another stimulus fails to trigger a ventricular depolarization.

pacemaker manufacturers use lithium iodine batteries to power pacemaker pulse generators.

A number of factors affect the pacing threshold of cardiac tissues (Table 5-4.) The pacing threshold rises within the first few weeks or months post-implant (acute phase). Subsequently, the pacing threshold declines to a stable level (chronic phase) which may remain steady for years or the lifetime of the lead (Figure 5-12). The maximum threshold achieved in the acute phase is correlated with the maximum local inflammation and size of the fibrous cap around the electrode ("virtual electrode") (Figure 5-15). The tim-

TABLE 5-4. Factors affecting cardiac stimulation threshold

Myocardial factors

Fibrosis or local area of scar or infarction (increases threshold)

Antiarrhythmic drugs (generally increase threshold)

Electrolyte imbalance (variable effect)

Lead/electrode factors

Maturity of electrode-tissue interface

Distance of electrode from excitable tissue (increased distance means higher threshold)

Unipolar versus bipolar electrode (unipolar electrode has slightly lower threshold (larger anode))

Electrode material and size (smaller electrodes result in lower threshold)

Electrode size (smaller size results in lower threshold)

Lead insulation (breaks in insulation result in current leaks and increases stimulation threshold)

Solid versus porous electrode (porous electrodes result in lower threshold)

Steroid leads (reduce acute and chronic threshold)

Lead fixation (lower early threshold with passive fixation leads)

Anodal or cathodal stimulus (lower threshold with cathodal stimulation)

ing and duration of the acute and chronic phase may be highly variable. Typically, this decline in chronic threshold is associated with a decline in the size of the virtual electrode as well as a reduction in the local inflammatory reaction. As mentioned above (Figure 5-11), the use of steroid-eluting leads results in a significant decline in the pacing threshold seen during both the acute and chronic phases. Potent Na^+ channel blocking drugs, such as flecainide, may increase the pacing threshold.

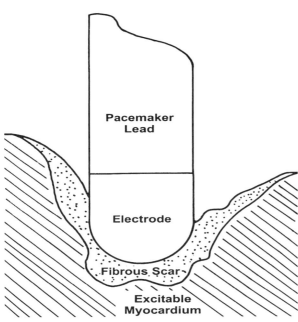

The cardiac stimulation threshold is defined as the minimal cathodal stimulus which is able to maintain consistent capture of the heart when delivered during late diastole. The strength-duration curve forms the basis for understanding the relationship between pulse duration and the cardiac stimulation threshold. The critical feature of this relation is that the threshold current, voltage, charge, and energy vary as a function of pulse duration, although not in linear fashion (Figure 5-16). An understanding of this relationship assists in optimal programming of the output parameters of pulse generators to ensure an adequate safety margin of stimulation without excessive and unnecessary battery drainage. The *rheobase* is the voltage or current stimulation threshold at an infinitely long pulse duration. For example, if the rheobase voltage is 2.0 V there will be no pulse width, no matter how long, which will result in tissue stimulation when output voltage is programmed to less than 2.0 V. The *chronaxie time* is the pulse duration at a voltage or current stimulation threshold twice the rheobase (Figure 5-17). Both the voltage and current thresholds decrease with an increase in pulse duration (Figure 5-17) reaching the rheobase value at a pulse duration of approximately 1.0 msec. Setting pulse duration greater than this value does not result in a significant further decline in the current or voltage threshold. Therefore, programming pulse width beyond values near rheobase will result in excessive battery drainage without reduction in threshold. The charge threshold steadily increases with an increase in pulse duration in almost a linear fashion (Figure 5-17). Charge ($I \times t$) threshold shares the most direct relationship to bat-

FIGURE 5-15. Schematic diagram on relationship between the pacemaker lead, electrode, and underlying fibrous and excitable tissue. The thickness of the fibrous scar "cap" overlying the electrode defines the extent of the virtual electrode

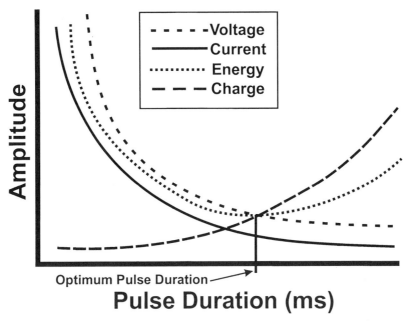

FIGURE 5-16. Schematic diagram illustrating strength-duration curves. The magnitude of energy, charge, voltage and current at the stimulation threshold are displayed as a function of pulse duration. The optimum pulse duration occurs at the lowest energy which generally occurs at a pulse duration of approximately 0.5 ms. Adapted from [46].

tery capacity (the battery is really nothing more than a reservoir of charge). Battery life will be longest when the minimal charge is expended to reach the pacing threshold. Energy (I x V x t) increases at very short and very long pulse widths. The energy threshold is at its minimum at a pulse duration of 0.4 - 0.5 ms. The optimal pulse duration is generally at the point of lowest energy which corresponds fairly closely to the chronaxie times (pulse duration at twice rheobase).

While measurement of threshold using charge, current, or energy is preferred, because pulse generators deliver constant voltage, only voltage threshold is easily obtainable. Construction of voltage threshold strength-duration curves involves determination of the voltage stimulation threshold at various pulse durations. The rheobase voltage can be approximated by programming the longest pulse width possible (generally 1.8 - 2.5 ms) and then finding the voltage stimulation threshold. Next, the chronaxie can be determined by doubling the rheobase voltage and then sequentially reducing the pulse width. The chronaxie time will be the pulse width at which rheobase voltage x 2 is the stimulation threshold. In general, the chronaxie time will normally be approximately 0.4 - 0.5 ms. Programming of very long pulse widths should be avoided if possible because they result in dramatic increases in pacing impedance (Figure 5-18). Electrical pacing using excessively long pulse widths results in more rapid battery depletion because of the increased charge required for threshold stimulation compared to shorter pulse widths (Figure 5-16).

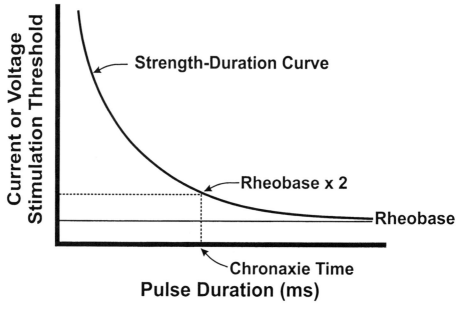

FIGURE 5-17. Schematic diagram of current or voltage strength-duration curve. The rheobase is the amplitude of the threshold stimulation voltage or current at an infinitely long pulse duration. The chronaxie time is
the pulse duration at a threshold stimulus which is double the amplitude of the rheobase. The chronaxie time
approximates the most efficient pulse duration for tissue stimulation. Adapted from [46].

For final settings, the pacemaker should *not* be programmed to the threshold voltage. Instead, a voltage increment, termed the *safety factor*, is added to the measured
threshold voltage so as to provide a margin for error in case the threshold voltage varies
over time, during a normal day-to-day activities, or changes in medications.

$$Safety\ Factor\ =\ \frac{Pulse\ Generator\ Output - Threshold\ Value}{Threshold\ Value}\ x\ 100$$

Immediately upon implantation the pulse generator voltage output should be programmed to five times the voltage threshold because the stimulation threshold may increase five-fold within the first one to two months after implantation (Figure 5-12). In
the chronic phase, the normal physiological variation in threshold is generally up to 50%.
Therefore, the pulse generator output in the case of a chronically implanted endocardial
lead should be programmed at twice the threshold value (100% safety factor).

Lithium iodine batteries are now routinely used in newly manufactured pacemaker
pulse generators. Lithium iodine batteries have a voltage of 2.8 V. The battery voltage
is dependent upon the chemistry of the half cells, and is independent of the physical size
of the battery. In order to provide outputs greater than 2.8 V, the pulse generator circuitry must include a voltage multiplier. The impact on battery longevity is significant,
sometimes reducing the battery life by half.

Lithium iodine cells have a characteristic rate of depletion with the output voltage
declining only gradually initially but more rapidly as it nears the time of replacement

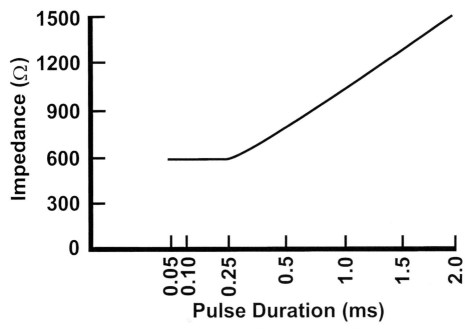

FIGURE 5-18. Pacing impedance increases dramatically with increases in pulse width. As seen here, impedance can more than double over the programmable pulse width options available in most pulse generators. Because shorter pulse widths produce cause much lower pacing impedances, shorter pulse widths are more efficient for stimulation. Adapted from [46].

(Figure 5-19). The *beginning-of-life* (*BOL*) output voltage of a new lithium iodine cell is approximately 2.8 V. As the battery is depleted the voltage declines and the internal resistance increases such that at battery *end-of-life* (*EOL*) the voltage is 1.8 V and the internal impedance increases dramatically. Manufacturers recommend replacement of the pulse generator before EOL. In general, the *elective replacement interval* (or *indicator*) (*ERI*) is at an output voltage of approximately 2.0 to 2.2 V.

The capacity of a battery is determined by the amount of charge it is capable of delivering. Everything else remaining constant, the larger the battery capacity the longer the battery life. A battery can be thought of as a reservoir of charge. When an electrical circuit is closed, the charge will flow from the reservoir because of the potential (voltage) difference. Charge will continue to flow until the reservoir is depleted. The amount of charge present in the reservoir at the beginning can be calculated by multiplying the rate of charge flow (current, I, in amperes) and the time required to deplete the reservoir (t, in hours). The *ampere-hour rating* of a battery reflects its charge capacity. The lithium iodine batteries in current use have a widely variable charge capacity ranging from approximately 0.8 to 3.5 ampere-hours with a resultant longevity ranging from four to 15 years. These numbers should be viewed as estimates only. In general, a battery may still contain charge but as output voltage and current falls with battery depletion the cell may become useless to operate the pulse generators basic circuitry. Therefore, especially in pacemakers with numerous advanced options requiring additional special circuitry and maintenance of stored data in memory, useful battery life may be significantly less than

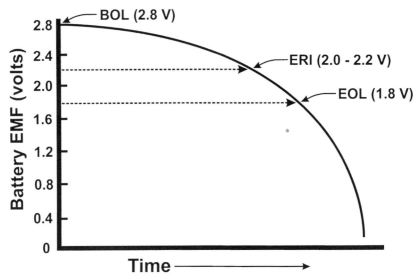

FIGURE 5-19. Schematic diagram illustrating battery depletion behavior of a lithium iodine battery. BOL, beginning of life; EMF, electromotive force; ERI, elective replacement indicator; EOL, end-of-life; V, volts.

predicted. A number of factors affect the longevity of a pulse generator battery (Table 5-5.) Pulse generator longevity can be estimated as follows:

$$\textit{Pulse Generator Longevity (in hours)} = \frac{\textit{Battery Capacity (in amperes-hours)}}{\textit{Continuous Battery Drainage (in amperes)}}$$

where continuous battery drainage is the amount of current required for the moment-to-moment sensing, pacing, miscellaneous circuit operation, and self-discharge. Most often

TABLE 5-5. Factors affecting battery longevity

Non-programmable factors

    Battery capacity and self-discharge

    Efficiency of pacing circuit

    Efficiency of sensing circuit

    Output impedance

Programmable factors

    Pacing rate

    Output voltage

    Duration of pulse width

    Proportion of time engaged in pacing

longevity is expressed in years which can be obtained by dividing the longevity in hours by 24 (hours/day) and 365 (days/year).

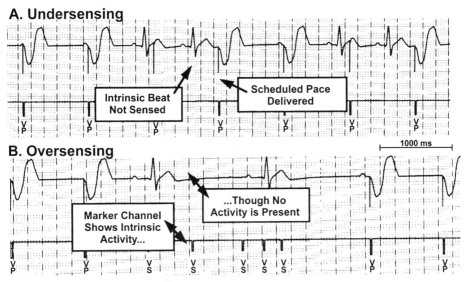

FIGURE 5-20. Comparison of undersensing (panel A) and oversensing (panel B). During undersensing an intrinsic beat is undetected by the pacemaker's sensing circuit, while during oversensing the sensing circuit detects non-cardiac electrical activity. See text for discussion. Courtesy of Medtronic, Inc.

5.3.4 SENSING OF CARDIAC SIGNALS

Normally, pacemakers are programmed to deliver a pacing impulse only if the heart fails to generate an intrinsic spontaneous depolarization. *Sensing* is the ability of the pacemaker system to detect or "see" when a native or spontaneous cardiac activation occurs. Accurate sensing ensures the pacemaker will not fail to detect a normal atrial or ventricular depolarization (*undersensing*), or will detect extracardiac electrical activity, mistaking it for a normal atrial or ventricular activation (*oversensing*) (Figure 5-20). The *intrinsic deflection* is the local electrogram inscribed by the depolarization wavefront passing immediately beneath the electrode(s). A single chamber pacemaker system that oversenses non-cardiac electrical activity in the atrium or ventricle will inappropriately fail to deliver pacing stimuli. Depending upon how it is programmed, a dual chamber system that oversenses in the atria may result in inappropriate rapid pacing in the ventricle. Proper sensing is also crucial because pacemaker timing cycles are triggered, set, and reset by accurate sensing of the intrinsic deflection (see "Pacemaker Timing Intervals" on page 213.)

Pacemakers sense cardiac depolarizations by measuring the potential difference
between the anode and cathode. A bipolar
intracardiac electrogram represents the
wavefront of depolarization passing beneath
the closely-opposed pair of electrodes. An
intracardiac bipolar electrogram recorded in
the ventricle is of much shorter duration than
the QRS complex recorded by the surface
ECG (Figure 5-21). In a sense, the surface
ECG recording of QRS complex represents
the sum total of all the intracardiac electrograms inscribed from different areas of the
ventricles at different times. Two critical
characteristics of the electrogram are the *amplitude* (measured in millivolts) and the *slew
rate* (measured in volts/sec) (Figure 5-22).

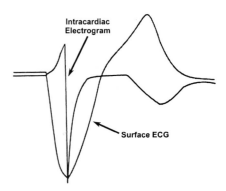

FIGURE 5-21. Schematic illustration of the difference between an intracardiac ventricular electrogram and the QRS complex recorded by a
surface ECG lead. See text for details.

The amplitude of an atrial electrogram may range up to 7-8 mV, but usually is between
2-4 mV. The magnitude of the ventricular electrogram may be as much as 25 mV, but is
typically 4-15 mV. The slew rate for atrial and ventricular depolarization is typically $\geq$
0.5 V/sec and $\geq$ 0.75 V/sec, respectively.

The best analogy for understanding the sensing circuit of a pacemaker is to consider
a person standing behind a fence. The height of the fence will determine how much the
observer will be able to see on the other side of the fence. If the fence is very high, the
viewer may only see the sky. If the fence is lower, tall trees may come into view. If the
fence is very low, the observer may see everything, including buildings, people, and low-

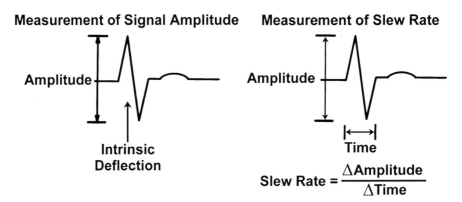

FIGURE 5-22. Optimal positioning of the pacemaker lead is the crucial step in implantation of a pacing system. During implantation of a pacemaker lead, measurements should be made of the amplitude and slew rate
of the intrinsic deflection. The intrinsic deflection is the local electrogram inscribed by the depolarization
wavefront passing immediately beneath the electrode. Strictly speaking, the slew rate is the maximum rate of
voltage change (dV/dt). Other parameters measured at lead implantation include the pacing threshold and
pacing resistance (impedance).

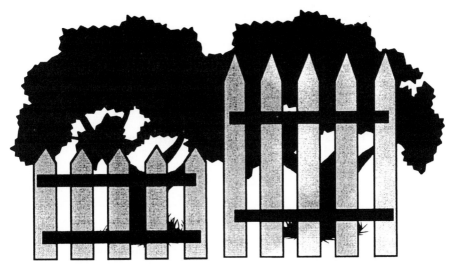

FIGURE 5-23. A pacemaker sensing circuit is analogous to an observer looking over a fence. The higher the fence the less that can be seen by the viewer on the other side of the fence. If the fence is low (high sensitivity), most of the tree can be seen. If the fence is high (sensitivity low), less of the tree can be seen. Courtesy of Medtronic, Inc.

lying plants and bushes (Figure 5-23). Similarly, in a pacemaker system if the fence is very high (very low sensitivity setting) only very large amplitude electrical signals will be detected. If the fence is very low (very high sensitivity setting), even very small amplitude signals will be sensed (Figure 5-24). The programmable sensitivity setting in the pulse generator corresponds to the height of the fence. The sensitivity setting, in turn, is in units of millivolts. The higher the millivolt setting, the higher the fence and the lower the sensitivity. The lower the millivolt setting, the lower the fence and the higher the sensitivity (Figure 5-24). A programmed value of 5 mV means that the pacemaker system will only "see" signals with amplitudes $\geq$ 5 mV. A sensitivity setting of 1.25 mV means that the system will "see" all signals with a magnitude $\geq$ 1.25 mV.

Optimally, the sensitivity setting should be adjusted to avoid inappropriate sensing of non-cardiac electrical noise while at the same time reliably detecting normal cardiac activity. If the system is failing to sense normal intrinsic cardiac activity, the fence must be lowered (increase the sensitivity). If the sensitivity setting is programmed to a very low millivolt value, even small amplitude signals will be detected. If the pacemaker system is sensing unwanted signals, the fence should be raised (make the system less sensitive). The unwanted signals most commonly sensed include T-waves, "far-field" R-waves (ventricular activation sensed in the atrial channel), electromagnetic interference (EMI), or biological noise such as myopotentials from skeletal muscle.

Factors that may affect sensing include lead polarity (unipolar versus bipolar), lead integrity, or EMI. With *unipolar sensing*, the cathode and anode are positioned far apart (Figure 5-25). Therefore, unipolar sensing results in detecting a large potential difference but at the expense of detecting non-cardiac signals originating anywhere in the pathway between the anode and cathode. Consequently, the unipolar system may sense

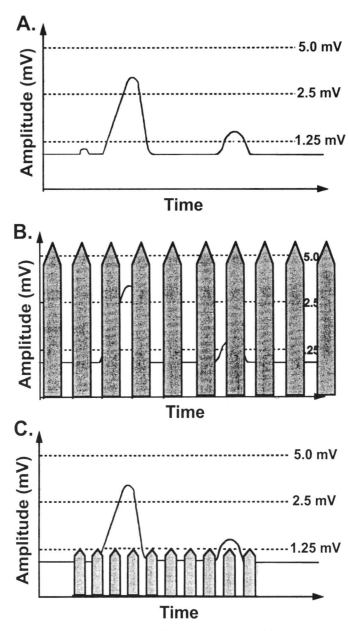

FIGURE 5-24. In the pacemaker sensing circuit the programmable sensitivity settings are in units of milli-volts. Panel A: Typical settings are 1.25, 2.5, and 5.0 mV. Panel B: If a sensitivity of 5.0 mV is programmed, all signals less than 5 mV in amplitude will be hidden by the fence (undersensing). Panel C: If a sensitivity is programmed to 1.25, even very small signals are no longer hidden by the fence. However, in this case the very high sensitivity setting (low fence) means that unwanted signals such as the T-wave are detected by the sensing circuit. Courtesy of Medtronic, Inc.

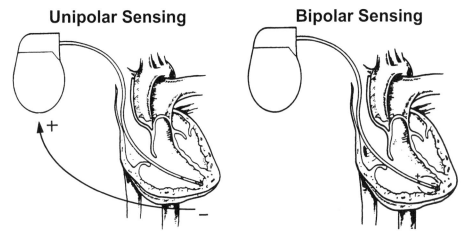

FIGURE 5-25. Bipolar and unipolar sensing. With unipolar sensing, the potential difference is measured between a cathode and anode that located far apart. This may result in detection of non-cardiac signals (oversensing). With bipolar sensing, both the cathode and anode are located only millimeters apart inside the heart. Oversensing is much less likely with a bipolar electrode system. Courtesy of Medtronic, Inc.

spurious signals such as muscle noise or EMI near the implant site of the pulse generator. On the other hand, with *bipolar sensing* the anode and cathode are closely opposed and reside entirely inside the heart (Figure 5-25). Therefore, the potential difference recorded is smaller but far-field, non-cardiac noise is of a much smaller amplitude and very unlikely to be detected. Closely spaced bipolar electrodes are optimal to limit the recording of only intracardiac electrical activity.

A breech of the lead insulation may cause both undersensing and oversensing. Undersensing can occur when the inner and outer conductor coils are continuously in contact. In this situation, intrinsic cardiac signals are attenuated at the sense amplifier. If sufficient attenuation occurs, the signal amplitude may be less than the programmed sensitivity setting. Oversensing can occur when the inner and outer conductor coils make intermittent contact. In this case, signals may be incorrectly interpreted as P- or R-waves.

A conductor fracture can also cause both under- and oversensing. Oversensing will occur when the severed ends of the wire intermittently make contact ("make or break" fracture). This erratic contact generates spurious potentials that are interpreted by the pacemaker as P- or R-waves. Undersensing occurs when the fracture is complete without intermittent contact. In this case, of course, all sensing function is lost using that lead.

In summary, the sensing circuit amplifies, filters, and either processes or rejects signals (Figure 5-26). After amplification, the unwanted components of the incoming signal is selectively attenuated with a bandpass filter. The absolute value component makes positive and negative signals equivalent. The reversion circuit adjusts the baseline to eliminate noise. The processed signal is compared with a reference voltage by the level detector to determine if the signal exceeds the programmed sensing level. Signals with magnitudes less than the sensing level are discarded as noise. Finally, signals with

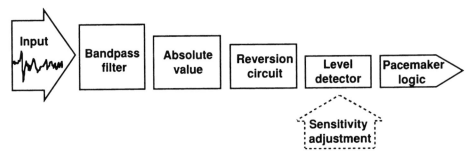

FIGURE 5-26. Schematic diagram summarizing the pacemaker sensing circuit. See text for details. Courtesy of Medtronic, Inc.

amplitudes greater than the sensitivity threshold are passed along to the pacemaker logic where timing intervals and marker channels are initiated.

5.3.5 INTERFERENCE WITH NORMAL PACEMAKER OPERATION

A number of environmental factors may interfere with normal pacemaker operation including electromagnetic interference from a variety of sources, transthoracic defibrillation, shock wave lithotripsy, and ionizing radiation.

Electromagnetic interference (EMI) results from electromagnetic fields located outside the patient's body. Signals with a frequency of 50 – 60 Hz are most frequently associated with pacemaker interference. EMI may result in oversensing (Figure 5-27), a transient pacing mode change (noise reversion) (Figure 5-28), or non-transient reprogramming (power on reset). Oversensing can occur because sensed EMI signals may be interpreted as P- or R-waves. In dual chamber systems programmed to sense in the atri-

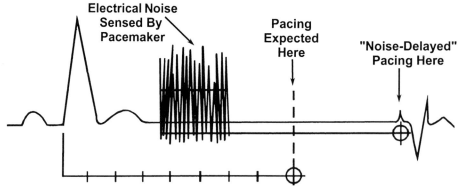

FIGURE 5-27. Oversensing resulting from detection of electromagnetic interference (EMI) inhibits pacing. A sensed ventricular event (first complex) triggers the start of a timing cycle. Sensing of EMI noise restarts the timer and the noise is interpreted as intrinsic activity. Because of this, the expected pacing output is inhibited. After cessation of the EMI, a pacing interval is delivered as expected after the new timing cycle elapses. Courtesy of Medtronic, Inc.

Continuous refractory sensing will cause pacing at the lower or sensor-driven rate

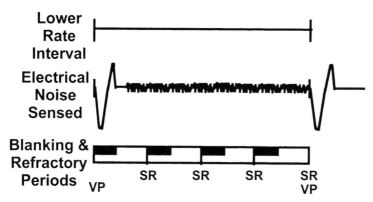

FIGURE 5-28. Schematic diagram illustrating noise reversion behavior. The portion of the refractory period after the end of the blanking period is referred to as the "noise sampling period." A sensed event during this period will initiate a new refractory and blanking period. If events continue to be sensed during the noise sampling period, a new refractory period will be repeatedly generated. Eventually, the device will pace at the programmed lower rate since the lower rate timer is not reset by events sensed during the refractory period. This behavior is known as *noise reversion*. In rate-responsive pacing modes, noise reversion will cause pacing at the sensor-driven rate. SR, sensed R-wave; VP, ventricular pacing. Courtesy of Medtronic, Inc.

um and pace in the ventricle, EMI sensed by the atrial channel could trigger ventricular pacing at rates as high as the programmed upper rate limit ("tracking" behavior). Unless the pacemaker is an asynchronous mode, pacing may be inhibited if EMI is sensed in single chamber pacing systems or in the ventricular channel of dual chamber systems. If EMI is sensed continuously for relatively long periods (greater than the duration of the programmed lower rate cycle length), noise reversion may occur with pacing stimuli delivered only at the lower rate limit (or at the sensor driven rate in the case of pacemakers programmed to a rate-responsive mode). EMI may lead to inadvertent reprogramming of pacing parameters, usually to an asynchronous mode. The device may revert to a backup mode termed *power-on-reset*, or simply "reset". If power-on-reset is triggered, the resultant pacing parameters may be identical to those that occur at battery end-of-life. To determine whether the pulse generator is in power-on-reset mode or at battery end-of-life, the battery voltage should be measured and an attempt made to reprogram the device back to the original parameters. Power-on-reset mode would be indicated by the ability to reprogram the device and the finding of a battery voltage greater than the end-of-life voltage. The default power-on-reset parameters vary with the manufacturer and whether a "full" or "partial" reset occurs. Unless the pacemaker is actually reprogrammed to another pacing mode by the EMI, eliminating the EMI or moving away from its source will usually return the device to its previous pacing mode.

Potential sources of EMI are numerous (Table 5-6.) Electrocautery devices used during surgical procedures as well as radiofrequency catheter ablation generators may trigger transient asynchronous or inhibited pacemaker operation during the duration of the EMI exposure. As a precaution, during these procedures, the current path should be kept as remote as possible from the pulse generator and pacemaker leads. In particular, direct contact between the ablation catheter and the implanted pacemaker lead should be avoided. Inhibition of pacing in pacemaker-dependent patients can be avoided by temporary reprogramming to the DOO or VOO/AOO modes (or application of a magnet over the pulse generator implantation site). In the case of electrocautery, problems can generally be completely avoided by using bipolar electrocautery forceps.

Transthoracic defibrillation may damage the pacemaker circuitry. To minimize this possibility, one should position the defibrillator paddles as far away as possible from the pulse generator (at least six inches) and use the lowest clinically appropriate defibrillation energy. In most modern pacemakers, protective thyristors help shield the pacemaker circuitry from electrical damage during external defibrillation procedures up to 360 – 400 watt-seconds.

TABLE 5-6. Possible sources of electromagnetic interference (EMI)

Electrocautery or diathermy
Transthoracic defibrillation
Extracorporeal shock-wave lithotripsy
Therapeutic ionizing radiation
Radiofrequency ablation
Transcutaneous electrical nerve stimulation (TENS)
Magnetic resonance imaging (MRI)
High-powered radio & television transmitters
High powered radar systems (airport radar)
High-powered engines & motors, including airplane engines
Subway breaking systems
Arc welders
Department store anti-theft devices

Likewise, shock wave lithotripsy can damage a pulse generator. Because the shock wave may synchronize with atrial output and inhibit ventricular output, lithotripsy may prevent ventricular pacing in dual chamber modes. The shock wave may stimulate or even damage the pressure-sensitive piezoelectric crystal in adaptive-rate pacemakers utilizing this sensor; this may trigger inappropriate rapid pacing. To minimize this possibility, the lithotripsy focal point should be greater than six inches from the pulse generator and the dual chamber devices should be reprogrammed to the ventricular demand mode.

Diagnostic radiation and fluoroscopy do not affect pacemaker function. However, high-energy ionizing radiation sources used to treat certain cancers (such as cobalt 60 or gamma rays) may cause permanent damage to the semiconductor circuitry, necessitating replacement of the pulse generator. Ionizing radiation has been reported to cause "runaway" with pacing at excessive rates or loss of output. To avoid potential problems, therapeutic radiation should not be focus directly at the area of the pulse generator. If patients require radiotherapy in the vicinity of the pacemaker lead shielding should be placed over the implant site.

Magnetic and radiofrequency fields produced by magnetic resonance imaging (MRI) machines may increase ventricular pacing beyond the rate limit, result in total inhibition of pacing output, initiate pacing at random rates, or trigger asynchronous pacing. In addition, magnetic fields may activate magnet mode operation, causing asynchronous pacemaker operation. Finally, the strong magnetic fields present in a MRI machine may damage the pacemaker. Therefore, if a clinician refers a pacemaker patient for a MRI procedure they should be closely monitored during the study and the programmed parameters verified after the procedure.

Transcutaneous electrical nerve stimulators (TENS) may interfere with pacemaker function, including inhibition of demand pacemaker operation. If patients require this treatment care should be taken to place the TENS electrodes as close to each other and as far from the pacemaker/lead system as possible. Cardiac monitoring during TENS use is strongly recommended and, if not possible, the clinician should reconsider its use.

Once outside the hospital environment patients should be instructed to avoid a number of other possible EMI sources. Very close association to electromagnetic fields produced by extremely high voltage transmission lines may generate sufficient EMI to interfere with pacemaker operation. Some specialized communication equipment such as microwave transmitters, linear-powered amplifiers, or some high-powered, poorly-shielded amateur transmitting equipment may emit enough EMI to interfere with some pacemakers. However, most of these systems that are professionally built and maintained will not disturb pacemaker function. Some commercial electrical equipment such as arc welders, induction furnaces, and resistance welders may generate adequate EMI so as to disrupt normal pacemaker operation for patients in very close proximity. In general, household appliances (including microwave ovens), electrical tools, and radio/ television equipment should not affect pacemaker operation. In those rare cases where function is disrupted, moving away from the source of the EMI will allow the resumption of normal pacemaker behavior.

There is some evidence suggesting a possible adverse interaction between hand-held cellular telephones and permanent pacemaker systems. The potential adverse effects may be either due to the radiofrequency signal generated or the magnet within the telephone handset. The possible effects include inhibition of demand pacing or asynchronous pacing when the telephone is in close proximity (within six inches (15 cm)) to the pulse generator. Because of the possibility of this interaction, device manufacturers have made some general recommendations regarding the use of cellular telephones by patients with pacemakers. They include maintaining a minimum separation of six inches (15 cm) between a hand-held cellular telephone and the implanted device. While most hand-held telephones transmit at less than three watts, portable and mounted cellular telephones often transmit at greater than three watts. When using these devices the antenna should be kept 12 inches (30 cm) from the pulse generator to avoid the potential for interaction. In addition, the patient should be instructed to hold the phone to the ear contralateral to the implanted device. Finally, patients should not carry the phone a pocket near the pulse generator even when it is merely turned ON in the standby mode because some cellular telephones emit signals in this listening mode.

5.3.6 RATE-RESPONSIVE PACING

The original indication for pacemaker therapy was complete AV block with syncope. As indications broadened to include patients with sinoatrial node dysfunction the vexing problem facing device manufacturers was (and continues to be) the development of a truly "physiological" rate-responsive pacemaker that robustly responds to the metabolic needs of patients with chronotropic incompetence. Although definitions vary, most authorities would agree that chronotropic incompetence implies an inability to increase the sinus rate to 70% of the maximum predicted heart rate for age. Many studies have documented the importance of chronotropic competence during exercise [24-30].

Rate-responsive (also known as *rate-modulated* or *adaptive-rate*) pacemakers provide patients with the ability to increase heart rate when the sinus node cannot produce the appropriate rate (Figure 5-29). If metabolic needs increase, adaptive-rate pacemakers are designed to respond with an increase in heart rate thereby producing additional cardiac output. The critical component of a rate-responsive pacemaker system is a *sensor* that transduces changes in a patient's metabolic need into electrical signals that trigger a change in the pacing rate. The "ideal" sensor is, of course, the sinus node. However, patients with sinoatrial node dysfunction or chronotropic incompetence lack a normal sinus node response to increased metabolic demands. Consequently, they need an artificial sensor to trigger an increase in pacing rate in response to an increased demand for cardiac output. A number of sensors are currently available or in clinical investigation (Table 5-7.) Optimally, the sensor-driven rate should closely match the predicted response of a normal sinus node to an equivalent increase in metabolic need. In an attempt to mimic normal sinus node behavior, sensors have been developed which respond to a variety of electrical, chemical, and physical stimuli. Most currently available pacing systems use either a *motion (activity) sensor* or a *minute ventilation sensor*.

Motion sensors operate using either a piezoelectric crystal which deforms in response to mechanical movement and generates a proportional electrical current, or an ac-

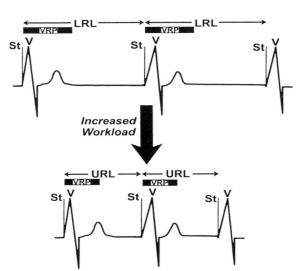

FIGURE 5-29. A ventricular rate-responsive pacemaker will pace the ventricle at rates between the programmed lower rate limit and the upper rate limit. The exact pacing rate at any particular time will be governed by the magnitude of the triggering signal originating from the sensor. The appropriateness of the pacing rate will depend upon the accuracy of the sensor in assessing the metabolic needs. Motion sensors are unable to sense true metabolic needs and therefore may respond with an inadequate rate increase if the sensor is insufficiently stimulated by the patient's movement. To partially overcome this limitation, sensors – including motion sensors – can be programmed to increase their "sensitivity" and "responsiveness".

celerometer (Figure 5-30). An accelerometer, which also senses body motion, is an integrated circuit located on the pacemaker's electronic circuit board. The accelerometer responds to activity in the frequency range of typical physiologic activity (1–4-Hz) (Figure 5-31). An algorithm translates the measured acceleration into a rate increase above the lower rate limit. Unlike the piezoelectric-based sensor, the accelerometer is not in contact with the pacemaker case; therefore, the rate-response resulting from pressure applied to the pulse generator is negligible.

TABLE 5-7. Pacemaker sensors currently available or in clinical investigation

Sensor Signal	Sensor
Mechanical	
Body activity (motion)	Piezoelectric crystal
	Accelerometer
Peak endocardial acceleration	Endocardial accelerometer
Temperature	Thermistor
Electrocardiogram	
QT interval	Unipolar lead
Depolarization gradient	Bipolar lead
Impedance	
Respiration rate	Auxiliary lead
Minute ventilation	Bipolar lead
Stroke volume	Multipolar lead
Pre-ejection interval	Multipolar lead
Impedance contractility	Multipolar lead
Special	
dP/dt	Pressure sensor
O_2 saturation	Light-emitting diode and optical sensor

Adapted from [31].

Motion sensors are the most commonly used sensors because they are simple, responsive, and don't require any special lead systems. However, there is one significant limitation to motion sensors; namely, they are not specific for increased metabolic need. Body motion is only loosely correlated with metabolic demand. For example, activity associated with greater use of the upper body, arms, and shoulders will generate a greater response by the motion sensor than equally demanding exertion associated predominant-

A. Piezoelectric Sensor

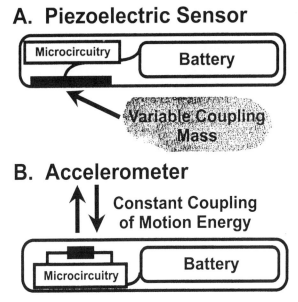

B. Accelerometer

FIGURE 5-30. Schematic diagram illustrating the physical principles involved in piezoelectric and accelerometer sensors. In both situations, mechanical forces are converted into electrical signals. Panel A: The piezoelectric sensor is bonded to the inside of the pacemaker case. The surrounding connective, muscle and fat tissues transmit the variable mechanical forces of vibration associated with patient motion to the pacemaker case (and associated piezoelectric crystal). The extent of contact and coupling of this mechanical vibration is highly variable. Panel B: In the case of the accelerometer, the sensor is mounted directly to the microelectronic circuit board within the pacemaker case. The accelerometer detects the anterior-posterior movement of the patient's body in space (typical frequency 1 – 4-Hz). Unlike the piezoelectric sensor, the accelerometer is insensitive to mechanical forces exerted on the pacemaker case. Adapted from [31].

ly with lower body movements. In the former case the motion sensor will trigger a robust pacing response while in the latter case the patient may be significantly limited by lack of an appropriate increase in pacing rate. However, it is generally agreed that accelerometers provide a better, more reliable response to motion, particularly in the anterior-posterior direction, than the piezoelectric sensor.

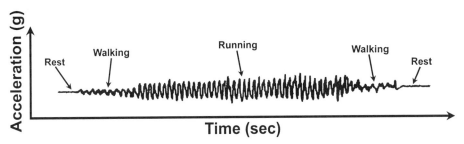

FIGURE 5-31. Illustration showing example of accelerometer behavior using 4-Hz low-pass filter in response to anterior-posterior motion. Each amplitude corresponds to an anterior-posterior step by the patient using an accelerometer 4-Hz low-pass filter. The increase in amplitude and frequency from walking to running is clearly seen, while at rest there is virtually no accelerometer output. Adapted from [31].

Because of this limitation, some pacemaker manufacturers have focused on developing a sensor that responds to minute ventilation (Figure 5-32). Minute ventilation (MV) is the volume of air introduced into the lungs in one minute,

$$MV = TV \times RR$$

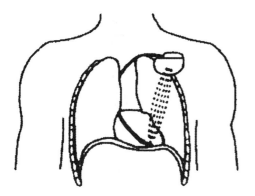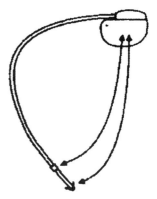

FIGURE 5-32. The minute ventilation sensor measures the change in electrical impedance between the pacemaker case and an intracardiac electrode. An increase in tidal volume and respiratory rate increases the transthoracic impedance which, in turn, increases the sensor-driven pacing rate. Courtesy of Medtronic, Inc.

where TV is the tidal volume and RR is the number of respirations in one minute. Minute ventilation very closely tracks oxygen consumption and therefore is an excellent physiological sensor. These sensors may measure either the frequency of cyclic changes in thoracic impedance during inspiration and expiration (thereby estimating respiratory rate) or the tidal volume (estimated by the magnitude of the changes in impedance), or both frequency of respiration and tidal volume. To determine the thoracic impedance a very low amplitude (subthreshold) constant current pulse is emitted from the proximal electrode of an atrial or ventricular lead and the voltage drop between a distal electrode on a pacemaker lead and the metallic can of the pulse generator is measured. Using Ohm's law the thoracic impedance can thus be calculated. An increase in TV or RR will result in an increase in thoracic impedance which is translated into an increase in pacing rate.

While an excellent sensor, there are some circumstances in which minute ventilation does not provide accurate information. For example, coughing, speaking and even simple arm movements may result in inappropriate activation of the sensor. An inappropriate tachycardia may also occur in some patients with congestive heart failure and Cheyne–Stokes breathing, making this condition, as well as chronic lung disease and asthma, relative contraindications to use of these devices. Pacing systems using a minute ventilation sensor will also have a shortened battery life resulting from the charge consumed by the frequent current pulses emitted for continuous measurement of the thoracic impedance.

5.4   Pacemaker Operation, Programmability & Timing Cycles

5.4.1   PACING MODE NOMENCLATURE

The purpose of an implanted pacemaker system is to do one or more (or all) of the following:

- Sense atrial activity
- Pace the atrium
- Sense ventricular activity
- Pace the ventricle

The pacemaker system accomplishes these tasks using implanted electrodes in the atrium, ventricle, or both (Figure 5-33).

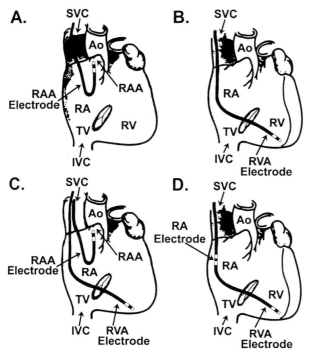

FIGURE 5-33. A pacemaker system is designed to perform one or more of the following tasks: atrial sensing, atrial pacing, ventricular sensing, ventricular pacing. A number of pacing and sensing combinations are possible depending upon the number and positioning of electrodes within the heart. Panel A: A single electrode is implanted in the right atrial appendage (RAA). This would allow for atrial sensing and pacing. Panel B: A single electrode is implanted at the right ventricular apex (RVA). This would allow for ventricular sensing and pacing. Panel C: Separate electrodes are implanted in the RAA and RVA. This would permit sensing and pacing in both the atrium and ventricle. Panel D: A single lead is implanted with a proximal pair of electrodes residing in the right atrium (RA) used for bipolar atrial sensing and the distal electrode in the RVA is used for ventricular pacing and sensing. Ao, aorta; IVC, inferior vena cava; RV, right ventricle; SVC, superior vena cava; TV, tricuspid valve.

In order to sense and pace the atrium a bipolar or unipolar electrode must be implanted in the atrium. In order to sense and pace the ventricle a bipolar or unipolar electrode must be implanted in the ventricle. If sensing and pacing of both the atrium and ventricles is desired, then electrodes must be implanted in both the atrium and the ventricles. Recently, a number of manufacturers have produced a single lead system that allows bipolar or unipolar sensing of atrial activity and bipolar pacing and sensing in the ventricle. With this lead the proximal sensing electrode(s) that is/are positioned in the atrium need not be in close contact with atrial endocardium; the electrode is designed to record far-field atrial (but not ventricular) activity.

A nomenclature has been developed by a joint committee of the North American Society of Pacing & Electrophysiology (NASPE) and the British Pacing & Electrophysiology Group (BPEG) [32,33] to describe the sensing, pacing, and programmability functions of pacemaker systems (Table 5-8.) The pacing mode code consists of up to five

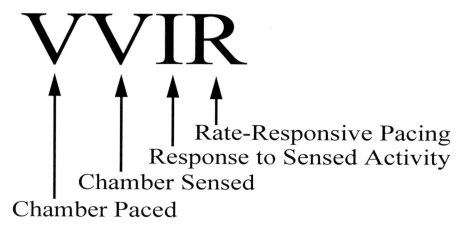

FIGURE 5-34. Example of four-letter pacing mode code used to describe the programmed pacing and sensing capabilities of a pacemaker system. In the example shown here, VVIR indicates that only the ventricle will be paced and sensed (first and second positions). In response to a sensed ventricular depolarization ventricular pacing will be inhibited (third position). The device is programmed to deliver rate-responsive pacing meaning that an internal sensor in the pacing system will cause a gradual increase in the ventricular pacing rate as the patient's level of exertion increases.

letters used to indicate the pacing, sensing, and some programmable options of the pacing system. In general, however, only the first four letters are commonly used (Figure 5-34). The first letter is used to indicate which cardiac chamber(s) is/are paced (V, ventricle, A, atrium, D, dual (both A and V), while the second letter is used to denote which chamber(s) is/are sensed (A, V, D (both A and V), or O (neither A or V). The third letter indicates how the pulse generator responds to sensed activity, and is designated T (triggered), I (inhibited), D (both triggered and inhibited), or O (not applicable). The fourth letter, if used, indicates whether the pulse generator has special programming options. At present, this fourth position is generally only used to indicate if the pulse generator can be programmed to deliver rate-responsive pacing. The abbreviations used and a description of each of the pacing modes most commonly used are discussed in Table 5-9.

5.4.2 PACEMAKER TIMING INTERVALS

In most cases, pacemaker timing intervals are reported in milliseconds. The exception to this general rule is the upper and lower rate limits; they are often expressed in pulses per min. Rates and intervals are interconvertable. To convert the rate (per minute) into an interval (in milliseconds): :

$$Interval \text{ (ms)} = \frac{60,000}{Rate \text{(per min)}}$$

To convert from an interval to rate

$$Rate \text{ (per min)} = \frac{60,000}{Interval \text{ (ms)}}$$

TABLE 5-8. Pacemaker code formulation of the North American Society of Pacing & Electrophysiology and British Pacing and Electrophysiology Group

Position	I	II	III	IV	V
Category	Chamber(s) Paced	Chamber(s) Sensed	Response to Sensed Event	Programmability, Rate Modulation	Special Antiarrhythmic Functions
Letters Used	V, ventricle	V, ventricle	T, triggered	P, limited programmability	O, none
	A, atrium	A, atrium	I, inhibited	M, multiprogrammability	P, antitachycardia pacing
	D, dual (A & V)	D, dual (A & V)	D, dual	C, communicating	S, shock
	O, none	O, none	O, none	O, none	D, dual (P & S)
				R, rate modulation	
Manufacturers Designation Only	S, single (A or V)	S, single (A or V)			

Modified from [32,33]

TABLE 5-9. Explanation of commonly used pacing modes

1st Letter (Chamber paced)	2nd Letter (Chamber sensed)	3rd Letter (Mode of response to sensed beat)	4th Letter (Programmable features available)	Description
A	O	O	–	Asynchronous atrial pacing; no atrial sensing.
A	A	I	–	Atrial pacing on demand; output inhibited by sensed atrial signals.
A	A	I	R	Atrial pacing on demand; output inhibited by sensed atrial signals. Atrial pacing rates can decrease and increase in response to sensor input, up to the programmed sensor-based upper limit of the rate.
V	O	O	–	Asynchronous ventricular pacing; no ventricular sensing
V	V	I	–	Ventricular pacing on demand; output inhibited by sensed ventricular signals.
V	V	I	R	Ventricular pacing on demand; output inhibited by sensed ventricular signals. Ventricular pacing rates can decrease and increase in response to sensor input, up to the programmed sensor-based upper limit of the rate.
V	D	D	–	Paces the ventricle; senses in both the atrium and the ventricle; synchronizes with atrial activity and paces the ventricle after a programmable AV interval up to the programmed upper limit of the rate.
D	D	I	–	Paces and senses in both the atrium and the ventricle; the only response to a sensed P- or R-wave is inhibition. No tracking of intrinsic atrial activity.
D	D	I	R	Paces and senses in both the atrium and the ventricle; the only response to a sensed P- or R-wave is inhibition. Atrial and ventricular pacing rates increase and decrease independently in response to sensor input. AV synchrony may not be achieved.
D	D	D	–	Paces and senses in both the atrium and the ventricle; paces the ventricle in response to sensed atrial activity up to the programmed upper limit of the rate.
D	D	D	R	Paces and senses in both the atrium and the ventricle. Atrial and ventricle pacing rates can decrease and increase in response to sensor input, up to the programmed sensor-based upper limit of the rate.

A, atrial; AV, atrioventricular; D, dual (both A and V); I, inhibited; O, none; R, rate-adaptive; V, ventricular. Adapted from [34]

The common timing intervals used when describing and discussing pacemaker operation and behavior are summarized in Table 5-10.

TABLE 5-10. Abbreviations and acronyms of pacemaker timing intervals

Abbreviation	Definition
P	Native atrial depolarization
A	Atrial-paced event
R	Native ventricular depolarization
V	Ventricular-paced event
A-R	Time interval between an atrial-paced event and a native ventricular depolarization
A-V	Time interval between an atrial-paced event and a paced ventricular event
P-R	Time interval between a native atrial depolarization and a native ventricular depolarization (due to normal AV conduction)
P-V	Time interval between a native atrial depolarization and a paced ventricular event
LRI	Lower rate interval
MTRI	Maximum tracking rate interval; usually expressed in pulses/min, but convertible to cycle length in milliseconds
MSRI	Maximum sensor-based rate interval; usually expressed in pulses/min, but convertible to cycle length in milliseconds
HRI	Hysteresis rate interval
AVI	Programmable AV interval; time between a sensed or paced atrial event and the subsequent delivery of a ventricular pacing stimulus in a dual chamber pacemaker system
SAVI	Programmable *sensed* AV interval; time between a sensed atrial event and the subsequent delivery of a ventricular pacing stimulus in a dual chamber pacemaker system
PAVI	Programmable *paced* AV interval; time between a paced atrial event and the subsequent delivery of a ventricular pacing stimulus in a dual chamber pacemaker system
RA-AVI	Rate-adaptive AV interval
VSPI	Ventricular safety pacing interval
AEI	Atrial escape interval; time interval between a sensed or paced ventricular event and a subsequent atrial-paced event (also known as the V-A interval)
RP	Refractory period
ARP	Atrial refractory period
VRP	Ventricular refractory period
PVARP	Post-ventricular atrial refractory period
TARP	Total atrial refractory period (TARP = PVARP + AVI)
BP	Blanking period
ABP	Atrial blanking period
VBP	Ventricular blanking period
PVABP	Post-ventricular atrial blanking period
PAVBP	Post-atrial ventricular blanking period

Single chamber timing cycles. Operation of single chamber pacemakers usually involves up to five timing intervals: *lower rate interval* (LRI), *refractory period* (RP), *blanking period* (BP), *maximum sensor-based rate interval* (in rate-responsive pulse generators) (MSRI), and the *hysteresis rate interval* (HRI) (Figure 5-35). If the pacing lead is implanted in the atrium, the RP refers to the atrial refractory period (ARP). If the pacing lead is implanted in the ventricle, the RP refers to the ventricular refractory period (VRP).

The LRI is the programmed lowest rate at which the pacemaker will pace (Figure 5-35). Usually it is expressed as pulses per minute, but it can be denoted as a cycle length in milliseconds (e.g., 100 pulses/min is equivalent to 600 ms). The LRI timer is restarted by either a paced or non-refractory sensed event.

The RP is designed to prevent inhibition of pacing by cardiac or non-cardiac events (Figure 5-35). During the RP, the pacemaker "sees", but is unresponsive to any electrical signals. During this period the LRI timer is not restarted in the event of oversensing. T-wave oversensing may occur in the VVI or AAI modes if the VRP or ARP, respectively, are too short. In the AAI mode, the pacemaker may even sense the ventricular depolarization (far-field R-wave) if

A. Lower Rate Interval

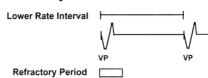

B. Refractory Period

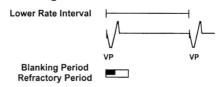

C. Blanking Period

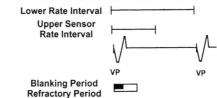

D. Maximum Sensor Rate Interval

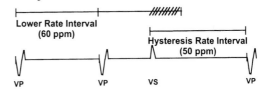

E. Hysteresis Rate Interval

FIGURE 5-35. Single chamber timing intervals. Panel A: Lower rate interval. Panel B: Refractory period. Panel C: Blanking period. Panel D. Upper sensor rate interval. Panel E: Hysteresis rate interval. Single chamber pacing systems can be implanted in the atrium or ventricle. In this example, implantation in the atrium is presumed. VP, ventricular paced event; VS, ventricular sensed event. See text for details. Courtesy of Medtronic, Inc.

the ARP is not long enough. The RP is restarted only by a paced, non-refractory, or refractory sensed event.

A paced or sensed event will initiate a BP (Figure 5-35). Blanking is the method by which multiple detections of a single paced or sensed event by the sense amplifier is prevented. This ensures that the pacemaker will not detect its own pacing stimuli or a triggered or spontaneous depolarization. During this period, the pacemaker is "blind" to any electrical activity. Although the BP is typically about 100 ms, in some pacemaker models the BP is dynamic with the duration dependent upon the strength/duration of the paced or sensed signal. The portion of the RP after the BP ends is referred to as the *alert period* or the *noise sampling period*. As previously discussed (Figure 5-28), continuous sensing of noise, such as EMI, during this period will repeatedly reset the RP timer. In turn, this results in noise reversion behavior causing asynchronous lower rate pacing (because the LRI timer is not restarted by events sensed during the RP).

The MSRI is the shortest interval (highest rate) that the pacemaker will pace as dictated by the sensor in rate-adaptive pacemakers (Figure 5-35). Adaptive rate pacing is discussed in more detail elsewhere (see "Rate-Responsive Pacing" on page 208.)

Hysteresis allows the sensed intrinsic rate to decrease to a level below the programmed lower rate before pacing resumes at the lower rate (Figure 5-36). Hysteresis provides the capability to maintain the patient's own intrinsic rate as long as possible, while pacing at a faster rate (the programmed LRI) if the intrinsic rate falls below the HRI. The hysteresis rate is always slower than the programmed lower rate. The LRI timer is initiated by a paced event, while the HRI timer is started by a non-refractory sensed event. As seen in Figure 5-35, the LRI is programmed to 60 pulses/min (1000 ms), while the HRI is set at 50 pulses/min (1200 ms). In this example, the patient is paced at 60 pulses/min until an intrinsic depolarization occurs. At that point the HRI timer is started at an interval of 1200 ms. During that hysteresis interval the patient fails to have another sensed spontaneous event and so a ventricular pacing stimuli is delivered when the HRI timer elapses. If instead, another sensed event had occurred within the 1200 ms, the HRI timer would have been restarted, allowing another 1200 ms interval before any ventricular pacing would occur.

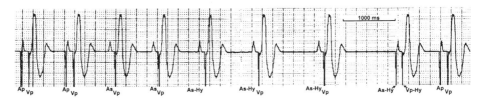

FIGURE 5-36. Example of rate hysteresis in the atrial channel of a dual chamber pacing system. The programmed LRI is 850 msec. while the HRI is 1500 msec. When the sinus rate is greater than 850 but less than 1500 msec, only atrial sensing occurs (even the though the programmed LRI is 850 msec). If the sinus cycle length increases beyond 1500 msec, atrial pacing resumes at the LRI (850 msec). By using the hysteresis option, the patient benefits from sinus rhythm for extended periods until the rate drops below a programmed rate even lower than the LRI (the HRI), whereupon atrial pacing resumes at the programmed LRI. Ap, atrial pace, As, atrial sense, Ap-Hy, atrial pace at hysteresis rate, As-Hy, atrial sense at hysteresis rate, Vp, ventricular pace, Vp-Hy, ventricular pace at hysteresis rate. Courtesy of Guidant/CPI, Inc.

Dual chamber timing cycles. Dual chamber pacemaker systems can exhibit four different behaviors: atrial and ventricular sensing, atrial and ventricular pacing, atrial sensing and ventricular pacing, and atrial pacing and ventricular sensing (Figure 5-37).

In general, timer activity is initiated either by sensing an intrinsic deflection or the delivery of a pacing stimulus. Depending upon the locations of the atrial and ventricular sensing electrodes, the atrial or ventricular intrinsic deflections may occur at the onset,

Atrial Pace, Ventricular Pace   **Atrial Sense, Ventricular Pace**

Atrial Pace, Ventricular Sense   **Atrial Sense, Ventricular Sense**

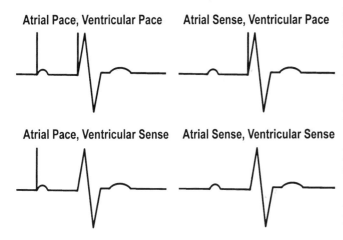

FIGURE 5-37. In the DDD mode the pacing system can exhibit four different pacing/sensing behaviors: 1) atrial and ventricular pacing; 2) atrial sensing and ventricle pacing; 3) atrial pacing and ventricular sensing; 4) atrial and ventricular sensing. Atrial or ventricular pacing is inhibited if spontaneous atrial or ventricular activity is sensed. After a sensed or paced atrial event ventricular pacing will occur after the programmed AV delay unless ventricular activation occurs spontaneously or secondary to normal AV conduction. A, atrial; V, ventricular

during, or even at the end of the inscription of the P- or R-waves on the surface ECG. It should not assumed that atrial or ventricular timing intervals begin with the onset of the P- or R-waves. In most cases, atrial pacing leads are implanted in the right atrial appendage and ventricular leads in the right ventricular apex. Therefore, timing cycles are normally based upon sensing or pacing by electrodes located at these positions. In a dual chamber pacing system, the AV interval begins with either sensing of the intrinsic deflection in the atrial channel or delivery of an atrial pacing stimulus by the pacemaker. The AV interval ends either with sensing intrinsic deflection in the ventricular channel or delivery of a ventricular pacing stimulus by the pulse generator (Table 5-11.) Since the atrial lead is normally located in the right atrial appendage, by the time the atrial lead "sees" a spontaneous atrial depolarization, right atrial activation is already well advanced. Similarly, since left ventricular activation normally precedes right ventricular activation, by the time the lead in the right ventricular apex senses a depolarization, normal left ventricular activation is also well along, especially in patients with a right bundle branch block.

TABLE 5-11.   AV intervals vary with atrial and ventricular pacing and sensing and lead location

A-sense, V-sense: Interval from sensed atrial depolarization to sensed ventricular depolarization

A-sense, V-pace: Interval from sensed atrial depolarization to ventricular pacing stimulus

A-pace, V-sense: Interval from atrial pacing stimulus to sensed ventricular depolarization

A-pace, V-pace: Interval from atrial pacing stimulus to ventricular pacing stimulus

In dual chamber pacemaker systems, the LRI is the lowest rate at which the pacemaker will pace the atrium in the absence of intrinsic atrial activity (Figure 5-38). Generally, the LRI is expressed as pulses per minute but, as with single chamber timing, the lower rate can be converted to an interval measurement in milliseconds (the A–A interval), which represents the longest time period between the delivery of pacing stimuli in the atrium.

In most recently manufactured pacemakers there are two AV intervals (AVI) that are programmable: the *sensed AV interval* (SAVI) and the *paced AV interval* (PAVI) (Figure 5-39). The SAVI is usually programmed to a shorter duration than the PAVI to allow for the difference in interatrial conduction time between intrinsic and paced atrial events. The purpose of the AV interval is to allow the appropriate amount of time to optimize ventricular filling after atrial contraction thereby enhancing the so-called "atrial kick" component of cardiac output. The distinction between the PAVI and SAVI is designed to ensure that the left atrial component to left ventricular filling remains the same regardless of whether bi-atrial activation proceeds from an intrinsic right atrial depolarization or a right atrial paced event.

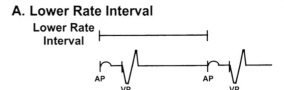

A. Lower Rate Interval

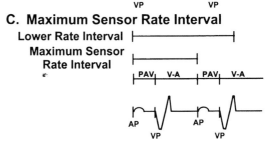

B. Maximum Tracking Rate Interval

C. Maximum Sensor Rate Interval

FIGURE 5-38. Rate-related timing intervals in dual chamber pacing systems. See text for details. Courtesy of Medtronic, Inc.

To understand this, consider the difference between atrial depolarization by normal sinus activation compared with activation from a paced atrial event. The cycle starting with the intrinsic right atrial activation uses the normal conduction pathway(s) to activate the left atrium, while the cycle starting with a paced right atrial activation may not proceed to the left atrium using the normal pathway(s). Consequently, a longer interatrial conduction time may occur after an atrial paced event compared to a spontaneous sinus event. Therefore, the PAVI is usually programmed to a value greater than the SAVI.

The *atrial escape interval* (AEI), also known as the *ventriculoatrial* (VA) *interval*, is defined as the longest time period that is allowed to elapse after a paced or sensed ventricular event before an atrial pacing stimuli is delivered (Figure 5-39). If a spontaneous atrial depolarization occurs before fulfillment of the AEI timer, an atrial stimulus will not be delivered. While the LRI and PAVI are programmable intervals, the AEI is not a programmable option. However, because of the relationship between the AEI, PAVI, and the LRI (LRI = AEI + PAVI), the AEI can be easily calculated.

The *maximum (or upper) tracking rate interval* (MTRI) represents the fastest ventricular pacing rate in response to sensed spontaneous atrial depolarizations (Figure 5-

A. AV Intervals

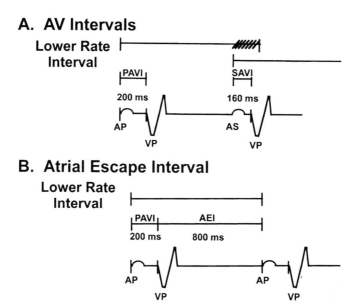

FIGURE 5-39. Atrioventricular and ventriculo-atrial timing intervals in dual chamber pacemaker systems. See text for details. Courtesy of Medtronic, Inc.

38). During "tracking" behavior (Figure 5-37, atrial sense, ventricular pace), for each sensed spontaneous atrial depolarization (not occurring within the atrial refractory period), the pacemaker delivers a ventricular pacing stimulus after the programmable AV delay (SAVI). If the rate of spontaneous atrial depolarizations becomes excessive, as would occur during atrial flutter or fibrillation, uncontrolled tracking could result in dangerously fast ventricular pacing. To avoid this, the maximum atrial rate that will result in triggered ventricular pacing (MTRI) can be programmed to a safe level. For example, in a patient prone to the development of atrial tachyarrhythmias, the MTRI may be programmed to 120 pulses/min, thereby avoiding the potential for ventricular pacing at rates above that level. Patients with chronotropic incompetence that lack the normal exercise-induced increase in sinus rate cannot benefit from tracking behavior that requires sinus activity for the triggering signal. The *maximum (or upper) sensor-based rate interval* (MSRI) is the maximum rate of atrial and ventricular pacing in response to the maximum rate trigger signal emitted from the rate-responsive sensor within the pacemaker (Figure 5-38). *Mode switching* is a programmable option available in most new pulse generators that remedies many of the problems associated with tracking of very high atrial rates (see "Mode switching" on page 239).

The *post-ventricular atrial refractory period* (PVARP) is the period of time after a sensed or paced ventricular event during which the atrial channel is refractory (Figure 5-40). During this period (and after completion of the blanking period), atrial events that are sensed do not initiate a SAVI. The purpose of the PVARP is to prevent sensed P-waves resulting from retrograde conduction, far-field R-waves, or atrial premature depolarizations from initiating a SAVI that could trigger inappropriate high-rate ventricular pacing.

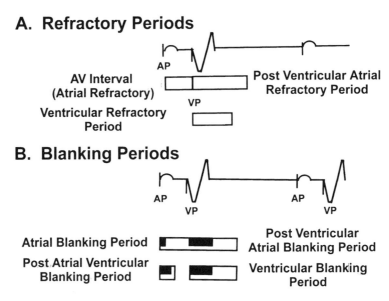

A. Refractory Periods

AP

AV Interval
(Atrial Refractory)

VP

Ventricular Refractory
Period

Post Ventricular Atrial
Refractory Period

B. Blanking Periods

AP   AP
VP   VP

Atrial Blanking Period

Post Atrial Ventricular
Blanking Period

Post Ventricular
Atrial Blanking Period

Ventricular Blanking
Period

FIGURE 5-40. Refractory periods in dual chamber pacing systems. See text for details. Courtesy of Medtronic, Inc.

The *ventricular refractory period* (VRP) is primarily designed to prevent oversensing and self-inhibition by spontaneous or paced ventricular activations and their associated T-waves (Figure 5-40). The VRP timer is started by a sensed or paced ventricular event. In the absence of a VRP, a sensed T-wave inscribed after the blanking period would reinitiate the AEI timer. Ventricular events occurring during the noise sampling portion of the VRP (following the blanking period) are detected but they do not restart the AEI interval. The atrial channel is refractory to sensed or paced events detected during the PAVI or SAVI, thereby avoiding the initiation of another AV interval.

Dual chamber pacing systems programmed to the DDD or DDDR modes often have four different blanking periods (Figure 5-40). As with single chamber pacing systems, blanking is the method to prevent multiple detections of a single paced or sensed event by the sense amplifier. Generally, blanking periods are not programmable; however, some newer pacemakers offer this capability for some of the blanking periods. An *atrial blanking period* (ABP) that varies from 50 - 100 ms is initiated each time the atrial channel paces or senses. This is to prevent the atrial channel from sensing its own pacing stimulus or P-wave (spontaneous or pacing-induced). The *post-ventricular atrial blanking period* (PVABP) is initiated by a sensed or paced ventricular event. The PV-ABP is designed to prevent sensing of far-field R-wave or ventricular pacing stimulus (*crosstalk*) by the atrial lead. A ventricular blanking period (VBP), usually 50 - 100 ms in duration, occurs after a ventricular sensed or paced event. It prevents oversensing of the ventricular pacing impulse or the spontaneous or pacing-induced R-wave. Finally, there is a *post-atrial ventricular blanking period* (PAVBP) that is designed to prevent crosstalk of the atrial pacing stimulus by the ventricular channel. This period may be

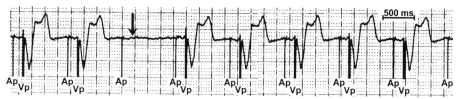

FIGURE 5-41. Example of crosstalk inhibition of ventricular pacing. With ventricular blanking programmed OFF, the third atrial pacing pulse (Ap) is sensed by the ventricular channel, inhibiting ventricular pacing (Vp) (downward arrow). Ventricular blanking after delivery of the atrial stimulus prevents crosstalk. Courtesy of Medtronic, Inc.

programmable in some models, but it should generally be set short (<40 ms) in order to insure that ventricular events that occur early in the AVI, such as premature ventricular depolarizations, are sensed. If the PAVBP is programmed to an excessively long duration, conducted ventricular events may go undetected causing the pulse generator to deliver a ventricular pacing stimulus after expiration of the AVI timer. Although unlikely, this stimulus could be delivered during a vulnerable period of the ventricular repolarization, potentially triggering a ventricular tachyarrhythmia. Ventricular blanking does not occur coincident with sensed spontaneous P-waves because the small amplitude these signals does not result in far-field sensing by the ventricular channel.

Crosstalk. Crosstalk is a phenomenon whereby one pacing channel senses the pacing stimulus delivered by the other channel (Figures 5-41 & 5-42). Crosstalk can result in inappropriate inhibition of pacing output by the sensing channel. For example, the ventricular channel could detect the far-field signal of the atrial pacing stimulus, even with normal sensitivity settings. Should this occur, ventricular pacing could be inhibited with potentially disastrous results. Ventricular blanking after delivery of an atrial pacing stimulus is one method used to address the problem of crosstalk (Figures 5-42 & 5-43). If the ventricular channel is "blinded" for a brief period of time immediately after delivery of the atrial stimulus crosstalk inhibition will be prevented.

A second method to manage the problem of crosstalk is with *ventricular safety pacing* (Figure 5-44), also known as "non-physiologic AV delay" or the "110-msec phenomenon". The ventricular safety pacing interval (VSPI), which is initiated by an atrial pace event, is generally 110 ms in duration. The first portion of the VSPI consists of the BP (generally about 25-30 ms). After the BP ends, any event sensed by the ventricular channel will trigger delivery of a ventricular pacing stimulus after the 110 ms period elapses. The logic behind VSPI is straightforward but often misunderstood. If a ventricular event is sensed within this 110 msec window it is assumed that this could not be the result of normal AV conduction of an atrial depolarization because it is too brief an interval. Instead, it is assumed that this sensed ventricular event either represents crosstalk, other electrical noise, or a ventricular premature depolarization. Rather than possibly mistakenly failing to deliver a ventricular pacing stimulus, the pulse generator will pace, possibly unnecessarily. If on the other hand, the sensed event is truly physiologic (rapid but normal AV conduction or a coincidentally-timed ventricular premature depolarization), pacing at the end of the 110 ms window ensures that the pacing stimulus will fall within

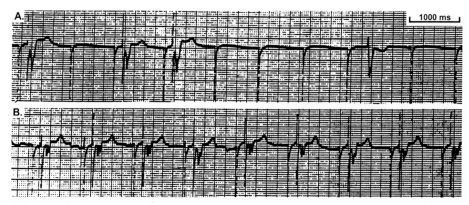

FIGURE 5-42. Intentional induction of crosstalk by programming a high atrial output, a high ventricular sensitivity and a short blanking period in a pacemaker lacking safety pacing option. Panel A: with a blanking period of 13 ms, sensing of the high amplitude atrial output in the ventricular channel results in inhibition of ventricular pacing. Panel B: crosstalk inhibition is avoided by increasing the blanking period to 50 ms. Courtesy of St. Jude/Pacesetter, Inc.

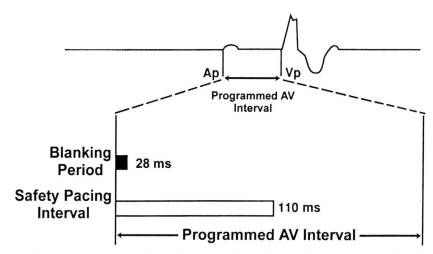

FIGURE 5-43. Schematic illustration showing relationship between the ventricular blanking and safety pacing intervals. The ventricular blanking period occupies the first 28 ms following delivery of the atrial pacing stimulus. The safety pacing interval follows the blanking period and elapses 110 ms after the delivery of the atrial pacing stimulus. See text for details. Courtesy of Medtronic, Inc.

the absolute refractory period of the ventricle. Ventricular safety pacing may also occur if there is atrial undersensing of a normal P-wave. If a scheduled atrial pacing event is delivered shortly after an unsensed P-wave, normal AV conduction and ventricular activation may occur before expiration of the PAVI timer and within the 110 msec window, triggering ventricular safety pacing. Ventricular safety pacing can be recognized on the surface ECG by the 110 msec interval between the atrial and ventricular pacing artifacts (Figure 5-44). Other methods to manage crosstalk include increasing the PAVBP, program the sensing polarity from unipolar to bipolar (if possible), decrease ventricular sen-

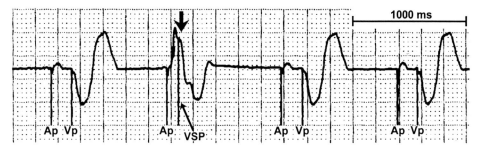

FIGURE 5-44. Example of ventricular safety pacing (VSP). Ventricular safety pacing occurs because a ventricular premature depolarization is sensed during the AV interval (downward arrow). The interval between Ap and VSP is 110 ms. Ap, atrial pacing stimulus; Vp, ventricular pacing stimulus. Courtesy of Medtronic, Inc.

sitivity (increase the millivolt setting), and reduce the atrial output amplitude or pulse width (within the acceptable output safety margin).

Upper rate behavior. One of the most difficult concepts for novices to understand is the upper rate behavior exhibited by a dual chamber pacemaker when the intrinsic atrial rate approaches or exceeds the maximum tracking rate. When this occurs, 1:1 tracking behavior is no longer possible and the pacing system will exhibit so-called Wenckebach and/or 2:1 blocking behavior (Figure 5-45). These blocking operations are designed to

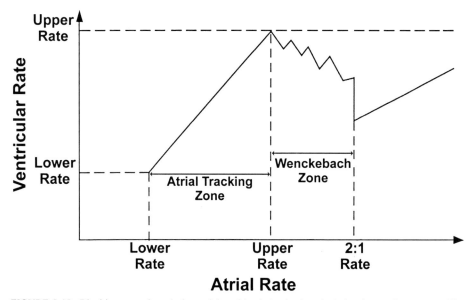

FIGURE 5-45. Blocking operations during atrial tracking behavior in a dual chamber pacing system. The jagged line represents Wenckebach operation characterized by lengthening of the AVI that occurs as the atrial rate exceeds the upper rate limit. If the atrial rate continues to increase, 2:1 block will develop. 2:1 block occurs when the P-P interval decreases until it is equal to the total atrial refractory period (TARP), which is the sum of the programmed AV interval and the post-ventricular atrial refractory period (PVARP). During 2:1 block, every other P-wave falls within the PVARP and fails to initiate the SAVI timer. Courtesy of Medtronic, Inc.

prevent 1:1 tracking of atrial tachyarrhythmias. To understand Wenckebach and 2:1 blocking behavior, the significance of the *total atrial refractory period* (TARP) must be appreciated. TARP defines the shortest P-P interval that the pacing system will track before blocking behavior occurs. The TARP interval is the sum of the SAVI and the PVARP and represents the total time period during which the atrial channel is in a refractory period (Figure 5-46).

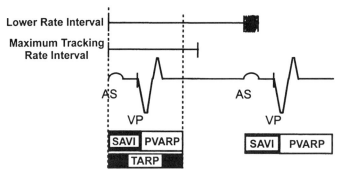

FIGURE 5-46. The total atrial refractory period (TARP) is the sum of the AV interval (SAVI) and the post-ventricular atrial refractory period (PVARP). The TARP is the highest rate (shortest interval) at which the pacemaker will track intrinsic atrial activity before 2:1 blocking behavior develops. AS, atrial sensing, VP, ventricular pacing. Courtesy of Medtronic, Inc.

Pacemaker Wenckebach has the characteristic Wenckebach pattern of gradual prolongation of the P-R (AV) interval until eventually a spontaneous atrial event falls within the PVARP, thereby preventing reinitiation of the AVI timer. Lacking initiation of an AVI interval, a ventricular pacing stimulus is not delivered following the preceding atrial depolarization (Figure 5-47). The MTRI is the atrial rate at which the pacemaker will exhibit Wenckebach behavior (Figure 5-48).

Pacemaker 2:1 block is characterized by sensing of two spontaneous atrial activations with the delivery of only one ventricular pacing stimulus. This pattern develops because every other P-wave is detected during the PVARP (Figures 5-49, 5-50 & 5-51). The P-P interval at which the pacemaker will exhibit 2:1 behavior is determined by the TARP (= SAVI + PVARP). If the P-P interval is less than the TARP, 2:1 ventricular pacing will occur. To determine the rate at which the pacemaker will exhibit 2:1 ventricular pacing behavior, simply convert the TARP interval to a rate; the atrial rate at which 2:1 block occurs is 60,000/TARP.

If the programmed MTRI is greater than the TARP interval, the pacemaker will initially exhibit Wenckebach behavior for a number of pacing cycles before 2:1 block develops with further increases in the atrial rate. If the MTRI is less than the TARP, 2:1 ventricular pacing will occur first before upper rate ventricular pacing can be achieved and without the initial development of Wenckebach behavior. Take the example where the MTRI is 120 pulses/min (500 ms), the PVARP is 350 ms, and the SAVI is 200 ms. In this case the TARP is 550 ms (350 ms + 200 ms) which is greater than the MTRI of 500 ms. Therefore, as the P-P interval decreases, the 2:1 blocking interval (550 ms, 109 pulses/min) will occur before the MTRI (500 ms, 120 pulses/min) is reached. Wenckebach pacing behavior will not occur. As another example consider the case where the MTRI is 100 pulses/min (600 ms), the PVARP is 350 ms, and the SAVI is 150 ms. In this case the MTRI of 600 ms is greater than the TARP of 500 ms. Therefore, in this sit-

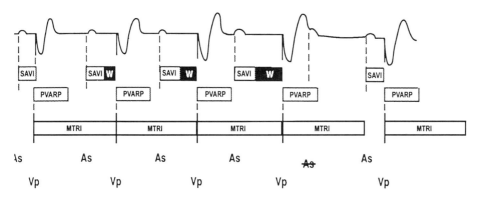

FIGURE 5-47. Schematic diagram illustrating Wenckebach operation during atrial tracking behavior in a dual-chamber pacemaker. Starting from the left side of the figure, the pacemaker senses an atrial depolarization (As) which initiates the SAVI timer. Because no spontaneous ventricular event occurs at the expiration of the SAVI, a ventricular stimulus (Vp) is delivered which starts the PVARP interval. A second intrinsic atrial event is detected after the PVARP timer elapses starting another sensed SAVI. This time when the SAVI times out, MTRI has not yet expired. Delivery of a pacing stimulus at this time would violate the inviolable MTRI. Consequently, the ventricular pace has to be delayed until the end of the MTRI at which time the stimulus is delivered. The amount of this delay is often termed the Wenckebach interval (W). This pattern of sensing a P-wave, starting the SAVI, waiting for the MTRI to elapse, and pacing the ventricle repeats until a P-wave falls within the PVARP, preventing the initiation of a SAVI and the delivery a pacing stimulus. The amount of the Wenckebach interval increases during each cycle, gradually lengthening the interval from the P-wave to the ventricular pacing stimulus. Once a P-wave falls within the PVARP, the pacemaker continues to look for the next sensed P-wave and the pacemaker Wenckebach cycle begins again. As, atrial sense; Vp, ventricular pace. For other abbreviations see Table 5-10. Courtesy of Medtronic, Inc.

uation the Wenckebach behavior would occur at a P-P interval of 600 ms (100 pulses/min) and continue until the P-P interval was 500 ms (120 pulses/min). At higher atrial rates 2:1 ventricular pacing would occur. Patients poorly tolerate the sudden and dramatic decrease in the ventricular pacing rate associated with a transition from 1:1 to 2:1 tracking behavior. Far preferable is the transition to a gradual decline in ventricular rate associated with initial Wenckebach behavior which, if the atrial rate continues to accelerate, is followed by the development of 2:1 atrial tracking. To summarize, 1) 1:1 atrial

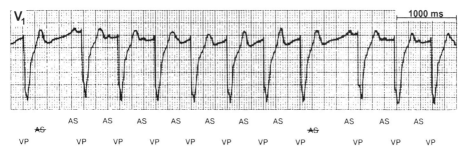

FIGURE 5-48. ECG recording showing pacemaker Wenckebach operation during rapid atrial activity. AS, atrial sensing, VP, ventricular pacing. Courtesy of Medtronic, Inc.

tracking will occur whenever the atrial rate is less than the maximum tracking rate (assuming TARP is < MTRI); 2) Wenckebach behavior will occur when the P-P interval (in

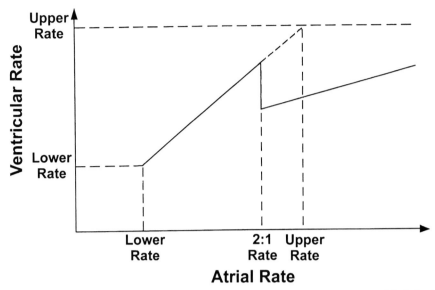

FIGURE 5-49. Schematic diagram illustrating 2:1 blocking operation in a DDD-programmed dual chamber pacemaker. If the pulse generator has the upper rate programmed to a rate higher than the 2:1 block rate (determined by the total atrial refractory period (TARP) = PVARP + AVI) then 2:1 block will occur before the upper rate is achieved. See text for details. Courtesy of Medtronic, Inc.

ms) exceeds both the MTRI and the TARP; and 3) atrial rates greater than the TARP cause 2:1 pacing behavior. In order to ensure that Wenckebach pacing occurs before 2:1 behavior, make the TARP interval less than the MTRI either by decreasing the duration of the PVARP or the SAVI, or program a rate-adaptive AVI.

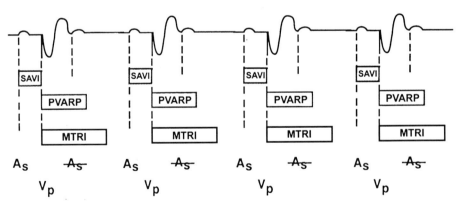

FIGURE 5-50. Schematic diagram illustrating 2:1 block operation in a dual-chamber pacemaker programmed to the DDD mode. Starting on the left side of the figure, the sequence begins with a sensed P-wave that initiates a SAVI. After expiration of the SAVI timer a ventricular pacing stimulus is delivered which starts the PVARP interval. The next P-wave falls within the PVARP; therefore, a SAVI is not initiated. The subsequent P-wave occurs after expiration of the PVARP so a SAVI is started and a ventricular stimulus is delivered when the SAVI times out. This pattern continues with every other P-wave triggering a ventricular-paced event resulting in a 2:1 block pattern. As, atrial sense; Vp, ventricular pace. For other abbreviations see Table 5-10. Courtesy of Medtronic, Inc.

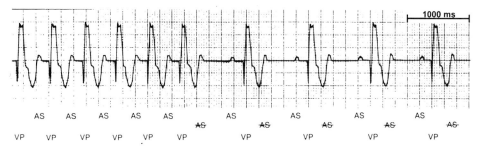

FIGURE 5-51. ECG recording showing 2:1 block operation during rapid atrial activity in a dual-chamber pacemaker. Marker channel displayed at·bottom of the figure. AS, atrial sense; VP, ventricular pace. Courtesy of Medtronic, Inc.

In a patient with a normal cardiac conduction system and normal autonomic nervous system, the AV conduction time (P-R interval) decreases as the heart rate increases and increases as the heart rate decreases. Pulse generators that have a programmable *dynamic* or *rate-adaptive AV interval* (RA-AVI) can mimic the normal physiologic behavior of the P-R interval (Figure 5-52). The RA-AVI results in a decrease in the SAVI or PAVI as the spontaneous or sensor-driven atrial rate increases (Figures 5-53 & 5-54). With higher intrinsic atrial rates, the SAVI will decrease, which reduces the TARP, and permits 1:1 tracking to occur up to the MTRI. As the sensor-driven atrial pacing rate increases, there is a proportional reduction in the duration of the PAVI, resulting in an increase in the duration of the AEI. Consequently, there is an increase in the duration of the atrial sensing window allowing more time for sensing closely-coupled intrinsic atrial events.

FIGURE 5-52. The rate-adaptive AV interval (RA-AVI) mimics the normal physiologic response of the P-R interval to exercise-induced increase in heart rates As shown here, without RA-AVI the P-P interval is greater than the TARP and 2:1 block would occur at the atrial rate of 133/min (450 ms) (panel A). With RA-AVI programmed ON, the TARP is greater than the P-P interval and 1:1 tracking can occur at the atrial rate of 133/min. Courtesy of Medtronic, Inc.

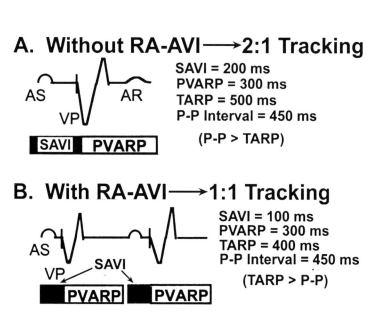

A. Without RA-AVI ⟶ 2:1 Tracking

SAVI = 200 ms
PVARP = 300 ms
TARP = 500 ms
P-P Interval = 450 ms

(P-P > TARP)

B. With RA-AVI ⟶ 1:1 Tracking

SAVI = 100 ms
PVARP = 300 ms
TARP = 400 ms
P-P Interval = 450 ms

(TARP > P-P)

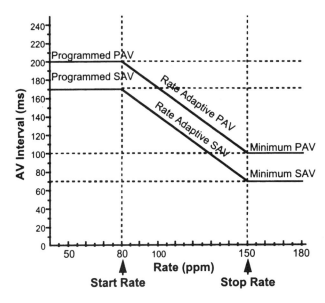

FIGURE 5-53. Graphic illustration depicting the operation of rate-adaptive AV interval. Both the paced AV interval (PAV) and the sensed AV interval (SAV) decrease with increasing rates. For the PAV, the adaptation is based upon the sensor-driven rate. For the SAV, the adaptation is based upon the intrinsic atrial rate. The rate-adaptive AV interval has three programming requirements, in addition to the SAV and the PAV: 1) the start rate, which determines the rate at which the rate-adaptive AV interval is initiated, 2) the stop rate, which determines the rate at which the minimum SAV and PAV is reached and, 3) the minimum AV interval, which is the shortest SAV and PAV permitted. Courtesy of Medtronic, Inc.

Consider the following example to illustrate the benefit of the RA-AVI option. Assume the MTRI is 140 pulses/min (429 ms), the SAVI is 150 ms, and the PVARP is 320 ms. In this situation, the TARP is 470 ms which is greater than the MTRI. Therefore, for atrial rates greater than 127/min (470 ms), 2:1 blocking behavior will occur and ventricular pacing at the MTRI is not possible. If however, the RA-AVI option is activated and the minimum SAVI is programmed to become 100 ms when the atrial rate reaches 120/min, then to TARP becomes 420 ms (143 pulses/min) which is less than the MTRI. Therefore, MTRI pacing can occur and Wenckebach operation, rather than 2:1 block, is triggered when the P-P interval first exceeds the MTRI.

Programming a dual chamber pacemaker from the DDD mode to the adaptive-rate pacing mode DDDR also can help prevent precipitous drops in the ventricular rate in response to rapid intrinsic atrial rates (Figure 5-55). If the sensor-driven rate is set slightly lower than the maximum atrial tracking rate, the fallback rate when the P-P interval exceeds the TARP will not be the 2:1 rate, but instead, will be the sensor-driven rate with the AV interval the PAVI instead of the SAVI (Figure 5-55). If the TARP is 400 ms and the MTRI is programmed to 150 pulses/min (400 ms) when the P-P interval exceeds 400

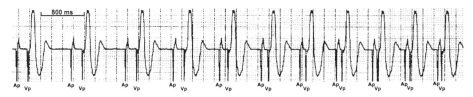

FIGURE 5-54. Example of dynamic or rate-responsive AV interval in a rate-responsive dual chamber pacing system. Note that the PAVI is 200 msec during LRI pacing (60 pulses/min). With an increase in atrial and ventricular pacing resulting from sensor activation, the PAVI progressively shortens to 80 msec at a pacing rate of 100 pulses/min. Courtesy of Guidant/CPI, Inc.

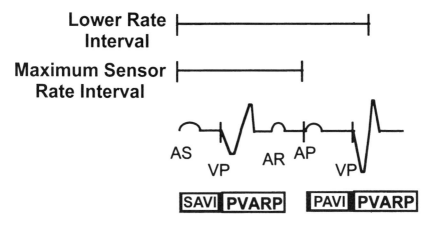

Lower Rate Interval

Maximum Sensor Rate Interval

AS VP AR AP VP

SAVI | PVARP   PAVI | PVARP

FIGURE 5-55. Benefit of adaptive-rate pacing (DDDR mode) to prevent a precipitous drop in heart rate due to upper rate behavior. Courtesy of Medtronic, Inc.

ms, the ventricular pacing rate will suddenly decline from 150 pulses/min to 75 pulses/min. However, if the MSRI is set at 120 pulses/min (500 ms), the fallback rate after the P-P interval exceeds 400 ms will be 120 pulses/min, rather than 75 pulses/min.

Comparison of atrial- and ventricular-based timing. Two different timing modes are used in dual chamber pacemaker systems: *V–V timing* and *A–A timing* (Figure 5-56). In V–V timing, an atrial depolarization that conducts to the ventricular before the expiration of the AV interval timer results in inhibition of ventricular pacing and immediate reinitiation of the AEI timer. This earlier than expected activation of the ventricle effectively shortens the AV interval causing the entire V–V interval (which is the sum of the AEI and the AV interval) to be reduced by an amount equal to the difference between the programmed AVI and the actual (reduced) AV conduction time. Therefore, the atrial pacing rate may be less than the programmed rate or, in fact, may vary as intrinsic AV conduction time varies. In A-A timing, an atrial depolarization that activates the ventricle before expiration of the PAVI timer also results in inhibition of ventricular pacing and initiation of the AEI timer. However, unlike the situation with V-V timing, the duration of the AEI is not fixed; instead, it is increased by an amount equal to the difference between the programmed PAVI and the actual duration of the reduced AV conduction time (Figure 5-56). This ensures that the atrial pacing rate remains constant at the programmed LRI instead being reduced as with V-V timing. A-A timing is most important at higher rates. Consider a pacemaker programmed to an upper rate of 130 pulses/min (460 ms) and with a PAVI greater than the actual spontaneous AV conduction time by 30 ms. If the pacemaker system were operating under V-V timing rules, the entire V-V interval at the upper rate would be shortened by 30 ms, resulting in an atrial pacing rate of 140 pulses/min. If A-A timing rules were in place, variability of the AEI would ensure that the atrial pacing interval would remain constant (Figure 5-56).

A. Atrial-Based Timing

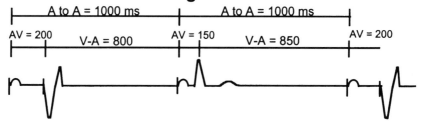

B. Ventricular-Based Timing

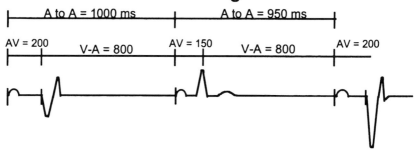

FIGURE 5-56. Comparison of atrial-based (A-A) and ventricular-based (V-V) timing. See text for details. Courtesy of Medtronic, Inc.

5.4.3 PACING MODES

Asynchronous (fixed-rate) pacing (VOO, AOO, DOO modes). In asynchronous (fixed-rate) pacing there is no sensing of spontaneous or pacing induced activity in any cardiac chamber. For example, a pulse generator programmed to the VOO mode delivers a pacing stimuli through a ventricular lead at a pacing cycle length equal to the programmable LRI, regardless of any spontaneous ventricular activity that may occur (Figure 5-57). In the VOO mode there is no VRP and sensing of spontaneous ventricular activity is inhibited during the entire duration of the LRI. Likewise pulse generators programmed to the AOO or DOO modes deliver pacing stimuli to the atrium (AOO) or atrium and ventricle (DOO) at a fixed cycle length LRI. If there is any spontaneous cardiac electrical activity, asynchronous pacing will result in competition between pacing-induced activation of the heart and any spontaneous depolarizations that may occur. Because of this, asynchronous pacing is almost never used for long-term pacing even though it is a programmable option in modern pulse generators. Asynchronous pacing is the mode of pacing performed when a strong magnet is applied over the implanted pulse generator (magnet application inhibits sensing). Some pulse generators revert to this pacing mode in response to sensing electrical noise or an electrical shock (for example from a defibrillator).

Noncompetitive (demand) pacing (VVI, AAI, VVT, AAT modes). In a demand pacing mode, the pulse generator is inhibited by electrical signals sensed within the chamber it

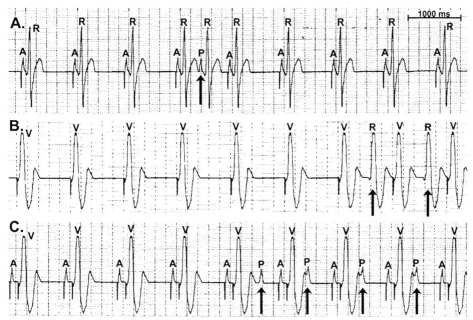

FIGURE 5-57. AAO (panel A), VOO (panel B), and DOO (panel C) modes. When pacing in these asynchronous or fixed-rate pacing modes, pacing stimuli are delivered at the programmed lower rate cycle length to the atrium (AOO), ventricle (VOO), or both (DOO). Sensing is inhibited during the entire pacing cycle. Consequently, spontaneous atrial or ventricular activations fail to inhibit atrial or ventricular pacing, respectively (upward arrows) Thus, competition can occur between any spontaneous rhythm and the paced rhythm occurring at the programmed lower rate. As a result, a stimulus may be delivered during a vulnerable period within cardiac diastole. Although uncommon, this asynchronous pacing could trigger an atrial or ventricular arrhythmia; therefore, this pacing mode is used infrequently. Application of a magnet over the pulse generator will temporarily activate the SOO or DOO mode. Electromagnetic interference (radiofrequency signals, electrocautery, or defibrillator shocks) may reset a pacemaker to the SOO or DOO mode. Some pacemakers also reset to these modes at end-of-life. For abbreviations see Table 5-10. Courtesy of Guidant/CPI, Inc.

is pacing, thereby avoiding competition between electrical pacing and spontaneous activation of the cardiac chamber. With ventricular demand pacing (VVI or VVT), sensing and pacing occurs in the ventricle (Figures 5-58 & 5-59). In both the VVI and VVT modes, the ventricle is paced at the LRI cycle length as long as there is no spontaneous electrical activity sensed in the ventricle outside of the VRP. In the VVI mode, ventricular pacing is inhibited by a spontaneous ventricular activation occurring during the *noise-sampling* or *alert period*, which is the time period between successive VRPs, while during VVT pacing a ventricular stimuli is delivered into any spontaneous ventricular depolarization that is sensed. In both modes ventricular sensing is inactive during the VRP. Because of the unnecessary triggered ventricular pacing when in the VVT mode, this mode is considered obsolete. VVI pacing is indicated for patients with chronic atrial fibrillation or other atrial tachyarrhythmias with associated symptomatic slow ventricular response.

In atrial demand pacing (AAI or AAT), the atrium is paced and the ventricle is activated by conduction of the depolarization wavefront from the atrium through the normal conduction system (Figures 5-58 & 5-59). In the AAI mode, atrial pacing is inhibited by

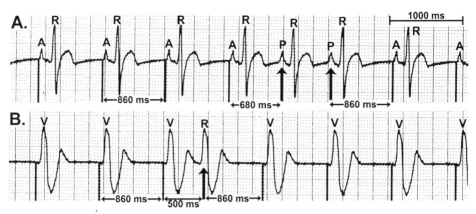

FIGURE 5-58. AAI (upper panel) and VVI (lower panel) modes. In these demand modes, pacing stimuli are delivered at the programmed lower rate limit cycle length (in this case 860 ms) unless delivery is inhibited by spontaneous activity that is sensed in the atrial channel (AAI) or ventricular channel (VVI) during the alert period. Unlike VOO or AOO pacing, during VVI or AII pacing the pulse generator will only deliver stimuli if a spontaneous depolarization is not sensed before the lower rate limit timer elapses. Consequently, there is no competition between pacemaker-derived activations and spontaneous depolarizations. If a spontaneous depolarization is sensed during the alert period (upward arrows), the lower rate limit timer is reset. A pacing stimuli is not delivered until the lower rate timer elapses. Sensing is inhibited during the respective refractory periods. The pulse generator is blinded to a spontaneous depolarization occurring during the refractory period. Therefore, the lower rate timer is not reset in this situation and a pacing stimuli will be delivered "on time" (unless inhibited by another spontaneous depolarization occurring during the alert period). For abbreviations see Table 5-10. Courtesy of Guidant/CPI, Inc.

a spontaneous atrial activation occurring outside of the ARP; during the ARP sensing is prevented. In the AAT mode, an atrial stimuli is delivered at the time a spontaneous atrial depolarization is sensed. In both AAT and AAI modes, atrial pacing is performed at the programmed LRI cycle length if there is no spontaneous atrial activity sensed during the period when sensing is occurring (after termination of the ARP and before delivery of the next pacing stimuli at the LRI cycle length). AAI and AAT pacing is only an option in patients with intact atrioventricular conduction. If there is spontaneous atrial activity, AAT is an inefficient pacing mode because the delivery of pacing stimuli immediately upon sensing of a spontaneous atrial depolarization will result in unnecessary pacing and accelerated battery depletion; therefore it is considered obsolete. AAI pacing is a very good option for patients with isolated sinoatrial node dysfunction and normal AV conduction; it is contraindicated in patients with frequent or chronic atrial fibrillation or atrial tachyarrhythmias.

Synchronous atrioventricular pacing (VAT, VDD modes). In these pacing modes (sometimes termed P-synchronous pacing or A-sense, V-pacing) any spontaneous sensed atrial depolarization triggers the delivery of a ventricular pacing stimulus. In both VAT and VDD modes, this "tracking" of atrial activity triggers subsequent ventricular pacing after a programmable delay. The difference between these modes is that with VAT pacing, sensing is not performed in the ventricle potentially resulting in competition between spontaneous ventricular activity and uninhibited ventricular pacing at the same rate as the spontaneous activity in the atrium. In VDD mode (Figure 5-60), sensing occurs in both the ventricle and atrium; consequently, ventricular pacing is inhibited if spontane-

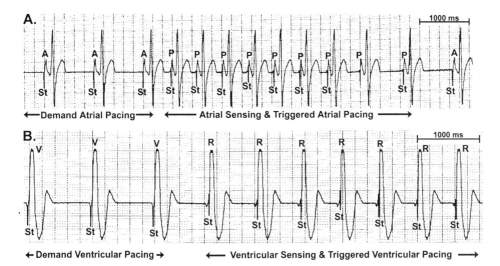

FIGURE 5-59. AAT (panel A) and VVT (panel B) modes. In the absence of sensed events, pacing pulses are delivered to the atrium (AAT) or ventricle (VVT) at the lower rate limit. Sensed spontaneous atrial or ventricular depolarizations will trigger the delivery of a pacing stimulus by the atrial channel (AAT) or ventricular channel (VVT) immediately upon sensing the spontaneous event. If at all, the AAT and VVT modes should only be used for diagnostic purposes. These modes allow verification of appropriate sensing by observing a pacing spike on the surface ECG during any spontaneous depolarization. However, with the wide availability of pulse generators with an internal event marker circuit that provides verification of sensing, the use of the AAT and VVT modes is generally no longer necessary. AAT and VVT pacing is not recommended for ambulatory use because in the event of oversensing of non-cardiac electrical activity, triggered inappropriate pacing could result. For abbreviations see Table 5-10. Courtesy of Guidant/CPI, Inc.

ous ventricular activity is sensed at a rate equal to, or greater than, the sensed atrial activity. As a result, the chance that a uninhibited pacing stimulus will trigger a ventricular tachyarrhythmia by exciting the ventricular myocardium during a vulnerable period is minimized. For these reasons, VAT pacing is considered obsolete and VDD is the preferred mode. In these pacing modes, a programmable option allows setting the maximum rate of 1:1 tracking of atrial rate preventing ventricular pacing at very high rates in patients who develop an atrial tachyarrhythmia.

Sequential atrioventricular pacing (DVI mode). With the DVI mode (Figure 5-61), pacing occurs sequentially in the atrium and, after a programmable AVI, in the ventricle. Because there is no sensing in the atrium, the atrial pacing stimulus is delivered at a programmable interval after a sensed or paced ventricular event even if spontaneous atrial activity is occurring at a rate faster than the programmed atrial pacing rate. Consequently, the potential exists for competition between spontaneous and paced atrial activity, resulting in the possibility for pacing-induced provocation of reentrant atrial tachycardias or fibrillation. DVI pacing preserves AV synchrony when the spontaneous atrial rate is less than the programmed atrial rate. At atrial rates greater than the programmed rate AV synchrony is lost because of the inability to sense atrial activity.

Soon after its development it became apparent that the DVI mode had a significant potential problem resulting from far-field sensing of the atrial pacing stimulus by the

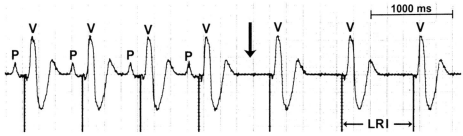

FIGURE 5-60. VDD mode. In the VDD mode, only the ventricle is paced, but both chambers are sensed. The most common use for VDD pacing is to "track" spontaneous atrial activity (P-synchronous pacing, left-half of rhythm strip). Ventricular stimuli are delivered after a sensed atrial event at a programmable delay (which triggers a SAVI timer). With the onset of sinus arrest or exit block (downward arrow), no spontaneous atrial activity is sensed and the pulse generator responds by pacing the ventricle at the programmed LRI. It should be added that in some pulse generators programmed to the VDD mode that the ventricular rate is permitted to dip below the LRI to promote AV synchrony, since atrial sensed events are accepted up to the end of the LRI. Therefore, it will pace at rates as low as the LRI + SAVI. Because there is no atrial pacing in the VDD mode, there is no PAVI timer in this mode. For abbreviations see Table 5-10. Courtesy of Guidant/ CPI, Inc.

ventricular channel. The manufacturers dealt with this problem by introducing a brief blanking period into the pacemaker's timing circuit immediately following delivery of the atrial stimulus. During this blanking period the sensing circuit of the ventricular channel is inactive. Through this means, the patient with AV conduction block is protected from inhibition of ventricular pacing by far-field sensing of the atrial stimulus. Although DVI pacing is rarely used, programming to this mode may be an option when atrial sensing is undesirable, as for example during pacemaker-mediated tachycardia which develops during VDD or DDD pacing. DVI pacing may also be useful in some patients with symptomatic sinus bradycardia and AV conduction block. DVI mode

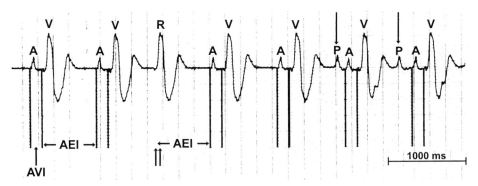

FIGURE 5-61. DVI mode. With DVI pacing both the atrium and ventricle are paced but sensing only occurs in the ventricular channel. The atrial stimulus is delivered at a defined interval (AEI) after a previous sensed or paced ventricular event. In the absence of AV conduction, the ventricular channel will deliver a pacing stimulus after a programmable delay (AVI). The lower rate interval (LRI) cycle length is the sum of the AEI and the AVI. A sensed spontaneous ventricular event (double upward arrows) resets the AEI timer and inhibits atrial and ventricular pacing. The next atrial paced event occurs after the newly reset AEI timer elapses. Note that on the right side of rhythm strip, spontaneous atrial activity develops (downward arrows) but is not sensed by the atrial channel. As a result, asynchronous atrial pacing continues and competes with the spontaneous atrial rhythm. Ventricular pacing continues at the LRI. For abbreviations see Table 5-10. Courtesy of Guidant/CPI, Inc.

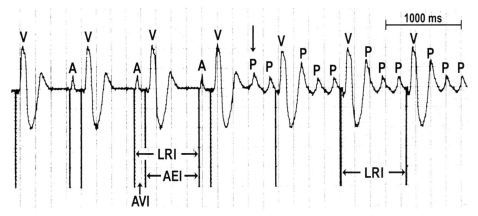

FIGURE 5-62. DDI mode. In the DDI mode, pacing and sensing occur in both the atrium and ventricle. The response to a sensed spontaneous atrial or ventricular event is inhibition. As seen on the left-half of the rhythm strip, if the spontaneous atrial and ventricular rates are less than the lower rate interval (LRI), atrial and ventricular pacing occurs at the LRI, with the ventricular stimulus delivered at a programmable interval (AVI) after delivery of the atrial stimulus. With the onset of atrial flutter (right-half, downward arrow), atrial pacing is inhibited and, in the absence of AV conduction, ventricular pacing occurs at the LRI without tracking the rapid atrial activity. For abbreviations see Table 5-10. Courtesy of Guidant/CPI, Inc.

should not be used in patients who have normal sinus node function or atrial tachyarrhythmias.

Inhibited pacing of atrium and ventricle (DDI). In DDI mode (Figure 5-62) there is pacing and sensing in both the atrium and ventricles; however, the only response to a sensed spontaneous atrial or ventricular activation is inhibition. When the pacemaker senses atrial activity it does not deliver a pacing stimulus in the atrium and initiation of the SAVI timer is prevented. Consequently, the pulse generator is prevented from delivering a ventricular stimulus in response to a spontaneous atrial depolarization (the ventricular channel will not "track" rapid atrial activity). The AVI timer only starts after a paced atrial event (PAVI). Therefore, synchronous AV pacing only occurs when the atrium is paced or during sinus rhythm when AV conduction is intact (and the programmed atrial pacing rate is less than the sinus rate). DDI(R) pacing can be thought of as AAI(R) with VVI(R) backup. When programmed to the DDI mode the pacemaker will never pace faster than the programmed lower rate. As a result, the patient will not have rate adaptation unless there is sinus node chronotropic competence and normal AV conduction. DDI (or DDIR) pacing may be useful in selected patients with paroxysmal atrial tachyarrhythmias in whom inappropriate 1:1 "tracking" of rapid atrial rates could result in equally rapid ventricular pacing. Newer dual chamber pulse generators have algorithms that allow "on-the-fly" *mode switching* from a tracking mode (DDD) to a nontracking mode (VVI or VVIR) in response to sensed spontaneous atrial activity above a certain programmable rate (See "Mode switching" on page 239). Following resolution of the atrial tachyarrhythmia, the pulse generator will resume its previous DDD program. This technology will almost certainly replace the use of the DDI mode.

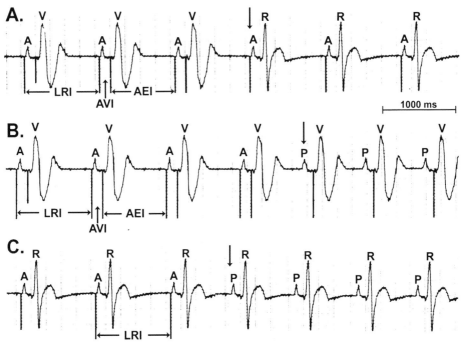

FIGURE 5-63. The spectrum of DDD operation. Panel A: Atrial and ventricular sequential pacing is performed at the LRI cycle length (atrial and ventricular pacing operation). During LRI pacing, each subsequent atrial pacing stimulus is delivered at a fixed interval (AEI) after sensing a ventricular pacing event. The ventricular pacing stimulus is delivered at a programmable fixed interval (AVI) after an atrial pacing event. If spontaneous AV conduction and ventricular activation occurs after the atrial pacing stimulus is delivered (atrial synchronous pacing, downward arrow) and before the AVI timer elapses, delivery of the ventricular stimulus is inhibited (atrial pacing and ventricular sensing operation). Panel B: Again, AV synchronous pacing is occurring at the LRI cycle length (left-half of rhythm strip). With an increase in the spontaneous atrial rate above the programmed LRI the pacemaker operation spontaneously changes to P-synchronous pacing (downward arrow) (atrial sensing and ventricular pacing operation). Under these conditions, the ventricle is no longer paced at the LRI cycle length; instead, the ventricular rate is driven by the P-P cycle length. Panel C: Atrial synchronous pacing is performed at the LRI cycle length (left-half of rhythm strip). With an increase in the spontaneous atrial rate to a point above the programmed LRI, atrial pacing is inhibited and the pacemaker operation changes to atrial sensing and ventricular sensing (downward arrow). For abbreviations see Table 5-10. Courtesy of Guidant/CPI, Inc.

Universal atrioventricular pacing (DDD mode). In the DDD mode sensing and pacing both occur in the atrium and ventricle. Because this dual sensing and pacing capabilities, DDD pacemaker systems can exhibit four different pacing/sensing behaviors, depending upon the presence or absence of spontaneous atrial or ventricular activity (Figures 5-37 & 5-63). In patients with intact atrioventricular conduction but sinus bradycardia, atrial pacing with ventricular sensing may occur. Atrial events, both sensed and paced, initiate an AVI timer. In the absence of a sensed spontaneous ventricular activation within the AVI period, delivery of a ventricular pacing stimulus is triggered at the end of the AVI. If a spontaneous ventricular depolarization is sensed during the AVI period, the ventricular channel is inhibited from delivering a pacing stimulus. In patients with intact AV conduction and normal sinus rhythm at rates greater than the lower rate limit, both atrial and ventricular pacing is inhibited (assuming the AV conduction time is less than the programmed AVI.

Many studies have demonstrated the short- and long-term hemodynamic benefits AV synchronous pacing compared with single chamber ventricular pacing. AV synchrony, especially in patients with non-compliant left ventricles due to underlying structural heart disease, may result in a 20% – 30% boost in end-diastolic and stroke volumes with a corresponding improvement in cardiac output [29,30,35-40].

Adaptive-rate pacing (AAIR, VVIR, DDIR, DDDR). A rate-responsive or adaptive-rate pacemaker system requires a sensor that can transduce changes in a patients metabolic need into electrical signals that trigger a change in the pacing rate. Ideally, the sensor should mimic the response of the normal sinus rate to increased demands for cardiac output. In a sense the DDD pacemaker in a patient with normal sinoatrial node function is the "ideal" rate responsive pacing system because it uses the patient's own sinus node as the sensor; as the sinus rate varies so does the ventricular pacing rate. Assuming that the rate of atrial activity is accurately reporting the patient's metabolic needs, with DDD pacing the ventricular rate will follow in a 1:1 fashion (up to a certain programmable rate). However, in patients lacking a normal sinus node response an artificial sensor must be included as part of the implanted device. Sensors have been developed that respond to a variety of electrical, chemical, and physical stimuli. In the United States the only currently available sensors respond to motion or minute ventilation.

Single chamber rate-responsive pacing is identical to non-rate-responsive pacing with the exception that the pacing rate is driven by a sensor (Figure 5-64). At baseline sensor activity, the device will pace at the lower rate limit. The sensor determines whether or not a rate increase is indicated and adjusts the rate accordingly. With an increase in sensor activity, the pulse generator will respond with a faster pacing rate up to the programmed upper rate limit. The highest rate the pacemaker is allowed to pace is determined by the MSRI. In AAI(R) mode, the atrial refractory period must be programmed to a long enough duration to avoid sensing far-field R- and T-waves. Therefore, the refractory period in AAI(R) mode must be greater than the VVI(R) mode, usually about 400 ms. Manufacturers have employed sensors in both single chamber pulse generators (AAIR, VVIR) as well as dual chamber units (DDDR, DDIR) (Figure 5-64).

Adaptive-rate pacing is not limited by refractory periods. Programming a long refractory period in combination with a high maximum sensor rate may result in asynchronous pacing during refractory periods because the combination can cause a very small sensing period (alert period), or none at all. For example, an AV delay set at 200 ms combined with a PVARP of 300 ms will result in asynchronous atrial pacing at sensor-indicated rates above 120 pulses/min in dual chamber adaptive-rate pacemakers. In adaptive-rate single chamber pacemakers, a programmed refractory period of 500 ms will result in asynchronous pacing at sensor-indicated rates above 120 pulses/min.

Mode switching. Patients with dual chamber pacemakers programmed to a physiologic tracking mode, such as DDD or DDDR, may have undesirable rapid ventricular pacing

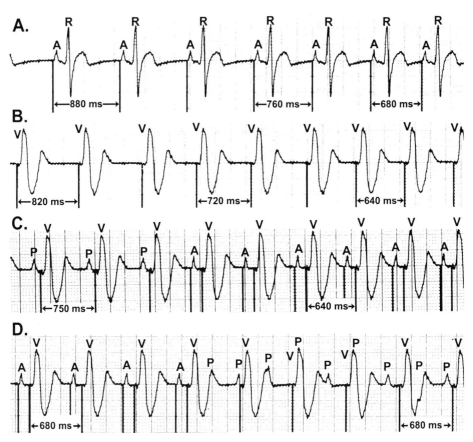

FIGURE 5-64. Spectrum of adaptive-rate pacing operations. Panel A: In the AAIR mode, the sensor-driven atrial pacing rate increases (shortening of the A-A cycle length) with increasing workload. A similar response is seen in the sensor-based ventricular pacing rate using the VVIR mode (Panel B). Panel C: P-synchronous pacing at a ventricular rate of 80 pulses/min (left-half) transitions into sensor-driven pacing in the DDDR mode (right-half). Both the atrium and ventricle are paced at a rate of 95 pulses/min. That this is in fact sensor-based pacing in the DDDR mode is confirmed because the atrial pacing rate is greater than the programmed lower rate. Panel D: Sensor-driven AV sequential pacing is occurring at 88 pulses/min (left-half). With the development of atrial tachycardia (P-P interval = 400 ms) at a rate greater than the programmed upper rate limit of the pulse generator, the pacemaker operation changes such that atrial sensing is inhibited and demand ventricular pacing occurs at the programmed lower rate limit. In other words, during spontaneous rapid atrial rates the DDIR-programmed pacemaker functions as if it were programmed to the VVI mode. For abbreviations see Table 5-10. Courtesy of Guidant/CPI, Inc.

during episodes of paroxysmal supraventricular tachycardias such as atrial flutter, tachycardia, or fibrillation (Figure 5-65). One method used to manage this possibility is to utilize the TARP to trigger 2:1 ventricular pacing in response rapid atrial rates. A second option is to program different values for the MTRI and the MSRI. If the MTRI is set low and the MSRI is set high, fast tracking of atrial tachyarrhythmias will be avoided while still permitting high sensor-driven pacing rates. A third option is to use *mode switching* (Figure 5-66). Mode switching can be used to prevent tracking of paroxysmal atrial tachyarrhythmias in the DDD, DDDR, or VDD modes. When the pacemaker detects a

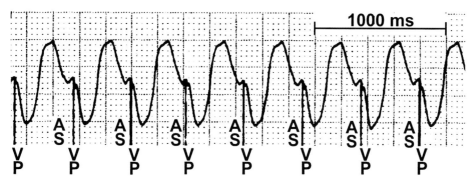

FIGURE 5-65. High rate ventricular pacing resulting from tracking paroxysmal supraventricular tachycardia. Patients with dual chamber pacing systems and supraventricular tachyarrhythmias have traditionally been managed by using the TARP to set a low 2:1 block rate or programming separate maximum tracking rate and upper sensor-driven rate. AS, atrial sense; VP, ventricular pace. Courtesy of Medtronic, Inc.

spontaneous atrial rate greater than a programmable rate, the pacemaker resets its atrial tracking mode to a non-tracking *fallback mode* (Figure 5-66). In most pacemakers that have the mode switching option, the fallback mode is either usually DDI(R), VVI(R), or VDI(R). As a result, even during a mode switch episode, ventricular rate-responsive pacing can occur. After cessation of the atrial arrhythmia and with a decline of the atrial rate below the mode switching trigger rate, the pacemaker returns to the originally programmed mode. The advantage of mode switching is ventricular pacing is transiently uncoupled from atrial events only during the period of the paroxysmal tachycardia; the pacemaker need not be programmed permanently to a non-tracking mode.

Although mode-switching algorithms vary among manufacturers, in general, four parameters may require programming to effectively institute mode-switching behavior. These include: 1) the spontaneous atrial rate at which mode-switching will be triggered, 2) the new non-tracking pacing mode triggered by the atrial tachyarrhythmia (the fall-

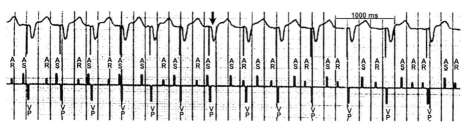

FIGURE 5-66. Mode switching in response to atrial tachyarrhythmia. Mode switch can be used to prevent tracking of paroxysmal atrial tachycardias in the DDD(R), DDD, and VDD modes. When the pacemaker detects a supraventricular tachycardia the device switches from the programmed atrial tracking mode to a non-atrial tracking mode until the atrial arrhythmia ceases (downward arrow). When the atrial arrhythmia terminates, the mode switch episode terminates and the pacemaker responds by returning to the original synchronous mode. As shown here, at the onset of an atrial arrhythmia the pacemaker compares a mean atrial interval (MAI), a running average of the A-A interval, to the current A-A interval. If the A-A interval is shorter than the MAI, the MAI is shortened by 24 ms. If the A-A interval is longer than the MAI, the MAI is lengthened by 8 ms. When the MAI reaches the interval corresponding to the mode switch detection rate interval, the pacemaker switches from the DDDR to the DDIR mode. AS, atrial sense, AR, atrial refractory sense; VP, ventricular pace. Courtesy of Medtronic, Inc.

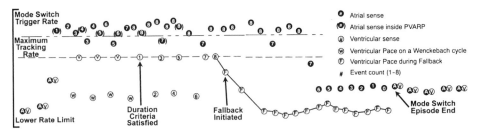

FIGURE 5-67. Illustration of mode-switching behavior in a dual chamber rate-responsive pacemaker (Guidant Discovery). A paroxysmal tachyarrhythmia with atrial rate greater than the programmed trigger rate results transient automatic reprogramming of the pacemaker to a non-tracking fallback mode (VDIR) after the duration criteria are satisfied (8 atrial activations above the triggering rate). Five seconds after termination of the supraventricular arrhythmia, atrial-sensing, ventricular-pacing resumes as the device automatically restores the original pacing mode (DDDR). Courtesy of Guidant/CPI, Inc.

back mode), 3) the required duration of atrial activity above the triggering rate after which a mode-switch episode begins (triggering the onset of fallback mode pacing) and, 4) time required to reach the fallback mode pacing rate (either the programmed lower rate limit or sensor-based pacing rate) once duration criteria have been satisfied (fallback time). The shorter the fallback duration and fallback time, the quicker atrial tracking will be terminated after the onset of an atrial tachyarrhythmia and the faster the original tracking mode will be restored after termination of the atrial arrhythmia. The pacemaker will continue to pace in the fallback mode at the sensor-indicated rate or the programmed lower rate until the atrial arrhythmia terminates. Upon termination of the arrhythmia, or when the atrial rate decreases below the mode-switch triggering rate, the mode-switch episode terminates and the original tracking mode is restored (Figure 5-67).

5.4.4 PACEMAKER SELECTION

In general, patients with isolated symptomatic SA node dysfunction should receive either an atrial single chamber rate-responsive pacing system (AAIR-programmable) or a dual chamber DDDR-programmable system (Figure 5-68). The use of single chamber atrial systems in these patients has been very popular among some physicians. The concern, of course, is that the patient's conduction system disease will progress to include AV block or the AV conduction system will fail accommodate the faster atrial rates resulting from sensor-driven pacing. Patients with SA node dysfunction along with paroxysmal atrial fibrillation or flutter should receive a dual chamber system with mode-switching capability. Individuals with isolated symptomatic AV block and normal SA node function should be implanted with either a dual chamber pacing system or a single lead system allowing atrial sensing and ventricle pacing and programmable to the VDD mode (Figure 5-69). Patients exhibiting both SA node dysfunction and AV block are best managed with a dual chamber DDDR-programmable system. Those patients with symptomatic bradycardia and chronic atrial fibrillation should receive a single chamber rate-responsive ventricular system. Finally, there are many physicians who believe that chronically ill, debilitated, and inactive patients with very rare and brief episodes of symptomatic

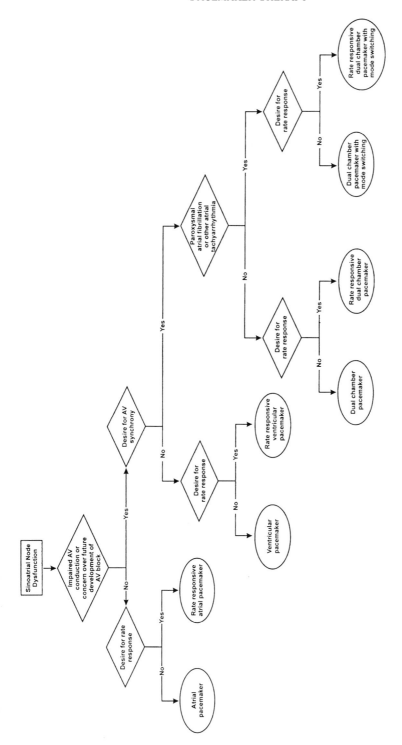

FIGURE 5-68. Algorithm for selection of appropriate pacemaker system in patients with sinoatrial node dysfunction. AV, atrioventricular. Adapted from [23].

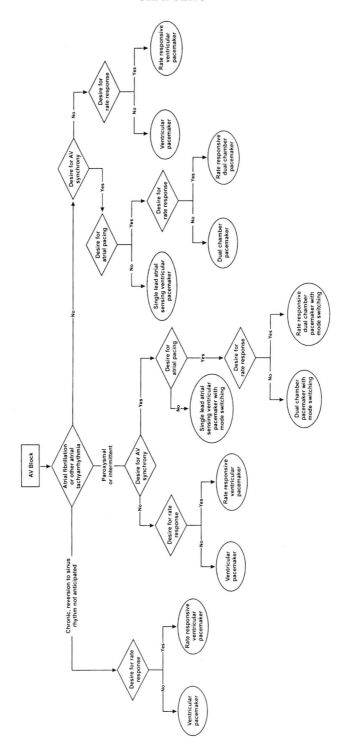

FIGURE 5-69. Algorithm for selection of appropriate pacemaker system in patients with AV block. AV, atrioventricular. Adapted from [23].

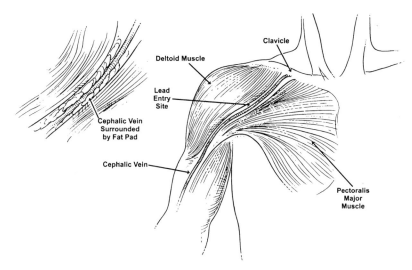

FIGURE 5-70. This cephalic vein lies in a fat pad located between the deltoid muscle and pectoralis major muscle. The groove at the junction of these two muscles can often be visualized and is generally palpable in the infraclavicular region. Using these landmarks, a surgical incision can be made over this area allowing access to the vein using simple blunt dissection techniques. After visualization of the vein, entry can be achieved directly and the pacemaker lead passed into the lumen. The generator pocket can be created through this same incision, also using blunt dissection. The axillary vein is located about 1–1.5 cm caudal to the cephalic vein and can be entered easily using radiopaque contrast-guided vein puncture.

bradycardia (either due to SA node dysfunction of AV block) are optimally and cost-effectively managed with a simple single chamber ventricular system.

5.5 Pacemaker Implantation

The purpose of this section is to discuss the general principles of implantation. Pacemaker implantation can only be mastered by working hands-on under the guidance of an experienced operator.

The right and left infraclavicular areas are acceptable sites for the subcutaneous pulse generator pocket. The incision for the pocket should generally be made midway between the ends of the clavicle and about 2-cm caudal to it. Normally, in right hand dominant patients the transvenous system is implanted in the left infraclavicular region. While a right-sided approach provides a more direct route to the right heart, most implanters find using the left side permits slightly easier atrial and ventricular lead placement. (Pediatric patients, or those requiring an epicardial lead system, usually have the pulse generator implanted within an anterior mid-abdominal subcutaneous pocket). For typical transvenous insertion using an infraclavicular approach, venous access is achieved either through the axillary, cephalic, or subclavian veins (Figure 5-70). The simplest access is achieved using contrast-guided puncture of the axillary vein. Injection of radiopaque contrast into an ipsilateral peripheral arm vein allows fluoroscopic visualization of the axillary vein as it courses over the first or second rib. Implantation using

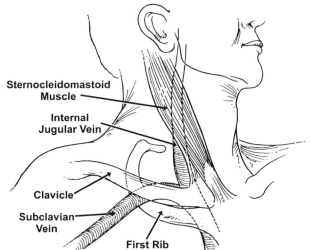

Sternocleidomastoid
Muscle

Internal
Jugular Vein

Clavicle

Subclavian
Vein

First Rib

FIGURE 5-71. Regional anatomy of the right neck and clavicular area. Patients in which insertion of the permanent transvenous pacing leads through the axillary or cephalic vein is not possible will require lead insertion through the subclavian vein. Because the subclavian vein commonly passes between the clavicle and the first rib, the leads are a risk of suffering a crush or abrasion injury over time. This may result in insulation breakage or fracture of the conductor resulting in malfunction of the pacing system and necessitating a revision of the lead system.

the axillary vein or cutdown to the cephalic vein is preferred over the subclavian approach because both the former techniques avoid the risk of chronic lead damage due to a crush injury between the bony clavicle and margin of the first rib (Figure 5-71) [41]. In some cases the cephalic vein route is not possible, usually due to small vein size or inability to advance the pacing lead through a tortuous vein lumen. In these cases, contrast-guided axillary vein puncture should be performed with lead insertion into the venous system accomplished using a peel-away sheath introducer system (Figure 5-72).

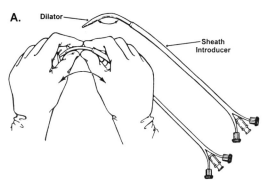

A. Dilator — Sheath Introducer

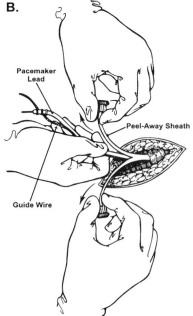

B. Pacemaker Lead — Peel-Away Sheath — Guide Wire

FIGURE 5-72. Pacemaker lead implantation through the axillary or subclavian vein using a peel-away sheath introducer system. After venipuncture, a J-guide wire is inserted through the needle into the vein lumen. Thereafter a peel-away sheath introducer containing a dilator (panel A) is passed over the guide wire into the vein. Removal of the dilator allows passage of the pacemaker lead through the sheath introducer into the vein lumen after which the sheath is withdrawn from the vein and "peeled apart", leaving the lead within the vein lumen (panel B). If an atrial and ventricular lead are to be implanted it is usually optimal to initially perform two separate venipuncture, using guide wires and two separate peel-away sheaths. Courtesy of Guidant/CPI, Inc.

In general, the atrial lead should be secured in the right atrial appendage using active fixation, while the ventricular lead should be positioned at the right ventricular apex using either passive or active fixation (Figure 5-73). In many patients who have undergone cardiac surgery, the right atrial appendage has been removed requiring active fixation of the atrial lead in another atrial location. An active fixation lead can be secured in the ventricular septum if pacing thresholds are elevated at the right ventricular apex especially in patients who have suffered a myocardial infarction in this region.

At the time of lead implantation a number of parameters should be measured to assess the adequacy of lead position (Table 5-12.) Using a *pacing system analyzer*, the intracardiac signal amplitude, impedance, slew rate, and the voltage, current, and pulse-width pacing thresholds are measured during the implantation procedure (Figure 5-22). The pacing analyzer delivers pacing pulses and contains sensing circuitry identical to the sensing and pacing characteristics of the pulse generator. Therefore, the analyzer can be used to assess the sensing and pacing capabilities of the pacing leads after they are positioned at the desired location within

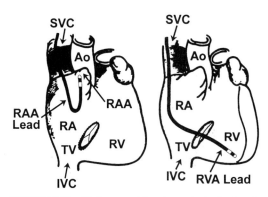

FIGURE 5-73. Optimum atrial and ventricular lead positioning for a dual chamber pacing system. The atrial J-lead ideally should be situated in the right atrial appendage (RAA) and the ventricular lead should be positioned at the right ventricular apex (RVA). Ao, aorta; IVC, inferior vena cava; RA, right atrium; RV, right ventricle; SVC, superior vena cava; TV, tricuspid valve

the heart but before they are connected to the pacemaker generator. Ideally, the amplitude of the intracardiac R-wave should be greater than 5.0 mV with a ventricular voltage pacing threshold preferably less than 1.0 V at a pulse width of 0.5 ms. The magnitude of the intracardiac P-wave should be greater than 2.0 mV with a voltage threshold less than 1.5 V at a pulse width of 0.5 ms. The pacing impedance varies with the particular lead but is generally between 400 and 1200 Ω. The slew rate for atrial and ventricular depolarization is typically greater than 0.5 V/sec and 0.75 V/sec, respectively.

TABLE 5-12. Pacemaker implantation measurements

Stimulation threshold
Sensing threshold
Slew rate
Pacing impedance
Retrograde conduction

Following implantation of a new pacing system, a chest x-ray should be obtained to rule-out a pneumothorax and document lead position. In addition, a 12-lead ECG should be obtained during ventricular pacing to confirm that the QRS morphology exhibits a left bundle branch block pattern, as would be expected during right ventricular pacing. Most implanting physicians recommended limitation of ipsilateral arm movement for a few weeks after the implantation to reduce the changes of lead dislodgment.

Short- and long-term complications associated with pacemaker implantation and therapy are summarized below in Table 5-13.

TABLE 5-13. Common complications associated with pacemaker implantation

Early Complications	Late Complications	Early or Late Complications
Pain/ecchymoses	Skin erosion	Lead dislodgment
Pneumothorax	Skin adherence	Pacemaker-related arrhythmias
Hematoma/seroma formation	Foreign body rejection	Twiddler's syndrome
Cardiac perforation	Lead-related thrombosis	EMI or myopotential oversensing
Pericardial effusion/tamponade	Pulse generator migration	Infection
Intraoperative lead damage	Therapeutic radiation damage	Pacemaker syndrome
Subcutaneous emphysema	Pacemaker failure	Pacemaker allergy
Thoracic duct injury	High thresholds/exit block	Pulse generator malfunction
Air embolism	Lead fracture/insulation break	Loose lead/connector block interface
Brachial plexus injury	Early battery depletion	Nerve & muscle stimulation
Subclavian artery puncture		

EMI, electromagnetic interference. Adapted from [42].

5.6   Pacemaker Follow-up

During routine follow-up of pacemaker patients – and especially if anomalous pacing behavior or suspicious symptoms develop – the clinician should obtain a focused clinical history and perform a *pacemaker system evaluation*. In this case, the operative words are "pacing system", not just "pacemaker", because the pacing system is comprised of the pulse generator, the lead(s) connecting the pacemaker to the heart, and the patient. All three components of the pacing system should be evaluated at the time of follow-up. The appropriateness of the current programmed parameters should also be assessed in each patient. In all cases, the pacemaker should he programmed so as to optimize the physiologic function for the patient. In general, follow-up after a new implant of a complete system should be within 7-10 days to assess the wound healing and then again in about 3 and 6 months to assess the pacing threshold(s) and program the chronic output settings for the system. In-office follow-up for chronic stable systems need be only 2-3 times per year. Some clinicians recommend transtelephonic monitoring periodically between these office visits. Follow-up intervals may need to be reduced as battery end-of-life is approached. The discussion that follows outlines the components of a complete evaluation of the pacing system (Table 5-14.) However, in many routine follow-up visits a more limited follow-up evaluation may be indicated. No didactic discussion can substitute for hands-on experience.

5.6.1 CLINICAL ASSESSMENT

The evaluation begins with a history and limited physical examination. The history is geared to detect any symptoms that may suggest a malfunction or suboptimal programming of the pacing system. Specifically, the clinician should question the patient concerning symptoms of pacemaker syndrome, palpitation, dizziness, syncope or symptoms similar to those that lead to implantation of the pacemaker. One should inquire as to fever or systemic symptoms that may reflect an infection. Symptoms localized so the pacemaker pocket such as pain and swelling should be the subject of specific concern.

TABLE 5-14. Summary of elements involved in complete pacemaker follow-up

Clinical assessment

Surface ECG

Documentation of programmed parameters

Evaluation of pacing threshold

Evaluation of sensing function

Measured data (lead impedance, battery status, intrinsic signal amplitude)

Intracardiac electrograms

Trending data

Histograms and event counters

Analysis of detected arrhythmias

Review of programmed special functions

Ancillary testing

Final interrogation and printed report

The physical examination includes the basic vital signs followed by an examination of the pacemaker pocket for signs of swelling, erythema, tenderness, increased warmth, fluctuance, skin erosion, or drainage. Neck vein examination may reveal high venous filling pressure, possible signs of local venous obstruction, or evidence for retrograde conduction with cannon A waves or AV dissociation. Venous obstruction may also result in venous distention and swelling of the ipsilateral arm. If there are symptoms of congestive heart failure, a detailed pulmonary and cardiac examination may be indicated.

5.6.2 ELECTROCARDIOGRAPHY

An EGG rhythm strip is obtained along with measurements of the free-running and magnet rates of the pacemaker. Measurements of the pacing rate, pacing interval (cycle length), pulse duration, and AV interval (dual chamber systems) should be obtained. If atrial and ventricular capture cannot he confirmed on a single lead rhythm strip, recording of other leads, or a complete 12-lead ECG, may be necessary. Because the first sign of battery depletion is reflected in a change in the magnet rate or behavior, the pacing cycle length during demand mode and after magnet application should be measured. Generally this is accomplished most easily using a commercially available digital counter.

5.6.3 INTERROGATION

Interrogation and *programming* of the pacemaker is performed using an electronic programming device equipped with a wand placed over the implanted pulse generator. Communication with the pacemaker is accomplished using coded radiofrequency signals that can unlock or change each programmable parameter. In addition, data from the pacemaker such as the current status of the programmed parameters and stored data such as electrograms and battery status can be retrieved by decoded radiofrequency signals emitted from the pacemaker and collected by the telemetry wand. Pacemaker interrogation will provide: 1) programmed parameters; 2) measured data include battery status and lead impedances; 3) ECG/EGM and event marker channels; 4) diagnostic information. In almost all systems, the programmer itself can display at least one surface ECG lead during pacemaker system evaluation, and newer devices can also display intracardiac electrograms from the atrial or ventricular channel. Most new pacing systems can

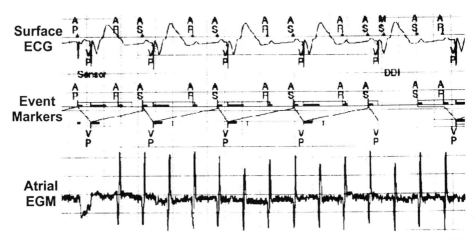

FIGURE 5-74. Example of programmer printout showing atrial electrograms, event markers, and surface ECG during a mode-switch episode in a Medtronic, Inc. Kappa series pacemaker. Event markers provide useful diagnostic information, especially in cases of possible pacing system malfunction. See text for further discussion. Courtesy of Medtronic, Inc.

also display *telemetry event markers* which identify how the pacemaker itself interprets intrinsic cardiac and pacemaker-related events. The event markers typically provide information concerning when the pacemaker has detected intrinsic atrial or ventricular events and when it delivers atrial or ventricular pacing stimuli (Figure 5-66). In addition, in most current devices, marker data includes information about sensor, mode-switching, and other special behaviors (Figure 5-74). The event markers appear as abbreviated annotations (Figure 5-75) on the programmer screen and at the bottom of the hard-copy printout that also typically displays recordings of a surface ECG lead and an atrial and/or ventricular intracardiac electrogram(s).

AS	Atrial Sensed	Ns	Sense Amp Noise
AP	Atrial Paced	FB	During A-Tachy Response
VS	Ventricular Sensed	MT	Atrial Tracked at MTR
VP	Ventricular Paced	PVP→	PVARP after PVC
S	Sensed (Single chamber)	PMT-B	PMT Detection and PVARP
P	Paced (Single Chamber)	Output↓	Threshold New Parameters Active
Hy	Hysteresis Rate	ATR↑	A-Tachy Sense Count Up
PVC	PVC after Refractory	ATR↓	A-Tachy Sense Count Down
( )	During Refractory	ATR-FB	Fallback Started
Sr	Sensor	ATR-Dur	Onset Started
↑	Rate Smoothing Up	ATR-End	Fallback Ended
↓	Rate Smoothing Down	TN	Noise Indication
→	Inserted after AFR	REFR	Refractory Interval
Tr	Trigger Mode	Caliper	Screen Caliper Location

FIGURE 5-75. Example of abbreviations used for event marker annotations by Guidant Discovery series pacemakers. Modern pacing systems not only provide information about sensed and paced atrial and ventricular events, but also information concerning special functions such as mode-switching, rate-smoothing, and noise behavior. Courtesy of Guidant/CPI, Inc.

5.6.4 NATIVE RHYTHM

It is appropriate to evaluate the patient's intrinsic rhythm at the time of each follow-up evaluation because the conduction system disease that was the original indication for pacing may evolve over time. In particular it is important to determine if the patient is patient is pacemaker dependent (Figure 5-76). Although there is no uniformly accepted

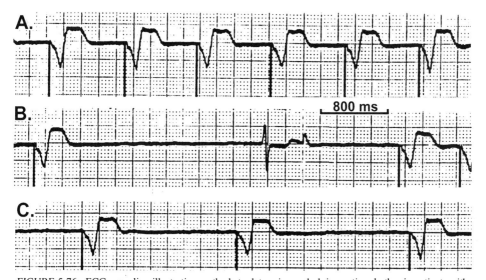

FIGURE 5-76. ECG recording illustrating methods to determine underlying native rhythm in patients with pacemakers. Panel A: VVI paced rhythm. Panel B: Transient complete inhibition of pacing output reveals an inadequate escape rhythm. Panel C: Transient programming to a rate of 30 pulses/min results in sustained pacing without appearance of a faster escape rhythm. Given these responses, this patient should be classified as pacemaker dependent. Courtesy of St. Jude/Pacesetter, Inc.

definition of pacemaker dependency, most electrophysiologists consider a patient to be pacemaker dependent if a hemodynamically stable intrinsic escape rhythm is not present upon abrupt cessation of pacing or abrupt decrease in the pacing rate. Thus, if there were an unexpected total failure of the pacing system such as a component failure, lead dislodgment, or development of high pacing thresholds resulting in loss of capture, it could he anticipated that the patient will have an immediate and dramatic symptom such as syncope. Patients noted to exhibit 100% pacing during routine follow-up may or may not be pacemaker dependent. Total pacing may merely indicate that the intrinsic rate is slower than the programmed pacing rate. Patients who are pacemaker dependent by the above definition may still develop a viable intrinsic rhythm after gradual slowing of the pacing rate; however, after abrupt cessation of pacing function an escape rhythm may not develop before significant hemodynamic consequences. Patients that exhibit pacemaker dependence may require more frequent or intense follow-up and early intervention with system revision or replacement at the first sign of a pacing system problem.

There are two methods to establish pacemaker dependence. One option is to transiently inhibit the pacing function using a special inhibit mode which can be activated from the programmer. It is important to note that total inhibition by any technique is not always safe, particularly if the patient does not have an adequate escape rhythm. A second approach, more commonly used, is to slow the pacing rate to an arbitrary low level while continuously recording an ECG rhythm strip, noting the appearance of an intrinsic escape rhythm faster than the pacing rate. If the pacemaker is in a tracking mode (DDD, VDD) and exhibits P-V pacing it must first be programmed to a non-tracking mode (VVI, DDI), otherwise there may be no visible decrease in the effective paced rate when a lower rate limit is programmed. Most commonly, a temporary rate of 30 pulses/min is used, although a faster rate may he selected if the patient does not tolerate this low rate, even when lying supine. If the patient is still paced at this slow rate, that patient should be considered pacemaker dependent.

5.6.5 SENSING THRESHOLD

The programmable sensitivity of a pacemaker is defined as the smallest amplitude signal (in millivolts) that can be sensed. A "high" sensitivity means that the pacemaker is capable of sensing a very low amplitude signal. Thus, the ability of the pacemaker to detect a 1-mV signal means it has a higher sensitivity than does a pacemaker that can detect a 2-mV signal. The sensing threshold is defined as the least sensitive programmable setting (largest millivolt value) at which normal sensing is consistently demonstrated during the period of observation of the patient's spontaneous intrinsic rhythm. If normal sensing is demonstrated even at the least sensitive programmable setting available in the pacemaker, this value is nevertheless taken as the sensing threshold, even if the amplitude of the actual signal is significantly larger.

The sensing threshold is not the same as the actual amplitude of the endocardial electrogram that can be measured using a pacing system analyzer at the time of lead implantation or pulse generator replacement, or recorded from a telemetered electrogram. Many pacing systems have the capability of telemetering the actual signal from inside the heart to the programmer and then providing a hard-copy printout of calibrated signal.

Although, it has been proposed that the peak-to-peak amplitude of this signal be taken as the sensing threshold in strictest terms this is not correct. The ability of a pacemaker to sense a given signal involves more than just the amplitude of the electrogram. The incoming signal is processed by a special filter with respect to frequency content and slew rate and is also amplified. The resultant signal is not the same as the recorded or telemetered electrogram. While there may be a close correlation between the telemetered electrogram and the non-invasively determined sensing threshold, the telemetry and the sensing amplifiers utilize different filters. The sense amplifier is designed to minimize oversensing of the low-frequency signals, including cardiac repolarization. Consequently, the peak-to-peak amplitude of the telemetered electrogram will generally not be the same as the sensing threshold. However, the telemetered intracardiac electrogram is valuable in identifying signals not visible on the surface ECG but nevertheless detected by the pacemaker. Furthermore, it facilitates the evaluation of retrograde conduction and can be used to calculate the slew rate and evaluate the quality of the sensed signal.

The sensing threshold can be determined non-invasively by progressively reducing the sensitivity of the pacemaker until the intrinsic depolarization is no longer detected. In the case of total pacing, this first requires a temporary reduction in the paced rate to a rate that is slower than the intrinsic rhythm. If there is no intrinsic rhythm, the sensing threshold cannot be obtained. The sensing threshold can be performed using the semiautomatic sensing test feature available in most modern programming systems. The surface ECG is monitored while the event markers are telemetered from the pacemaker. When the signal of interest is no longer detected the P- or R-marker will disappear from the marker channel recording even though a spontaneous P- or R-wave will be clearly observed on the monitored ECG rhythm. While marker channel notations make determination of sensing threshold somewhat easier, it is certainly not necessary because loss of sensing is heralded by a change in pacing function (in general, an inappropriate delivery of pacing stimuli) that can be detected on the surface ECG. The techniques used to determine the sensing threshold varies with different pacing modes and the rate of the intrinsic spontaneous activity. The following discussion details the programming changes that need be made to evaluate sensitivity in a variety of clinical settings.

VVI(R) or AAI(R) modes. To determine the sensing threshold, reduce the pacing rate below the intrinsic rate. As the sensitivity of the pacemaker is progressively decreased, loss of sensing will be identified by competition between the pacemaker and the native rhythm.

DDD(R) mode. In this situation, decrease the pacing rate so that P-V, P-R, or AV pacing will occur at the lower rate. In the case of AV pacing, a sensing threshold cannot be performed. If P-R pacing behavior (atrial and ventricular sensing) is present, both atrial and ventricular sensing thresholds can be determined immediately by progressive reduction of the atrial or ventricular sensitivity. To determine the sensing threshold in the atrium, reduce the atrial pacing rate below the intrinsic rate. As the sensitivity of the atrial channel is progressively decreased, loss of atrial sensing will be identified by competition between the pacemaker and the native atrial rhythm. To evaluate ventricular sensing when the atrial and ventricular pacing is inhibited, progressively reduce the ventricular sensitivity until a ventricular stimulus is delivered at the end of the programmed AV interval. In a dual chamber system, this will occur within either the terminal portion of the QRS complex, the ST segment, or the T-wave. In the case of a bipolar output configuration, ECG identification of the bipolar stimulus may be very difficult. If possible, program the pacemaker to the unipolar output configuration to facilitate identification of the pacing stimulus. If P-V pacing activity is present, the atrial sensing threshold can be directly assessed without further programming changes by noting the appearance of atrial pacing activity as the atrial sensitivity is progressively reduced. However, to assess ventricular sensing in the case of P-V pacing, increase the AV interval to the maximum. If this results in P-R pacing behavior, then evaluate the ventricular sensing threshold. If there is still P-V pacing but the patient has a hemodynamically stable intrinsic rhythm, program the pacemaker to VVI mode and then to a temporary rate that is slower than the patient's own rhythm (e.g., use temporary 30 pulses/min), following which the semiautomatic sensitivity test can be utilized.

Once the sensing threshold is determined, the final sensitivity setting of the ventricular and/or atrial channels needs to he programmed. A margin of safety of at least twofold is recommended to allow for potential fluctuations in signal amplitude with changes in posture and metabolic factors. This may be further modified based upon a number of clinical factors. If the patient has atrial and ventricular ectopic activity, one may need to program the pacemaker to a very sensitive level so as to ensure that ectopic depolarizations are appropriately detected. On the other hand, an excessive increase in the sensitivity may predispose to oversensing, especially in the unipolar sensing configuration. If the sensitivity is increased, the incidence of oversensing of myopotentials should he carefully evaluated in patients with a pacemaker system utilizing unipolar sensing. In a pacemaker dependent patient, one may elect to reduce the ventricular sensitivity to the safest level in order to minimize oversensing problems.

5.6.6 CAPTURE THRESHOLDS

The capture threshold of the atrium or ventricle is the lowest output setting of the pacemaker that results in stable and consistent atrial or ventricular depolarization, respectively. If even one stimulus of a series at a given output fails to capture the cardiac chamber, that output setting is considered to be subthreshold. Strictly speaking, capture thresholds may be expressed in terms of pulse amplitude (volts or milliamperes) and duration (milliseconds), as well as pulse energy (microjoules) or pulse charge (microcoulombs) (see "Basic Concepts & Biophysical Aspects of Pacing" on page 175.) However, the only two parameters that the clinician can independently regulate are the voltage amplitude and pulse duration. Capture threshold is defined by the programmable output options of the pacing system. If capture is consistent at the lowest available output pulse amplitude and duration of the pulse generator, this output is accepted us the capture threshold for the system even if the threshold were determined to be lower by an invasive assessment through the pacing leads using a pacing system analyzer.

The ability to capture the myocardium is defined by a strength-duration curve (Figure 5-77). Pacemaker stimuli with very brief pulse durations that fall to the left of the curve will be ineffective at producing capture even at the highest pulse amplitude. On

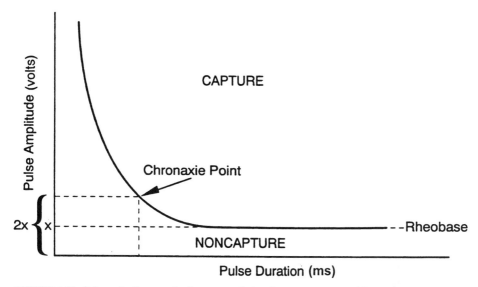

FIGURE 5-77. Schematic diagram of voltage strength-duration curve. Any combination of pulse duration and amplitude lying below or to the left of the curve will fail to result in capture. Any combination of pulse duration and amplitude lying above or to the right of the curve will produce capture. The terms chronaxie and rheobase were previously defined (see "Basic Concepts & Biophysical Aspects of Pacing" on page 175.) Courtesy of St. Jude/Pacesetter, Inc.

the other hand, using combinations of pulse amplitude and duration that fall above the strength-duration curve results in reproducible cardiac capture.

In order to understand the rationale for final programming of the pacemaker output, it is valuable to appreciate the energy threshold. Recall (Table 5-3.) that energy is the product of voltage, current, and pulse duration:

$$Energy = Volts \times Current \times Pulse\ Duration$$

Substituting Ohm's Law produces:

$$Energy = \frac{Volts^2 \times Pulse\ Duration}{Resistance}$$

While doubling the pulse duration will only double the delivered energy, doubling the pulse amplitude will quadruple the energy delivered. On the other hand, halving the pulse amplitude will reduce the delivered energy fourfold while halving the pulse duration will decrease the energy only by a factor of two. If the energy strength-duration curve is constructed, an interesting curve results (Figure 5-78). At very short pulse durations, the energy required to pace the heart is extremely high due to squared voltage term in the above equation. The amount of energy necessary to trigger cardiac activation progressively decreases and reaches a minimum as the pulse duration approaches the chronaxie point. As the pulse duration increases beyond the chronaxie, there is a progressive rise in energy threshold as the voltage threshold approaches the rheobase. As the rheobase is approached, the threshold voltage does decrease, but the rate of decrease dramatically slows. Consequently, the decline in threshold voltage does not compensate for the progressive increase in the pulse duration, resulting in a progressive increase in the energy threshold. Once the rheobase is reached, the effective voltage fails to decrease further even at greater pulse durations, resulting in a steep increase of the energy threshold as the pulse duration is increased further. From the standpoint of both battery efficiency and providing the best output safety margin in all directions, the optimum pulse duration setting is near the chronaxie point. Programming an output voltage setting two-fold greater than voltage threshold at the chronaxie point provides the recommended safety margin. In most pacing systems, the chronaxie is commonly between 0.4 to 0.6 ms, which explains why the nominal pulse duration setting in most pulse generators is approximately 0.5 ms.

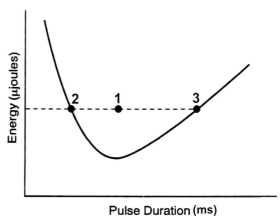

Pulse Duration (ms)

To determine the voltage threshold, the semi-automatic capture threshold test should be used when available. This is especially valuable in determining the pacing threshold in pacemaker-dependent patients. The test begins at a specified starting value for pulse width and amplitude and the device incrementally reduces either the pulse width (*pulse width threshold*) or pulse amplitude (*pulse amplitude threshold*) until capture is lost. The automatic test sequence returns the system to its baseline pre-test output immediately after terminating the test, ensuring that a pacemak-

FIGURE 5-78. Plot of energy threshold as a function of pulse duration. The nadir of the curve closely approximates the chronaxie point. The delivered energy corresponding to a 100% margin of safety at the chronaxie pulse duration (point #1) is just the threshold at both a narrower (point #2) and wider (point #3) pulse duration. See text for further discussion. Courtesy of St. Jude/Pacesetter, Inc.

er-dependent patient will not have any significant period of asystole. In pacing systems lacking the capability for semi-automatic threshold testing, threshold testing to the point of loss of capture is usually inappropriate. Therefore, in these patients many clinicians choose to only reduce the voltage output slightly to confirm that there remains a good margin of safety. In order to assess the capture threshold not only must the pulse generator deliver pacing stimuli, but also there must be clear evidence of pacing stimuli-induced depolarization. Thus, if the ventricular stimulus merely deforms the early phase of a natively conducted R-wave (*fusion* or *pseudofusion*), capture cannot be assumed to have occurred. Consequently, verification of capture usually requires some programming changes especially if inhibition of pacing and/or fusion is noted. Some examples are discussed below.

AAI(R) and VVI(R) modes. To assess atrial or ventricular capture in a single chamber pacing system, program the pacemaker to a rate that is faster than the intrinsic rate.

As the output voltage is progressively reduced, capture will eventually fail, resulting in a slower escape rhythm. In pacemaker-dependent patients, the semi-automatic threshold testing option should be used to avoid long periods of asystole after loss of capture.

DDD(R) mode. To assess atrial capture, program the pacemaker to a rate that is faster than the intrinsic rate and maximize the AV interval. This results in either P-R pacing or AV pacing with ventricular pseudofusion. As the output voltage is progressively reduced, atrial capture eventually fails. Since there will not be any atrial depolarization to conduct to the ventricle the pacemaker will deliver a ventricular pacing stimulus after expiration of the lower rate interval. The presence of a paced ventricular depolarization can also serve as a marker for loss of atrial capture in cases where atrial pacing-induced depolarization is poorly seen on the surface ECG.

If the patient is capable of exhibiting ventriculo-atrial conduction and the PVARP is sufficiently short, the atrial capture threshold test performed while in the DDD mode may initiate a pacemaker-mediated tachycardia associated with retrograde conduction following the first ventricular paced beat occurring after the loss of atrial capture. ECG and event marker recording during the onset of this arrhythmia may allow the accurate measurement of the VA conduction time. In turn, this may guide the programming the appropriate PVARP duration so as to prevent future episodes of pacemaker-mediated tachycardia.

To assess ventricular capture when the system is inhibited (P-R pacing operation) one needs to shorten the AV interval. Commonly, the shortest AV interval allowed by the system is chosen in order to assure complete ventricular capture (avoid fusion). When capture fails as the output is progressively reduced there will be restoration of intact AV conduction signaled by the reappearance of the native QRS complex.

In the setting of P-V pacing, assessment of ventricular capture is straightforward given access to one of the semiautomatic capture test functions. This is especially helpful when the patient is known to have pacemaker-dependent complete heart block.

Assessing atrial capture in a dual chamber pacemaker programmed to the DDD(R) mode is no more difficult but often presents more of an intellectual challenge. If the atrial rate is sufficiently slow, the lower rate of the pacemaker is programmed to a rate faster than the intrinsic atrial rate. When atrial capture is present, there will be stable AV pacing because the sinus or intrinsic atrial mechanism is overdriven and suppressed. When atrial capture is lost, a slower escape rhythm will be noted, often displaying cycles of AV and P-V pacing.

It is important to compare the results of threshold testing with threshold measurements obtained during prior evaluations. A rise in the pacing threshold may be normal such as that see during lead maturation in the weeks following implant. A late increase in pacing threshold may indicate a developing problem with either the lead itself or at the electrode-myocardial interface. In a patient with a chronic pacing system who does not complain of any potential pacemaker-related symptoms, programming a higher output and increasing the frequency of pacing system monitoring may be prudent. Additionally, in some patients securing a chest radiograph and/or ambulatory ECG monitoring may be indicated to further evaluate lead integrity. If the pacing thresholds are stable (unchanged thresholds at two successive evaluations at least three months apart), the voltage outputs are programmed to reduce current drainage from the battery (consistent with at

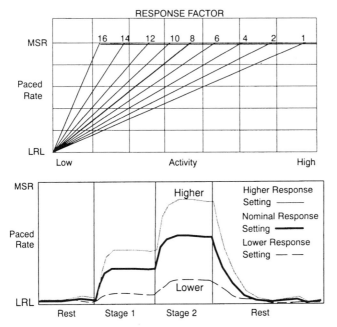

FIGURE 5-79. Schematic diagrams illustrating the sensor response factor (slope) parameter. Top panel: Example of the relationship between the programmed response factor setting and the rate response of the pacemaker. Bottom panel: Effects of response factor settings in a theoretical two stage exercise test. Increasing the response factor (slope) increases the pacing rate at a given level of activity. See text for further discussion. Courtesy of Guidant/CPI, Inc.

least two-fold safety margin), thereby maximizing pacing system longevity. Some clinicians program a voltage output setting to three times the voltage threshold in patients that are pacemaker-dependent. In general, the pulse duration should never be programmed to a value less than 0.2 ms, even if possible, because the voltage strength-duration curve is very steep at very short pulse durations. Consequently, small changes in voltage threshold, even those occurring normally throughout the day, may lead to a loss of capture.

5.6.7 SENSOR PROGRAMMING & FOLLOW-UP

In rate-responsive or adaptive-rate pacing modes, a sensor (such as an accelerometer) attempts to detect increases in the patient's metabolic needs and increases the pacing rate accordingly. Patients implanted with an adaptive-rate pacemaker for treatment of chronotropic incompetence may need adjustment of the sensor and the pacing response to sensor activation. The sensor can be programmed to either the *active* or *passive* (monitor-only) mode. In most pacing systems, the clinician must adjust four programmable sensor parameters: 1), slope or response factor, 2) sensor threshold, 3) reaction time, 4) recovery time. The sensor *response factor* or *slope* parameter determines the pacing rate that will occur above the programmed lower rate at various levels of patient activity. As seen in Figure 5-79, the pacing rate is faster at a particular level of activity when the response factor is programmed to a higher level (note the increase in slope of the lines). Programming a higher slope will enable the rate to reach the maximum sensor-driven rate with a lower level of activity than would be required with a lower slope value. The pacing rate will be limited either by the detected level of activity or by the programmed maximum sensor rate. If the detected activity level results in a steady-state rate below

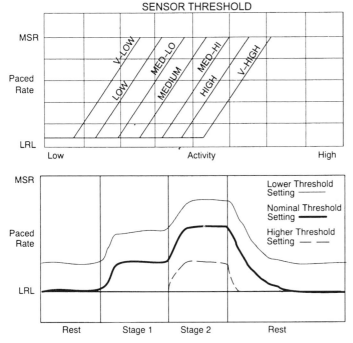

FIGURE 5-80. Schematic diagrams illustrating the sensor threshold parameter. Top panel: Example of the relationship between the sensor threshold setting and the rate response behavior of the pacemaker. Bottom panel: Effects of sensor threshold settings in a theoretical two stage exercise test. Decreasing the sensor threshold increases the response. See text for further discussion. Courtesy of Guidant/CPI, Inc.

the maximum sensor rate, the pacing rate can still increase when the detected activity levels increase. The steady-state rate is independent of the reaction and recovery times (see below).

The *sensor threshold* is a programmable parameter that sets the minimum level of sensor activation that must occur before it will trigger any sensor-driven pacing (Figure 5-80). This means that in the case of a motion sensor, such as an accelerometer or piezoelectric crystal, the sensor must detect a certain level of movement before it will initiate sensor-based pacing. To measure acceleration, for example, both the frequency and the amplitude of the sensor signal are evaluated during signal processing. Signal frequency reflects how often an activity occurs, while signal amplitude reflects the force of the motion. The sensor threshold prevents the pacemaker from increasing the rate due to low-intensity exertion that would not ordinarily trigger an increase in sinus rate. The sensor threshold prevents increases in pacing rate inappropriate for the level of exertion. Ideally, the clinician should attempt to program a sensor threshold level that would mimic the normal sinus rate for the various levels of activity normally engaged in by the patient. In general, a high setting will require a higher level of exertion to trigger the onset of sensor-driven pacing, while a lower setting will result in sensor-based pacing at lower levels of activity.

The *reaction time* is a programmable parameter that determines how rapidly the pacing rate will rise to a new higher pacing level in response to an incremental increase in sensor activation (Figure 5-81). In essence, the value selected for the reaction time will determine the time required for the sensor-driven pacing rate to reach the maximum

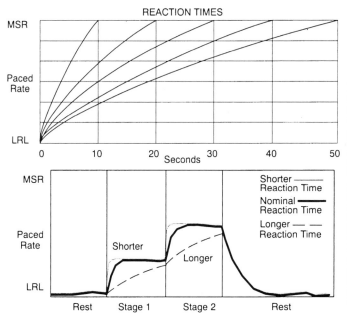

FIGURE 5-81. Schematic diagrams illustrating the sensor reaction time parameter. Top panel: Example of the relationship between the reaction time and the paced rate depending upon the programmed reaction time setting. Bottom panel: Effects of sensor reaction time settings in a theoretical two stage exercise test. Decreasing the reaction time value results in a more rapid increase in pacing rate during exercise. See text for further discussion. Courtesy of Guidant/CPI, Inc.

sensor-driven rate when the sensor is abruptly maximally activated. Reaction time affects only the time required for a rate increase to occur. A short reaction time will allow the pacing rate to increase rapidly in response to patient activity. A long reaction time will result in a slower increase in the pacing rate.

The *recovery time* parameter determines the time required for the sensor-driven paced rate to decrease from the maximum sensor rate to the programmed lower rate in the absence of any sensor activation (Figure 5-82). In essence, the value selected for the recovery time will determine the time required for the sensor-driven pacing rate to decrease from the maximum sensor-driven rate to the programmed lower rate when the maximally-activated sensor abruptly changes to the inactivated state. This feature is designed to prevent an abrupt decline in pacing rate concurrent with the conclusion of pacing activity. A shorter recovery time will allow the pacing rate to decrease more rapidly after cessation of or lowered level of exertion. A longer recovery time will force a slower decrease in the pacing rate with a decline in the level of activity. Recovery time affects only the rate of deceleration of the pacing rate and is independent of other parameters.

During the period following implantation many clinicians elect to program the sensor function to the "passive" or "monitor" mode during which heart rate data is logged by the event counters and trend monitoring circuitry. Pulse generators with trend monitoring capabilities can provide rate and sensor trends and allows sensor evaluation based upon information stored in the pulse generator memory. Devices equipped with histogram and counter functions can report the total number and percentage of paced and sensed events,. In addition, depending upon the pacemaker model, event counters can be used as well to collect statistics on various other types of events, such as number of

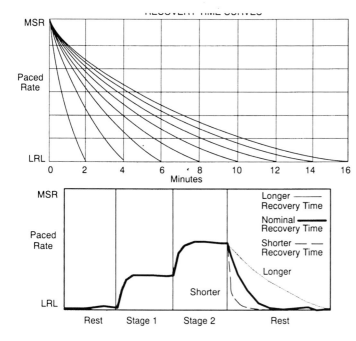

FIGURE 5-82. Schematic diagrams illustrating the sensor threshold parameter. Top panel: Example of the relationship between the recovery time setting and the rate response behavior of the pacemaker. Bottom panel: Effects of sensor recovery time settings in a theoretical two stage exercise test. A shorter recovery time will allow the pacing rate to decrease more rapidly after cessation of or decline in patient's level of exercise. See text for further discussion. Courtesy of Guidant/CPI, Inc.

mode-switch episodes, ventricular premature depolarizations or episodes of ventricular or atrial tachyarrhythmias. Rate histogram data can be extracted from the device during the follow-up period and correlated with patient activity. In addition, many modern pacemakers also record data concerning projected sensor response and sensor-driven pacing rates, even when the sensor is programmed to the monitor mode. This data allows the clinician to estimate in advance what sensor-driven rate would result from the patient's routine activity. This can allow the clinician to adjust the sensor parameters (slope, sensor threshold, reaction and recovery times) so as to provide the optimum sensor-driven rate for the patients various activities, i.e., the physician may be able to "fine-tune" sensor-driven behavior based upon the patient's behavior.

5.6.8 MEASURED DATA, BATTERY STATUS & GENERATOR END-OF-LIFE

Some physicians recommend that at the time of the first office evaluation, and once a year thereafter, that telemetered atrial and ventricular electrograms be recorded and printed for the permanent record. These recordings serve as a baseline for future comparison should problems develop such as undersensing, oversensing, or possible lead malfunction. It is often helpful to print the electrograms at 25, 100, and 400 mm/sec. This allows for calculation of slew rates and provides a better view of the morphology of morphology of the intrinsic deflection. Most current devices also allow on-demand measurement of the intrinsic P- and R-wave amplitude, either on a digital read-out or by measuring the peak-to-peak amplitude on a calibrated paper printout. Some devices will automatically make these measurements daily and store the information in memory for later downloading and analysis. Obviously, measurement of the magnitude of intrinsic signals necessitates the patient exhibiting spontaneous electrical activity; amplitude measurements cannot be obtained if the patient is entirely paced during the testing period.

Most current devices also permit real-time on-demand measurements of lead impedance. Lead impedance measurements are only available for a given cardiac chamber if pacing is enabled for that chamber. The pacing impedance test can be used as a relative measure of lead integrity over time. In addition, lead integrity can be ascertained with pacing measurements.

Battery status can be assessed either through programmer telemetry or by using a manually applied magnet over the implanted pulse generator. In many modern pulse generators, the current battery voltage, battery impedance, and even an estimate of battery longevity can be determined on-demand or are automatically measured by the device once-a-day. In addition, most current devices will indicate if end-of-life or replacement time has been reached, sometimes even with programmable audible tones. Some devices directly measure battery impedance and voltage, while others assess battery status by the time required to charge a capacitor.

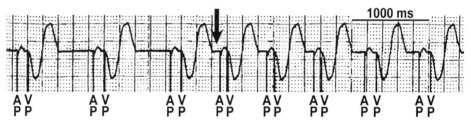

FIGURE 5-83. Effect of magnet application on pulse generator behavior. In this case, application of the magnet (downward arrow) results in asynchronous atrial and ventricular pacing at a rate of 100 pulses/min (cycle length = 600 ms) for three cycles with a paced AV interval of 100 ms. Following this, DOO pacing continues at a rate of 85 pulses/min (cycle length = 705 ms) using the programmed AV interval. Courtesy of Guidant.

Battery status can also be determined by applying a magnet stronger than 70 gauss over the pulse generator. This method is usually required in older devices with the inability to provide digitally-displaced status indicators. The magnet actuates a switch within the pacemaker, thereby converting it to an asynchronous mode (DOO or SOO) with a fixed pacing rate (and fixed AV interval if in DOO mode) that varies with manufacturer and pulse generator model. Magnet application causes asynchronous pacing at a designated "magnet rate" (Figure 5-83). Magnet operation varies between different manufacturers and device models, but usually involves a temporary rate change and a transient output change when the magnet is applied. For example, magnet application may result in the delivery of three stimuli at a rate of 100 pulses/min, followed by a *magnet rate* of 85 pulses/min. In dual chamber devices, the AV interval may be adjusted to an arbitrary duration, usually 100 ms, during magnet application. The pacemaker remains in the magnet mode (asynchronous pacing) as long as the magnet is applied over the pulse generator. The magnet rate at the elective replacement time of the device is different, and generally lower, than the basic magnet rate. Many older pacemakers use the programmed lower rate as the magnet rate and the magnet rate decreases gradually as the battery is depleted until it reaches the elective replacement time. When the elective re-

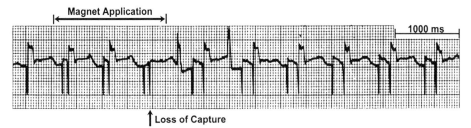

FIGURE 5-84. ECG rhythm strip showing effects of magnet application. After application of the magnet, asynchronous AV pacing is performed with a paced AV interval of 100 ms. The pulse widths of the third atrial and ventricular pacing stimuli are reduced 50% of the programmed level. Note that neither atrial nor ventricular capture occurs at the reduced pacing output, indicating that the atrial and ventricular pacing outputs are less than twice the pulse width threshold. Courtesy of Medtronic, Inc.

placement time is reached, about 3 more months of battery life normally remain before end-of-life is reached. After ERI is reached and EOL is approached, any number of programmable pacemaker functions may become unavailable in order to conserve energy. Programmable functions that may become unavailable include adaptive-rate pacing, stored electrograms, rate and sensor trending/histograms, rate-smoothing, mode-switching, and event markers. When EOL is reached most pacemakers, even dual chamber systems, revert to single chamber operation (usually VVI at some base rate, often 50-60 pulses/min). As battery depletion continues, the pacing output is reduced, reprogramming is no longer possible and telemetry is often unavailable beyond EOL.

Application of the magnet is also used to perform the *threshold margin test* (Figure 5-84). After application of the magnet, one or more pacemaker pulses (usually the second or third) are delivered with the voltage amplitude or pulse width reduced by 25%, 50%, or even 75% of the programmed values. For example, some new pulse generators reduce the output by 25% on the third pulse, 50% on the fifth pulse and 75% on the seventh pulse after magnet application. These magnet operations allow the clinician to quickly assess the pacing threshold safety margin and battery status of the device. In order to determine the specific magnet operation of any particular pulse generator, the technical manual should be consulted.

5.6.9 SPECIAL PACEMAKER FUNCTIONS

Many new pacemakers now provide a number of special diagnostic and therapeutic functions (Table 5-15.) For example, some devices provide the capability to record atrial and ventricular arrhythmias based upon programmable criteria, or in response to triggering the device by patient intervention (using magnet application over the device). In other cases, chronically implanted pacemakers can be used to performed programmed electrical stimulation for arrhythmia induction in selected patients requiring this procedure. In most cases, these "bells and whistles" provide little additional benefit and may dramatically accelerate battery drainage and shorten the usable device of the life. Therefore, caution should be exercised to only utilize options that are necessary for optimum therapy of the patient.

TABLE 5-15. Standard & special features available in some modern pacemaker systems

Diagnostic features	Therapy features
P- & R-wave amplitude measurements	Multiple pacing modes
Event counters	Programmable rate, output, sensitivity, & refractory periods
Semi-automatic threshold tests	Rate-responsive pacing
Sensor trending	Mode switching
Rate histograms	Dynamic or rate-related AV delay
Real-time intracardiac electrogram	PVARP extension after a VPD
Event markers	Rate smoothing
Automatic stored intracardiac electrograms	Sensor rate hysteresis
Patient-triggered stored electrograms	Sensed and paced AV delay
High-resolution rate trending	Ventricular safety pacing
Beat-to-beat trending	Non-competitive atrial pacing
	Rate drop response
	Automatically adjustable PAVI, SAVI, and TARP
	Automatic sensitivity adjustment
	Automatic threshold measurement & output adjustment

PVARP, post-ventricular atrial refractory period; VPD, ventricular premature depolarizations

5.6.10 ANCILLARY TESTING

In selected patients with suspected pacemaker system malfunction or symptoms possibly related to a pacemaker-related problem, certain ancillary tests my be useful. A postero-anterior and lateral chest x-ray should always be obtained post-implant to document lead position and rule out a potential pneumothorax. In addition, during the follow-up period, a chest x-ray can rule-out any change in lead position and may either show frank lead damage or developing signs of potential lead failure in pacing systems showing evidence of lead malfunction. An x-ray may show conductor discontinuity suggesting a conductor fracture or conductor deformity as it crosses between the clavicle and first rib or between an excessively tight tie-down ligature.

An exercise treadmill test may be useful in selected cases to assist in programming the sensor parameters. In most cases, however, sensor programming can be accomplished based upon the patient's usual daily activities using trending and histogram data.

Ambulatory ECG recording may prove helpful in diagnosing pacemaker malfunctions, especially under- or oversensing. The capability for patient triggered electrogram recording in response to symptoms may prove useful in this regard as well.

5.6.11 FINAL INTERROGATION & DOCUMENTATION

At the end of the evaluation the pulse generator should be interrogated one last time and the final programmed parameters carefully reviewed. A final report should be printed and placed in the patient's permanent record. Some clinicians prefer also to give a copy of the final printout to the patient. A copy for the patient may prove useful should the patient require evaluation at an outside facility.

5.7   Pacemaker Troubleshooting

Troubleshooting and remediation of a possible pacemaker malfunction must be approached in a systematic fashion. It is crucial to precisely identify and completely define the scope of the problem. Only after that can corrective steps be taken. Pacemaker system malfunctions usually come to attention either because: 1) the patient develops suspicious symptoms or, 2) evidence of pacing system misbehavior is noted on an ECG recording.

Common ECG findings suggestive of a pacemaker malfunction include: 1) inappropriate failure to deliver pacemaker output, 2) failure of a pacemaker output stimulus to activate atrial or ventricular tissue (failure to capture), 3) inappropriate delivery of a pacemaker stimulus (undersensing), and 4) inappropriate pacemaker rate.

Symptoms potentially the result of a pacemaker system malfunction include near-syncope, syncope, fatigue, dyspnea, or palpitations. Similar symptoms may also occur in pacemaker patients due to suboptimal programming, or may be totally unrelated to the pacemaker system. Therefore, it is crucial to clinically evaluate the patient as well as investigating the pacemaker system when troubleshooting a potential pacemaker malfunction.

5.7.1   ECG EVIDENCE OF PACING SYSTEM MALFUNCTION

Potential pacemaker problems that can be identified on an ECG can generally be assigned to five categories (Table 5-16.)

TABLE 5-16.   Classification of potential pacing system malfunctions

Undersensing
Failure to deliver output/oversensing
Failure to capture
Pseudomalfunction

Undersensing. Causes of undersensing (Figures 5-20 & 5-85) are summarized in Table 5-17. Insulation breaks may cause undersensing if the insulation break results in a failure of intrinsic cardiac signals to reach the sense amplifier and failure of the cardiac signal amplitude to meet the sensitivity requirement. Conductor fracture may cause an open circuit. If intrinsic signals fail to cross the conductor fracture, undersensing will occur. The primary cause of conductor fracture is the chronic stress imposed on the lead body as a result of its implantation in the subclavian region between the rigid bone structures of the first rib and the clavicle (subclavian crush damage). Conductor fracture can often be diagnosed by an increase in pacing impedance. During lead maturation, fibrotic

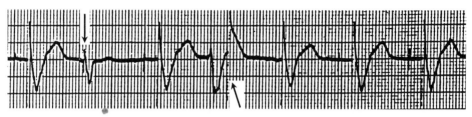

FIGURE 5-85. An example of pseudopseudofusion and undersensing resulting from a ventricular premature PD) occurring during the blanking period in a dual chamber pacing system programmed to the DDD mode. The downward arrow denotes a pseudopseudofusion beat in which an ineffective atrial stimulus is delivered coincidentally into the onset of a ventricular premature depolarization. The intrinsic deflection of this VPD occurs after the blanking period and is normally sensed thereby inhibiting the ventricular output. The upward arrow highlights a VPD that occurs within the ventricular blanking period following the intrinsic deflection. Therefore, this VPD is not detected and a ventricular stimulus is ineffectively delivered near the end of the spontaneous ventricular activation   Courtesy of St. Jude/Pacesetter, Inc.

growth near the electrode reduces the magnitude of the intrinsic signal recorded by the pacemaker system by 20% - 50%, increasing the chances of undersensing (depending upon the programmed sensitivity setting). Steroid-eluting leads have been shown to minimize fibrous growth, thereby reducing the chances of undersensing. Lead dislodgment usually occurs early in the life of the pacemaker before the lead has become fixed to the endocardial tissue by the development of the fibrotic scar. The primary causes of lead dislodgment are suboptimal lead positioning or inadequate fixation of the lead body at the time of implant, or inappropriate post-implant activity by the patient, especially excessive overhead arm movement. Lead dislodgment occurs in approximately 2% - 3%

TABLE 5-17. Causes of undersensing

| Lead dislodgment |
| Poor lead position |
| Lead failure (insulation break or conductor failure) |
| Low-amplitude Intracardiac signal |
| Magnet application |
| Environmental electrical noise |
| Pacemaker refractory period |
| Inappropriate programming of sensitivity |

of implants. Changes in the magnitude of the native cardiac signal may be caused by myocardial infarction, change in medications, and severe electrolyte imbalance. Finally, undersensing may result if the magnitude of the intrinsic signal is less then the programmed sensitivity setting.

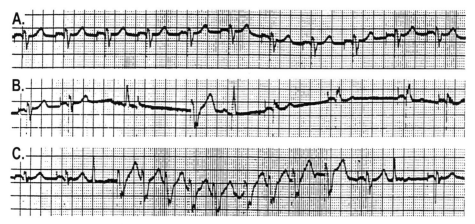

FIGURE 5-86. Example of oversensing in the ventricular and atrial channels of a dual chamber pacing system programmed to the DDD mode. Panel A: baseline AV pacing. Panel B: ventricular channel senses myopotentials resulting in inhibition of ventricular pacing. Panel C: myopotentials are detected by the atrial channel resulting in triggered ventricular pacing at the maximum tracking rate of 130 pulse/min. Courtesy of St. Jude/Pacesetter, Inc.

Failure to deliver output. Failure to deliver expected pacemaker output has a number of potential causes (Table 5-18.) The most common cause of output failure is oversensing

TABLE 5-18. Causes of failure to deliver pacemaker output

Oversensing

Total battery depletion

Lead fracture

Lead disconnection

Pacemaker component failure

Crosstalk

(Figures 5-20 & 5-86). Causes of oversensing are summarized in Table 5-19. Typically, oversensing may be caused by lead failure (disruption of insulation or "make-and-break" fracture), poor connection at the connector block, and electrical interference. Insulation failure, which is the most common cause of oversensing, occurs when myopotentials are detected by the pacemaker lead through the insulation break. As discussed above, myopotential oversensing is of greater concern with unipolar sensing than with bipolar sensing (see "Sensing of Cardiac Signals" on page 199.) A lead conductor fracture may cause oversensing as the frayed ends of the conductor wires "make-and-break" contact, producing intermittent transient voltage signals. Oversensing may also occur if the lead pin is loose in the connector block ("header"), resulting in spurious, non-physiological signals as the lead pin "rattles-around" within the connection port of the connector block.

Finally, oversensing may occur if electromagnetic interference (EMI) signals are incor-

TABLE 5-19. Causes of pacemaker oversensing

Biological signals
T-wave sensing by ventricular channel
Far-field P-wave sensing by ventricular channel
Far-field sensing of ventricular depolarization by atrial channel
Sensing of concealed extrasystoles by atrial or ventricular channels
Sensing of somatic muscle potentials (e.g., pectoral, diaphragmatic)
External electromagnetic interference (EMI)
Electrocautery or diathermy
Nuclear magnetic resonance
Electrical defibrillation current
Transcutaneous nerve stimulators
Radio and television transmitters
Arc-welding equipment
Internally-generated interfering signals
Afterpotentials generated by pacing stimuli
Spurious potentials originating within the generator (autointerference)
Intermittent contact of inactive leads or metal electrode parts
Electrolysis of old metal leads or metal components

rectly interpreted as P- or R-waves. Sources of EMI are discussed elsewhere (see "Interference with Normal Pacemaker Operation" on page 204.)

Crosstalk is a special type of oversensing in which the output stimulus of one pacemaker channel is sensed by the other channel resulting in inappropriate inhibition of the pacing output from this channel (Figures 5-41 & 5-42). Most modern pacemakers are shipped with nominal settings that include generous blanking periods in the atrial and ventricular channels. That, along with the introduction of safety pacing, has made crosstalk an infrequent or non-existent problem in most current pacing systems (Figures 5-40, 5-43, 5-44 & 5-87). However, in some cases, it may be necessary evaluate a device for the presence of crosstalk. To screen for crosstalk, program the pacemaker to the desired output and sensitivity settings and then increase the lower rate to a level that is faster than the intrinsic atrial rate. In addition, shorten the AV interval to a value that is shorter than that seen during the patient's intrinsic AV conduction. These changes will result in AV sequential pacing. If there is no crosstalk, there will be stable AV pacing. If crosstalk is present, one of two possible rhythms may result: atrial pacing with inhibition of ventricular output (which is of no consequence if AV nodal conduction is intact) or atrial pacing followed by ventricular standstill in patients with complete AV block and no escape rhythm. If crosstalk is demonstrated, increasing the blanking period will usually eliminate it. This is particularly important in those patients who predominantly exhibit AV pacing. However, a long blanking period may increase the chance of competition in those patients with frequent ventricular ectopy; consequently, the blanking period should be as short as possible. In selected patients with high grade AV block as their indication for pacing, it may be useful to screen for crosstalk in selected patients. However, enabling safety pacing has all but eliminated the problem of crosstalk-induced inhibition of ventricular pacing. The most common cause of safety pacing is late cycle

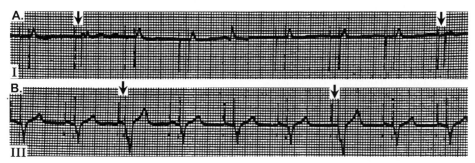

FIGURE 5-87. Example of ventricular safety pacing resulting from crosstalk in a dual chamber pacemaker programmed to the DDD mode. Panel A: lead I. Panel B: lead III. Downward arrows mark pacing cycles with short PAVI (100 ms) consistent with ventricular safety pacing. Normal PAVI is 160 ms. Courtesy of St. Jude/Pacesetter, Inc.

ventricular depolarizations that coincides with the crosstalk sensing or detection (safety pacing) window. While a ventricular stimulus will be triggered in response to this detection, it should not be misinterpreted as undersensing. In addition, because the stimulus is delivered a time when the ventricular myocardium is refractory (from the ventricular premature depolarization), it will not result in ventricular activation. If crosstalk is known to be absent but then develops in an otherwise chronic stable pacing system, an insulation defect involving the atrial lead should be suspected. This may allow crosstalk because the insulation break will reduce the stimulation impedance and increase the current amplitude; the ventricular channel may detect the larger amplitude stimulus.

TABLE 5-20. Causes of failure to capture

Lead dislodgment or perforation
Lead insulation break
Lead conductor fracture
Poor connection at the connector block
Exit block
Metabolic abnormalities
Battery depletion
Inappropriate low-energy output settings
Pacemaker stimulus delivered during refractory period of cardiac tissue

Failure to capture. Possible causes of failure of pacing stimuli to capture the myocardium are summarized in Table 5-20. Insulation break can cause capture failure because electric current is lost to non-cardiac tissues through the insulation break. Other less common causes of non-capture include Twiddler's syndrome, severe electrolyte abnormalities (especially hyperkalemia), myocardial infarction near the stimulation electrode, drug therapy, battery depletion, exit block of the stimulus pulse at the electrode-tissue interface. Lack of pacemaker output can be caused by poor connection to the connector block, lead failure (especially conductor fracture, but also insulation break), battery depletion, and, very rarely, circuit failure (pulse generator malfunction).

Pseudomalfunctions. Represent ECG findings that appear to result from malfunction of the pacemaker system but in reality are normal pacemaker operation. Pseudomalfunctions are classified under the following categories: 1) pacing rate; 2) AV interval/refractory periods; 3) mode; and 4) sensing.

Pseudomalfunctions due to pacing rate changes are more common than ever, especially since incorporation of special functions in pacemakers such as sensor-driven pacing and mode-switching. Rate changes that may result from normal device operation are summarized in Table 5-21.

TABLE 5-21. Causes of pseudomalfunctions due to pacing rate changes

Magnet operation
Timing variations (A-A timing versus V-V timing)
Upper rate behavior (Wenckebach and 2:1 block)
Electrical reset
Battery depletion
Sensor-driven rate behavior
Intervention behavior for pacemaker-mediated tachycardia
Misinterpretation of special pacing functions

Magnet application causes asynchronous pacing at a designated "magnet rate" (Figure 5-88). Some pacemaker telemetry wands have a a built in electromagnet that can be switched "on" or "off". In these cases, magnet operation of the pacemaker can occur after placement of the wand over the pulse generator (see "Pacemaker Follow-up" on page 248.) Unless the operator appreciates this, the magnet-induced pacing behavior may be misinterpreted as a pacing system malfunction.

Timing variations may also cause pseudomalfunctions. If a device uses an atrial-based timing algorithm, it will maintain a stable atrial rate regardless of any intrinsic AV conduction that may occur. Ventricular-based timing will result in a stable ventriculoatrial interval (AEI) that will permit paced rates greater than the lower rate limit if intrinsic AV conduction occurs.

As mentioned above, during Wenckebach operation there is gradual prolongation of the P-V interval until a P-wave is not followed by the delivery of a ventricular pacing stimulus. Pacemaker Wenckebach occurs when the intrinsic atrial rate exceeds the upper rate limit. Since the ventricular pacing rate cannot exceed the MTRI, the SAVI is increased until the MTRI timer elapses and a ventricular pacing stimulus can be delivered

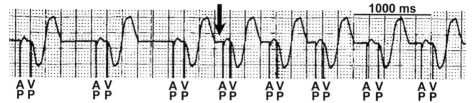

FIGURE 5-88. Example of magnet operation in a dual chamber pacing system. After application of the magnet (downward arrow), atrial and ventricular pacing is performed at a rate of 100 pulses/min for three cycles with a paced AV delay of 100 ms. Thereafter AV pacing is performed at the magnet rate of 85 pulses/min and the programmed AV delay. AP, atrial pace; VP, ventricular pace. Courtesy of Guidant/CPI, Inc.

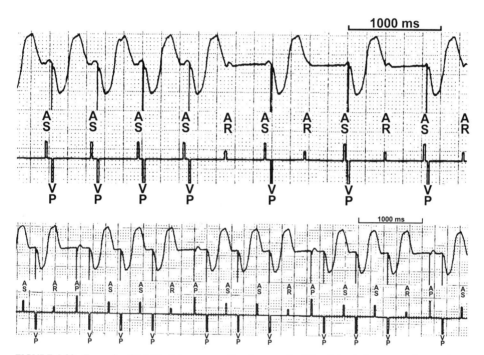

FIGURE 5-89. Example of 2:1 block (upper panel) and pacemaker Wenckebach (lower panel) operations. Analysis of the marker channel in each case makes it clear that these rhythm strips do not illustrate a malfunction of the pacing system. AS, atrial sense; AP, atrial pace; AR, atrial refractory sense; VP, ventricular pace. Courtesy of Medtronic, Inc.

(Figure 5-89). An atrial sensed event eventually falls within the refractory period and, therefore, is not followed by a ventricular pace. Similarly, 2:1 block behavior, which occurs when the P-P interval is less than the TARP, results in a dramatic drop in pacing rate (Figure 5-89). Both upper rate behaviors may be misinterpreted as pacemaker system malfunction.

Electrical reset usually results in rate change and (often) a mode change. Reset may occur due to exposure to EMI – including electrocautery, defibrillation, and radiof-

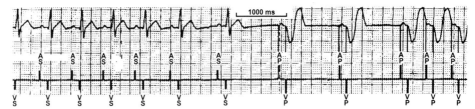

FIGURE 5-90. Some pacemakers include a rate drop response feature. This programmable option allows pacing at a high rate when an episodic sudden decrease of heart rate occurs. This option may be useful in selected patients with medically refractory, neurally-mediated syncope with a predominant bradycardia component (vasovagal). Patients exhibiting syncope primarily due to vasodilation (vasodepressor) are unlikely to receive significant benefit from this therapy option. Medical therapy is the primary treatment for neurally-mediated syncope. Even the rare patient requiring pacemaker therapy usually also require medical therapy. Courtesy of Medtronic, Inc.

requency current – causing reversion to the device's "back-up" mode. The settings in back-up mode may be similar or identical to those that occur at the ERI or EOL of the device. Therefore, it is crucial not to mistake end-of-life behavior with resetting, nor should resetting or battery depletion be interpreted as a pacemaker malfunction. In general, a device that has been reset can usually be programmed back to the original parameters, while a device at EOL generally cannot be reprogrammed.

Finally, sudden rate changes may occur due to special programmable options including: 1) PMT disruption by PVARP extension; 2) rate-responsive pacing; 3) rate hysteresis; 4) rate drop response; 5) mode switching; 6) sleep function (Figures 5-90, 5-91 & 5-92). If any of these behaviors are observed they may be incorrectly interpreted as a system malfunction by the unsuspecting clinician.

Pseudomalfunctions due to changes in AV intervals/refractory periods is also not uncommon. Atrioventricular intervals and refractory periods may appear anomalous due to: 1) safety pacing (Figure 5-93); 2) blanking; 3) rate-responsive AV delay (Figure 5-94); 4) response to ventricular premature depolarizations (VPD response) (Figure 5-94);

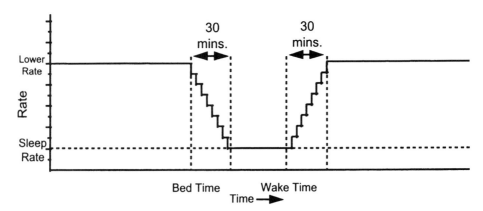

FIGURE 5-91. Programmable sleep function behavior designed to preserve battery life by reducing the lower pacing rate during sleep time. A gradual rate decrease to the sleep rate (below the programmed lower rate) is observed as the programmed bedtime approaches. The lower rate gradually increases at the programmed wake time. Courtesy of Medtronic, Inc.

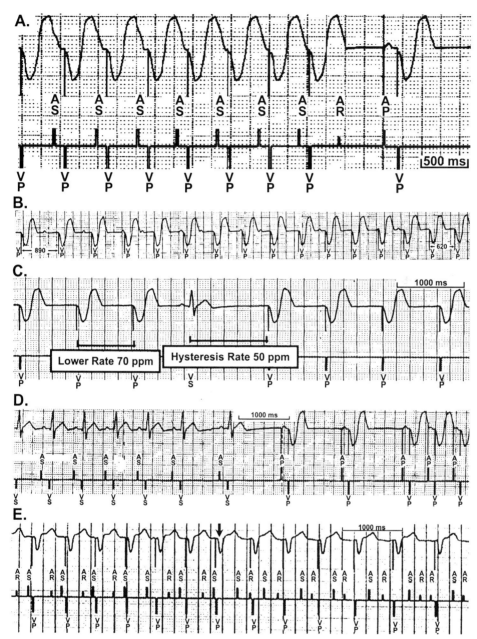

FIGURE 5-92. Examples of special programmable functions resulting in rate changes that may be misinterpreted as a pacing system malfunction. Panel A: intervention for pacemaker-mediated tachycardia (PVARP extension); Panel B: rate-responsive pacing (VVIR mode) with increase in rate from 67 pulses/min to 97 pulses/min; Panel C: hysteresis; Panel D: sudden rate-drop response that is often beneficial in neurally-mediated syncope; Panel E: mode-switching (downward arrow) in response to atrial tachyarrhythmia. AS, atrial sense; AP, atrial pace; AR, atrial refractory sense; VP, ventricular pace; VS, ventricular sense. Courtesy of Medtronic, Inc.

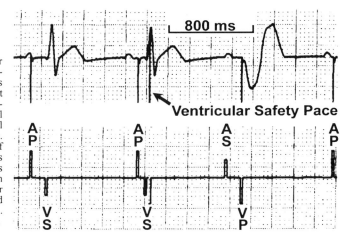

FIGURE 5-93. Ventricular safety pacing. In this example, atrial undersensing is occurring (P-wave not sensed) resulting in inappropriate delivery of an atrial pacing stimulus. The atrial pace initiates a PAVI timer. During the first 110 ms of the PAVI a spontaneous ventricular activation is sensed which results in delivery of a ventricular pacing stimulus at the end of the 100 ms interval. Courtesy of Medtronic, Inc.

5) non-competitive atrial pacing behavior (Figure 5-94); and 6) sensor-varied PVARP (duration of the PVARP shortens as the sensor-driven pacing rate increases); 7) automatic AV and TARP adjustment to minimize pacemaker Wenckebach or 2:1 upper rate behavior.

Pseudomalfunctions due to a change in pacing mode have also been observed. A change in pacing mode may be caused by: 1) battery depletion; 2) electrical reset; 3) mode switching (Figure 5-92); 4) noise reversion (Figure 5-95).

Pseudomalfunctions can also occur secondary to presumed sensing malfunctions. Recall that in demand mode, the delivery of a pacing stimulus is prevented if a intrinsic depolarization is detected. Depending upon the location of the sensing lead and the origin of the spontaneous depolarization, the lead may not detect the spontaneous depolarization until myocardial activation is almost complete. The lead can only report the occurrence of an atrial or ventricular depolarization as the wavefront passes beneath the sensing electrode (intrinsic deflection). Consequently, the pacemaker may still appropriately deliver a pacing stimulus even though the ventricle has been almost completely activated. This stimulus may or may not result in capture and propagation of a second depolarization wavefront. For example a ventricular *fusion* beat occurs when ventricular activation results from dual activation of the ventricles from both the pacing stimuli as well as the intrinsic depolarization The resulting QRS complex has a hybrid morphology somewhere between a completely paced QRS complex and QRS complex generated from intrinsic activation. In the case of a ventricular *pseudofusion* beat, ventricular activation occurs entirely from an intrinsic depolarization; however, a coincidentally-time ineffective pacing stimulus is delivered into the QRS complex. This pacing stimulus may mistakenly be assumed to have contributed to ventricular activation because of its timing. However, the clue that this ventricular depolarization is not a true fusion beat, but rather a pseudofusion beat in which the pacing stimulus is ineffective is that the morphology of the QRS complex is identical to a native spontaneous complex, and is distinctly different than the hybrid fusion complex (Figure 5-96).

FIGURE 5-94. Example of pseudomalfunctions due to changes in AV intervals or refractory period. Normally, the P-R interval decreases as the heart increases and increases as the heart rate decreases. The rate-adaptive AV delay (panel A) can be programmed to mimic the normal physiologic response of the P-R interval to increasing heart rates. A pacemaker cannot distinguish a ventricular premature depolarization (VPD) from any other spontaneous ventricular depolarization. Pacemakers with VPD response (panel B) define a VPD as a ventricular sensed event following a sensed or paced ventricular event without any intervening atrial event. If the VPD response is activated a sensed VPD results in extension of the PVARP in order to prevent sensing any resulting retrograde P-wave. The extended PVARP and resultant resetting of the VA timer may be mistaken as a pacing system malfunction. Non-competitive atrial pacing (NCAP) (panel C) prevents atrial pacing from occurring too close to the relative refractory period, which may trigger atrial arrhythmias. If NCAP is implemented, the scheduled atrial pace is delayed (downward arrow) until 300 ms has elapsed since the refractory-sensed P-wave (upward arrow) has occurred. To keep the ventricular rate from experiencing the same delay the ensuing PAVI is shortened. Ap, atrial pace; Ar, atrial refractory sense; As, atrial sense; PAVI, paced AV interval; Vp, ventricular pace; Vs, ventricular sense. Courtesy of Medtronic, Inc.

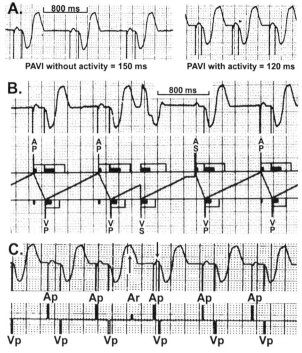

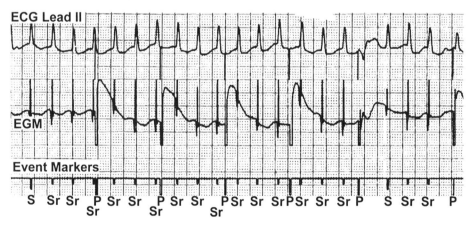

FIGURE 5-95. Example of noise reversion behavior. This is a single chamber ventricular pacemaker in a patient who develops ventricular tachycardia. The repeated sensing of ventricular events during the ventricular refractory period (Sr) triggers noise reversion behavior with ineffective delivery of ventricular pacing stimuli (P) at the programmed lower rate interval. S, non-refractory sense event. Courtesy of Medtronic, Inc.

5.7.2 SYMPTOMS & SIGNS SUGGESTIVE OF PACEMAKER MALFUNCTION

Signs and symptoms suggestive of a potential pacemaker malfunction or inappropriate programming need to be investigated systematically. The clinician should be careful to obtain a thorough history including the date of implant, implantation data (thresholds, lead impedance, P- and R-wave amplitudes), indication for pacing therapy, and lead and generator information. A complete description of the patient's symptoms should be obtained to ensure that the symptoms are indeed a consequence of the pacing system.

The patient should be questioned concerning possible exposure to EMI, electrocautery, radiation, defibrillation, cardioversion, high energy ultrasound, or external sources such as heavy-duty electrical equipment. In addition, medication changes that may increase pacing thresholds and potentially lead to patient symptoms include class IA, IC, and III antiarrhythmic drugs. Some corticosteroids, such as prednisone, may actually reduce pacing thresholds. Daily activities, such as exercise, eating, and sleeping, are associated

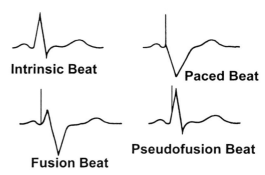

FIGURE 5-96. Schematic example of ventricular fusion and pseudofusion. A ventricular fusion beat has a hybrid QRS morphology sharing attributes of both spontaneous and totally-paced QRS complexes. A pseudofusion beat exhibits a QRS morphology characteristic of a spontaneous QRS complex that is distorted by a superimposed pacing stimulus; the stimulus fails to capture the already-activated ventricular myocardium.

with (generally) small changes in pacing thresholds. A focused clinical examination may proved useful in establishing a diagnosis of pacing malfunction. Specifically, upper body isometric or isotonic exercises may confirm myopotential sensing. Palpation of the pulse generator pocket and lead may identify an insulation break, conductor fracture, or loose connection at the connector block. These maneuvers are particularly valuable because many sensing and pacing problems are intermittent and may only occur under unique conditions.

A number of signs and symptoms may occur in patients with pacemakers and may indicate pacemaker malfunction or suboptimal programming including: 1) muscle stimulation; 2) palpitations; 3) pacemaker syndrome; 4) pacemaker-mediated tachycardia; 5) shortness of breath due to inappropriate rate response settings.

Muscle stimulation may be caused by inappropriate electrode placement, break in lead insulation, or unipolar pacing. Diaphragmatic stimulation may occur because of inappropriate lead placement near the diaphragm or right phrenic nerve, or because of pacing through a thin-walled right ventricle. Diaphragmatic activation may be described as a "hiccup" by the patient. Programming a lower output may eliminate the diaphragmatic stimulation. Optimally, testing the lead position at implant by pacing at an output of 10 volts is normally an adequate indicator of possible post-implant problems with diaphragmatic stimulation. If no diaphragmatic stimulation is experienced when pacing at 10 volts, it is unlikely that diaphragmatic stimulation will develop post-implant. A break in the lead insulation may result in skeletal muscle activation near the site of the break. Not uncommonly, the skeletal muscle involved is the pectoralis or deltoid, near the site of implant or the pulse generator pocket. Current flow through the insulation breech is responsible for the skeletal muscle activation. Patients with unipolar pacing systems may experience muscle stimulation near the pulse generator. This can occur with a unipolar system because the output current flows between the cathode in the heart and the pulse generator case which functions as the anode (Figure 5-25).

Palpitations (uncomfortable sensing of one's own heartbeat) may occur in patients as a result of tracking an atrial tachyarrhythmia, undersensing, oversensing, or failure to pace (see above), pacemaker-mediated tachycardia, or pacemaker syndrome (Table 5-22.) All these possibilities may need to be investigated in pacemaker patients complaining of palpitations.

TABLE 5-22.   Signs and symptoms associated with the pacemaker syndrome

Symptoms associated with pacemaker syndrome

   Weakness, fatigue, lassitude

   Near-syncope and syncope

   Psychological changes (anxiety, malaise, apprehension)

   Dyspnea, orthopnea and cough

   Chest pain

   Neck and abdominal pulsations

Physical and objective findings associated with pacemaker syndrome

   Congestive heart failure and frank pulmonary edema

   Cannon A waves

   Systemic hypotension

   Increase in vascular resistance & decline in cardiac output and arterial pressure

Pacemaker syndrome.   Pacemaker syndrome has been described as an assortment of symptoms related to the adverse hemodynamic impact from the loss of AV synchrony. This syndrome is caused by: 1) loss of atrial capture or sensing in a dual chamber system; 2) programming extremely long duration AV intervals in a dual chamber system; 3) development of 2:1 pacing (upper rate behavior); 4) single chamber pacing (VVI); 5) absence of a pacing rate increase with exercise. The pacemaker syndrome is most common in patients treated with VVI pacing. In patients with sinus rhythm, VVI pacing results in a loss of AV synchrony with the resultant elimination of the atrial contribution to left ventricular filling with a corresponding reduction of cardiac output. In some patients these changes may produce a variety of symptoms and physical findings which together have been termed the pacemaker syndrome (Table 5-22.) Fundamentally, relief from the pacemaker syndrome is usually achieved by the restoration of AV synchrony. Management often requires reprogramming the device to an AV synchronous pacing mode or, depending upon the cause, adjustment of the atrial sensitivity or output, rate-response parameters or upper rate options (including TARP). Single chamber ventricular systems may have to be upgraded to a dual chamber system to provide this capability (or a single chamber system allowing atrial sensing and ventricular pacing using the VDD mode).

Retrograde conduction & pacemaker-mediated tachycardia (PMT). There are two situations that can result in pacemaker-mediated tachycardia: 1) retrograde conduction or 2) high rate atrial tracking caused by atrial flutter or fibrillation, or by atrial oversensing (Figure 5-97). A dual chamber pacemaker system, in essence, adds a second artificial AV conduction system in the heart which runs parallel to the patient's native AV conduction system. Just as patients with Wolff-Parkinson-White syndrome may develop a circus movement tachycardia by using their normal AV conduction system and their accessory AV conduction system, some patients with a dual chamber pacemaker system programmed to the DDD mode may develop a sustained tachycardia using the two parallel AV pathways. Specifically, this may occur if the pacemaker patient has ventriculoatrial conduction using the normal AV conduction pathway. Pacemaker-mediated tachycardia is a (usually) rapid ventricular paced rhythm that is sustained by ventricular events that conduct retrograde to the atrium (Figure 5-92, panel A). Up to 40% of patients with anterograde AV block, and 60% of patients with sinoatrial node dysfunction, are capable of ventriculoatrial conduction [43-45]. However, in addition to retrograde conduction, the development of PMT requires that retrograde activation must occur outside of the refractory period of the atrial channel, thereby initiating a SAVI timer.

Most commonly, PMT is initiated by a premature ventricular depolarization which then conducts retrograde from the ventricle to the atrium (Figure 5-98). If the retrograde activation of the atrium occurs after the refractory period of the atrial sensing circuit has elapsed and before the next spontaneous or paced atrial depolarization, it will be sensed by the atrial channel. This sensed atrial event will trigger the AVI timer culminating in

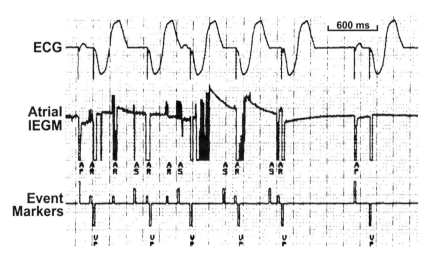

FIGURE 5-97. High rate atrial tracking, either due to supraventricular tachyarrhythmias or atrial oversensing of myopotentials or extraneous noise (above), may cause pacemaker syndrome. IEGM, intracardiac electrograms. Courtesy of Medtronic, Inc.

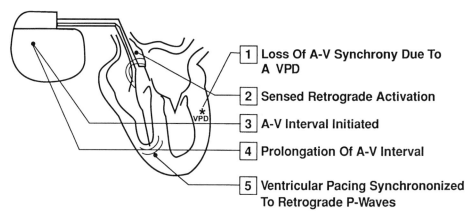

1	**Loss Of A-V Synchrony Due To A VPD**
2	**Sensed Retrograde Activation**
3	**A-V Interval Initiated**
4	**Prolongation Of A-V Interval**
5	**Ventricular Pacing Synchrononized To Retrograde P-Waves**

FIGURE 5-98. Illustration of mechanism of development of pacemaker-mediated tachycardia by a ventricular premature depolarization (VPD). VPDs may conduct retrograde to the atrium. If the retrograde P-wave is sensed outside the PVARP, an SAVI timer is initiated. A ventricular paced event will occur after expiration of the SAVI timer, unless this would violate the upper tracking rate limit. If the MTRI timer has not expired, the SAVI is prolonged until MTRI timer is satisfied, after which a ventricular pacing stimulus is delivered. Should conduction again be possible within the normal ventriculoatrial conduction pathways, this paced ventricular activation may cause another retrograde atrial activation. If this cycle continue, a sustained tachycardia will result. Similar mechanisms are responsible for pacemaker-mediated tachycardia occurring secondary to atrial oversensing (Figure 5-99), atrial undersensing (Figure 5-100), atrial premature depolarizations (Figure 5-101), and failure of atrial capture (Figure 5-102). Courtesy of Medtronic, Inc.

delivery of a paced ventricular activation (assuming no spontaneous ventricular depolarization occurs). This paced ventricular depolarization may then again conduct retrograde and, if sensed by the atrial channel, may trigger another paced ventricular activation. Should this sequence continue, a sustained tachycardia may result. PMT can also occur with a loss of AV synchrony caused by: 1) atrial oversensing of, for example, electromagnetic interference (Figure 5-99), atrial undersensing (failure to sense a spontaneous atrial depolarization) (Figure 5-100), a premature atrial depolarization (Figure 5-101), loss of atrial capture (Figure 5-102), or magnet application.

There is a relatively simple method to determine if the patient can sustain conduction in a retrograde direction. The classic method is to program the pacemaker to the VVI mode at a rate that is faster than the intrinsic atrial rate and then look for the presence or absence of a retrograde P-wave falling within the ST segment or T-wave of the paced ventricular beat. However, it is often difficult to detect a retrograde P-wave in this portion of the cardiac cycle. Consequently it is usually very helpful to simultaneously view the intracardiac atrial electrogram and marker channels. The interval between the ventricular stimulus and the atrial electrogram represents the retrograde conduction time, which can be accurately measured by recording these signals at a rapid speed or using electronic calipers that are often included in modern pacemaker programmers. If retrograde conduction is demonstrated, the VVI rate should be increased to the proposed maximum tracking rate to determine if retrograde conduction can be sustained at this rate.

In older pacemaker models, disruption of the pacemaker-mediated circus tachycardia can be accomplished by inhibition of atrial sensing (by application of a magnet over the pulse generator or reprogramming the device to a mode which prevents atrial sensing

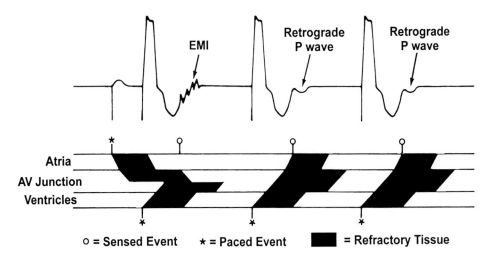

FIGURE 5-99. Retrograde conduction resulting from atrial oversensing. Sensing of electromagnetic interference (EMI) following a ventricular paced event may trigger initiation of a SAVI timer, resulting in a successive ventricular paced event. Should this ventricular activation be conducted retrograde and the retrograde P-wave be detected outside of the PVARP, ventricular pacing would again be triggered. Pacemaker-mediated tachycardia could be maintained as long as repeated retrograde conduction continues. Courtesy of Medtronic, Inc.

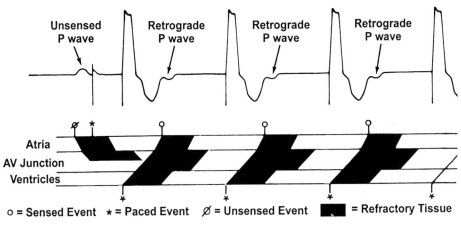

FIGURE 5-100. Retrograde conduction resulting from atrial undersensing. See text for further discussion. Courtesy of Medtronic, Inc.

(e.g., VVI, DVI, etc.) using the external programming system). Also, increasing the duration of the PVARP may prevent induction of pacemaker-mediated tachycardia. Under these conditions, a premature ventricular depolarization which conducts retrograde to the atrium may then result in activation of the atrium during the refractory period of the atrial sensing circuit. In this case, retrograde atrial depolarization will not be sensed and consequently it will not trigger a subsequent ventricular paced depolarization.

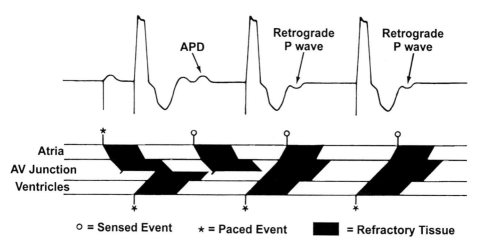

FIGURE 5-101. Retrograde conduction can develop secondary to an atrial premature depolarization. See text for further discussion. Courtesy of Medtronic, Inc.

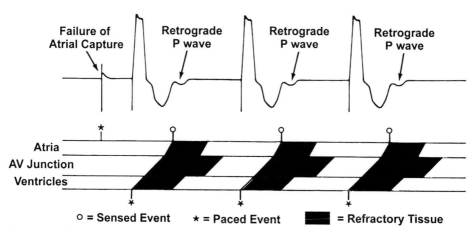

FIGURE 5-102. Mechanism of retrograde conduction resulting from loss of atrial capture. Failure of atrial activation allows a paced ventricular event to conduct retrograde to the atria. If sensed outside the PVARP, it could trigger another paced ventricular event. Pacemaker-mediated tachycardia could be maintained as long as repeated retrograde conduction continues. Courtesy of Medtronic, Inc.

In many newer pacemaker models a number of automatic programmable features are available to manage or prevent PMT. One common method is extension of the PVARP after the pacemaker senses a ventricular premature depolarization (Figure 5-103). Generally, a ventricular premature depolarization is defined as two consecutive ventricular events without an intervening atrial event. When the PVARP extension option is activated, a pacemaker-defined ventricular premature depolarization triggers an extension of the PVARP, for example to 400 ms (unless the PVARP is already programmed to that value). This extension of the PVARP means that P-waves conducted retrograde to the atrium generally will fall within the extended refractory period, thereby preventing the initiation of the SAVI timer (Figure 5-103).

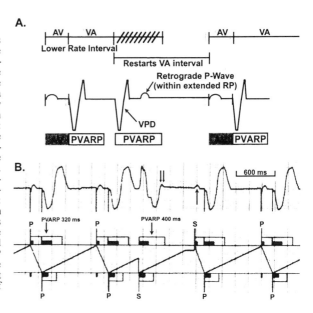

FIGURE 5-103. Many pacemakers incorporate a special programmable feature allowing automatic extension of the PVARP following the detection of a ventricular premature depolarization (VPD). In general, a VPD is defined as the second of any two ventricular events without an intervening atrial event. Panel A: When a VPD occurs and retrograde atrial activation results, the retrograde P-wave falls within the extended refractory period (RP). Therefore, a SAVI timer is not initiated and pacemaker-mediated tachycardia is prevented. Panel B: Example of PVARP extension from a baseline value of 320 ms to 400 ms after a VPD. The retrograde P-wave which results (double downward arrow) falls within the extended RP and does not trigger a SAVI. The event is a spontaneous sinus beat (upward arrow). Courtesy of Medtronic, Inc.

A second method available in some pacemakers to manage PMT involves extension of the PVARP after the onset of PMT (Figure 5-92). In general, pacemakers with this feature often determine the presence of PMT by detecting eight consecutive ventriculoatrial intervals (AEI) that meet the following three criteria: 1) duration less than 400 ms, 2) initiated by a paced ventricular event and, 3) end with a sensed atrial event. After the ninth paced ventricular event the PVARP will be increased to 400 ms, usually resulting in termination of the tachycardia.

5.7.3 REMEDIATION OF ANOMALOUS PACING SYSTEM BEHAVIOR

In general, the clinician has four options to manage pacing system malfunction or misbehavior: 1) reprogramming; 2) repositioning the lead; 3) replacing the lead(s) or pulse generator; 4) observation and watchful waiting. Reprogramming may often be used to correct oversensing, undersensing, and loss of capture. In some patients, sensing or pacing problems may be manageable by reprogramming from unipolar to bipolar. It may also provide a temporary solution in some cases of an insulation break. For example, in a pacemaker-dependent patient reprogramming to an asynchronous mode may be a short-term solution in a patient with oversensing. In other patients, reprogramming from unipolar to bipolar pacing may be an option. Programming changes can also allow optimization of AV intervals and rate response behavior. Repositioning the lead(s) may be necessary if a lead moves out of its original position and pacing or sensing is significantly compromised. In addition, management of skeletal muscle, diaphragmatic, or phrenic nerve stimulation may require lead repositioning. In rare cases, left ventricular pacing may be present due to lead misplacement in the left ventricle, either directly through the arterial system, or indirectly secondary to unintentional lead advancement through the interventricular septum at the time of implant. Rarely, the operator may mistakenly reverse the atrial and ventricular lead connection at the connector block. In this case lead repositioning is necessary, but only at the connector block. Replacing the lead or the pacemaker may be necessary when lead failure is confirmed, the battery is depleted, pacemaker syndrome occurs in a patient with a single chamber ventricular pacing system, passive fixation leads fail to remain in the appropriate position, or true pulse generator malfunction. Finally, some presumed malfunctions merely require observation and watchful waiting. For example, changes in drug therapy or a post-implant rise in pacing threshold may require no, or only minor, temporary reprogramming while the patient is followed closely in the outpatient clinic.

References

1. Hyman AS: Resuscitation of the stopped heart by intracardial therapy. *Arch Intern Med* **46**:553, 1930.
2. Hyman AS: Resuscitation of the stopped heart by intracardial therapy. II: Experimental use of an artificial pacemaker. *Arch Intern Med* **50**:283, 1932.
3. Mond HG, Sloman JG, Edwards RH: The first pacemaker. *PACE Pacing and Clinical Electrophysiology* **5**:278, 1982.
4. Zoll PM: Resuscitation of the heart in ventricular standstill by external electric stimulation. *N Engl J Med* **247**:768, 1952.
5. Callaghan JC, Bigelow WG: An electrical artificial pacemaker for standstill of the heart. *Ann Surg* **134**:8, 1951.
6. Leatham A, Cook P, Davies JG: External electric stimulator for treatment of ventricular standstill. *Lancet* **2**:1185, 1956.
7. Folkman MJ, Watkins E: An artificial conduction system for the management of experimental complete heart block. *Surg Forum* **8**:331, 1957.
8. Weirich WL, Gott VL, Lillehei CW: The treatment of complete heart block by combined use of a myocardial electrode and an artificial pacemaker. *Surg Forum* **8**:360, 1957.
9. Lillihei CW, Gott VL, Hodges PC, et al.: Transistor pacemaker for treatment of complete atrioventricular dissociation. *JAMA* **172**:2006, 1960.
10. Furman S, Robinson G: The use of an intracardiac pacemaker in the correction of total heart block. *Surg Forum* **9**:245, 1958.
11. Furman S, Schwedel JB: An intracardiac pacemaker for Stokes-Adams seizures. *N Engl J Med* **261**:943, 1959.
12. Senning A: Cardiac pacing in retrospect. *Am J Surg* **145**:733, 1983.
13. Glenn WWL, Mauro A, Longo E, et al.: Remote stimulation of the heart by radiofrequency transmission. *N Engl J Med* **261**:948, 1959.
14. Glenn WW, Furman S, Gordon AJ, et al.: Radiofrequency-controlled catheter pacemaker. Clinical application. *N Engl J Med* **275**:137-40, 1966.
15. Hunter SW, Roth NA, Bernardez D, et al.: A bipolar myocardial electrode for complete heart block. *J Lancet* **79**:506, 1959.
16. Stephenson SE, Edwards WH, Jolly PC, et al.: Physiologic P-wave cardiac stimulator. *J Thorac Cardiovasc Surg* **38**:604, 1959.
17. Abrams LD, Hudson WA, Lightwood R: A surgical approach to the management of heart block using an inductive coupled artificial cardiac pacemaker. *Lancet* **1**:372, 1960.

18. Chardack WM, Gage AA, Greatbatch W: A transistorized, self-contained, implantable pacemaker for the long term correction of complete heart block. *Surgery* **48**:643, 1960.

19. Battye CK, Weale FE: The use of the P wave for control of a pacemaker in heart block. *Thorax* **15**:177, 1960.

20. Furman S, Hayes DL, Holmes DR: *A Practice of Cardiac Pacing*. Armonk, New York: Futura, 1993.

21. Griffin JC, ed. *Cardiac Pacing*. Philadelphia: W. B. Saunders, 1992.

22. Ellenbogen KA, ed. *Cardiac Pacing*. Boston: Blackwell Scientific, 1992.

23. Gregoratos G, Cheitlin MD, Conill A, et al.: ACC/AHA Guidelines for Implantation of Cardiac Pacemakers and Antiarrhythmia Devices: Executive Summary--a report of the American College of Cardiology/American Heart Association Task Force on Practice Guidelines (Committee on Pacemaker Implantation). *Circulation* **97**:1325-35, 1998.

24. Batey RL, Sweesy MW, Scala G, Forney RC: Comparison of low rate dual chamber pacing to activity responsive rate variable ventricular pacing. *Pacing Clin Electrophysiol* **13**:646-52, 1990.

25. Hargreaves MR, Channon KM, Cripps TR, et al.: Comparison of dual chamber and ventricular rate responsive pacing in patients over 75 with complete heart block. *Br Heart J* **74**:397-402, 1995.

26. Lau CP, Tai YT, Leung WH, et al.: Rate adaptive pacing in sick sinus syndrome: effects of pacing modes and intrinsic conduction on physiological responses, arrhythmias, symptomatology and quality of life. *Eur Heart J* **15**:1445-55, 1994.

27. Buckingham TA, Janosik DL, Pearson AC: Pacemaker hemodyr.amics: clinical implications. *Prog Cardiovasc Dis* **34**:347-66, 1992.

28. Sulke N, Chambers J, Dritsas A, Sowton E: A randomized double-blind crossover comparison of four rate-responsive pacing modes. *J Am Coll Cardiol* **17**:696-706, 1991.

29. Kruse I, Arnman K, Conradson TB, Ryden L: A comparison of the acute and long-term hemodynamic effects of ventricular inhibited and atrial synchronous ventricular inhibited pacing. *Circulation* **65**:846-55, 1982.

30. Karlof I: Haemodynamic effect of atrail triggered versus fixed rate pacing at rest and during exercise in complete heart block. *Acta Med Scand* **197**:195-206, 1975.

31. Alt E: What is the ideal rate-adaptive sensor for patients with implantable cardioverter-defibrillators: lessons from cardiac pacing. *Am J Cardiol* **83**:17D-23D, 1999.

32. Bernstein AD, Camm AJ, Fletcher RD, et al.: The NASPE/BPEG generic pacemaker code for antibradyarrhythmia and adaptive-rate pacing and antitachyarrhythmia devices. *Pacing Clin Electrophysiol* **10**:794-9, 1987.

33. Bernstein AD, Camm AJ, Fisher JD, et al.: North American Society of Pacing and Electrophysiology policy statement. The NASPE/BPEG defibrillator code. *Pacing Clin Electrophysiol* **16**:1776-80, 1993.

34. Kusumoto FM, Goldschlager N: Cardiac pacing. *N Engl J Med* **334**:89-97, 1996.

35. Hartzler GO, Maloney JD, Curtis JJ, Barnhorst DA: Hemodynamic benefits of atrioventricular sequential pacing after cardiac surgery. *Am J Cardiol* **40**:232-6, 1977.

36. Samet P, Bernstein WH, Nathan DA, Lopez A: Atrial contribution to cardiac output in complete heart block. *Am J Cardiol* **16**:1-10, 1965.

37. Samet P, Castillo C, Bernstein WH: Hemodynamic sequalae of atrial, ventricular, and sequential atrioventricular pacing in cardiac patients. *Am Heart J* **72**:725-9, 1966.

38. Samet P, Castillo C, Bernstein WH: Hemodynamic consequences of atrial and ventricular pacing in subjects with normal hearts. *Am J Cardiol* **18**:522-5, 1966.

39. Reiter MJ, Hindman MC: Hemodynamic effects of acute atrioventricular sequential pacing in patients with left ventricular dysfunction. *Am J Cardiol* **49**:687-92, 1982.

40. Greenberg B, Chatterjee K, Parmley WW, et al.: The influence of left ventricular filling pressure on atrial contribution to cardiac output. *Am Heart J* **98**:742-51, 1979.

41. Parsonnet V, Roelke M: The cephalic vein cutdown versus subclavian puncture for pacemaker/ICD lead implantation. *PACE* **22**:695-697, 1999.

42. Furman S, Hayes DL, Holmes DR. Pacemaker complications. *A Practice of Cardiac Pacing*. Armonk, NY: Futura Publishing Company, 537-569: 1993.

43. Akhtar M, Damato AN, Batsford WP, et al.: A comparative analysis of antegrade and retrograde conduction patterns in man. *Circulation* **52**:766-78, 1975.

44. Levy S, Corbelli JL, Labrunie P, et al.: Retrograde (ventriculoatrial) conduction. *Pacing Clin Electrophysiol* **6**:364-71, 1983.

45. van Mechelen R, Hagemeijer F, de Boer H, Schelling A: Atrioventricular and ventriculo-atrial conduction in patients with symptomatic sinus node dysfunction. *Pacing Clin Electrophysiol* **6**:13-21, 1983.

46. Furman S, Hayes DL, Holmes DR. Basic concepts. *A Practice of Cardiac Pacing*. Armonk, NY: Futura Publishing Company, 29-88: 1993.

CHAPTER 6

IMPLANTABLE CARDIOVERTER-DEFIBRILLATOR THERAPY

The treatment options for patients with ventricular tachyarrhythmias may include antiarrhythmic drugs, catheter ablation, and cardiac surgery (Figure 6-1). Treatment with catheter ablation or antiarrhythmic drugs alone are generally more effective in patients with structurally normal hearts and idiopathic forms of monomorphic ventricular tachycardia. On the other hand, implantable cardioverter-defibrillators have become the first-line treatment for patients with structural heart disease who have ventricular tachyarrhythmias and no reversible cause, such as atherosclerotic coronary artery disease with prior myocardial infarction and primary or secondary cardiomyopathy.

Implantable cardioverter-defibrillators, otherwise known as ICDs, are electronic devices that are used to treat ventricular tachyarrhythmias. The initial ICD systems, first available in the early 1980's, only delivered a high energy electric shock in the event that the heart rate increased above an arbitrarily-programmed, rate. Not only did these early devices lack programmability, they also required an open thoracotomy procedure for implantation of epicardial defibrillation patches. In the intervening years considerable advances have been made in programmability, availability of multiple shock energies for low energy cardioversion or high energy defibrillation, introduction of antitachycardia

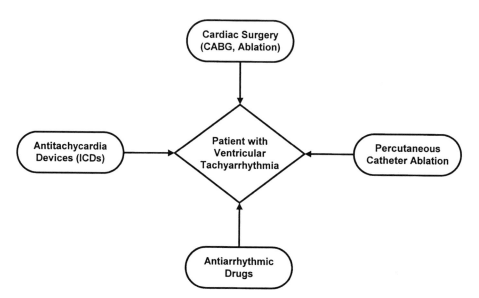

FIGURE 6-1. Spectrum of treatment options for patients with ventricular tachyarrhythmias.

pacing options to allow overdrive pace-termination of ventricular tachycardia, and the development of new transvenous lead systems obviating the need for the open thoracoto-my. Most recently, combination ICD systems have become available that allow atrial and ventricular defibrillation in addition to dual chamber pacing. Because of continuous reduction in size, ease of implantation, increase in programmable options, and dual chamber capabilities, the indications for ICD use have evolved beyond the initial indica-tion of recurrent episodes of sustained ventricular tachycardia or ventricular fibrillation refractory to medical therapy.

In general, the pacing technology available in the latest ICD devices is identical to that found in stand alone pacemaker generators. Therefore, readers is referred to the pre-vious chapter "Principles of Pacemaker Therapy" on page 173 for a complete discussion of the device treatment of bradyarrhythmias. In this section, our focus will be entirely upon the antitachyarrhythmia capabilities of these devices.

6.1 Historical Perspectives

The concept of electrical shocks for termination of ventricular tachyarrhythmias is an old idea, with the first documented report dating from the time of the American Revolution. The initial report comes from Abilgard who shocked a chicken into lifelessness; the bird was revived and returned to normal after repeating the shock [1]. It was not until 1899, however, that Prevost & Batelli discovered that a capacitor discharge could terminate ventricular fibrillation [2,3]. This was confirmed by Wiggers in 1940 [4] and Gurvich and Yuniev in 1946 [5,6]. These latter investigators extended earlier work by finding that damping and prolonging the capacitor discharge by adding a small inductance to the circuit increased its effectiveness [5,6]. In 1956, Zoll used alternating current for tran-sthoracic defibrillation in humans [7]. Finally, in the early 1960s, Lown introduced the damped capacitor discharge to replace alternating current defibrillators [8].

The idea of "automatic defibrillation" is a much more recent concept. Despite the countless detractors of the efficacy and wisdom of this approach [9], the technology was virtually single-handedly developed and promoted by Michel Mirowski at the Sinai Hos-pital of Baltimore and later at the Johns Hopkins University School of Medicine [10-16]. The process was "automatic" because the tachyarrhythmia was detected and electrical therapy administered by a pre-programmed electronic device without the necessity of human intervention. The historical milestones in the development of the ICD are dis-cussed below and outlined in (Table 6-1.)

In the late 1960s while living in Israel, Mirowski conceived of the idea for an im-plantable, automatic defibrillator after the sudden death of his colleague and friend, Dr. Harry Heller. The initial design [10] involved detection of ventricular fibrillation indi-rectly by noting the loss of the phasic right ventricular pressure recording using a right ventricular pressure sensor. The loss of the phasic pressure wave triggered the charging of capacitors to 2500-V from a battery. The capacitors were subsequently discharged be-tween an electrode incorporated into the right ventricular catheter and a subcutaneous patch electrode located over the anterior chest. In early prototypes, the amount of energy delivered ranged from 10–50-J. Likewise, the detection and charging ranged from 15-50 seconds. Mirowski, and his collaborator Morton Mower, subsequently showed that defibrillation in dogs could be accomplished by a single integrated electrode system without the need of any subcutaneous, extrathoracic patch [11]. The finding that ventricular fibrillation could be successfully converted by energies as low as 3-J allowed for the development of a prototype miniaturized device that could deliver 10-J [12]. It was small enough to be implanted because the capacitor size required to administer 10-J shocks was relatively small. The Mirowski group continuously experimented with new sensors, including a right ventricular catheter that detected both R-waves as well as right ventricular mechanical activity using a strain gauge device incorporated into the catheter [12]. Therefore, the early prototype devices were envisioned as transvenous devices which would deliver relatively low energies for termination of ventricular fibrillation (up to 10-J) and which would use the pulsatile right ventricular pressure wave, or contractile activity of the heart, as an indicator of ventricular fibrillation.

TABLE 6-1. Early historical milestones in the development of the implantable-cardioverter defibrillator

Year	Historical Event
1960	Mirowski conception of miniaturized, fully-implantable automatic defibrillator
1969	First experimental prototype (automatic, external)
1969	First successful transvenous defibrillation
1973	Mirowski & Mower partnership with Medrad
1976	First canine implant of fully implantable automatic ICD
1979	Formation of Intec Systems, offshoot of Mirowski/Mower/Medrad
1980	First human implant of automatic ICD at Johns Hopkins Hospital
1982	Addition of cardioverting capabilities
1983	First human implant of Medtronic transvenous cardioverter (not defibrillator, low energy shock only)
1985	FDA approval of Medrad/Intec ICD for human use
1986	Medrad/Intec ICD technology acquired by Cardiac Pacemakers, Inc. (CPI)
1988	First partially programmable ICD (CPI Ventak 1550) approved
1990	Development & implantation of first transvenous devices
1991	First ICD approved with low energy cardioversion option (CPI Ventak 1600)
1993	First tiered-therapy device approved (Medtronic PCD)
1993	FDA approval of transvenous lead systems

By 1972 Mirowski & Mower needed an infusion of capital and engineering expertise to move the prototype to the next level. They first approached Medtronic, Inc., which initially showed some interest, but subsequently declined to develop a commercial model of the device. Subsequently, the Mirowski group joined forces with Stephen Heilman, a physician and engineer, who had founded a company called Medrad in Pittsburgh. Medrad was engaged primarily in the manufacture of power injectors for angiographic procedures; however, the subsidiary that eventually evolved, Intec Systems, fostered the development of a commercial device and guided it through the US Food & Drug Administration approval process.

The first implantable prototype was significantly different from the early breadboard models. Firstly, it was realized that higher energies than 5–15-J would be required to reliably defibrillate patients with diseased hearts. The implantable prototype, therefore, involved direct placement of an epicardial patch on the cardiac apex (requiring a thoracotomy). This was used in conjunction with a transvenous lead positioned in the superior vena cava. Secondly, reliable sensing of ventricular fibrillation is essential. The original sensors that involved the recording of pressure or contractile activity were abandoned and the Medrad/Intec engineers developed a sensing system for ventricular fibrillation based on a probability density function (PDF). The PDF defines ventricular fibrillation as a rhythm that lacks any significant isoelectric periods. Thirdly, more rapid defibrillation was required. The original commercial device allowed detection, capacitor charging, and shocking within 15-20 sec. Finally, ancillary equipment and instrumentation was developed which allowed the non-invasive evaluation of the device and its operational readiness. This new device, small enough to be implanted in humans, was tested and worked remarkably well in a series of five dogs [14].

On February 4, 1980, the first human implant of an ICD (Intec Systems AID device) was performed in a 57-year old woman. The results of implantation in the first three patients were reported by the Mirowski group in a landmark paper [16]. The implanted device weighed 250-gm and occupied a volume of 145-cm³ and was hermetically-sealed in a titanium case. One defibrillating electrode was placed transvenously in the superior vena cava while the other defibrillating electrode was in the shape of a cup that fit over the cardiac apex extrapericardially. The device was able to deliver up to four consecutive shocks before having to recycle by sensing about 35-sec of a normal rhythm. The shock energy was programmed at the factory with the first two shocks at 25-J and the latter two shocks at 30-J.

Subsequent improvements in the original device evolved over the ensuing years, the first of which involved the incorporation of rate determination and R-wave synchronization capabilities into the device to effectively treat ventricular tachycardia as well as ventricular fibrillation. Other improvements have followed including the development of entirely transvenous lead systems, low energy cardioversion, antibradycardia and antitachycardia pacing capabilities, and internal storage of intracardiac tachyarrhythmia electrograms.

6.2   Indications for ICD Therapy

As with any therapeutic approach, physicians should be aware of the indications and contraindications for implantation of these devices (Table 6-2.) The reader should be cautioned that the indications for ICDs are controversial and continuously evolving based upon recent studies [17-20]. Furthermore, while these are general guidelines, each patient's clinical situation is unique and should be evaluated as such.

Patients with severe systemic disease, multi-organ failure, cardiogenic shock, or metastatic cancer or a terminal illness that will lead to their death within months should probably not be considered for an ICD, even if they have one of the indications cited above. This is because their ventricular arrhythmia is unlikely to be the limiting factor in their life expectancy. Patients having ventricular tachycardia or ventricular fibrillation storm also should not receive and ICD at least until the their incessantly recurrent ventricular tachycardia or ventricular fibrillation is better control after the appropriate medical or surgical therapy.

TABLE 6-2. Indications for implantation of cardioverter-defibrillators

Indicated	Uncertain or Possible Indication	Not Indicated
Cardiac arrest due to VF or VT not due to a transient or reversible cause.	Cardiac arrest presumed to be due to VF when EP testing is precluded by other medical conditions.	Syncope of undetermined cause in a patient without inducible sustained ventricular tachyarrhythmias.
Spontaneous sustained VT.	Severe symptoms attributable to sustained VT while awaiting cardiac transplantation.	Incessant VT or VF.
Syncope of undetermined origin with clinically relevant, hemodynamically significant sustained VT or VF induced during EP testing when drug therapy is ineffective, not tolerated, or not preferred.	Familial or inherited conditions with a high risk for life-threatening VT or VF such as long QT syndromes or hypertrophic cardiomyopathy.	VT or VF resulting from arrhythmias amenable to surgical or catheter ablation, including atrial arrhythmias associated with the Wolff-Parkinson-White syndrome, right ventricular outflow tract VT, idiopathic left ventricular VT, or fascicular VT.
NSVT with CAD, prior MI, or LV dysfunction, and inducible sustained VT during electrophysiology testing.	Recurrent syncope of undetermined cause in the presence of LV dysfunction and inducible VT during EP testing when other causes of syncope have been excluded.	Sustained VT or VF due to a transient or reversible cause such as acute ischemia/infarction, drugs, trauma, toxic/metabolic disturbance, or electrolyte imbalance.
		Significant psychiatric illness that may be aggravated by device implantation or may preclude systematic follow-up.
		Terminal illness with life expectancy $\leq$ 6 months.
		Patients with CAD & LV dysfunction undergoing coronary bypass surgery without clinical or inducible VT.
		Patients with NYHA class IV heart failure who are not candidates for heart transplantation.

CAD, coronary artery disease; EP, electrophysiology; LV, left ventricular; MI, myocardial infarction; NSVT, nonsustained ventricular tachycardia; VF, ventricular fibrillation; VT, ventricular tachycardia.
Adapted from [21].

6.3   Basic Concepts of Defibrillation

The basic electrical principles of defibrillation are reviewed in this section. Although fairly complete, excellent discussions are available for further reading from which much of the present discussion is derived [22,23].

6.3.1 CARDIOVERSION VERSUS DEFIBRILLATION

Electrical *cardioversion* is defined as the delivery of a pulse of electrical current synchronized to the occurrence of a ventricular depolarization (QRS complex). In contrast,
electrical *defibrillation* is defined as the delivery of a non-synchronized electrical current
pulse. In this case, the electrical shock is delivered randomly during the cardiac cycle.
Delivery of a synchronized shock is preferred in patients with an organized tachyarrhythmia, such as monomorphic ventricular tachycardia, in order to avoid the potential for
shock-induced ventricular fibrillation. Conversely, for patients with ventricular fibrillation (which typically exhibits QRS complexes of variable amplitude), a high-energy,
non-synchronized shock is preferred in order to avoid any delay in the delivery of the
shock that may occur while the defibrillator sensing circuit searches for a QRS complex.

6.3.2 THEORIES OF DEFIBRILLATION

Despite the fact that electrical defibrillation has been used clinically for over 40 years,
there is still considerable debate regarding the mechanisms by which an electrical current
pulse terminates fibrillation. At the cellular level, the current flows around and through
cardiac cells, thereby altering transmembrane potential gradients. Most investigators
agree that at the macroscopic level defibrillation requires that a certain amount of current
density reach the myocardium (atrial or ventricular). However, currently, two theories
have been proposed to explain the mechanism of defibrillation: 1) critical mass hypothesis and 2) critical voltage gradient or current density hypothesis. These two theories are
not necessarily incompatible and, in fact, may be complimentary.

   Critical mass hypothesis. This theory proposes that maintenance of sustained fibrillation requires involvement of a critical mass myocardium [24]. Successful defibrillation is accomplished only when the electrical shock depolarizes a sufficient amount of
tissue to reduce the fibrillating mass below the critical value. Support for this proposal
has been obtained from computerized mapping studies [25-27].

   Critical voltage gradient or current density hypothesis. This theory proposes that a
critical voltage gradient or current density must be reached throughout the entire myocardium (not just a critical mass) for defibrillation to be successful. If the global gradient
is inadequate, the subthreshold current density will reinitiate fibrillation [28-33]. According to this theory, shocks of insufficient defibrillation magnitude succeed in terminating all activation wavefronts but simultaneously reactivate regions of myocardium
during their vulnerable period. Consequently, new depolarization wavefronts are created
and reinitiate fibrillation. To the observer, the fibrillation is unaffected, but in reality it is
terminated and simultaneously re-induced. One possible mechanism to explain the
defibrillating effects of high, but not low energy shocks, is that higher energy shocks
prolong the refractory period significantly more than low energy shocks [34]. The inability of the depolarization wavefront to propagate across these zones of increased refractoriness may be the mechanism responsible for the termination of fibrillation.

6.3.3 DEFIBRILLATION PARAMETERS

An understanding of the basic electrical principles of defibrillation is helpful in order to appreciate the functioning of implantable defibrillators. At the ultimate level of single cardiac cells, defibrillation is the result of the influence of electrical fields on transmembrane electrical properties. At the macroscopic level of the whole heart, the defibrillation requirements follow an average current law for both monophasic defibrillation shocks and the first phase of biphasic shocks. These requirements also obey the same type of strength-duration curve that succinctly describes the activation of the heart by electrical pacing stimuli (Equation 6-2). As will be discussed below, the *defibrillation strength-duration curve* is defined by the *chronaxie* pulse duration and the *rheobase* current. The rheobase current is the defibrillation threshold (DFT) at a current of infinite duration. The chronaxie duration is that pulse duration which requires a doubling of the rheobase current for successful defibrillation. Whereas the rheobase current is a physiological parameter, another parameter, termed the *effective current*, is an electronic parameter that quantifies defibrillator output. The effective current expresses the ICD output in terms of its defibrillation capability as defined by the strength-duration curve. The effective current is useful since it is a measure of the ICD output that directly relates to the defibrillation requirements of the heart, i.e., the rheobase. *Energy* is the most popular parameter used by electrophysiologists to quantify the defibrillation efficacy of ICDs. However, energy is a meaningful dosage unit for defibrillation only when resistance, capacitance, and pulse duration are all fixed, a condition that is normally satisfied.

Defibrillation strength-duration curve, rheobase, and chronaxie
During cardiac pacing, very low amplitude current pulses (microamperes) are delivered to the heart to initiate action potential propagation thereby triggering cardiac contraction. Similarly, cardiac defibrillation results from the delivery of very high amplitude current pulses (amperes) to terminate atrial or ventricular fibrillation. Just as a current of sufficient magnitude is required to initiate cardiac pacing (the *pacing threshold current*), there is a minimum current required to ensure successful cardiac defibrillation (the *defibrillation threshold current*). Consequently, just as the current threshold for cardiac pacing is defined by a strength-duration curve (Figures 5-16 & 5-17), the current threshold for cardiac defibrillation is also defined by a strength-duration curve (Figure 6-2). The simplest type of current waveform is a rectangular pulse (Figure 6-3). In the case of a true rectangular current pulse, the average current (I_{AVE}) delivered during the pulse is simply the maximum amplitude of the current pulse, because the current amplitude is constant during the extent of the pulse. The *defibrillation rheobase* (I_R) is the current amplitude at an infinitely long pulse duration that results in successful defibrillation at least 99% of the time. The rheobase current is essentially the DFT expressed as a current at a standardized (infinite) pulse width. There can be no current less then the rheobase that will successfully defibrillate the heart, regardless of the duration of the current pulse. Therefore, the rheobase current is the minimally effective current that will defibrillate the heart and it is sometimes also termed the effective current, or I_{EFF} [35]. The *defibrillation chronaxie* is the shortest pulse duration that results in successful defibrillation at

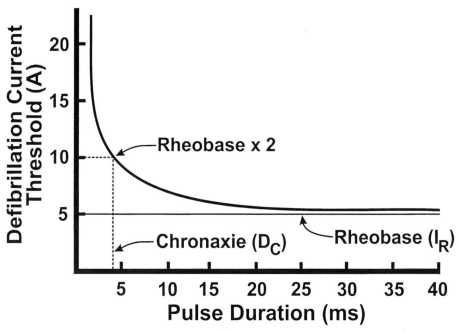

FIGURE 6-2. Example of defibrillation strength-duration curve. The rheobase current (I_R) is the average current required for defibrillation at an infinitely long pulse duration. At the chronaxie pulse duration (D_C) the successful defibrillation current is twice I_R. See text for additional discussion. Adapted from [36].

twice the defibrillation rheobase current. Experimental studies suggest that the defibrillation chronaxie in humans is approximately 2–4-msec [36]. The typical range for the defibrillation rheobase in humans is 2.3–5.6 A [36]. As seen in Figure 6-3, for rectangular current pulses, the lowest energy requirement occurs when the duration equals the chronaxie time. This is analogous to the reduced energy during cardiac pacing with the use of shorter duration, higher current pulses. Determining the minimum defibrillation current at very long pulse duration (e.g. 40-msec) closely approximates the rheobase current. Then, the minimal pulse duration that results in successful defibrillation can be determined at twice the rheobase, yielding the chronaxie pulse duration.

As seen in Figure 6-3, the rheobase current is related to an intrinsic parameter of the defibrillation pulse, termed the *average current*. From experimental and theoretical studies, a simple mathematical relationship has been derived that describes the relationship between the average current (I_{AVE}) of a successful defibrillation pulse and the rheobase current (I_R):

$$I_R = \frac{I_{AVE}}{1 + \dfrac{D_C}{D}} \qquad \text{(Eq 4)}$$

where D is the pulse duration of the effective rectangular pulse and D_C is the chronaxie pulse duration. From this equation it is clear that the rheobase current is simply the aver-

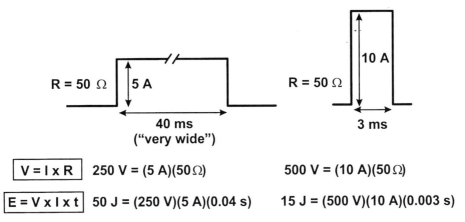

FIGURE 6-3.   Effect of duration current pulse on the energy necessary for defibrillation using a rectangular current pulse. Chronaxie time is 3-msec, and the impedance is fixed at 50-W. Using very long pulse durations (left side), the average current required for defibrillation (the rheobase) is 5-A. At the chronaxie pulse duration, the average current required for defibrillation is 10-A (right side). For rectangular current pulses, the lowest energy requirement occurs when the pulse duration equals the chronaxie time. See test for additional discussion.

age current divided by a duration correction factor. The average current of a pulse is the best measure of its effectiveness when compared to other pulses of the same width regardless of shape [37,38].

The maximum rheobase current that a given pulse can satisfy is referred to as the *effective current*, I_{EFF}. While the rheobase is a physiological parameter that quantifies the heart's defibrillation requirements, I_{EFF} is an electronic parameter that quantifies the output of the defibrillator. However, both parameters are based upon the average current:

$$I_{EFF} = \frac{\text{Average Current}}{\text{Duration Correction}} = \frac{I_{AVE}}{1 + \dfrac{D_C}{D}} \tag{Eq 5}$$

The effective current of a pulse simply measures its average current corrected for the duration. Effective current is useful because it is a measure of the ICD output that directly relates to the defibrillation requirements of the heart, i.e., the rheobase.

While simpler theoretically, the use of rectangular current pulses in ICD pulse generators is not practical because it would require a large power supply. Instead ICD devices employ the *capacitive discharge waveform* (Figure 6-4). While not a rectangular waveform, the strength-duration curve nevertheless still applies in so far as capacitive pulses of longer duration require a lower average current for successful defibrillation than pulse durations near the chronaxie. ICD devices function by the charging of a capacitor using current from a battery, and then discharging the charge from the capacitor into the patient's heart using the lead system. During discharge, the exponentially-decaying current flows through a series resistance that includes the lead system and the cardiac and non-cardiac tissues lying between the negative and positive poles of the lead conductors. In general, the peak voltage produced by maximum charging of the capaci-

FIGURE 6-4. Typical monophasic capacitive discharge waveform (truncated exponential). Time course of the voltage decay follows an exponential curve that is truncated after a pre-specified time period (pulse duration) or upon attainment of a capacitor voltage that yields the desired tilt. Represented here is a discharge of a 140-μF capacitor into a 50-Ω impedance. The initial voltage is 750-V and with a 65% tilt the voltage would be truncated at 263-msec after a duration of approximately 7-msec. The calculated average current is 9.75-A and the calculated effective current is 7.0-A. This means that this pulse will defibrillate any patient with a rheobase threshold ≤ 7.0-A. Adapted from [36].

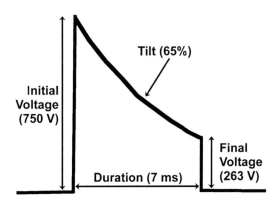

tors is 700–800-V. In modern ICDs, lower current shocks can be administered by charging the capacitor to lower voltages. This *charge voltage* is also referred to as the *initial voltage* or *leading edge voltage*. Typically, the capacitor is discharged over an arbitrary period of time (the pulse duration) after which the terminal portion of the decaying current pulse is truncated. The capacitor voltage at the moment of truncation is termed the *final* or *trailing edge* voltage. The tilt, or overall rate of decay of the current pulse can be calculated by knowing the initial and final capacitor voltages:

$$Tilt = \frac{V_i - V_f}{V_i} \qquad \text{(Eq 6)}$$

The average current resulting from a capacitive discharge can be calculated as:

$$I_{AVE} = \frac{C \cdot (V_i - V_f)}{D} \qquad \text{(Eq 7)}$$

where V_i is the initial (leading edge) voltage and V_f is the final (trailing edge) voltage. Therefore, by substitution of Equation 6 into Equation 7 the average current is:

$$I_{AVE} = \frac{C \cdot V_i \cdot Tilt}{D} \qquad \text{(Eq 8)}$$

There is a logarithmic relationship between tilt, duration, and resistance:

$$Tilt = 1 - e^{(-D)/(RC)} \qquad \text{(Eq 9)}$$

or, solving for pulse duration, it becomes:

$$D = -R \cdot C \cdot \log_e(1 - Tilt) \qquad \text{(Eq 10)}$$

(where tilt is expressed as a ratio and not as a percentage). Although Equation 10 seems to imply that increasing the tilt (steeper rate of decay of current pulse) increases the average current, in reality the average current actually decreases with increasing tilt because the duration increases faster as a function of tilt. Therefore, assuming capacitance is fixed, the duration required to achieve a desired tilt can be determined once the resistance of the defibrillation circuit is measured (usually by delivering a test shock). This calculated duration basically represents the time required for the capacitor voltage to decline from its initial value to the value required to produce the desired tilt percentage. The average current produced by a capacitive discharge pulse decreases rapidly as the capacitor voltage decreases. Therefore, extending the pulse duration to "deliver more energy" is usually of limited benefit with capacitive discharge shocks.

By combining Equation 5 and Equation 8 and rearranging, the effective current, I_{EFF}, can be expressed as a function of the leading edge voltage and pulse duration:

$$I_{\text{EFF}} = \frac{C \cdot V \cdot Tilt}{D + D_C} \qquad \text{(Eq 11)}$$

Substituting Equation 9 for tilt yields (for a fixed pulse duration):

$$I_{EFF} = \frac{C \cdot V \cdot (1 - e^{(-D)/(RC)})}{D + D_C} \qquad \text{(Eq 12)}$$

Substituting Equation 10 for a tilt-based pulse gives:

$$I_{EFF} = \frac{C \cdot V_i \cdot Tilt}{[-R \cdot C \cdot \log_e(1 - Tilt)] + D_C} \qquad \text{(Eq 13)}$$

Equation 12 can be used to calculate the effective current over a range of pulse durations. This provides another way to show what pulse duration yields the most effective current. As can be seen (Figure 6-5), the maximum effective current is achieved at a pulse width that is twice the chronaxie time. From this figure, note that the effective current rises rapidly for the first 3-msec of pulse duration. A large majority (>90%) of the effective current is attained within the first 3-msec of the pulse. Said differently, there is little additional benefit delivered from energy delivered after the chronaxie duration. The effective current declines after a duration of 6-msec. Consequently, current delivered after the first 6-msec is not only inefficient, it is, in fact, counterproductive. Therefore, optimal truncation of the exponentially-decaying capacitive waveform is mandatory for delivery of maximal effective current and successful defibrillation.

If at maximum output one ICD can deliver an effective current of 12-A and another ICD can deliver an effective current of 16-A, one can confidently say that the second device has a higher defibrillation capability than the first (assuming both devices deliver either monophasic or biphasic pulses), regardless of the voltage, capacitance value, and pulse duration. The same cannot be said for a simplistic parameter such as energy.

The first phase of a biphasic pulse (Figure 6-6) appears to behave similar to a monophasic shock. It follows the same hyperbolic strength-duration relationship as a monophasic shock [39,40]. This does not mean that the second phase is irrelevant because this phase appears to significantly reduce the electrical requirements of the first phase [41]. Clinical studies have shown a significant reduction in the DFT by using bi-

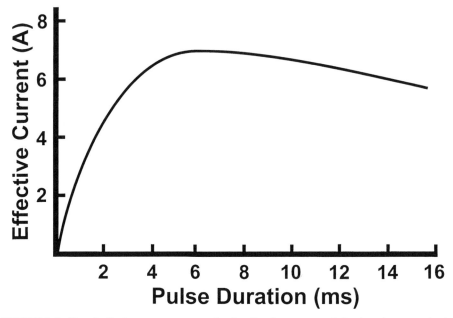

FIGURE 6-5. Plot of effective current versus pulse duration for a exponentially-decaying monophasic shock. Data shown assume a 140-µF capacitor charged to 750-V with a chronaxie time of 3-msec and an electrode resistance of 50-Ω. Note that the maximum effective current results using a pulse duration of 6-msec, which is twice the chronaxie pulse duration. Despite the fact that all points on the curve represent shocks with the same stored energy (39.4-J), there is nevertheless a significant range of defibrillation capability as measured by the effective current, because of varying pulse durations. Not all joules are created equal. Thus the DFT, as measured by energy, will be minimized with the shock duration corresponding to the apex of the curve. Adapted from [36].

phasic waveforms with each phase duration near the chronaxie [42,43]. A shock with the first phase at 3.5-msec (42% tilt) results in delivered energy thresholds that are half that observed with biphasic pulses using a conventional first phase pulse duration of 7-msec and 65% tilt. For calculations of average or effective current, the first phase must be used.

Energy as a parameter
Although energy, expressed in joules, is widely used among clinical electrophysiologists to quantify a defibrillation shock, in reality, energy is not directly linked to the defibrillation requirements of the heart. For example, consider the situation shown in Figure 6-7. Although the energy of the pulse (45-J) is well above the typical defibrillation energy threshold seen in patients, in reality this pulse has virtually no chance of successfully terminating ventricular fibrillation. This is because the average current of 0.3-A is well below the typical rheobase current (1–10-A). Thus the energy of the pulse does not predict its ability to defibrillate the heart, primarily because the energy of the pulse does not necessarily correlate with the average current of the pulse.

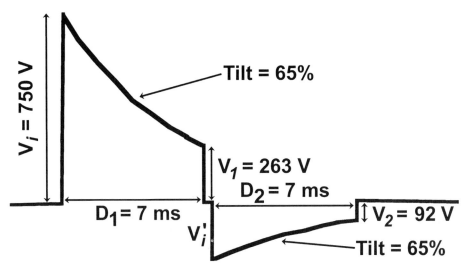

FIGURE 6-6. Example of a biphasic capacitive discharge waveform using a constant tilt of 65% in both the positive and negative phases. In the implementation illustrated here, the leading edge (initial) voltage of the second phase (V_i') is identical in absolute value to the trailing edge (final) voltage of the first phase (V_1). A single capacitor is used and the polarity of the capacitor discharge current is electronically inverted to produce the second phase. Not all manufacturers implement the biphasic pulse as shown here. Adapted from [36].

FIGURE 6-7. Energy is not necessarily a reliable measure of the defibrillation requirements of the heart. In this example, even though the energy is 45 J – well above the typical energy-based DFT – this rectangular shock has no chance of successfully terminating ventricular fibrillation because of the extremely low average current of 0.3 A. Typically, average currents of 1-10 A are required for successful defibrillation. It is only because of the extremely long pulse duration (10 sec) that this low average current results in such a high energy. This pulse duration is more than an order of magnitude greater than the typical pulse duration used in ICD devices.

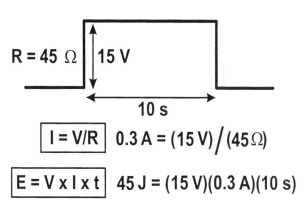

Nevertheless, energy is a popular parameter to use to describe defibrillation energy requirements at least partly because it is an easy parameter to measure. The *stored energy* (in joules) of a capacitive discharge is simply:

$$E_{Stored} = 0.5 \cdot C \cdot V_i^2 \qquad \text{(Eq 14)}$$

where C is the capacitance in farads and V_i is the initial or leading edge voltage.

Another term often used is "delivered energy". Unfortunately, there is no consistent definition of "delivered energy". Depending upon where it is measured, the delivered energy will vary dramatically. The highest delivered energy will be measured at the capacitor and can be calculated based upon the initial and final capacitor voltage as seen in Equation 15

$$E_{\text{Delivered}} = 0.5 \cdot C \cdot (V_i^2 - V_f^2) \qquad \text{(Eq 15)}$$

where, V_f is the final of trailing edge voltage. In general, the delivered energy (as measured at the capacitor) of an ICD shock is approximately 90% of the stored energy. However, if the delivered energy is measured at the lead set-screws in the connector block, the lead tips in the heart, or the actual energy delivered into the tissue, it will be less. While the delivered energy measured at the capacitor is generally 90% or more of the stored energy, the energy actually delivered "into the heart tissue" distal to the electrode tip may be only 10% of stored energy [44]. Thus, the use of energy, especially "delivered energy" is a very poor comparative indicator of defibrillation requirements.

The specific problems with the use of energy as a defibrillation parameter is that energy depends upon resistance, pulse width, and capacitance. Figure 6-8 illustrates the effect of resistance on the defibrillation energy threshold using a hypothetical rectangular pulse wave (more complicated calculations using a capacitive discharge are, however, qualitatively similar). Note that doubling the resistance from 50- to 100-Ω results in an increase in the required energy for defibrillation from 15-J to 30-J, while a fourfold increase in the pulse duration above the chronaxie produces a greater than 50% increase in the defibrillation energy.

Capacitance can also significantly affect the defibrillation energy threshold. Capacitors with lower capacitance deliver their bolus of charge faster than capacitors with higher capacitance. The fundamental reason for this stems from the fact that capacitors must discharge through a series resistance. The drainage of the charge from the capacitor through the series resistance is determined by the *time constant* of the circuit:

$$\tau = R \cdot C \qquad \text{(Eq 16)}$$

where τ is in μs when R is expressed in Ω and C in μF. The time constant of such an "RC circuit" represents the time required to drain 37% of the charge stored on the capacitor through the resistor. Assuming resistance is constant, the time constant increases as the capacitance increases. For example, if R = 50-Ω and C = 140-μF, τ = 7000-μs or 7-msec. On the other hand, if C = 180-Ω, τ would increase to 9-msec, assuming R remains constant at 50-Ω. Therefore, everything else being equal, an ICD with a higher capacitance should deliver a lower average current (I_{AVE}) and require a longer pulse duration to deliver the same effective current (I_{EFF}) than an identical system with a lower capacitance. This prediction is indeed borne out as seen in Table 6-3. The data in this table are based upon two ICD systems, one with capacitance of 120-μF and a second with capacitance of 180-μF, using the equations previously presented in this section. In each case, the charging voltage is 750-V, resistance is 50-Ω, chronaxie is 3-msec, and tilt is 65%. A higher capacitance will result in a higher stored energy DFT but will require a longer

A. Energy Dependence Upon Resistance

$I_R = 5\ A$
$D = D_C = 3\ ms$
$I_{AVE} = I_R(1 + D_C/D) = (5\ A)(1 + 3/3) = 10\ A$

$R = 50\ \Omega$
$V = I \times R = (10\ A)(50\ \Omega) = 500\ V$
$E = V \times I \times t = (500\ V)(10\ A)(0.003\ sec) = \boxed{15\ J}$

$R = 100\ \Omega$
$V = I \times R = (10\ A)(100\ \Omega) = 1000\ V$
$E = V \times I \times t = (1000\ V)(10\ A)(0.003\ sec) = \boxed{30\ J}$

B. Energy Dependence Upon Pulse Duration

$I_R = 3\ A$
$R = 50\ \Omega$
$D_C = 3\ ms$

$D = 3\ ms$
$I_{AVE} = I_R(1 + D_C/D) = (3\ A)(1 + 3/3) = 6\ A$
$V = I \times R = (6\ A)(50\ \Omega) = 300\ V$
$E = V \times I \times t = (300\ V)(6\ A)(0.003\ sec) = \boxed{5.4\ J}$

$D = 12\ ms$
$I_{AVE} = I_R(1 + D_C/D) = (3\ A)(1 + 3/12) = 3.75\ A$
$V = I \times R = (3.75\ A)(50\ \Omega) = 187.5\ V$
$E = V \times I \times t = 187.5\ V \times 3.75\ A \times 0.012\ sec = \boxed{8.4\ J}$

FIGURE 6-8. Example calculations illustrating the effects of resistance (panel A) and pulse duration (panel B) on energy. Unlike the situation in ICDs that utilize the truncated exponential waveform, for simplicity purposes these calculations are based upon a rectangular pulse wave. In the situation depicted in panel A, a rheobase current (I_R) of 5 A, a chronaxie (D_C) time and pulse duration (D) of 3-msec, yielding an average current (I_{AVE}) of 10-A. Note that increasing the resistance (R) from 50-Ω to 100-Ω results in a doubling of the defibrillation energy (E) threshold from 15-J to 30-J. This increase primarily results from a doubling of the required charging voltage (V) from 500-V to 1000-V. Currently available ICDs can only charge the capacitor to approximately 750-V. In situation depicted in panel B, increasing the pulse duration from the chronaxie duration of 3-msec to 12-msec results in a 56% increase in the defibrillation energy threshold from 5.4-J to 8.4-J. See text for additional discussion.

pulse duration to deliver the required effective current for defibrillation success. Everything else being equal, the larger capacitor will have an energy threshold approximately 20% greater than the device with the smaller capacitor. Consequently, this larger capacitance will require a larger physical volume for the same defibrillation capability. The larger stored energy requirement also reduces the number of shocks that an ICD can deliver. Advances in capacitor technology have allowed the design of smaller ICDs using significantly smaller capacitors (e.g., 90-μF) with improved longevity.

TABLE 6-3. Effect of capacitance on stored energy defibrillation threshold

Capacitance	Pulse Duration	Charging Voltage	Stored Energy	Average Current	Effective Current
120 μF	6. 3-msec	750-V	33.8-J	9.29-A	6.29-A
180 μF	9.4-msec	669-V	40.3-J	8.28-A	6.29-A

Adapted from [36].

Relationship between pulse duration and tilt

Ideally, during delivery of a defibrillation shock, the shock duration must be sufficiently long to discharge the capacitor while keeping the pulse duration near the chronaxie time. As seen in Figure 6-4, tilt and pulse duration are inextricably linked. Assuming resistance and capacitance are constant, an increase (or decrease) in pulse duration will necessarily result in an increase (or decrease) in tilt. Assuming capacitance is a constant, it can be seen from Equations 9 and 10 that tilt will tend to increase with increases in pulse duration but will decrease with increases in resistance. On the other hand, pulse duration will tend to increase with increases in resistance but will decrease with decreases in resistance. Because capacitance is a constant in ICD devices, resistance is the most important variable affecting tilt and pulse duration. If tilt is specified as constant, an increase in resistance will necessarily lead to increase in pulse duration (Figure 6-9). If pulse duration is specified as constant, an increase in resistance will necessarily cause a decrease in tilt. Device manufacturers may choose to specify the duration of a shock by fixing the time of the pulse (e.g., 6-msec) or the tilt (e.g., 65%). Each of these specifications will result in a different response to changes in resistance.

If a pure fixed pulse duration specification is implemented, the tilt will vary depending upon the resistance as seen in Figure 6-9. For example, if the pulse duration is fixed at 7.0-msec, the calculated tilt (Equation 9) would be 83%, at a resistance of 40-Ω (assuming a capacitance of 100-μF). If, however, the resistance increases to 150-Ω, this same pulse duration will yield a tilt of 37%. Assuming this capacitor is charged to 750-V in both cases, by Equation 15 the delivered energy will be 27.3-J when the tilt is 83% and 17.0-J when the tilt is 37%. From Equation 13, when the impedance is 40 Ω and the tilt is 83%, the effective current, I_{EFF}, is 6.2-A, while I_{EFF} is 2.8-A when the resistance is

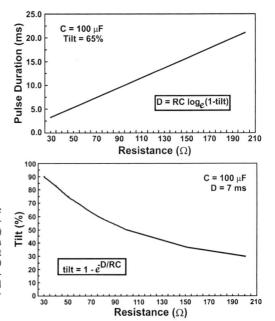

FIGURE 6-9. Relationship between resistance and pulse duration (fixed tilt = 65%) and resistance and tilt (fixed pulse duration = 7-msec) for a monophasic capacitive discharge. Data illustrated for a range of clinically relevant resistances. Capacitance is assumed to be 100 μF. Pulse duration plot calculated using Equation 10 (upper panel) and tilt plot constructed using Equation 9 (lower panel). See text for additional discussion.

150-Ω and the tilt is 37%.Consequently, with a fixed pulse width device, a dramatic increase in impedance significantly reduces the tilt and markedly reduces the effective current and the delivered energy, even though the stored energy is identical at 28.1-J (Equation 14). If I_{EFF} becomes less than the rheobase current, I_R, the shock will fail to defibrillate the patient. Therefore, as resistance increases, less current is delivered as tilt decreases because of the fixed pulse width. As typically implemented, fixed pulse duration devices allow the electrophysiologist to program the pulse width based upon the measured impedance (obtained from a test shock). Usually programming the pulse duration is only required at the time of initial implantation; however, this capability may prove useful in borderline cases where modest increases in resistance may compromise defibrillation efficacy.

Devices manufactured using a fixed tilt specification guarantee that a certain fixed amount of energy is delivered because the capacitor is always drained to a final fixed voltage level (see above discussion related to Equation 15). Fixed tilt devices have been termed "constant energy" devices, because the delivered energy – as measured at the capacitor – is constant regardless of the impedance (within a certain wide range of resistance values). Because pulse duration is proportional solely to resistance (when tilt and capacitance are fixed), fixed tilt devices may result in very long pulse durations with marked increases in resistance. As a consequence, the I_{EFF} may drop well below the minimum current required for successful defibrillation, I_R. For example, as seen from Figure 6-9, with a fixed tilt of 65% and a capacitance of 100-μF, the pulse duration is 4.2-msec when the resistance is 40-Ω, but the pulse width significantly increases to 15.7-msec when impedance increases to 150-Ω. Using Equations 12 or 13, this increase in pulse duration results in a dramatic decrease in I_{EFF} from 5.8-A to 2.5-A, even though the stored energy is identical at 28.1-J (Equation 14). If the rheobase current, I_R, is 4.0 A, this prolonged shock would fail to defibrillate the patient. Therefore, the problem with the fixed tilt approach is that the increase in pulse duration in response to an extreme increase in resistance (e.g., > 50-Ω) may compromise the safety margin for defibrillation. During a typical implantation procedure, the usual impedance is 30–50-Ω. An impedance of 150-Ω would be unusual and should suggest a partial or complete disruption of a lead conductor. With the impedance levels typically encountered in most clinical situations, "constant energy" devices have been widely used and have a proven track record of success.

6.4   Components of ICD Systems

An ICS is best viewed as a system consisting of a number of components as summarized in Table 6-4. These components are described in more detail below.

TABLE 6-4. Components of an ICD system

Pulse generator
High energy defibrillation
Low energy cardioversion
Anti-tachycardia pacing
Anti-bradycardia pacing
Event (tachyarrhythmias, electrograms, therapy history, etc.) recording and storage
Lead(s)
Atrial and ventricular sensing, pacing, and cardioversion/defibrillation
Programmer
Pacing system analyzer (PSA)*
External cardioverter-defibrillator (ECD)**

*PSA may be a standalone device or may be incorporated into the programmer. ** In most cases, defibrillation threshold testing is generally performed using the ICD generator itself, making a standalone ECD unnecessary.

6.4.1 EQUIPMENT

Pulse generators

The first ICDs implanted in the early 1980s weighed over 290 gm and had a volume greater than 160 cm³. Almost exclusively, those early devices required implantation in a subcutaneous or subrectus abdominal pocket. As with pacemakers, ICD size has decreased dramatically, allowing routine implantation in the pectoral region. Devices having a volume < 30 cm³ are on the horizon.

The ICD pulse generator consists of a number of major components (Figure 6-10) [45], including a sensing and amplification circuit, pacing output circuit, high voltage

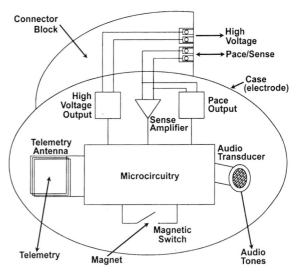

FIGURE 6-10. Major components and interfaces of an ICD pulse generator. See text for additional discussion. Adapted from [45].

output circuit, telemetry interface circuit, audio transducer, magnet-sensitive switch, an epoxy connector block ("header") that provides the entry ports for the lead pins, and a lightweight titanium ICD housing ("can") that also may function as an electrode and contribute to one of the pathways for the defibrillation current. The block diagram in Figure 6-11 summarizes the major internal components of an ICD pulse generator and are discussed in further detail below.

The goal of the amplification and sensing circuit, and its associated amplification circuit, is to assure R-wave detection. In general, two varieties of amplifier circuits have been employed: *automatic gain control* or *automatic threshold control*. Sensing is required for both tachycardia and bradycardia detection. Interpretation of tachycardia or

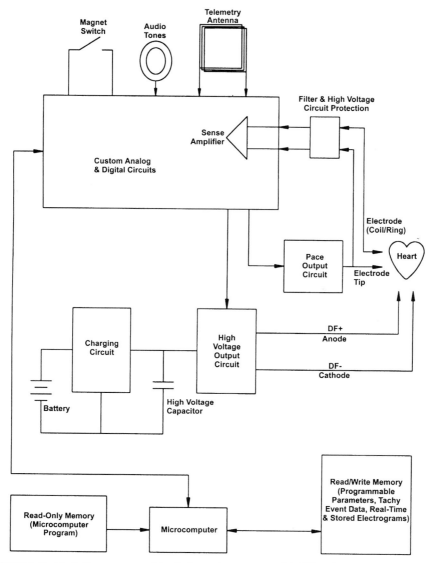

FIGURE 6-11. Block diagram summarizing the internal components of the ICD pulse generator. See text for additional discussion. Adapted from [45].

bradycardia rate data (i.e., detection) may be performed by the custom digital circuitry or the microcomputer software.

The high voltage output circuit includes the capacitor charging circuit, the high voltage storage capacitors, and the high voltage output switches. After the detection of a tachyarrhythmia (or by a direct command from the programmer), the microcomputer program (or custom digital circuitry) initiates charging the capacitor, in essence converting the low voltage in the battery or batteries (3 – 6-V) into a much larger voltage stored across the capacitor plates (approximately 750-V for maximum output). Maximum capacitor charging generally requires 5 – 10-sec. After completion of capacitor charge sequence, computer logic causes delivery of the charge bolus into the lead system, usually after confirmation establishes that detection rate criteria are still fulfilled.

The pacing output circuit, under the guidance of the microcomputer program and custom digital circuitry, delivers antitachycardia and antibradycardia pacing therapy in accordance with the programmed criteria.

Many ICD pulse generators incorporate an audio transducer allowing the generation and broadcast of a variety of audible tones. The type, quality, and cadence of the transmitted tones that are emitted provide a programmable diagnostic capability useful for patient safety or announce the development of potential device malfunctions. For example, battery depletion to level of the elective replacement time may be indicated by a series of characteristic beep tones. Manufacturers vary in the use of the audio transducer, but it has been widely in some devices as a quick means to assess sensing function and to inactivate and reactivate the device (see below).

The *magnetic reed switch* is a thin magnetic strip (resembling the reed from a woodwind musical instrument) that is sealed inside a slender glass cylinder along with another conducting strip. A sufficiently strong magnetic field will cause the strips to come in contact, thereby closing an electrical circuit. In addition to its role in ensuring the integrity of data transmission in some devices, closing the circuit with the switch also may inhibit arrhythmia detection (and therefore prevent the delivering of therapy), completely inactivate the device, or trigger the emission of audible tones. Tachycardia detection and therapy are suspended (but not programmed to inactive) in all currently available devices by application of the magnet over the pulse generator. Removal of the magnetic field immediately restores the normal (previously programmed) device function. Generally, antibradycardia pacing therapy is not inhibited by magnet application. Devices manufactured by Guidant/CPI, Inc. have traditionally incorporated the capability to program "off" the tachyarrhythmia detection and therapies, and not merely suspend this functions during the duration of magnet application. With these devices, application of the magnet causes the emission of audible beeping tones synchronous with intrinsic R-wave detection by the device. After applying the magnet continuously for 30-sec, the intermittent beeping tone changes to a continuous tone, indicates inactivation of tachyarrhythmia detection and therapies. At this point, removal of the magnetic field *will not* restore normal device function, i.e., arrhythmia detection remains "turned-off". After reapplication of the magnet, the continuous audible tone is emitted for 30-sec, after which normal device detection and normal device function is restored. This resumption of previously programmed function is heralded by the reappearance of the intermittent beeping tones that are emitted synchronous with sensed R-wave activity. Even in the Guidant/

CPI line of devices, this unique magnet operation can be programmed "off", thereby permitting these devices to exhibit magnet function similar to devices from other manufacturers.

Powering all the detection, therapy, and diagnostic, and housekeeping functions of the ICD is the *battery*. The demands upon an ICD battery are considerable, particularly when compared to those required of a pacemaker battery. The ICD battery not only must be capable of operating for long periods of time at low current drains for monitoring/ housekeeping functions, but in addition it must be able to abruptly deliver a high current pulse for capacitor charging if the patient develops a ventricular tachyarrhythmia. The power requirements of the ICD system typically include delivery of shocks, pacing (antibradycardia, antitachycardia), and a continuous current for background monitoring/ housekeeping functions (Table 6-5.)

TABLE 6-5. Example of power requirements for an ICD assuming worst case requirements.

Function	Charge Requirements	Assumptions
5 years background monitoring	0.43 A-h	10 µA drainage
5 years pacing (single chamber)	0.30 A-h	100% pacing
200 shocks	0.37 A-h	75% efficiency
Total	1.10 A-h	

A-h, ampere-hours (measure of total charge required). Adapted from [46].

Since 1992, ICDs have been powered by lithium/silver vanadium oxide (LiSVO) cells. The anode consists of pure lithium metal, while the cathode material is silver vanadium oxide. The unique chemical properties of the LiSVO cell result in a discharge curve that displays plateaus at various voltages and a general gradual decline in the voltage over time (Figure 6-12). The *beginning-of-life (BOL)* and *end-of-life (EOL)* voltages for the ICD battery are determined by the chemical constituents and the discharge curve. Significantly, the decline in voltage is not caused by an increase in internal cell resistance and, therefore, the cell's ability to rapidly deliver current to charge the capacitors (see below) is retained throughout the usable battery life. The typical unloaded cell voltage at BOL is approximately 3.2 – 3.3-V. An unloaded (or *open-circuit*) voltage of 2.5-V (manufacturer range 2.38 – 2.55-V) is the typical value for the *elective replacement indicator (ERI)*. However, because some devices contain two batteries in series, the ERI voltage is approximately twice the single battery level (5.0-V). A loaded (or *charging*) voltage of approximately 1.5-V, or an unloaded voltage of approximately 2.3 – 2.4-V, is termed end-of service or end-of life. Establishing the battery ERI involves an estimate of the remaining time before the pulse voltage declines below a level that can achieve defibrillation. Some manufacturers use a combination of parameters including loaded or unloaded voltage and the capacitor charge time to determine when ERI has been reached. The ERI quoted by the manufacturer may include a safety margin of approximately three months before EOL is reached (assuming no additional shocks).

Some ICD designs use dual battery sources: lithium/silver vanadium oxide for defibrillation shocks and lithium iodide for pace/sense and monitoring functions. While

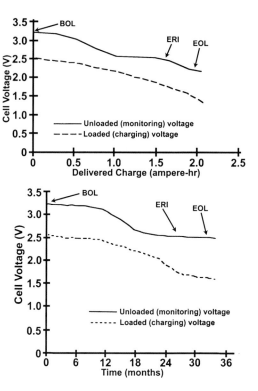

FIGURE 6-12. Discharge behavior of a lithium/silver vanadium oxide cell. Top panel illustrates a cumulative delivered charge test (performed over one-year) in a simulated ICD application that includes an exaggerated steady monitoring (background) current (consistent with 100% pacing at 15-V at a pulse width of 1-ms) and a defibrillation regimen of four-shocks delivered every two months. The cell is subjected to an extreme load to shorten the cell life to one-year. The voltage is plotted versus the cumulative charge delivered in ampere-hours. Bottom panel shows life test discharge results for a ICD battery in a simulated ICD application that includes the steady low-level monitoring current and monthly four-shock defibrillation regimens. Unloaded (monitoring) voltage refers to the voltage measured before capacitor charging, while the loaded voltage is the minimum voltage measured after the fourth charge. Adapted from [46].

the LiSVO cell offers high current for rapid capacitor charging, it only has one-half of the energy density of the standard lithium iodide cell used in pacemakers. Therefore, the use of this dual battery technology allows the energy dense lithium iodide cell to supply the heavy power requirements needed for monitoring, pacing, and sensing functions, reserving the LiSVO battery for the high voltage and current therapy functions.

While the battery is the power source for the entire ICD, the capacitor functions as a temporary energy storage component. Under control of the microprocessor, the high voltage charging circuit charges the capacitor. In fact the ICD must have two high power circuits in order to function. A charging circuit constructed with a specially designed power transformer, termed a "flyback" transformer, is used to convert the low voltage in the ICD battery (typically 3 – 6-V) to the much higher voltage (generally 750-V) required for defibrillation. After this high voltage is concentrated in the capacitor, a second high output switching circuit then transfers the energy to the heart. During the charging process, a load of charge is quickly stored in the capacitor within a few *seconds*; during the discharging process, however, this same load of charge must be delivered into the heart within only a few *milliseconds*. Whereas an ICD capacitor is charged to 750-V typically with current of 10-mA, it may be have to deliver a current pulse of over 30-A. The commonly used analogy is of a bucket that is slowly filled with water using a garden hose only to be quickly dumped out. The volume of water in the bucket corresponds to the total charge stored in the capacitor, while the volume of water moved per second represents the current.

Originally, capacitors used in ICDs were large and exclusively cylindrical in shape, but advances in technology have reduced their size, flattened their profile, and increased their charge-storing capacity ("energy density"), allowing for the production of smaller and thinner devices. ICDs have traditionally used aluminum-based electrolytic capacitors. These components are constructed using a permanent dielectric formed on the surface of a metal electrode; the other electrode is the (aluminum) electrolyte. The chief advantage of electrolytic capacitors is that they offer a very high capacitance and achieve a high energy density using only moderate voltages (e.g. 300 – 400-V). The major disadvantages of the aluminum electrolytic capacitor is that it degrades when not used. This degradation means that a considerably greater energy is required to charge the capacitor for the first time after a period of storage compared with the energy required immediately following a charge/discharge cycle. This phenomenon manifests itself as a prolongation of the charge time after a prolonged period of quiescence. In order to limit this degradation and minimize the charge time under clinical conditions, the capacitor is "reformed" on a regular schedule, generally every 3 – 4-months. In the past, this had to be done manually using the programmer; however, currently all devices perform this function automatically under programmable control. Basically, during the reforming process the capacitor is repaired electrochemically by performing a charge/discharge cycle (without shocking the patient). In so doing the behavior of the capacitor returns to normal. Although the automatic reforming process is still a default operation performed by most pulse generators, technological advances in capacitor design has meant that currently used capacitors actually require little reforming. In fact, because ICD batteries require periodic usage to maintain a low internal impedance (required to permit very rapid charging of the capacitor), the schedules for capacitor reforming recommended by the manufacturers in part represent these battery requirements.

Leads

The *lead* is that portion of the implanted device that transmits electrical impulses between the pulse generator and the heart. The *electrode* is the conductive portion of the lead and is designed to provide sensing, pacing, or defibrillation functions. There are three functional requirements for a defibrillation lead system: 1) defibrillation, 2) pacing, and 3) sensing. Leads permit the electrophysiologist to position the electrodes in an endocardial, intravascular, or extrathoracic location to perform these functions. Historically, the first ICD systems utilized epicardial patches that required a thoracotomy procedure for placement. For these early systems, sensing was performed using a two closely-spaced epicardial screw-in leads. However, with the development of a purely transvenous defibrillation system, implantation of ICD systems has reached a new level of safety and simplicity.

It is useful to think of any lead – pacemaker or defibrillator – as having five distinct components: 1) connector, 2) conductor, 3) insulator, 4) fixation mechanism, and 5) electrodes. Leads for ICDs are very similar to those used with pacemaker systems, except for some significant differences that are reviewed below. In general, the ICD lead system implanted will consist of one or more of the following components:

1. Integrated tripolar or quadripolar transvenous defibrillation lead including proximal and distal defibrillation coils and distal pace/sense electrodes. This single lead can provide all the functions necessary for a functional ICD system, including pacing, sensing, and defibrillation. The distal defibrillation coil may function as one the pace/sense electrodes along with the tip electrode (tripolar lead), or there may be a separate ring electrode between the tip electrode and distal defibrillation coil (Quadripolar lead). The tip of this lead is typically positioned at the right ventricular apex (Figure 6-13).

2. Transvenous defibrillation lead with a single defibrillation coil but without a pace/sense electrode. The tip of this lead is often positioned in the superior vena cava or innominate vein (Figure 6-14).

3. A subcutaneous array lead consisting of three long conductors, rather than a traditional "patch" electrode placed in the left lateral chest or left axillary positioned. This lead is typically used in conjunction with the main integrated transvenous defibrillation lead.

4. Transvenous bipolar pace/sense lead used for atrial or ventricular pacing and rate sensing. This lead may be used in the right atrium for pacing and sensing in a dual chamber ICD, or as a partial replacement lead for pacing and sensing function of an integrated right ventricular defibrillation lead that has lost function of the pace/sense electrodes.

5. Epicardial or subcutaneous defibrillation patch leads. Rarely used because almost ICD implants have acceptable DFTs using the transvenous route (Figure 6-14).

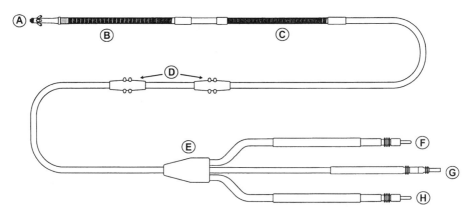

FIGURE 6-13. Schematic diagram of typical tripolar transvenous defibrillation lead. A: distal steroid-eluting pace/sense electrode (cathode); B: proximal pace/sense spring electrode (anode) and distal defibrillating spring electrode; C: proximal defibrillating spring electrode; D: anchoring sleeves; E: yoke; F: distal defibrillating electrode terminal (cathode); G: proximal and distal pace/sense electrode terminal; H: proximal defibrillating electrode terminal (anode). Courtesy of Guidant/CPI.

FIGURE 6-14. Commonly used lead/electrode systems. Panel A: subcutaneous lead with patch electrodes. Panel B: defibrillation lead system involving a right ventricular (RV) lead with pace/sense (P/S) electrodes and a long RV defibrillation electrode. A second transvenous lead is positioned in the right atrium (RA), superior vena cava (SVC), or rarely, the coronary sinus (CS). Panel C: an integrated transvenous lead incorporating distal P/S electrodes, distal (RV) defibrillation electrode, and a proximal (RA/SVC) defibrillation electrode. The bipolar P/S electrode may utilize separate tip and ring electrodes (as shown here), or more commonly, the tip electrode is paired with the distal defibrillation electrode. Adapted from [147].

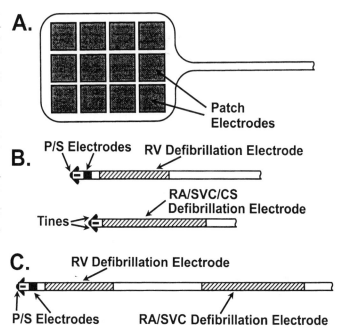

6. Epicardial screw-in sense leads. Rarely used because almost all ICD implants are performed via the transvenous route.

The sensing leads must allow the ICD to detect heart rates over a wide range, up to 400 beats/min. To accomplish this task, closely-spaced bipolar sensing electrodes are preferred over unipolar sensing. A bipolar configuration provides discrete localized sensing that is required for accurate rate counting, without the contamination of far-field signals (myopotentials or electromagnetic interference) that may be detected by a unipolar system. In addition to simple rate counting, some detection and discrimination capabilities of ICD devices require a morphological analysis of cardiac signals. To achieve this, a more global picture of cardiac activity is required and is usually attained by sensing between the proximal and distal defibrillation electrodes, or the tip electrode and distal defibrillation electrode.

The connector design must ensure that the lead is secured both mechanically and electrically to the pulse generator connector port and provide electrical isolation to the surrounding tissue. The manufacturers of the ICD generators and leads have agreed to conform to international design standards for the sizes of lead pins and connector ports, including the IS-1 standard for pace/sense lead interconnects, and the DF-1 standard for defibrillation lead interconnects.

Defibrillator conductors must carry very high peak currents. For example, while the maximum current a pacemaker lead is required to transmit is 15-mA, a defibrillation conductor may need to deliver 40-A. To deliver such high currents efficiently with limited voltage loss, low resistance conductors must be used. Two *composite* conductor de-

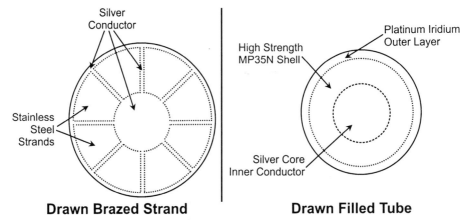

Drawn Brazed Strand   **Drawn Filled Tube**

FIGURE 6-15. Schematic diagram depicting cross-section of drawn brazed strand (DBS) composite wire and drawn filled tube (DFT) wire. The DBS construction consists of six stainless strands surrounded by a low resistance silver conductor in the middle, between strands, and on the outer surface. The DFT composite wire consists of a low resistance inner conductor (silver), a high strength shell (MP35N), and an optional noble metal outer layer (platinum iridium) for use as the electrode. See text for additional discussion.

signs have been widely used, including the *drawn brazed strand* and the *drawn filled tube* designs. These wires are usually manufactured with a combination of materials, including silver for high conductivity, along with stainless steel, MP35N (an alloy of nickel, cobalt, chromium, and molybdenum), or titanium in ensure high strength. Wires constructed using the drawn brazed strand technology combine six or seven strands of a metal of high strength (e.g., stainless steel) with a a strand of soft, but low resistance metal (e.g., silver) (Figure 6-15). Conductors created using the drawn filled tube technology are manufactured with a high strength outer shell of stainless steel, MP35N, or titanium (often coated in platinum/iridium) that surrounds an inner core of a highly conductive metal such as silver (Figure 6-15). Next, the drawn metal tube or drawn brazed strand wires are further formed into multifilar coils or twisted into small diameter cables to further increase flexibility or strength (Figure 6-16). Coiling also creates a lumen that allows for the passage of a stylet necessary to provide firmness and support to the lead while it is manipulated during the implantation procedure. Finally, to produce a lead with the three or four conductive pathways required for an integrated transvenous defibrillation lead, the conductor cables or coils are arranged concentrically, or in a parallel orientation (Figure 6-17), and encased in an insulating tube.

The insulator tubing must electrically isolate the conductors by providing a minimum of 50,000 Ω resistance to any current leakage. If insulation is inadequate, sensing signals will be attenuated and undersensing will occur. Microscopic pinholes can allow shunting of current during the 750-V defibrillation shock, possibly resulting in a failure to terminate the arrhythmia. Silicone rubber has been the most widely used insulation material for defibrillation leads, although polyurethane also has been used. Silicone is also used as a backing material for subcutaneous and epicardial patch leads.

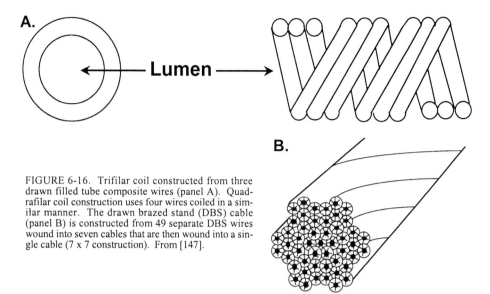

FIGURE 6-16. Trifilar coil constructed from three drawn filled tube composite wires (panel A). Quadrafilar coil construction uses four wires coiled in a similar manner. The drawn brazed stand (DBS) cable (panel B) is constructed from 49 separate DBS wires wound into seven cables that are then wound into a single cable (7 x 7 construction). From [147].

Fixation of the tip of an endocardial lead to selected region of cardiac tissue is accomplished using either flexible tines (passive fixation) or a rigid/retractable metallic helix (active fixation). Tined leads are most commonly used when fixation is required at the right ventricular apex, although an active fixation lead can also be used in this region. Active fixation leads also have the added advantage of permitting a greater choice of fixation sites in the ventricle or atrium. Subcutaneous (or epicar-

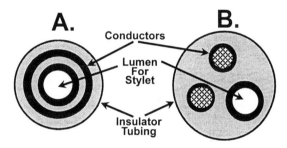

FIGURE 6-17. Cross-section of concentric and parallel lead conductor configurations. Panel A: two conductor concentric configuration. Panel B: three conductor parallel configuration consisting of two drawn brazed strand cables and a drawn filled tube coil containing a center lumen for passage of a guiding stylet. Adapted from [147].

dial) patch leads must be sutured securely in place in order to avoid crinkling of the electrode surface, reducing defibrillation efficacy.

The final component of the lead system are the electrodes. Defibrillator electrodes are commonly constructed using platinum/iridium. In general, implanted defibrillation electrodes have a system impedance of $30 - 55\ \Omega$. Impedance measurements higher than these should prompt repositioning or revision. Defibrillation electrodes must provide a large surface area to optimize current distribution to the widest area of myocardium. With the development of the biphasic waveform, patch electrodes are uncommonly needed. If additional defibrillating power is needed, it is more common to use a subcutaneous array lead, which is constructed of flexible three-fingered coiled electrodes that offer very low resistance and further reduces DFTs [47]. For additional information regarding lead technology, sensing, and pacing see the previous discussion ("Components of Implantable Pacing Systems" on page 183).

ICD programmer and test equipment

The programmer is the electrophysiologist's window into the functionality of the ICD, including its operation, programmable settings, and real time and stored data (Figure 6-18). Programmer function and the graphical display interface for the information vary considerably from manufacturer to manufacturer. The programming system allows the clinician to interrogate and program: 1) sensing and detection parameters, 2) a variety of antitachycardia therapies (antitachycardia pacing, low energy cardioversion and high energy defibrillation) in the ventricle (and atrium), 3) the typical single and dual chamber antibradycardia pacing parameters, and 4) a collection of diagnostic parameters. The programmer provides access to the real-time and stored electrogram data, tachyarrhythmia

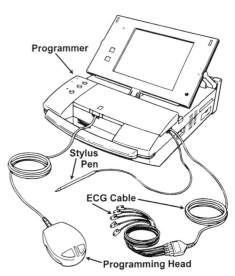

FIGURE 6-18. Typical components of an ICD programming system. Courtesy of Medtronic.

episodes, real-time marker telemetry and stored marker data, and therapy history. This latter capability ensures that the device is correctly interpreting and effectively treating a variety of supraventricular and ventricular tachyarrhythmias. The marker data indicates how the device interprets sensed events or intervals (Figure 6-19). The ICD attaches a notation to each event, and a dictionary of "marker codes" is available to interpret the marker annotations (Figure 6-20). Finally, the programmer provides the capability to perform electrophysiology studies using the device (Figures 6-21 & 6-22), induce tachyarrhythmias, assess DFTs, deliver directed emergent shocks, and abort impending or ongoing therapies.

For the telemetry interface to function, the programming head ("wand") must be placed within approximately 10-cm of the ICD pulse generator. Even though the communication link is referred to as an "RF link", data transmission is actually not a radio transmission because the two antennas are too close together for radio waves to be developed. Rather, data transfer is accomplished using inefficient transformer coupling with one winding in the pulse generator and the other in the programming wand. The mechanism of data transfer involves data-dependent modulation of a high frequency (approximately 100-kHz) carrier signal. The integrity and authentication of the data transmission must be assured using a variety of verification techniques. For example, some manufacturers include a magnet within the programming head along with the telemetry circuitry.

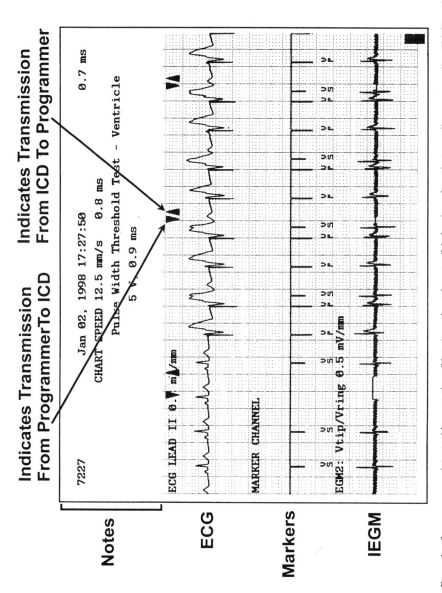

FIGURE 6-19. Example of programmer printout with annotations (Notes), marker telemetry (Markers), surface electrocardiogram recording (ECG), and intracardiac electrogram (IEGM), in this case from ventricular lead. Courtesy of Medtronic.

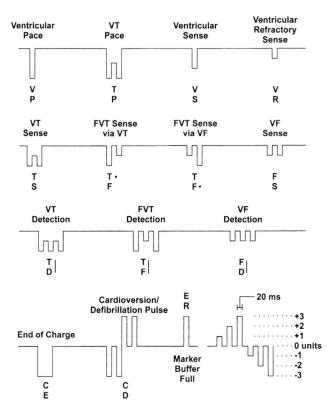

FIGURE 6-20. Example of marker telemetry symbols and annotations. These symbols and annotations are displayed on the printout or the programmer display and can provide real-time information concerning the moment-to-moment operation of the device and how the ICD is interpreting intracardiac signals. Courtesy of Medtronic.

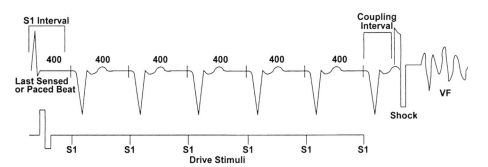

FIGURE 6-21. Schematic diagram illustrating shock during T-wave for induction of ventricular fibrillation (VF). A drive train of equally spaced bipolar pacing pulses (S1) are delivered through the pace/sense electrodes (usually 8-12 stimuli) followed by the delivery of a low energy shock (0.6 – 1.2-J) through the shocking electrodes at a programmable coupling interval. Ideally, the shock should be delivered during the latter portion of the ascending phase of the T-wave (coupling interval 270 – 320-ms). Courtesy of Guidant/CPI.

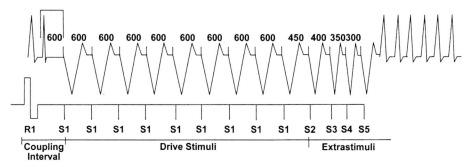

FIGURE 6-22. Schematic diagram illustrating programmed electrical stimulation (PES) capabilities of ICD devices. A drive train of equally-spaced pacing stimuli (S1) are delivered (usually 8-12) followed by the introduction of up to 4 extrastimuli (S2-S5) for initiation or termination of ventricular tachycardia. Courtesy of Guidant/CPI.

After application of the programming wand, the magnetic reed switch is closed before the ICD pulse generator will begin to assemble and execute commands coming from the programmer. This ensures that random spurious signals are not permitted to affect device function or alter the programmed parameters.

Many programming systems also include a pacing system analyzer (PSA) that is commonly used during pacemaker implantation procedures to measure intrinsic electrogram amplitudes and slew rates, as well as atrial and ventricular pacing thresholds and pacing impedances. A stand-alone PSA unit, or PSA circuitry integrated into the programmer, is similarly used during implantation of an ICD system. Originally, DFT testing was performed using an external cardioverter-defibrillator that (ideally) incorporated identical circuitry (particularly the capacitance) to that found in the ICD pulse generator. Presently, however, almost all DFT testing performed during the implantation procedure utilizes the ICD pulse generator itself for arrhythmia induction and termination (*device-based defibrillation testing*).

6.5   ICD Operation and Programmability

ICD systems are designed to provide antitachycardia and antibradycardia therapies. Antitachycardia therapies include: 1) antitachycardia pacing, 2) low or high energy cardioversion, and 3) defibrillation (Figure 6-23).

6.5.1   ICD FEATURES AND FUNCTIONS

As with pacemakers, ICD devices have a standardized code that describes – using shorthand notation – the capabilities of the device. However, unlike the situation with pacemakers, the NASPE/BPEG code is not commonly used to describe ICD function by electrophysiologists and the manufacturers. However, as ICD devices begin to provide antitachycardia and antibradycardia therapies in both the atrium and ventricle, this nomenclature may be more widely used (Table 6-6.)

FIGURE 6-23. Block diagram summarizing the basic operation of an ICD system. The ICD monitors cardiac rate and initiates pacing for bradycardia or one of three possible therapies for tachycardia (antitachycardia pacing, low or high energy cardioversion, or defibrillation). Not all therapy options need be programmed in each patient. In selected patients with hemodynamically stable tachyarrhythmias a stepwise treatment algorithm can be programmed, starting with antitachycardia pacing and progressing through low energy cardioversion to high energy defibrillation (or until the tachyarrhythmia is terminated). Safety features are incorporated by the device manufacturers to assure rapid progression to the most aggressive therapy (usually high energy defibrillation) if a less aggressive therapy causes acceleration of the tachycardia. For patients with fast, hemodynamically unstable tachyarrhythmias, immediate treatment with defibrillation is generally most appropriate. The remainder of this chapter discusses the details of tachyarrhythmia detection and programmable therapies.

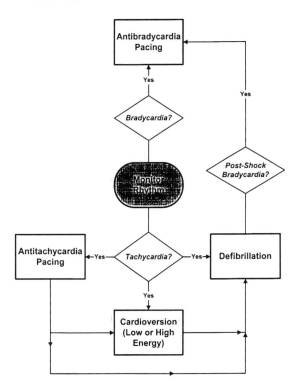

TABLE 6-6. NASPE/BPEG Defibrillator Code

Position I	Position II	Position III	Position IV
Shock Chamber	*ATP Chamber*	*Tachycardia Detection*	*ABP Chamber*
O = None	O= None	E = Electrogram	O = None
A = Atrium	A = Atrium	H = Hemodynamic	A = Atrium
V = Ventricle	V = Ventricle		V = Ventricle
D = Dual (A & V)	D = Dual (A & V)		D = Dual (A & V)

Tachycardia detection always utilizes electrogram analysis; this scheme proposes the possibility that future devices may also utilize hemodynamic parameters to provide further detection criteria. ABP, antibradycardia pacing; ATP, antitachycardia pacing. Adapted from [48].

ICDs incorporate an ever-increasing number of diagnostic and therapeutic features (Table 6-7.) Because each new generation of devices may include a number of new features, the electrophysiologist is obligated to review the manufacturer-supplied physician manual.

TABLE 6-7. Summary of standard and many of the advanced features of ICD systems

Category	Device Feature
Sensing/Detection	Multiple rate detection zones
	Sensitivity
	Automatic sensitivity gain control
	Atrial fibrillation rate threshold
	Ventricular & atrial rate comparisons during tachycardia
	Interval stability
	Sudden onset
	Sustained rate duration
Antibradycardia Therapy	Single & dual chamber pacing
	Rate-responsive pacing
	Mode-switching
	Rate-smoothing
	Sense and pace AV delays
	Variable AV delay
	Hysteresis
Antitachycardia Therapy	Antitachycardia pacing
	Tiered therapy
	Variable high energy defibrillation
	Synchronized low energy cardioversion
	Monophasic/biphasic waveforms
	Programmable tilt

EP, electrophysiology; ERI, elective replacement indicator; VF, ventricular fibrillation

TABLE 6-7. Summary of standard and many of the advanced features of ICD systems

Category	Device Feature
	Automatically variable tilt (constant energy)
Diagnostics & Follow-up	Stored ventricular &/or atrial electrograms
	Real-time ventricular &/or atrial electrograms
	Intracardiac electrograms (true bipolar; tip-to-coil; coil-to-coil)
	Stored & real-time event markers
	Antitachycardia therapies delivered & outcome
	Tachycardia event & therapy counters
	Event histograms
	Sensor and event trending
	Programmable magnet function
	Audible tones (ERI, charging, sensing/pacing, component failure)
	Battery status indicator
	Automatic capacitor reformation
	Antibradycardia diagnostic features (e.g., semiautomatic threshold testing)
EP testing options	"Shock-on-T-wave" VF induction
	High frequency (50 Hz) burst VF induction
	Programmed electrical stimulation
	Manual burst pacing
	Commanded shock
	Commanded antitachycardia pacing

EP, electrophysiology; ERI, elective replacement indicator; VF, ventricular fibrillation

6.5.2 TACHYARRHYTHMIA SENSING

The role of the *sense* circuit is to register the occurrence of successive cardiac depolarizations. *Detection* represents the higher level integration, processing, and interpretation of the sensed data after completion of all amplification and filtering. The purpose of the detection process is to either declare the presence or absence of a tachyarrhythmia. Ideally, the sense circuit functions by comparing the amplitude of an incoming cardiac waveform to a fixed reference voltage (*threshold*) using an electronic circuit termed a *comparator*. Should the amplitude of the input cardiac signal exceed the reference threshold voltage, the comparator outputs a digital pulse, registering a sensed event (Figure 6-24). No comparator signal is generated if the input cardiac signal fails to achieve the threshold voltage. This example oversimplifies the actual situation. In reality, cardiac signals must be amplified and filtered before any comparison is made to the reference voltage.

The use of a *fixed* reference threshold voltage in a sensing circuit works well for pacing systems, but it is inadequate for an ICD system. This is because an ICD is expected to deal with the much wider range of signal amplitudes present during ventricular fibrillation, as well as during sinus rhythm in the immediate post-shock period. The programmable, but fixed, threshold typically employed in the sensing circuits of pacemakers may be too high to permit detection of the re-duced signals occurring during ventric-ular fibrillation (i.e., sensitivity too low with resultant undersensing) [49]. The amplitude of R-waves during ventricu-lar fibrillation may be as low as 20% of the amplitude of the R-waves generat-ed during sinus rhythm [50]. The solu-tion to this problem is not to merely reduce the threshold reference voltage, because that only increases the likeli-

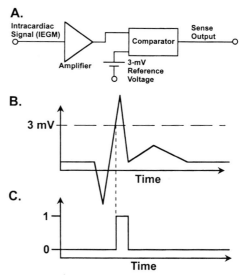

FIGURE 6-24. Schematic diagram illustrating opera-tion of an amplifier/comparator (panel A) in a sense circuit. In response to an intracardiac electrogram (IEGM) exceeding the threshold amplitude (3-mV) (panel B), the comparator outputs a digital pulse (panel C) registering a sensed event. Adapted from [146].

hood of T-wave oversensing. Instead, to ensure reliable sensing, ICD manufacturers use one of two automatic adjustment schemes, either *automatic threshold control* or *auto-matic gain control* (Figure 6-25). In the case of automatic threshold control, the compar-ator threshold level is decreased when the amplitude of the electrogram signal declines. With automatic gain control, the amplifier gain increases when the signal amplitude de-creases. Both of these automatic adjustment methods accomplish the same goal; namely, adapting the sensitivity of the sensing circuit to changing signal amplitudes.

6.5.3 TACHYARRHYTHMIA DETECTION

Rate detection zones
Detection of ventricular (or atrial) tachyarrhythmias primarily relies upon evaluation of the rate of ventricular (or atrial) depolarization as obtained from the rate sense amplifier and comparator circuit. The term "sensing" is generally reserved for the process of reg-istering the occurrence of a depolarization event. "Detection" refers to the higher level

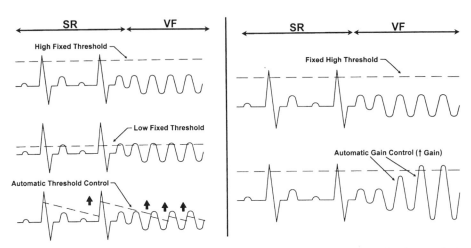

FIGURE 6-25. Schematic diagram illustrating of automatic threshold control and automatic gain control. A fixed threshold device may fail to sense low amplitude electrograms during fibrillation if the threshold is programmed too high (sensitivity too low with undersensing) (upper tracing in each panel). Conversely, if the reference threshold voltage is programmed too low, T-waves may be inappropriately sensed during sinus rhythm (SR) (sensitivity too high with oversensing) (left panel, middle tracing). During automatic threshold control (automatic threshold tracking) (left panel, lower tracing), the sensing circuit "finds" the lower amplitude signals occurring during ventricular fibrillation (VF) because the threshold level is progressively reduced. After registering a sensed event, the threshold voltage is reset to a higher level (upward arrows). During automatic gain control (right panel), the threshold reference voltage is fixed. Instead, the amplitude of the fibrillation signal is quickly amplified to match that occurring during sinus rhythm. See text for additional discussion. Adapted from [146].

interpretation of sensed data to determine if criterion are satisfied to declare the presence of a tachyarrhythmia. The primary method used by ICD devices for detection of arrhythmias is based upon the concept of multiple rate-defined detection zones (Figure 6-26). In general, the detection algorithms used in ICDs are based upon comparing the sensed R-R intervals to a programmable parameter known as a *rate zone limit* or *rate zone boundary* (Figure 6-26). If a sensed R-R interval resides within a programmed tachyarrhythmia zone, it triggers the execution of the detection algorithm. In its simplest form, detection involves incrementing a tachycardia zone *counter* each time the R-R interval criterion for that zone is satisfied. When the value of the counter reaches a certain programmable value, anti-tachycardia therapy is delivered as programmed for that zone.

The first step in the detection process involves measuring the intervals (*cycle length*), in milliseconds, between consecutive sensed cardiac depolarizations (atrial or ventricular). Each time a depolarization event is registered, the value of the timer is reset after calculating the elapsed time from the last sensed event, yielding the cycle length. Each cycle length interval that is detected will fall within one of the detection zones, as seen in Figure 6-26. An interval that falls within a tachycardia rate zone will increment a counter; each tachycardia zone has a separate counter. Depending the implementation of the detection algorithm, the counter may be incremented for that zone only, or for the zone of the current interval and all lower tachycardia rate zones. The advantage of this latter scheme is that tachycardia cycle lengths residing in more than one zone will probably be detected and treated sooner. Without simultaneously incrementing lower zone counters or adding additional zone count summation criteria, it is possible for rhythms to go undetected if adjacent cycle lengths alternately fall within different zones.

Each time a ventricular event is sensed, a timing interval, termed the *tachyarrhythmia sense refractory period*, is initiated. Signals detected during this refractory period are ignored by the detection algorithm. This prevents incorrect counting of device-filtered signals that typically have more waveform peaks than the original cardiac signal. Tachyarrhythmia sense refractory periods are generally < 200-msec in ICD devices. This refractory period may be programmable down to a minimum value corresponding to the device's non-programmable *blanking period*. Regardless, the sense refractory period should not be programmed to a value longer than half the cycle length of the rate boundary of the highest rate tachyarrhythmia sense zone. Otherwise, at certain tachycardia rates only every other spontaneous depolarization would fall inside the refractory period, resulting in the rate being counted at only one-half its true value.

The rate ranges that define the detection zones generally provide a direct linkage to the level of therapy aggressiveness. For example, the device may be programmed with a tachycardia zone for a very slow ventricular tachycardia, and fibrillation zone for a faster, more dangerous ventricular tachycardia, or ventricular fibrillation. The clinician may program the device to attempt anti-tachycardia pacing therapy and/or an attempt at low energy cardioversion for any tachycardia falling within the slower tachycardia zone. If those less aggressive therapies were unsuccessful at terminating the arrhythmia, therapy would progress to a high energy shock. However, in the faster tachycardia zone, the physician may only program high energy shock therapy. In general, ICD devices operate under the principle of *monotonic therapy aggression*. According to this principle, during any episode of ventricular tachycardia, the therapy delivered by an ICD will not revert to a less aggressive level (i.e., revert to a lower energy shock or anti-tachycardia pacing) even if the tachyarrhythmia slows and comes to reside within a lower rate detection zone. Therefore, a high energy shock may be delivered, for example, for a tachyarrhythmia that ordinarily would be treated with antitachycardia pacing if the tachycardia had been converted to a slower rate by the previous shock therapy.

FIGURE 6-26. Schematic diagram illustrating programmable therapy and detection zones in a typical tiered-therapy ICD device. The tachyarrhythmia detection algorithms for ICDs are designed to divide the range of possible ventricular rates (beats/min) or ventricular cycle lengths (msec) into non-overlapping zones. Different manufacturers use different terminology to define the boundaries of these zones, such as the fibrillation detection interval, fast tachycardia interval, tachycardia detection interval, tach A, or tach B. Consequently, the technical manual for each manufacturer must be consulted. Establishing these tachyarrhythmia zones permits the electrophysiologist to program different therapies for different tachycardias the patient may develop. Adapted from [144].

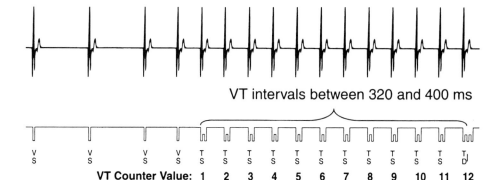

FIGURE 6-27. Example of ventricular tachycardia (VT) detection using the consecutive cycle length algorithm. When the R-R interval is less than the programmed VT detection interval, the ICD marks this event as a VT event and increments the VT detection counter. An episode of VT is declared when the VT detection counter reaches the programmed value (in this case 12). Using the consecutive cycle length criterion, the VT detection counter is reset to zero if any cycle length is measured that is greater than the VT detection interval before fulfillment of the detection criteria (i.e., 12 consecutive R-R intervals < the programmed VT detection interval). Because the VT detection counter can be reset to zero with a single R-R interval within the normal rate range, there may be delayed detection and treatment of VTs with rates at near the lower rate boundary of the VT zone. An R-R interval sensed in the fibrillation zone will not reset the counter. TD, tachycardia detection declared; TS, tachycardia sense; VS, (non-tachycardia) ventricular sense. Courtesy of Medtronic.

Duration requirements for detection

It is obviously desirable that an ICD not deliver therapy every time a single cycle length falls within a tachycardia detection zone. In order for a tachyarrhythmia to be recognized and assigned to a given rate zone, it must exhibit a minimum number of appropriate cycle lengths. This *duration criterion* for detection may be implemented using various algorithms. The two most commonly employed duration criteria are the *consecutive cycle length algorithm* (Figure 6-27) and the *X out of Y algorithm* (Figure 6-28). According to the consecutive cycle length algorithm, a specific programmable number of *consecutive* cycle lengths must fall within a tachycardia zone in order to trigger tachyarrhythmia detection. For each consecutive cycle length residing within the tachycardia zone the detection counter is incremented. When the counter reaches the detection threshold, the therapy delivery sequence is initiated. According to this algorithm, if a single cycle length falls within the normal rate zone the detection counter is reset to zero. While this type of algorithm increases the specificity of the algorithm, it may also delay detection for those tachyarrhythmias exhibiting cycle lengths very close to the lower border of the tachycardia detection zone. In this case, sporadic cycle lengths may fall outside the tachycardia zone resulting in reset of the detection counter. In general, this algorithm is used only for ventricular tachycardia zones and should be specifically avoided for ventricular fibrillation zones. Tachycardia zones using this algorithm should only be used for patients with hemodynamically stable monomorphic ventricular tachyarrhythmias.

Rapid, hemodynamically unstable monomorphic ventricular tachycardia, ventricular fibrillation, or polymorphic rhythms with potentially highly variable cycle lengths are best managed using the X out of Y algorithm. This criterion requires that only a certain

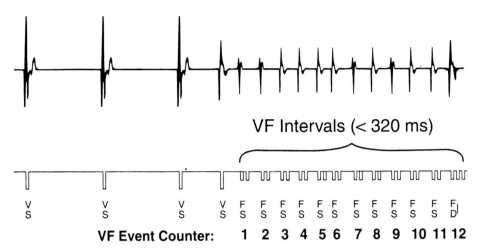

FIGURE 6-28. Example of X out of Y criterion for detection of ventricular fibrillation (VF). When a R-R interval is shorter than the programmed VF detection interval, the ICD marks that event as VF and increments the VF counter. An episode of VF is declared when the VF detection counter reaches the programmed value (in this cases 12 of the last 16 sensed events). In current ICD devices, the X to Y ratio always equals 75%. FD, fibrillation detection declared; FS, fibrillation sense; VS, (non-tachycardia) ventricular sense. Courtesy of Medtronic.

number of cycle lengths ("X") within a window of preceding cycle lengths ("Y") fall within the tachycardia rate zone in order to register detection of a tachyarrhythmia. The values of X and Y are generally both programmable. X out of Y algorithms use the concept of a "sliding window". Only the most recent Y cycle lengths are used in the analysis while all earlier cycle lengths are discarded. Thus the "window of cycle lengths analyzed "slides" with the appearance of each new cycle length. The detection counter is only reset to zero if Y consecutive cycle lengths all fall below the tachycardia rate zone.

In order to not prolong detection, an additional feature termed the *safety-net duration timer*, also commonly termed the *extended high rate* or *sustained high rate timers*, is usually incorporated into detection algorithms. Delayed detection may occur when the tachycardia rate varies slightly and tachyarrhythmia cycle lengths fall into more than one zone, one of which utilizes a consecutive cycle length detection algorithm. Therefore, the detection criterion of neither zone is quickly satisfied, delaying delivery of therapy. An example would be a rhythm whose cycle lengths wander between a tachycardia zone (consecutive cycle length criterion used) and a fibrillation zone (X out of Y criterion used). The safety-net duration timer begins when a potentially sustained tachyarrhythmia is initially declared. As long as the detection criteria timers have not been reset (i.e., a normal rate rhythm has not been sensed), the timer continues to run. Once the timer expires, tachyarrhythmia detection is declared. This declaration directs the delivery of therapy even if the cycle length detection criteria of each of zone are not individually satisfied.

A more common way to manage the problem of a tachycardia wandering between two zones is to use a *summation criterion* that adds the total tachyarrhythmia interval counts in the two neighboring zones (Figures 6-29 & 6-30). Therapy is delivered when

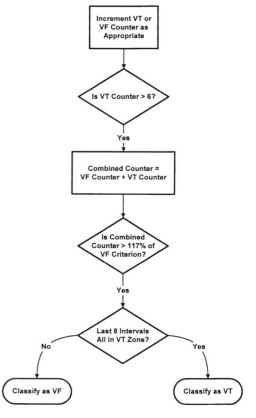

FIGURE 6-29. Flowchart summarizing the use of the summation criterion for ventricular tachycardia (VT) and ventricular fibrillation (VF) detection. The purpose of the summation criterion is to avoid the possibility of a tachyarrhythmia evading detection because its rate (R-R interval) wanders between the two tachyarrhythmia detection zones. To meet the VF or VT criteria, a specific number R-R intervals (e.g., 12) must fall within the respective VT and VF zones. For each R-R interval falling within the VT or VF zones, the VT or VF counters are incremented by one. The combined counter is the sum of the VT and VF counters. The 117% factor (actually equal to the fraction of 7/6) for the summation is chosen to be low enough to assure that there is minimal detection delay, yet it must be > 1 in order ensure that it does not come into play before satisfaction of normal VF criterion during a consistently high rate. Adapted from [144].

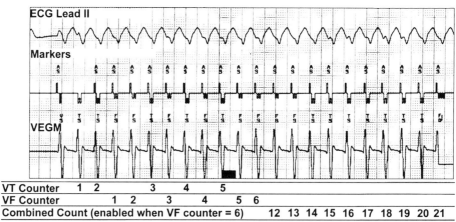

FIGURE 6-30. Illustration of use of summation algorithm (combined count). Delivery of therapy may be delayed if the cycle length of an arrhythmia fluctuates between the ventricular tachycardia (VT) zone (consecutive cycle length algorithm) and the ventricular fibrillation (VF) zone (X out of Y algorithm). In this example, VF detection resulted after early intervals were in the VT zone while later intervals satisfied VF detection criterion. VF (and not VT) was declared because not all of the last eight intervals satisfied VT criterion. FS, VF sense; TS, VT sense; VS, ventricular sense. Courtesy of Medtronic.

the timer expires or a critical summation total is attained, since in either case it is presumed that the arrhythmia has continued too long. In cases where detection is declared by the safety net timer or summation criterion, the tachycardia zone that directs therapy is generally determined by an average of preceding cycle lengths intervals. For example, if the average of the last few cycle lengths or a moving average of cycle lengths falls within the faster rate zone, the therapy delivered will be the therapy programmed for faster rate zone. In other cases, the algorithm will use the shortest detected cycle length to direct therapy generally resulting in the delivery of the most aggressive therapy (e.g., a shock instead of antitachycardia pacing).

Because even very rapid and dangerous ventricular tachyarrhythmias may self-terminate during the capacitor charging process, modern ICDs incorporate a *confirmation ("second look") algorithm* that is designed to confirm that the tachyarrhythmia is still continuing after the charging sequence. If after charging the high voltage capacitors, the confirmation algorithm recognizes that the arrhythmia has spontaneously terminated, the charge may not be delivered but rather is allowed to dissipate or is dumped to an internal load. This "second look" is performed in order to avoid the delivery of unnecessary therapy to a patient after spontaneous termination of the triggering tachyarrhythmia (Figure 6-31). Therefore, in these situations the therapy is termed *non-committed*. If a shock is *committed*, it is delivered regardless of whether the arrhythmia spontaneously terminates. Most devices employ non-committed therapies for tachycardia zones, but may only deliver committed therapy within the ventricular fibrillation zone, since it is highly dangerous and almost always sustains.

Detection enhancements & tachycardia discrimination
The original ICD detection algorithms employed rate-only criteria for detection of ventricular tachyarrhythmias. Because the ventricular rate during sinus and some supraventricular tachyarrhythmias may be greater than the programmed ventricular rate detection cut-off, inappropriate ventricular therapy could be delivered to a patient with a supraventricular tachyarrhythmia. In an attempt to alleviate this, ICD manufacturers have incorporated programmable options into the newest devices that are designed to increase the ability of the ICD to discriminate between supraventricular tachyarrhythmias and ventricular tachycardias. If the ventricular rate criterion is satisfied, these discrimination enhancements are designed to reduce the incidence of delivery of ventricular therapy to patient with supraventricular tachyarrhythmias. The enhancements that have been developed include: 1) *sudden onset*; 2) *interval stability*; 3) *atrial sensing and dual chamber detection*; and 4) *automatic morphology analysis*. Typically, these detection enhancements are employed together so as to increase specificity.

Sudden onset. Patients with slow ventricular tachycardia may have the problem of potential overlap of the ventricular rate during sinus tachycardia with the rate of the patient's clinical ventricular tachycardia. While therapy should be delivered for ventricular arrhythmia, it should not be delivered for sinus tachycardia. *Onset algorithms* are designed to discriminate between sinus tachycardia and ventricular tachyarrhythmias using the onset behavior of the rhythm. Sinus tachycardia has a gradual onset with no sudden

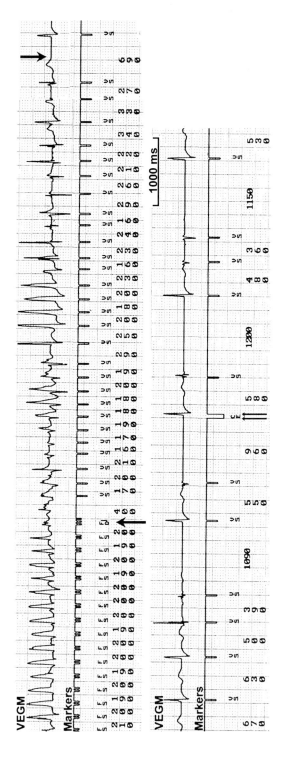

FIGURE 6-31. Example of "second look" phenomenon and non-committed defibrillation therapy. Stored electrogram shows spontaneous episode of ventricular fibrillation (VF) that terminates spontaneously (single downward arrow) before delivery of high energy shock therapy. Note that VF detection criteria are fulfilled (FD at single upward arrow). Capacitor charging is completed (CE, double upward arrow), but no shock is delivered because the "second look" sensing algorithm determines that the tachycardia has spontaneously resolved with resumption of a rhythm within the normal rate zone.

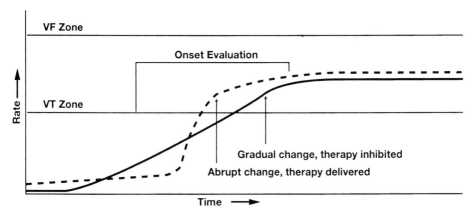

FIGURE 6-32. Graphical illustration of sudden onset criterion. The onset feature prevents delivery of therapy for a tachycardia that exhibits a gradual onset (solid line), even if the tachycardia satisfies the rate criterion. If the rate criterion is fulfilled and the onset was abrupt (dashed line), therapy would delivered for a presumed ventricular tachycardia. Courtesy of Guidant/CPI.

change in cycle length. Ventricular tachycardia, however, typically exhibits an abrupt onset with the first beat of tachycardia having a much shorter cycle length compared to the previous sinus cycle length (Figure 6-32).

Onset algorithms are based upon the evaluation of the change in cycle length (Figure 6-33). In order for a tachycardia to be declared ventricular as opposed to sinus, a measured change in cycle length, or *delta*, must exceed a programmed value. In general, the delta parameter is programmable in milliseconds, percent of previous cycle length, or in percent cycle length shortening. When described in percent cycle length shortening, the typical selections are numbers such as 10-50%. When the delta is described in terms of percent of previous cycle length, then typical selections encountered are 50-95%. When milliseconds are used, the programmable parameter values are in the range of 50–500-msec.

Onset algorithms may fail to detect a ventricular tachycardia that emerges during a sinus tachycardia. In addition, these algorithms will not discriminate between supraventricular and ventricular tachyarrhythmias of the same rate since both can have an equally sudden onset. Most devices back-up the onset algorithm with a separate sustained high rate duration criterion in case the sudden onset criterion is not fulfilled but the rate remains high for a programmable duration (measured in time interval or cycle lengths). Sudden onset algorithm should always be used in conjunction with a sustained high rate algorithm (Figure 6-34).

Interval stability algorithms. Atrial fibrillation is characterized by an irregular ventricular response whereas monomorphic ventricular tachycardia is typically characterized by regular R-R intervals. It is undesirable to deliver therapy to the ventricle in a patient with atrial fibrillation and a rapid ventricular response exceeding the lower boundary of the ventricular tachycardia rate zone (Figure 6-35). Stability algorithms attempt to capitalize on this difference by using cycle length variability analysis to discriminate be-

R-R Interval Sequence (I_n)

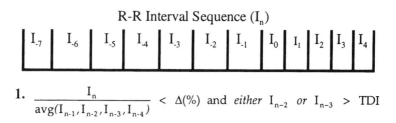

1. $$\frac{I_n}{avg(I_{n-1}, I_{n-2}, I_{n-3}, I_{n-4})} < \Delta(\%) \text{ and } either \ I_{n-2} \ or \ I_{n-3} > TDI$$

2. First, require 8 intervals < TDI cycle length (These 8 are designated above as I_0 to I_7 although the depicted interval sequence only goes to interval I_4 for readability.) Find maximum interval-to-interval difference in previous intervals; the shorter of these two intervals (generating this difference) is called the "pivot interval" (I_0 above). Then require:

$$1 - \frac{I_0}{I_{-1}} > \Delta(\%) \text{ and, in 3 out of the 4 intervals } \{I_0, I_1, I_2, I_3\},$$

$$1 - \frac{I_k}{avg(I_{-3}, I_{-4}, I_{-5}, I_{-6})} > \Delta(\%) \text{ where } k = 0,1,2,3$$

FIGURE 6-33. Example of commonly used onset algorithms (#1 and # 2 above). Onset algorithms are applied to a succession of tachycardia intervals which begin with I_0. The result of the onset algorithm is then compared to a programmable *delta* (Δ) parameter. These algorithms necessarily use various actual or average reference cycle lengths. Subsequent cycle lengths are compared to these reference values. The reference value may be the average of four consecutive cycle lengths (#1 and #2). In this case, the four cycle length average is continuously computed using a "sliding window" of, for example, the four cycle lengths preceding the current interval. Some algorithms are continuously performing these computations, while others wait until intervals begin to reside within the tachycardia zone (#2). The benefit of this approach is that battery charge is not expended to perform unnecessary calculations when the heart rate is below the tachycardia detection interval (TDI). Some algorithms are rather complicated such as # 2 in the figure. In this case, the algorithm first identifies the most abruptly shortened interval (compared with the previous one). Then, skipping the two intervals preceding the shortened interval, the four previous intervals are used to compute the reference average. I_n represents the R-R interval that has just been sensed and I_{n-1} is the immediately preceding interval, while I_{n-2} immediately precedes I_{n-1}, etc. *avg*, average. See text for additional discussion. Adapted from [144]

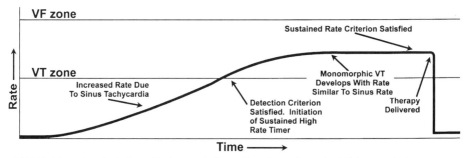

FIGURE 6-34. Hypothetical graphical example illustrating of use of sustained high rate criterion to ensure delivery of antitachycardia therapy in a patient who develops slow ventricular tachycardia during sinus tachycardia at rate very similar to the sinus rate.

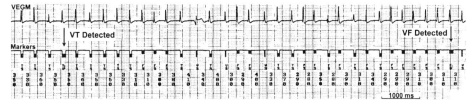

FIGURE 6-35. Stored electrogram recording of a patient with atrial fibrillation and rapid ventricular response (average 150 beats/min (400-ms)) detected as ventricular tachycardia (VT) and ventricular fibrillation (VF). The ICD is programmed to two zones: a VT zone with lower rate boundary of 140 beats/min (430-ms) and a VF zone with lower rate boundary of 188 beats /min (320-ms). No therapy is programmed for the VT zone. As seen, the atrial fibrillation is initially detected as VT (no therapy delivered). Eventually, with further acceleration of the ventricular response (right half of panel), the VF detection criterion is fulfilled and a high energy shock is delivered (not shown).

tween atrial fibrillation and monomorphic ventricular tachycardia (Figure 6-36). Stability algorithms are available only as a programmable option for tachycardia zones. The programmable stability parameter is generally specified in milliseconds with a typical range of 1–30-ms. For example, in a typical implementation, each tachycardia cycle length must not vary from its three predecessors by more than the programmable millisecond difference. If this variance is exceeded, atrial fibrillation is presumed to be the cause of the tachycardia and the detection counter is reset. In another algorithm, the running average of the last four cycle lengths must not exceed the most recent cycle length by more than a programmable millisecond value or the rhythm is declared unstable (i.e., atrial fibrillation). While useful, these algorithms must be programmed with caution to avoid non-detection of an irregular ventricular tachycardia, such as polymorphic ventricular tachycardia. In addition, a programmed value that ensures 100% detection of ventricular tachyarrhythmias will typically result in some inappropriate therapy delivery for even some episodes of atrial fibrillation. Finally, as with the onset algorithm, the stability criterion typically is governed by an extended or sustained high rate timer, ensuring

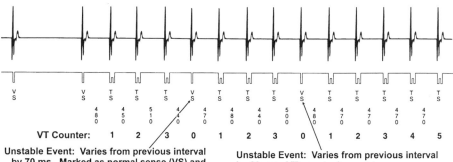

FIGURE 6-36. Example of operation of stability onset algorithm. When the stability criterion is activated, the ICD performs a beat-to-beat analysis of each measured interval falling within a ventricular tachycardia (VT) rate zone. An interval is judged unstable if the difference between that interval and any of the previous three intervals is greater than the programmed stability interval (in this case 50-msec). Otherwise, the interval is marked as stable. Each unstable interval resets the VT counter to zero. As implemented here, the ICD does not apply the stability algorithm until the value of the VT counter is at least three. Courtesy of Medtronic.

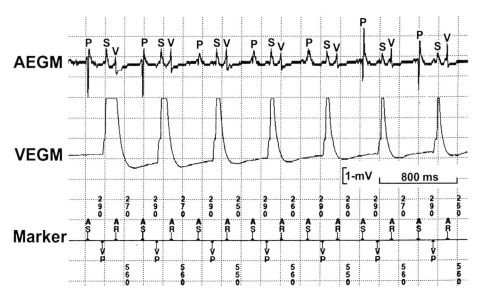

FIGURE 6-37. Example of crosstalk in patient with complete AV block and ventricular tachycardia implanted with an ICD system with dual chamber pacing capability. Antibradycardia pacing is programmed to the DDD mode with atrial sensitivity at 0.9-mV. P-V pacing is occurring with sensing of normal atrial activation (P) triggering ventricular pacing at 90 pulses/min (after an AV delay of 170-ms). Note that the atrial channel also senses the far-field ventricular pacing stimulus (S) as well as the resultant far-field ventricular depolarization (V) approximately 100-ms later. As seen on the marker recording, the pacing stimulus is not sensed because it occurs during the post-ventricular atrial blanking period (PVABP). However, the far-field ventricular depolarization is sensed, but it is detected during the programmed post-ventricular atrial refractory period (PVARP = 310-ms). Normally this may be corrected by reducing the sensitivity of the atrial channel, if possible. AS, normal atrial sense; AR, atrial sense during PVARP; VP, ventricular pace.

therapy delivery after a preset time even if the tachycardia is classified as unstable. This will avoid failure to deliver therapy for an irregular tachycardia at the expense of inappropriately delivering repetitive ventricular therapy for a non-ventricular arrhythmia.

Atrial sensing and dual chamber detection algorithm
Another capability to improve discrimination of tachyarrhythmias is atrial sensing. Dual chamber sensing requires two separate leads in the atrium and ventricle, or possibly, a single ventricular lead with atrial electrodes. Dual chamber ICDs use DDD(R) pacing to provide AV synchrony and optimize cardiac output as well as dual chamber detection algorithms to reduce inappropriate ventricular therapy for supraventricular tachyarrhythmias. Inappropriate detection and treatment of supraventricular tachyarrhythmias by ventricular-only detection algorithms during clinical studies have ranged up to 41% [51].

Crucial to the appropriate function of a dual chamber ICD system is avoidance of oversensing of spontaneous or paced atrial or ventricular events by the sensing electrodes in the opposite chamber (Figures 6-37 & 6-38). Oversensing of far-field R-waves by the atrial channel is avoided by post-ventricular atrial refractory and blanking periods. However, this interval must be minimized in an ICD device because the atrial rhythm must be reliably sensed during high ventricular rates. Long atrial blanking periods may preclude sensing of atrial tachyarrhythmias. Closely-spaced bipolar electrodes will min-

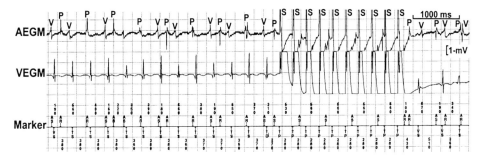

FIGURE 6-38. Example of atrial sensing of ventricular activation during ventricular tachycardia (VT) (same patient as depicted in Figure 6-37). Atrial sensitivity set at 0.9-mV. Left half of panel shows sinus rhythm (100 beats/min) occurring concomitantly with ventricular tachycardia (160 beats/min). The atrial channel is sensing the ventricular activation. Overdrive antitachycardia pacing is performed and terminates the VT (right half of panel). Atrial sensing of far-field ventricular signals is also recorded after termination of the VT (far right side of panel). AS, normal atrial sense; AR, atrial sense during PVARP; P, sinus P-wave; V, far-field ventricular depolarization recorded in atrial channel; TD, tachycardia detection; TP, tachycardia pace; TS, tachycardia sense; VP, ventricular pace.

imize far-field R-wave sensing while still permitting reliable P-wave sensing. In addition, sense amplifier blanking during delivery of pacemaker stimuli in the opposite chamber is important so as to avoid oversensing. However, the ventricular post-pace blanking and ventricular blanking after atrial pacing should be minimized so as assure adequate sensing of ventricular tachyarrhythmias that begin during paced rhythms, particularly near the programmed pacemaker upper rate limit.

The simplest dual chamber detection algorithm could assume the tachycardia is ventricular in origin if the ventricular rate is greater than the atrial rate. Therefore, if the atrial rate is greater than the ventricular rate, the rhythm would be presumed to supraventricular in origin. However, if atrial fibrillation and ventricular tachycardia occurred simultaneously (*double tachycardia*), or ventricular tachycardia developed after atrial fibrillation, this simple algorithm may fail to detect the ventricular tachycardia. Additionally, in cases where there is a 1:1 relationship between atrial and ventricular activation, this algorithm would fail to distinguish a supraventricular tachycardia with 1:1 AV conduction from a ventricular tachycardia with 1:1 ventriculoatrial conduction. Therefore, more sophisticated criteria must be used to distinguish between supraventricular and ventricular arrhythmias.

While dual chamber sensing capabilities are a relatively recent development in ICD systems, the first dual chamber discrimination algorithms were published as long ago as 1979 [52,53]. The P-P, P-R, R-P, and R-R intervals were analyzed in patients with supraventricular and ventricular tachyarrhythmias. If the ventricular rate was greater than the atrial rate, ventricular tachycardia was diagnosed. If the atrial rate was greater than the ventricular rate, the atrial rate was used to classify atrial fibrillation (>350 beats/min), atrial flutter (between 240 and 330 beats/min), and atrial tachycardia (<240 beats/min). For tachycardias with a 1:1 AV relationship, sudden onset was used to distinguish an abnormal paroxysmal tachycardia from sinus tachycardia that was defined as exhibiting a gradual onset. In a prospective analysis, this algorithm was highly successful at distinguishing ventricular from supraventricular arrhythmias.

A number of requirements are necessary in any clinically useful dual chamber detection algorithm. Only if dual chamber data can positively establish that a tachycardia with rates in the ventricular tachycardia or ventricular fibrillation zones is supraventricular in origin, should detection be prevented and therapy withheld. In addition, the algorithm must assure prompt detection of ventricular tachycardia or ventricular fibrillation during an ongoing supraventricular tachyarrhythmia, such as atrial fibrillation, where the atrial rate may exceed the ventricular rate.

Atrial and ventricular rate and comparison algorithms. The simplest dual chamber detection algorithm adds two enhancements, *atrial fibrillation rate threshold* and *ventricular rate > atrial rate*, to the preexisting single chamber algorithms. This algorithm is more sensitive than previously available onset and stability algorithms based solely on ventricular rate. The atrial fibrillation rate threshold enhancement is used in conjunction with the ventricular rate stability and onset algorithms as therapy inhibitors. The ventricular rate > atrial rate enhancement is an inhibitor override that uses the average atrial rate to overrule all therapy inhibitors including the ventricular rate onset or stability algorithms. Figure 6-39 is a block diagram summarizing the logic used in this dual chamber detection algorithm.

After initial detection by 8 of 10 fast R-R intervals, at least 6 of 10 R-R intervals must remain fast during the duration time to avoid resetting detection. At the end of the duration time, the last interval must be in the detection zone to complete ventricular rate detection. Once duration is met each therapy enhancement that is activated will provide diagnostic information. The onset algorithm searches backward in time to find a pivotal interval that defines the onset of the episode. A comparison of the intervals on both sides of this pivotal interval is made to assess whether the onset is sudden or gradual. The stability algorithm averages the R-R interval differences. A comparison is made between this average and the programmed stability threshold (in milliseconds) to decide whether the rhythm is stable or unstable. The atrial fibrillation rate threshold algorithm compares the 10 most recent P-P intervals to a threshold. The atrial fibrillation rate threshold criterion is met if 6 of 10 (and 4 of 10 thereafter) intervals are greater than the programmed atrial fibrillation rate threshold.

Once duration is met, the ventricular rate > atrial rate detection enhancement uses the average of the 10 most recent P-P and R-R intervals to determine which chamber has the faster rate. If the ventricular rate exceeds the atrial rate by 10 beats/min, the ventricular rate > atrial rate criterion is met. If the previously described inhibitors collectively recommend to inhibit therapy, they will be overruled if the ventricular rate > atrial rate criterion is met. The ventricular rate > atrial rate algorithm analyzes the average atrial and ventricular rates and does not compare the beat-to-beat timing of individual atrial and ventricular events. A sustained high rate duration timer will override the inhibitors if therapy has been withheld for a time equal to the programmable sustained high rate threshold. It is important to note that all enhancements are calculated and assessed concurrently and not sequentially. All diagnostic information from active therapy inhibitors and inhibitor overrides are used collectively to generate a final therapy decision (inhibit or do not inhibit). Figures 6-40, 6-41 and 6-42 provide examples of the clinical use of this algorithm.

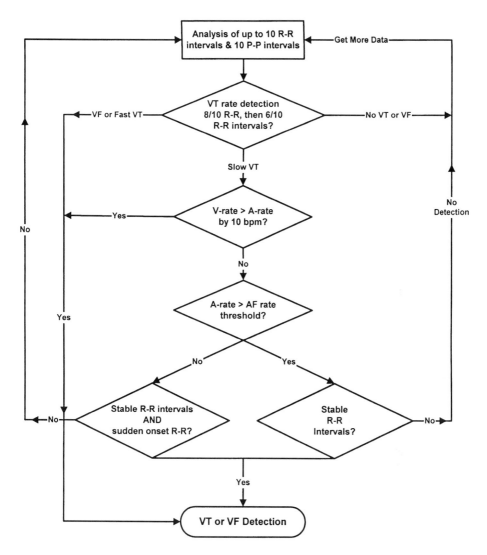

FIGURE 6-39. The simplest dual chamber detection algorithm modifies R-R interval stability and onset algorithms using atrial rate information. For each ventricular event, the 10 most recent P-P and R-R intervals are analyzed if ventricular rate detection initially finds 8 of 10 R-R intervals in the slow ventricular tachycardia zone and if at least 6 of 10 R-R intervals remain in the slow ventricular tachycardia zone. If the dual chamber analysis in the slow ventricular tachycardia zone finds that the ventricular rate is greater than the atrial rate by at least 10 beats/min, then detection occurs. Otherwise, if the atrial rate is greater than the atrial fibrillation rate threshold and the R-R intervals are not stable, then detection is withheld. If the atrial rate is not greater than the atrial fibrillation rate threshold, then detection still can be withheld if the R-R intervals are stable and there is sudden onset of the short R-R intervals. A, atrial, AF, atrial fibrillation; V, ventricular; VF, ventricular fibrillation; VT, ventricular tachycardia.

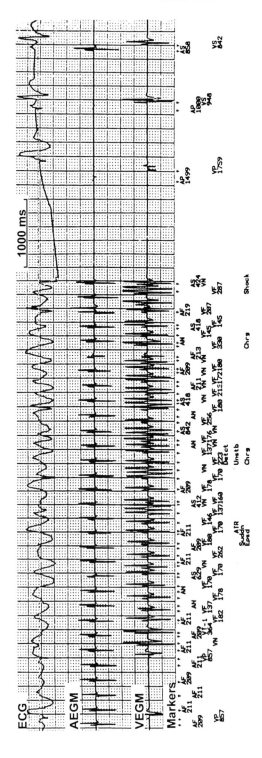

FIGURE 6-40. Real-time electrogram recording from a dual chamber ICD system showing ongoing atrial flutter and subsequent initiation of spontaneous ventricular fibrillation (VF) that was appropriately detected and terminated with an ICD shock. The atrial rhythm was sensed and atrial fibrillation markers show P-P intervals of about 210-msec. There is some atrial undersensing (AS) and atrial sensing within the noise window (AN) during ventricular fibrillation. Ventricular sensing as ventricular fibrillation with some sensing within the noise window (VN) resulted in initial 8 of 10 detection (Epsd), sudden onset (Suddn) and mode switch (ATR) during ventricular fibrillation detection (Detct). The rhythm was judged unstable (Unstb) and charging began (Chrg), was completed (Chrg) and the shock (Shock) was delivered appropriately. The first post-shock beat was paced in both chambers and sensing soon returned. Abbreviations: AEGM, intracardiac atrial electrogram; AF, atrial fibrillation; AFib, atrial fibrillation criteria satisfied; AN, atrial noise; AP, atrial pace; AS, atrial sense; ATR, atrial tachy response mode switch; Chrg, start/end of charge; Detct, detection criteria satisfied; ECG, surface electrocardiogram; Epsd, start/end of episode; Shock, shock delivered; Stb, stable; Suddn, onset-sudden; Unstb, unstable; V>A, V rate faster than A rate; VEGM, intracardiac ventricular electrogram; VF, ventricular fibrillation sense; VN, ventricular noise; VP, ventricular pace; VS, ventricular sense; VT, ventricular tachycardia sense; VT-1, VT-1 zone sense. Courtesy of Guidant/CPI.

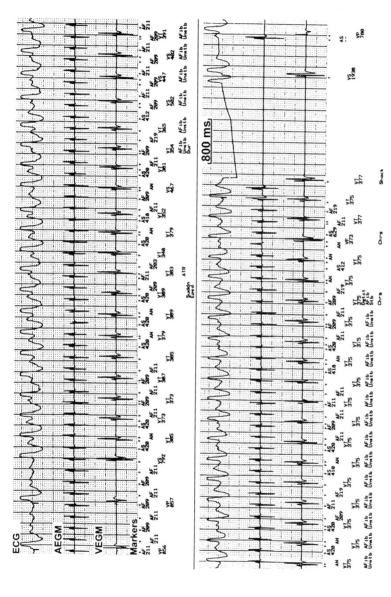

FIGURE 6-41. Real-time electrogram recording showing atrial flutter and spontaneous ventricular tachycardia (VT). Upper panel: sudden onset, mode switch, and duration criteria are satisfied for the unstable ventricular rhythm that was initially diagnosed as atrial fibrillation because both the atrial rate is faster than the atrial fibrillation rate threshold and the ventricular rate is unstable. The ventricular tachycardia was reliably sensed, initially detected (Epsd), sudden onset and mode switching occurred, and when the duration (Dur) expired, the unstable (Unstab) R-R intervals inhibited detection due to atrial fibrillation (AFib). Some atrial undersensing is occurring (note AS markers with 420-msec P-P intervals). On the lower panel the ventricular tachycardia became stable, was detected (Detct) and terminated with an appropriate shock. Abbreviations as in Figure 6-40. Courtesy of Guidant/CPI.

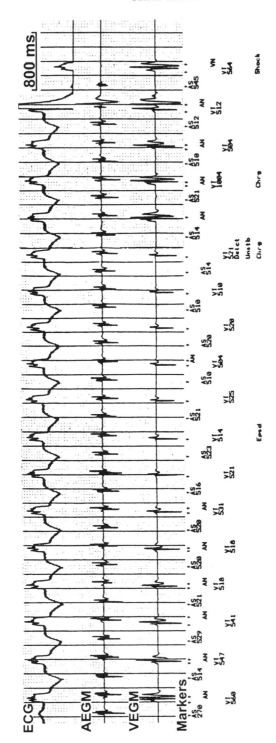

FIGURE 6-42. Two to one atrial flutter rhythms can result in relatively regular ventricular responses that may be inappropriately detected as ventricular tachycardia (VT), especially if there is undersensing of atrial activity. Eight VT beats met initial detection (Epsd) and after five more VT beats, VT was detected (Detct) despite the R-R intervals being unstable (Unstb). VT was incorrectly detected because every other P wave was not sensed or sensed as noise (AN), so the atrial fibrillation rate threshold was not met. Therefore, capacitor charging occurred and an inappropriate shock was delivered. VT detection would not have occurred if simple stability had been used; however, VT detection occurred because the additional criterion of atrial rate > atrial fibrillation rate is not satisfied due to P wave undersensing. The undersensed P waves are inscribed immediately following ventricular depolarizations and fall within the post-ventricular atrial blanking period. Abbreviations as in Figure 6-40. Courtesy of Guidant/CPI.

AV relationship and pattern matching algorithm. A dual chamber detection algorithm that uses pattern recognition of atrial and ventricular events and analysis of timing of atrial and ventricular events was first described in 1995 [51]. One well-developed algorithm utilizes the pattern and relationship of atrial and ventricular activity, along with the atrial and ventricular rates, to more accurately distinguish between supraventricular and ventricular tachyarrhythmias. Dual chamber ICDs implementing the *AV relationship and pattern matching* algorithm use four criteria to evaluate tachyarrhythmias including: 1) the *pattern* of the atrial and ventricular electrograms, 2) the atrial and ventricular *rates*, 3) the *regularity* of ventricular events and, 4) the presence or absence of *AV dissociation*.

Pattern refers the position of atrial events relative to ventricular events. The ICD examines R-R intervals over a series of cardiac cycles and assigns one of 19 "couple codes" to each pair of R-R intervals based upon the number, timing and relationship of neighboring atrial events (Figure 6-43). Zero, one, or more atrial events for each R-R interval are classified within the first half or second half of each R-R interval. If a P-wave occurs within 80-msec before, or within 50-msec after a ventricular event ("junctional zone"), then the P-wave should not be related to the ventricular event by either antero-grade or retrograde conduction. As the R-R intervals vary, the P-P intervals, P-R intervals, and R-P intervals may or may not change. As seen in Figure 6-43, P-waves may be in the junctional zone, the "anterograde zone" (from 50% of the R-R interval to 80-msec before the R-wave), or the "retrograde zone" (from 50-msec after the R-wave to 50% of the R-R interval). Any cardiac rhythm generates a series of couple code letters. The device analyzes the string of codes to determine if an arrhythmia matches a pattern suggesting a particular arrhythmia (i.e., supraventricular or ventricular tachycardias, ventricular fibrillation, or a simultaneous supraventricular and ventricular tachyarrhythmia). The string of letters is compared to a stored dictionary of letter sequences known to occur during specific tachyarrhythmias. The pattern matching occurs continuously in real-time and is analogous to a word processor spelling checker. Once ventricular tachycardia rate detection criteria are satisfied, a supraventricular tachyarrhythmia must be positively identified *on a continuous basis* in order for the ICD to withhold detection and therapy for ventricular tachycardia or fibrillation. As implemented, there are patterns for three groups of supraventricular arrhythmias: 1) sinus tachycardia, 2) atrial flutter and fibrillation, and 3) other supraventricular tachycardias with 1:1 AV conduction such as atrial tachycardia, AV nodal reentrant tachycardia, and AV reciprocating tachycardia.

Rate is the second criterion used in the AV relationship and pattern algorithm. The median ventricular (R-R) and atrial (P-P) intervals are calculated using the last 12 events. There is a programmable supraventricular tachycardia cycle length threshold ("SVT limit") below which the dual chamber detection algorithm is not activated and ventricular rate-only algorithms apply. The SVT limit is the minimum ventricular cycle length at which the AV pattern matching algorithm is operating; at ventricular cycle lengths less than the SVT limit, ventricular rate detection criteria take precedence. The SVT limit should not be programmed to a rate faster than the slowest boundary of the rate zone for ventricular fibrillation detection.

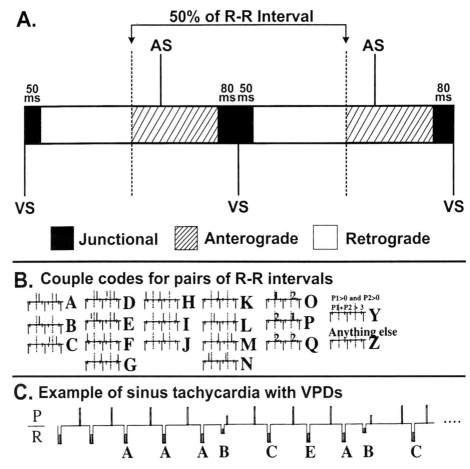

FIGURE 6-43. Principles of atrioventricular pattern matching algorithm. Panel A: schematic illustration of subintervals of the R-R interval that are used to distinguish different atrial and ventricular activation patterns. The junctional zone lies in the 130-msec interval surrounding a ventricular sensed event (VS). The anterograde P-wave is defined as occurring within a segment preceding the junctional interval, while a retrograde P-wave is declared if it falls within a segment after the junctional subinterval. AS, atrial sensed event. Panel B: for the last two R-R intervals the number and timing of P-waves are used to classify the current R-wave as one of 19 couple codes represented by letters of the alphabet. Panel C: example of use of couple codes in patient with sinus tachycardia and ventricular premature depolarizations (VPDs). See text for additional discussion Courtesy of Medtronic.

    An analysis of the regularity of ventricular cycle lengths is also performed. Regularity is one of the criterion used to define atrial fibrillation/atrial flutter and detect double tachycardias (simultaneous supraventricular and ventricular tachycardias). The regularity algorithm analyzes the most recent 18 R-R intervals. The rhythm is defined as regular if at least 75% of these R-R intervals fall within no more than two cycle length "bins" (Figure 6-44). The rhythm is declared to be irregular if 50% or less of the R-R intervals reside within two cycle length "bins". The atrial fibrillation counter increments by one when two or more atrial events occur within one R-R interval (Figure 6-45).

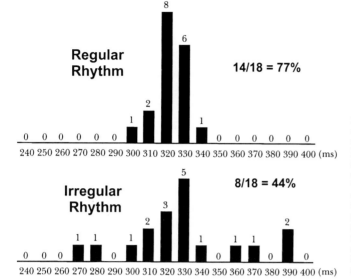

FIGURE 6-44. Regularity of ventricular activation is evaluated by comparing how often the two most common intervals occurred during the most recent 18 ventricular events. Regularity of R-R intervals is one of the criteria used to define atrial fibrillation/flutter and detect double tachycardias, such as ventricular tachycardia and atrial fibrillation. See text for additional discussion.

When the counter is ≥ six, the criterion for atrial fibrillation is fulfilled *provided* that all other detection rules for atrial fibrillation are satisfied (i.e., pattern matching, SVT limit, etc.). This counter increments to 10 and remains satisfied as long as the counter remains ≥ five.

Atrioventricular dissociation is the final criterion employed within AV relationship and pattern matching algorithm. A rhythm is classified as exhibiting AV dissociation if four of the most recent eight intervals exhibit either: 1) no atrial events within the R-R interval, or 2) an AV interval occurs that differs by more than 40-msec when compared with the average of the previous eight AV intervals. To minimize the potential for sensing far-field R-waves by the atrial channel, the algorithm employs a far-field R-wave discriminator designed to distinguish far-field ventricular depolarizations from true atrial depolarizations (Figure 6-46). A sensed far-field R-wave is deemed to be present if: 1) two atrial events are detected for each ventricular event, 2) a short-long pattern of atrial events are noted, and 3) either atrioventricular (P-R) intervals < 60-msec, or ventriculoatrial (V-A) intervals < 160-msec are consistently detected. The far-field R-wave criterion is satisfied if a far-field R-wave is identified in 10 of the most recent 12 R-R intervals.

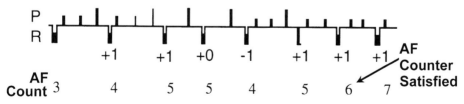

FIGURE 6-45. Atrial fibrillation counter increments by one when two or more atrial events occur within one R-R interval. After the counter reaches six, the rhythm can be classified as atrial fibrillation. See text for additional discussion. Courtesy of Medtronic.

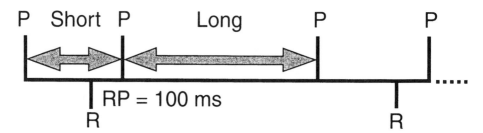

FIGURE 6-46. The far-field R-wave discriminator is designed to distinguish true atrial depolarizations from far-field sensing of ventricular activations. A sensed far-field R-wave is declared if three criteria are met: two atrial events are detected for each ventricular event, a short-long pattern of P-P intervals is observed, and consistent PR intervals < 60-msec or short RP intervals < 160-msec are noted. Courtesy of Medtronic.

Together, these building blocks of P-R pattern matching, rate, regularity, and AV dissociation combine to create a dual chamber detection algorithm as summarized in Figure 6-47. Figures 6-48, 6-49 and 6-50 provide clinical examples of the use of AV relationship and pattern matching algorithm.

Dual chamber detection and therapy. Implantable devices are available to permit detection and treatment of *both* supraventricular and ventricular arrhythmias. Figure 6-51 shows a block diagram of the three major stages of detection for both ventricular and atrial tachyarrhythmias. The ventricular tachyarrhythmia detection algorithm is identical to the dual chamber AV pattern and timing algorithm discussed above. For every ventricular event, the ventricular tachycardia and ventricular fibrillation detection algorithm always has the highest priority. If ventricular detection does not occur, then initial detection begins for an atrial tachyarrhythmia. The median P-P interval and the P-R pattern data are used to declare either atrial fibrillation, or atrial flutter/tachycardia. The atrial fibrillation and atrial flutter/tachycardia detection cycle lengths may be programmed to overlap (Figure 6-52). Atrial cycle length variability is used to discriminate between atrial flutter/tachycardia and atrial fibrillation in the zone of overlapping rates. The atrial rhythm is defined as irregular if the difference between the shortest and longest of the last 12 cycle lengths is more than 25% of the median atrial cycle length. If the atrial rhythm is regular for at least six of the last eight ventricular events, then the rhythm is declared to be atrial fibrillation, otherwise the ICD labels it atrial flutter/tachycardia. If no tachyarrhythmia is detected, the algorithm continues to collect more data. If either atrial fibrillation or atrial flutter/tachycardia is detected, then a programmable duration algorithm is applied to determine if the episode of atrial fibrillation or atrial flutter/tachycardia is sustained. When detection criteria are fulfilled, antitachycardia pacing and shock therapy are programmable.

Automatic electrogram morphology analysis. Device manufacturers have attempted from the earliest days of ICD devices to incorporate algorithms that will discriminate between ventricular and supraventricular arrhythmias based upon the *morphology* of ventricular electrograms. Early devices manufactured by Cardiac Pacemakers, Inc. employed a *probability density function* or *turning point morphology*. These algorithms

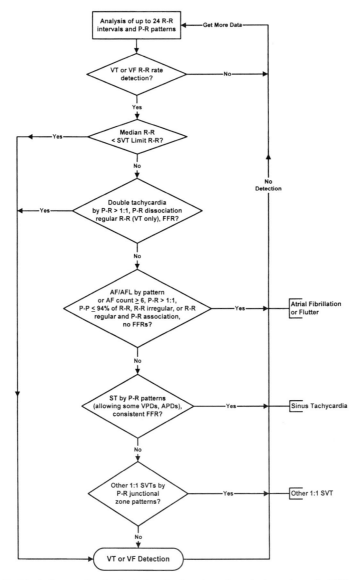

FIGURE 6-47. Block diagram showing logic flow for detection of ventricular tachycardia (VT) or ventricular fibrillation (VF) by dual chamber detection algorithm utilizing PR pattern matching, rate, regularity, and, AV dissociation parameters. It is assumed that all three SVT rejection criteria (sinus tachycardia (ST), atrial fibrillation (AF), or other 1:1 supraventricular tachycardias (SVTs)) are activated. Then R-R, P-P, R-P, and P-R data are analyzed after sensing each R-wave. If the ventricular rate-only detection criteria are not fulfilled, there is no detection. If R-R rate detection occurs, and the median R-R interval is less than the programmable supraventricular tachycardia R-R rate limit (SVT limit), then VT or VF is detected based on rate-only criteria. If not, the algorithm tests for evidence of double tachycardias in both chambers and, if found, VT or VF detection is declared. Should VT or VF still be undetected at this point, then the AF, ST, or other 1:1 SVT criteria can be sequentially applied and have the opportunity to withhold detection and therapy if they positively identify an SVT. If an SVT is not positively identified, then VT or VF are declared based on rate data alone and ventricular therapy is delivered. AFL, atrial flutter; APDs, atrial premature depolarizations; FFR, far-field R-waves; VPDs, ventricular premature depolarizations. Courtesy of Medtronic.

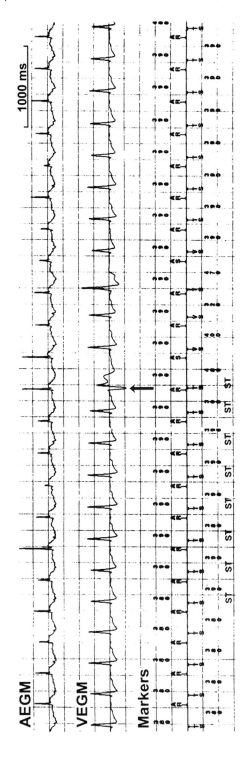

FIGURE 6-48. Appropriate detection of sinus tachycardia and avoidance of delivery of therapy for ventricular tachycardia (VT) in a patient with a dual chamber detection algorithm using AV relationship and pattern matching. The VT detection interval is 400-msec, which is identical to the sinus rate. After fulfillment of the ventricular tachycardia detection criterion (16 R-R intervals ≤ 400-msec), sinus tachycardia (ST) is appropriately declared based upon the pattern matching algorithm. The ST annotations end because the compensatory pause of 480-msec after the ventricular premature depolarization (upward arrow) resets the VT counter to zero. Detection of sinus tachycardia cannot occur again until the VT counter reaches 16 consecutive qualifying R-R intervals. AEGM, atrial electrogram; AR, atrial refractory sense; AS, atrial sense; ST, ventricular detection withheld because sinus tachycardia criterion satisfied; TS, ventricular tachycardia sense; VEGM, ventricular electrogram; VS, ventricular sense. Courtesy of Medtronic.

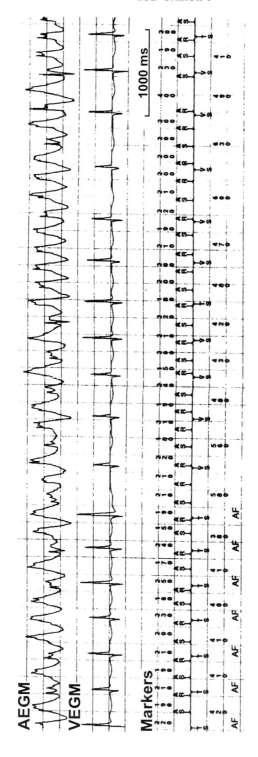

FIGURE 6-49. A stored tachycardia episode from ICD with dual chamber detection algorithm (AV pattern and timing) in a patient with atrial fibrillation (AF). Therapy for ventricular tachycardia (VT) is withheld because AF is recognized (see markers). On the left side of the recording, the AEGM recording shows AF and the VEGM recording shows the rapid ventricular response (VT detection zone programmed to ≤ 400-msec) with sensing of ventricular tachycardia (TS). On the right side the panel, the ventricular response slows and the consecutive counter for VT detection avoids inappropriate detection. Abbreviations as in Figure 6-48. Courtesy of Medtronic.

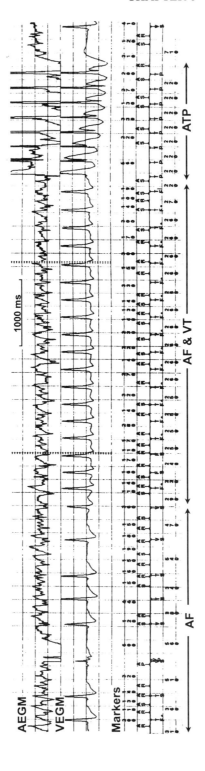

FIGURE 6-50. Stored tachycardia episode from a dual chamber ICD system showing a double tachycardia (atrial fibrillation (AF) and ventricular tachycardia (VT)). The ventricular tachycardia is appropriately detected and terminated by antitachycardia pacing (ATP). AEGM, bipolar atrial electrogram; AR, atrial refractory sense; AS, atrial sense; TF, fast VT sensed; TP, tachycardia pace; TS, slow VT sense; VEGM, ventricular electrogram (tip to shocking electrode); FS, ventricular fibrillation sense; VS, ventricular sense. Courtesy of Medtronic.

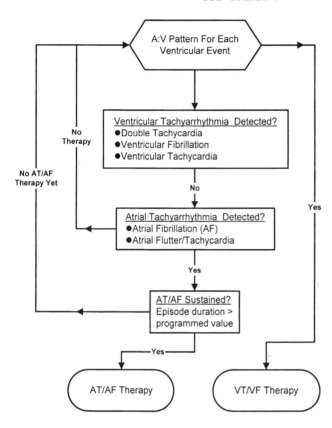

FIGURE 6-51. This diagram that explains the dual chamber detection algorithm has three major blocks. After each ventricular event, ventricular tachyarrhythmia detection (VT/VF) may result in ventricular antitachycardia pacing or shock therapy. If not, then preliminary atrial tachyarrhythmia (AT or AF), if detected leads to sustained detection of AT or AF for the programmed duration until atrial antitachycardia pacing or shock therapy. If neither ventricular nor atrial therapy begins, then the algorithm waits for the next ventricular event and the process repeats.

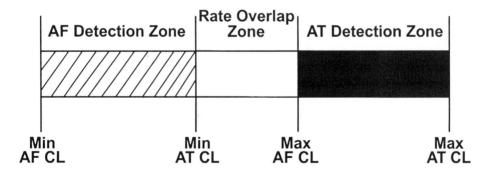

FIGURE 6-52. Atrial fibrillation (AF) and atrial tachycardia (AT) detection zones in dual chamber therapy device. The AF and AT detection zones may overlap. For atrial rhythms with median P-P intervals in this overlap zone, the irregularity of the P-P intervals determines whether detection is for AT or for AF. A typical AT detection zone might be 400-msec to 210-msec, while the AF detection zone may be from 280-msec to the atrial blanking period (normally about 100-msec).

used electrograms recorded from the shocking electrodes (or epicardial patch electrodes) to determine if there is a significant isoelectric period during cardiac activity. Ventricular tachyarrhythmias, particularly fast ventricular tachycardia or ventricular fibrillation, will typically lack any significant isoelectric period while supraventricular rhythms will typically retain a clear isoelectric period. While lacking specificity, these algorithms were utilized in selected patients with modest success.

Automatic electrogram morphology analysis should be employed only in patients with both supraventricular tachycardias and slow, hemodynamically well-tolerated ventricular tachycardias. This option should not be programmed in patients with fast or poorly tolerated ventricular tachycardias. In addition, caution should exercised if programming this feature in patients with ventricular tachycardia exhibiting relatively narrow QRS complexes, individuals with underlying bundle branch block, or patients with increases in QRS duration due to antiarrhythmic drugs. In general, these algorithms are only used during initial detection; they are not employed during re-detection, or if fibrillation rate criteria are met.

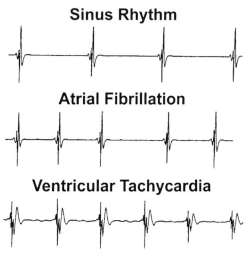

FIGURE 6-53. Example of differences in electrogram morphology recorded an ICD connected to a bipolar sensing lead in a patient with both atrial fibrillation and ventricular tachycardia. Courtesy of St. Jude/Ventritex.

The morphology of an intracardiac ventricular electrogram is determined by the direction of the depolarization wavefront and its orientation to the sensing electrodes. Wavefronts approaching the electrodes from different directions will produce electrograms with different morphologies (Figure 6-53). Except in patients with manifest accessory AV connections, supraventricular tachyarrhythmias conduct to the ventricles using the normal His-Purkinje conduction pathway. Therefore, from the standpoint of the ventricular sensing electrodes, the morphology of the ventricular intracardiac electrogram resulting from a supraventricular tachycardia should be identical to that produced by sinus rhythm. However, a tachyarrhythmia originating in the right or left ventricle will generate a depolarization wavefront that, statistically, is very likely to approach the right ventricular sensing electrodes from a different orientation and produce a different intracardiac electrogram morphology than that generated by a supraventricular rhythm. Rate-dependent aberrant AV conduction could cause a supraventricular tachycardia to inscribe a ventricular electrogram significantly dissimilar to that produced during normal sinus rhythm. Conversely, in situations where a ventricular tachycardia conducts through the ventricles using a route very similar to that traversed by a normally-conduct-

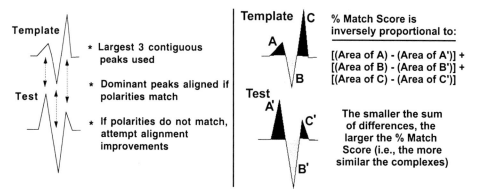

FIGURE 6-54. The electrogram discriminator feature is a high-speed dynamic template matching algorithm. Left Panel: The baseline template electrogram is compared to the test (tachycardia) electrogram; electrograms are aligned and peaks are compared. Right panel: The morphology score is derived from the sum of differences of the aligned baseline and tachycardia electrograms. The greater the similarity the higher the resultant percentage match score. Courtesy of St. Jude/Ventritex.

ed impulse (e.g., high fascicular origin), the resultant morphology of the ventricular electrogram may be similar to that inscribed during normal ventricular activation.

As implemented by one manufacturer, QRS *morphology detection* algorithm involves a measurement of the width of the QRS complex as recorded between the tip sensing electrode and a defibrillation electrode or between two defibrillation electrodes. A QRS complex is defined by a minimum slew rate. Ventricular tachycardia is declared when the QRS duration (measured in complexes that meet the slew rate threshold) increases beyond a programmed threshold for X out of Y intervals. Tachycardia discrimination involves comparison of a stored template electrogram obtained during the baseline rhythm to a intracardiac ventricular electrogram detected during ventricular rates greater than the programmed rate cut-off. A scoring system is used to assess the equivalence of electrograms recorded at baseline and during tachycardia (Figure 6-54). The morphology of tachycardia test electrograms are compared in real-time to the stored baseline template electrogram. As a result of this comparison, a percentage score is generated representing the degree of similarity between the test and baseline template electrograms. The smaller the difference between the tachycardia and baseline electrograms, the higher the percentage match score (Figure 6-55). The critical feature of the electrogram discrimination algorithm is the requirement that the physician set the threshold for acceptance of the baseline and test electrograms as being equivalent. Tachycardia electrograms with morphology scores equal to, or exceeding, the threshold percentage level are classified as matching the baseline template, preventing delivery of therapy (Figure 6-56). Tachycardia electrograms with morphology scores less than the programmed threshold percentage are defined as different from the baseline template electrograms, resulting in the delivery of the programmed therapy (Figure 6-57).

Another morphology analysis algorithm involves a simple measurement of the width of the ventricular electrogram (*electrogram width criterion*). The ICD measures the durations of preceding QRS complexes and compares them to a programmable threshold. The ICD will declare the tachycardia as ventricular if a sufficient number of

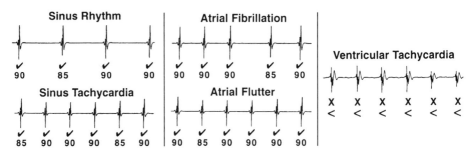

FIGURE 6-55. Ventricular electrograms generated during supraventricular tachyarrhythmia (top four panels) have morphology scores greater than or equal to the percentage match threshold (85%). Electrograms generated during ventricular tachycardia (bottom panel) do not match the template and have a morphology match score less than 85%. Courtesy of St. Jude/Ventritex.

measured complexes are wide. Measurements of QRS duration are made using electrograms recorded between the tip of the transvenous electrode in the right ventricle and the adjacent long shocking electrode (*far-field EGM*). As implemented by the manufacturer, the ICD identifies the start and end points of a sensed QRS complex using a *slew threshold* parameter that is based upon the rate of change of the amplitude of the inscribed electrogram during ventricular activation. As the rate of the change of the amplitude increases above a programmable threshold, the ICD marks that point as the onset of the QRS. As the rate of change of the amplitude decreases near the end of the QRS complex below the programmed threshold value, the ICD marks that latest point as the end of ventricular activation. The QRS duration is defined as the time period in milliseconds between these two points. Higher slew thresholds tend to yield narrower (and generally

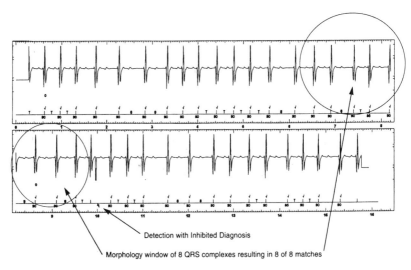

FIGURE 6-56. Stored bipolar ventricular electrogram during atrial fibrillation. Electrograms recorded during periods when ventricular rate exceeded the rate cut-off were classified as similar enough to the stored baseline electrogram to inhibit the delivery of therapy. Courtesy of St. Jude/Ventritex.

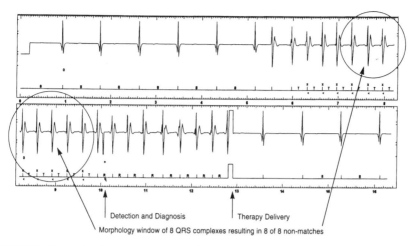

Detection and Diagnosis   Therapy Delivery

Morphology window of 8 QRS complexes resulting in 8 of 8 non-matches

FIGURE 6-57. The ventricular electrograms recorded during ventricular tachycardia are scored as different from the baseline electrograms resulting in the delivery of therapy. Courtesy of St. Jude/Ventritex.

more predictable) QRS duration measurements, while lower slew thresholds tend to result in the measurement of wider (and generally more variable) QRS width durations (Figure 6-58). The ICD compares the measured QRS duration to the to the programmed width threshold to determine whether a measured QRS complex should be declared as wide or narrow (Figure 6-59). As most commonly implemented, the ICD measures the QRS duration of each new beat. After satisfaction of rate criteria for tachycardia, the tachycardia is defined as ventricular if six of the last eight QRS complexes are scored as wide (Figure 6-60)

Activation of multiple detection criteria. ICD systems usually allow activation of multiple detection enhancements, including onset, stability, atrial sensing with dual chamber detection, and morphology analysis. While the use of combination criteria increases the specificity (avoids false positive detection), it decreases sensitivity and may risk the failure to detect a potentially life-threatening ventricular tachyarrhythmia. The safety-net high rate timer should, of course always be employed with these detection enhancements. The use of advanced detection criteria alone or in combination should generally

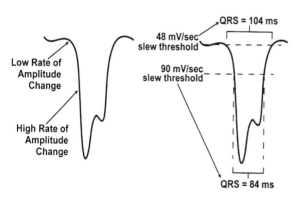

FIGURE 6-58. Example showing the variability of the measured QRS duration depending upon the chosen slew rate threshold. Higher slow thresholds yield narrower QRS widths, while lower slew thresholds result in the measurement of a wider QRS duration. In this example programming a 48-mV/sec slew threshold yields a QRS duration measurement of 104-msec, while a 90-mV/sec slew threshold results in a QRS width duration of 84-msec. Ideally, one should program the lowest slew threshold that yields predictable and stable QRS width measurements during sinus rhythm. Courtesy of Medtronic.

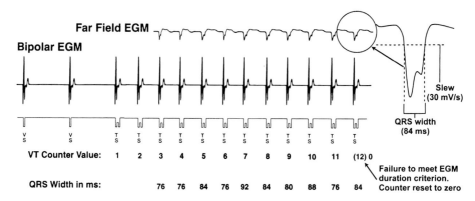

FIGURE 6-59. Effect of slew threshold on rhythm classification. TS, tachycardia sense; VS, (non-tachycardia) ventricular sense. Width threshold programmed to 88-msec. See text for details. Courtesy of Medtronic.

only be used for patients with hemodynamically stable ventricular tachycardia and should not be programmed in tachycardia zones designed to detect and treat fast and unstable ventricular tachyarrhythmias.

Post-therapy detection
After delivery of an antitachycardia therapy the key issue to be determined is whether the arrhythmia has been terminated. Post-therapy detection consists of two components: 1) a criterion to determine if a normal rate has been restored thereby defining the *end of episode*, and 2) a re-detection algorithm. Depending upon the particular implementation, the end of episode may be established when a certain consecutive number of cycle lengths falls below the lowest rate boundary of the lowest tachycardia rate zone, when X out of Y programmed intervals fall below the lowest rate zone, or after expiration of a

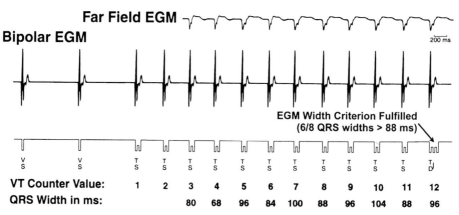

FIGURE 6-60. Example of satisfaction of electrogram width criterion. Width threshold programmed to 88-msec. TD, tachycardia detection fulfilled; TS, tachycardia sense; VS, (non-tachycardia) ventricular sense. See text for details. Courtesy of Medtronic.

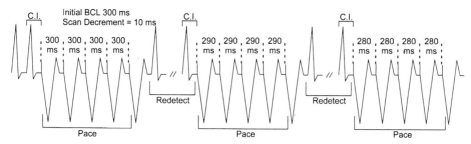

FIGURE 6-61. Schematic diagram illustrating the technique of antitachycardia pacing. Overdrive pacing of a ventricular tachycardia is performed using a stimuli cycle length of 300-msec. After failure to terminate the tachycardia, a second drive train of five pacing stimuli is delivered at a cycle length of 290-msec. This train is also unsuccessful, resulting in the delivery of a third drive train at a cycle length of 280-msec. The coupling interval (CI) (the interval between the last spontaneous beat and the delivery of the first pacing stimuli) may be independently programmed or be equal to the cycle length of the pacing stimuli delivered during the train. This decrementation of the coupling interval from one drive train to the next is termed *decremental scanning*. Courtesy of Guidant/CPI.

specific time period without re-detection of a tachyarrhythmia. Once end of episode is established, resumption of tachyarrhythmia would lead to re-initiation of the standard therapy protocol for that zone. On the other hand, if end of episode cannot be confirmed, the pre-programmed therapy protocol for that zone resumes. For example, if antitachycardia pacing had been the first therapy programmed for that zone and it had failed to terminate the arrhythmia, the device would proceed to deliver the second programmed therapy (e.g., low energy cardioversion). Many devices incorporate safety features into the re-detection algorithm such that if a previously delivered therapy accelerates a tachycardia, the current therapy protocol is aborted and maximal therapy is delivered (e.g. maximal high energy shock). This may occur even if the accelerated tachycardia would not otherwise immediately trigger such therapy based upon its rate alone. In addition, as already mentioned (principle of *monotonic therapy aggression)*, re-detection of a therapy-induced slower tachyarrhythmia will not result in initiation of a less aggressive therapy protocol than previously activated, even though by rate criteria this may be indicated.

6.5.4 ANTITACHYCARDIA THERAPIES

The *only* effective therapy for sustained ventricular fibrillation is an electrical counter-shock. However, organized tachyarrhythmias such as ventricular tachycardia often can be terminated by overdrive antitachycardia pacing (Figure 6-61), especially if the tachycardia rate is slow. Because monomorphic ventricular tachycardia is much more frequent than ventricular fibrillation, even in patients who suffered a cardiac arrest due to ventricular fibrillation, it is particularly important to have an understanding of the overdrive pacing options available in ICD devices. Thoughtful programming of this therapy may allow reliable termination of monomorphic ventricular tachycardias without the need to deliver painful shock therapies, thereby improving the patient's quality of life. However, the possibility that antitachycardia pacing may accelerate hemodynamically stable ventricular tachycardia to a more rapid unstable ventricular tachycardia or even ventricular fibrillation necessitates the availability of back-up high energy defibrillation.

Mechanism of pacing-induced termination of reentrant tachyarrhythmias

In order for antitachycardia pacing to terminate a reentrant tachyarrhythmia, the pacing stimuli must trigger a cardiac depolarization that conducts to and enters the reentrant circuit during the period of the excitable gap (see "Mechanisms of Cardiac Arrhythmias" on page 7 and "Concept of excitable gap" on page 121). In order to terminate the arrhythmia within the circuit, an appropriately timed paced depolarization must conduct in an antidromic fashion within the circuit, colliding with and extinguishing the oncoming reentrant wavefront. In addition, however, the wavefront conducting in the orthodromic direction within the circuit must encroach on refractory tissue leading to conduction block (Figure 6-62). If antidromic collision occurs, but orthodromic conduction is not

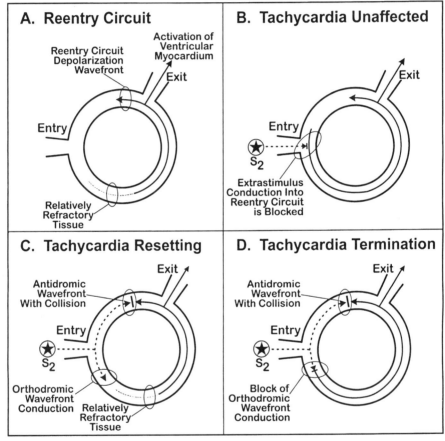

FIGURE 6-62. Mechanism of tachycardia termination by antitachycardia pacing. Panel A: Schematic diagram of hypothetical reentry circuit. Panel B: Failure of any conducted pacing stimuli to enter the reentry circuit during tachycardia leaves the tachycardia unaffected. Panel C: An extrastimulus enters the reentry circuit and conducts in both the antidromic and orthodromic directions. The antidromic wavefront collides with the oncoming tachycardia wavefront, thereby extinguishing it, while the orthodromic wavefront continues to circulate resetting and reinitiating the tachycardia. Panel D: An extrastimulus enters the reentry circuit and conducts in both the antidromic and orthodromic directions. The antidromic wavefront collides with and extinguishes the oncoming tachycardia wavefront, and conduction of the orthodromic wavefront is blocked by encroaching on refractory tissue; consequently, the tachycardia is terminated.

blocked, the tachycardia will be reset and continue to circulate. Among the factors influencing the ability to terminate a reentrant tachycardia with overdrive pacing include: 1) the "length" of the excitable gap, 2) distance of the pacing electrode from an entry point to the reentry circuit and, 3) rate of the tachycardia. Antiarrhythmic drugs may significantly effect the excitable gap as well as the rate of the tachycardia.

Types of antitachycardia pacing
Historically, *underdrive pacing* was the first pacing modality used to terminate reentrant tachycardias. Using this technique asynchronous pacing was performed at rates less than the tachycardia rate. As a result, pacing stimuli were introduced randomly during the diastolic period in the hope that one would succeed in conducting into the reentry circuit thereby terminating the arrhythmia. The success rate of underdrive pacing at terminating a tachycardia is extremely low.

While underdrive pacing proved a failure at reliably terminating tachycardias, it did illustrate the point that the delivery of *critically timed* extrastimuli during diastole was most successful at tachyarrhythmia termination. Because the rate of a tachycardia can vary in cycle length from one episode to the next, the need to automatically adjust the timing of the extrastimuli depending upon the cycle length of the tachycardia became apparent. These findings lead to the development of the programmed extrastimulation technique as a more reliable means to terminate arrhythmias. Programmed extrastimulation involves the delivery of one, or at most a few, pacing pulse(s) at a specific coupling interval following a spontaneous depolarization. By definition, when the extrastimuli (or the first stimulus of a train of pulses) is delivered progressively earlier in diastole relative to the previous spontaneous cycle length (decreased coupling interval), they are said to be *decrementally scanned* (Figure 6-61). *Incremental scanning* means that the extrastimuli are delivered later in diastole relative to the previous spontaneous depolarization (increased coupling interval). When *scanning* is used alone without qualifier, it generally refers to decremental scanning. Strictly speaking, "scanning" refers to decrementation (or incrementation) of the *coupling interval* (the interval between the last spontaneous beat and the delivery of the first pacing stimuli). Some manufacturers employ antitachycardia pacing algorithms that fix the coupling interval at some percentage of the tachycardia cycle length – even during subsequent drive trains delivered during a single tachycardia episode – and only decrement (or increment) the subsequent cycle lengths (after the coupling cycle length) in the pacing train.

The most common form of antitachycardia pacing is *burst* pacing (Figures 6-61 & 6-63). During burst pacing, multiple pulses are delivered (VOO mode) at fixed cycle lengths that are generally 60 – 90% of the tachycardia cycle length. Each burst attempt generally consists of less than 15 pulses. The number of burst attempts (i.e., separate drive trains for each tachycardia episode) that the physician should program will depend upon the hemodynamic stability of the tachycardia and the perceived risk of pacing-induced acceleration of the arrhythmia to a more dangerous arrhythmia. In most cases, less than 10, and often less than six attempts, are programmed. The rate of each burst attempt can be either at pre-determined fixed rate (*fixed burst*) or, more commonly, at a rate that is calculated based upon the rate of the tachycardia (*adaptive burst*) (Figures 6-

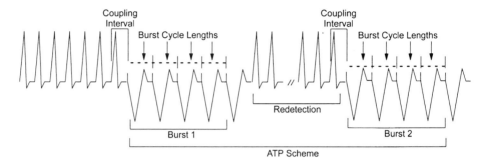

ATP Scheme

FIGURE 6-63. Schematic diagram of a a typical scheme of antitachycardia pacing (ATP). Antitachycardia pacing involves delivering a series of critically timed pacing pulses in an attempt to interrupt a reentrant tachycardia. Delivery of antitachycardia pacing is coupled to the last sensed event that fulfills detection criteria. Within an antitachycardia pacing scheme the user may define the following components: 1) the number of bursts delivered; 2) the number of pulses within each burst; 3) the coupling interval (i.e., the interval between the a tachycardia beat and the first pacing stimulus); 4) the burst cycle length and its characteristics; 5) the minimum pacing interval. These programmable variable can be used to produce at least four types of antitachycardia pacing therapy schemes: burst, ramp, scan, and ramp/scan. Shown in this figure is an adaptive burst antitachycardia pacing scheme. During adaptive burst pacing, pacing stimuli are delivered at a cycle length that is a percentage of the tachycardia cycle length (generally 60 - 95%). The first stimulus of the burst train is delivered following a sensed tachycardia beat at a coupling interval equal to the programmed percent of the calculated cycle length. Courtesy of Guidant/CPI.

64 & 6-65). Fixed burst pacing is generally not employed because the rate of a clinical tachycardia may vary widely from episode to episode even within the same patient. The most frequently utilized burst mode is adaptive, with the cycle length programmed to be 70 – 90% of the tachycardia cycle length. As mentioned above, the coupling interval of the first stimulus of the burst train may be equal to the programmed cycle length of the pacing stimuli (e.g, 70 – 90% of the tachycardia cycle length), or may be separately pro-

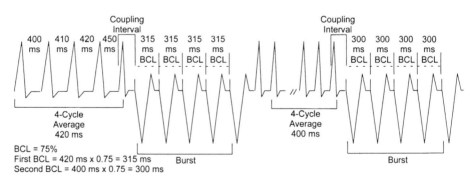

FIGURE 6-64. Schematic diagram illustrating simple adaptive burst antitachycardia pacing (ATP) regimen. A burst is a sequence of critically timed pacing pulses usually delivered at a rate faster than the patient's tachycardia. The onset of the first stimulus of each burst is determined by the programmed burst cycle length (BCL) in percent or milliseconds. The programmable burst cycle length intervals generally range from 50-95% (or 120–750-msec). As seen above, if the average cycle length of the ventricular tachycardia is 420-msec, and the BCL is programmed to 75%, the first, and subsequent, pacing stimuli are delivered at a BCL of 315-msec (75% of ventricular tachycardia cycle length). This first burst fails to terminate the tachycardia, and during re-detection the average of the last four beats preceding antitachycardia pacing is calculated to be 400-msec. Therefore, the second burst is delivered at a cycle length of 300-msec. The characteristic of adaptive burst pacing is that the BCL is dependent upon the tachycardia cycle length. Courtesy of Guidant/CPI.

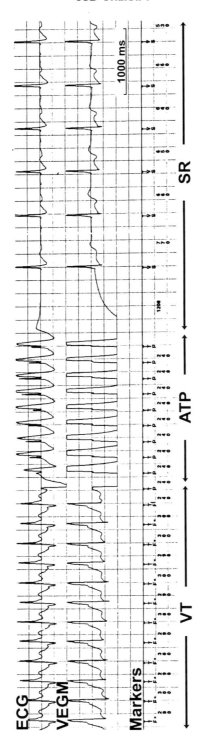

FIGURE 6-65. Real-time electrogram recording showing example of antitachycardia pacing-induced termination of ventricular tachycardia. Ventricular tachycardia at a rate of approximately 185 beats/min is terminated by overdrive pacing using an 10-pulse adaptive burst train. ATP, antitachycardia pacing; SR, sinus rhythm; TF, fast tachycardia sense; TP, antitachycardia pacing; VEGM, ventricular electrogram; VS, ventricular sense; VT, ventricular tachycardia.

grammable. Adaptive burst pacing assures that the overdrive pacing cycle length is a constant fraction of the tachycardia cycle length. Consequently, pacing stimuli are delivered at the same relative time during diastole, regardless of the absolute rate of the tachycardia.

Adaptive burst pacing with *scanning* is often more effective than simple adaptive burst pacing. In this regimen, the first burst rate is calculated as a percentage (e.g., 85%) of the average tachycardia cycle length. If the first adaptive burst train is unsuccessful, subsequent adaptive burst trains are delivered using a progressively decreasing (decremental scanning) or increasing (incremental scanning) cycle length. Typically, decremental scanning is utilized and the amount that the cycle length is decreased (*scanning step size*) during each successive burst is generally 5 – 30-msec (Figure 6-66).

Another variation on burst pacing is *adaptive ramp* pacing. In this regimen, during each burst attempt the cycle lengths between successive pacing stimuli vary. An *incremental ramp* produces bursts that progressively increase in cycle length after the first interval. On the other hand, *decremental ramp* produces bursts that progressively decrease

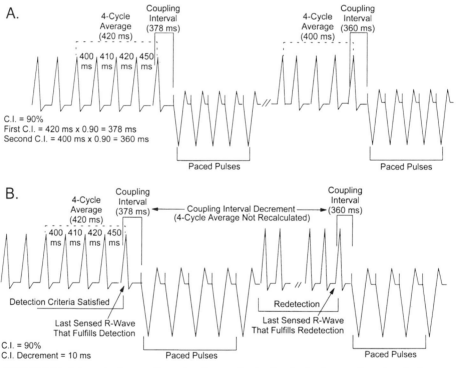

FIGURE 6-66. Schematic diagram illustrating the use of a simple adaptive burst regimen (panel A) versus the use of a programmable autodecremental coupling interval (panel B). In panel A, the first, and subsequent, pacing stimuli are delivered at a cycle length that is product of the cycle length of the tachycardia and the programmable burst cycle length percentage (90% in this example) (adaptive burst pacing). In panel B, the coupling interval between the first pacing stimulus and the preceding tachycardia beat of the first burst episode is determined by the programmable coupling interval percentage as in panel A. The coupling interval of the second (and subsequent) burst episodes decreases, according to the programmed decrement value in milliseconds (10-msec as shown here). Courtesy of Guidant/CPI.

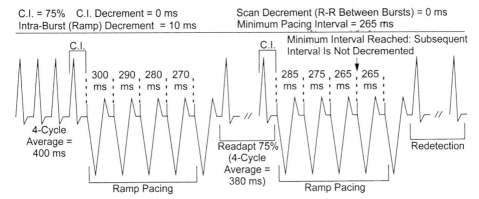

C.I. = 75%   C.I. Decrement = 0 ms   Scan Decrement (R-R Between Bursts) = 0 ms
Intra-Burst (Ramp) Decrement = 10 ms   Minimum Pacing Interval = 265 ms

FIGURE 6-67. Schematic diagram illustrating a decremental adaptive ramp pacing scheme. A decremental ramp scheme is defined as a burst in which each paced-to-paced interval within the burst is decremented. When programming a ramp pacing regimen, the intra-burst decrement must be programmed. The intra-burst decrement (in milliseconds) is the amount by which subsequent pacing intervals are decreased (until the programmable minimum burst pacing interval is reached). As each additional pacing stimulus is delivered, its interval is shortened by the programmed intra-burst (or ramp) decrement until the last paced pulse of the burst is delivered. The coupling interval in milliseconds between the first pacing stimulus and preceding beat of tachycardia during each ramp episode is the product of the programmable coupling interval percentage and the average cycle length of the tachycardia (generally the preceding four cycle lengths). Courtesy of Guidant/CPI.

in cycle length after the first interval (Figure 6-67). Decremental ramp pacing is most commonly used clinically. The amount of change in cycle length from stimuli-to-stimuli is termed the *intra-burst step size*. In addition, ramp pacing can be combined with scanning such that there is both an intra- and inter-burst decrement (increment). Other variations on ramp and scan pacing include the ramp/scan protocol (Figure 6-68) and the so-called "ramp+" regimen (Figure 6-69).

Decremental scanning or decremental ramp adaptive burst pacing can produce very rapid pacing rates, especially if several bursts and pulses per burst are used to treat a rapid tachycardia. Using clinical judgment, the electrophysiologist may decide that there is some maximum pacing rate beyond which further bursting attempts (or further decrement) are undesirable due to encroachment on tissue refractoriness or because of the po-

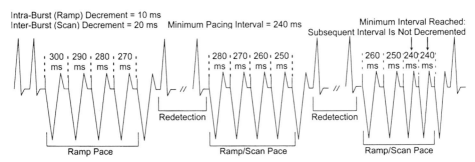

Intra-Burst (Ramp) Decrement = 10 ms
Inter-Burst (Scan) Decrement = 20 ms   Minimum Pacing Interval = 240 ms

FIGURE 6-68. Schematic of ramp/scan antitachycardia pacing regimen. During ramp/scan pacing there is both interburst and intra-burst decrement (or increment). No pacing stimuli are delivered at a cycle length below the programmed minimum. See text for additional discussion. Courtesy of Guidant/CPI.

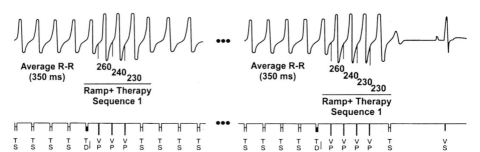

FIGURE 6-69. Schematic diagram illustrating enhanced ramp (ramp+) antitachycardia pacing protocol. The first pulse of each ramp+ sequence is delivered at a programmed percentage of the tachycardia cycle length, timed from the sensed event that fulfills detection (in this case 75%). The second pulse interval is calculated using a programmable percentage (less than that used to time the delivery of the first stimulus, in this case 69%). Any remaining pulses in the ramp episode are all delivered using a third calculated interval, again based upon a programmable percentage (in this case 66%). No pacing stimuli will be delivered at a cycle length less than the programmable minimum (in this case 230-msec). If the tachycardia is re-detected, the ICD applies the programmed percentages to the new cycle length to calculate the pacing intervals for the next ramp+ sequence. If a tachycardia is not terminated by a ramp+ sequence, one additional pacing pulse is added to each succeeding ramp. In this case, two ramp+ therapy sequences are delivered with the second therapy sequence resulting in tachycardia termination. TD, tachycardia detection criteria fulfilled; TS, tachycardia sense; VP, ventricular pace; VS, ventricular sense. Courtesy of Medtronic.

tential risk of accelerating a hemodynamically stable tachycardia into a faster and more dangerous tachyarrhythmia. All available devices allow programming of a maximum burst pacing rate or minimum burst cycle length. Antitachycardia pacing pulses are never delivered at less than the programmed minimum pacing interval. This minimum pacing interval is the same for all antitachycardia pacing therapies. If the calculated interval is shorter than the programmed minimum, the pulses are delivered at the programmed minimum interval. After each pacing sequence, the ICD must re-detect the original arrhythmia before it will deliver the next sequence. If a different arrhythmia is re-detected, or antitachycardia pacing therapy caused acceleration of the tachycardia, delivery of the remaining pacing sequences is cancelled and the ICD delivers the next programmed therapy for the current arrhythmia.

There are two commonly used approaches for calculating the rate of adaptive burst pacing during re-detection of a tachycardia following unsuccessful overdrive pacing therapy. One approach is to use the initially detected tachycardia rate to calculate the burst rate and subsequent scanned burst steps. Another algorithm recalculates the adaptive burst rate between each burst attempt. This latter approach readjusts to the faster tachycardia ensuring that pacing stimuli are delivered at the same relative time of cardiac diastole as occurred during the slower tachycardia.

An important parameter unrelated to timing of antitachycardia pulses is the pulse amplitude and pulse width. During a tachycardia it is important to pace with a high output to ensure capture and propagation of pacing stimuli. Typically, the pacing output of the antitachycardia and antibradycardia circuits of ICD devices are separately programmable, allowing the programming of high outputs for antitachycardia pacing and lower (but safe) outputs for potentially more frequent antibradycardia pacing, thereby maximizing battery longevity.

Effectiveness of antitachycardia pacing

Numerous studies have documented both the effectiveness of antitachycardia pacing therapy and the low risk for tachycardia acceleration [54,55]. In a group of patients in whom antitachycardia pacing therapy was deemed appropriate, pacing regimens were effective at terminating 94% of episodes, while antitachycardia pacing was unsuccessful in 5% of episodes and produced acceleration in 1% of episodes, requiring high energy shock for termination (Figure 6-70) [55]. Testing the efficacy of antitachycardia pacing is often very useful before programming the final pacing settings. This is often done either at the time of, or immediately following the implantation procedure, or as part of a pre-discharge device check. Using the non-invasive programmed stimulation capabilities of the device, monomorphic ventricular tachycardia can be induced

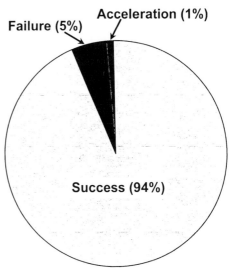

FIGURE 6-70. Pie chart summarizing the effectiveness of antitachycardia pacing in 17,115 episodes of spontaneous monomorphic ventricular tachycardia in 1040 patients implanted with the Ventritex Cadence ICD. Adapted from [148] with data from [55].

and a variety of antitachycardia pacing protocols can be assess for their efficacy at terminating the arrhythmia (Figure 6-71). Ideally, the clinical ventricular tachycardia should

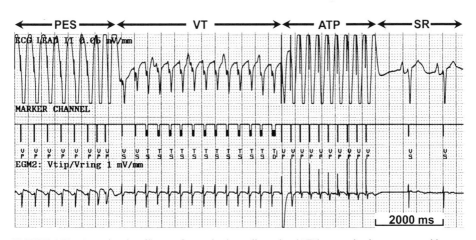

FIGURE 6-71. Assessing the efficacy of an antitachycardia pacing (ATP) at terminating monomorphic ventricular tachycardia (VT) in a patient with clinical VT who received a tiered-therapy ICD. Top tracing is surface ECG, middle tracing shows corresponding event markers, lower tracing displays intracardiac electrograms. Using the programmed electrical stimulation (PES) capabilities of the ICD, VT is induced, is appropriately sensed, and is terminated to sinus rhythm (SR) by adaptive burst pacing. VP, ventricular pace; VS, ventricular sense; TS, tachycardia sense; TD, tachycardia detection criteria fulfilled.

be induced and a overdrive pacing regimen found that reliably terminates.the arrhythmia without triggering acceleration. Although not always feasible, it is also preferable to perform testing of antitachycardia pacing with the patient on any cardioactive drugs they will be receiving, especially antiarrhythmic drugs. If any significant changes are subsequently made in the antiarrhythmic drug regimen, re-testing for effectiveness of antitachycardia pacing may be indicated. Likewise, if the patient experiences subsequent spontaneous episodes that are either ineffectively treated or accelerated to a more rapid tachyarrhythmia, reevaluation, re-testing, and reprogramming may be necessary.

Empiric approaches to programming of antitachycardia pacing
The therapeutic efficacy of antitachycardia pacing may be different for spontaneous (clinical) versus laboratory-induced ventricular tachycardias. Furthermore, some cardiac arrest survivors who have never experience a clinical ventricular tachycardia (nor have inducible ventricular tachycardia) may eventually develop monomorphic ventricular tachycardia. Because of these situations, some electrophysiologists have proposed empiric programming of antitachycardia pacing therapy in selected patients (Table 6-8.) One universal regimen successfully terminated 98.4% of ventricular tachycardia episodes in 162 patients with only a 1% incidence of ventricular tachycardia acceleration to ventricular fibrillation requiring defibrillation [56].

TABLE 6-8.   Proposed protocol for empiric ATP and LEC programming of ICD devices

Phase	Therapy	Attempts	Pulses	Coupling Interval	Decrement
1	decremental ramp	≤ 7	5-11	91% of VT CL	10-msec between pulses
2	adaptive burst	≤ 6	7	84% of VT CL	10-msec between bursts
3	LEC				

ATP, antitachycardia pacing; CL, cycle length; LEC, low energy cardioversion; VT, ventricular tachycardia. Adapted from [56].

6.5.5 Low Energy Cardioversion

In addition to antitachycardia pacing, synchronized low energy cardioversion is an available therapy option in ICD systems. Low energy cardioversion attempts to terminate a monomorphic tachycardia by simultaneously depolarizing a large region of myocardium, thereby rendering this tissue refractory and terminating the arrhythmia (Figure 6-72). While antitachycardia pacing is painless and has proven to be both highly effective for selected patients, low energy cardioversion (< 10-J) is both painful and has a high incidence of producing tachyarrhythmia acceleration [57] (Figure 6-73). In general, only very low energy shocks, usually less than 0.5-J, are perceived as painless by patients; however, these extremely low energy shocks are rarely successful at terminating ventricular tachycardia, especially in patients with significant reductions in left ventricular function [57]. A more realistic therapeutic low energy pulse of 2.5-J is 100,000 times

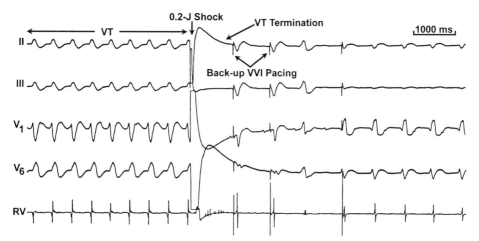

FIGURE 6-72. Termination of monomorphic ventricular tachycardia (VT) by a low energy synchronized cardioversion shock (0.2 J) from an ICD. Note the post-shock antibradycardia pacing. RV, right ventricular endocardial electrogram.

the energy of a painless pacing stimulus (approximately 25-μJ). Most patients experience a shock of this magnitude as indistinguishable from a high energy shock. As with antitachycardia pacing, the efficacy and safety of low energy cardioversion should be tested in selected patients using the non-invasive programmed stimulation capabilities of the device. Ideally, the clinical VT should be induced and the *cardioversion energy requirement* determined (i.e., the low energy shock energy that reliably terminates the arrhythmia without triggering acceleration). Only a relatively few patients will be identified that have clinical tachycardias that are safely and painlessly terminated with very low energy shocks, but are not terminated by any antitachycardia pacing regimen.

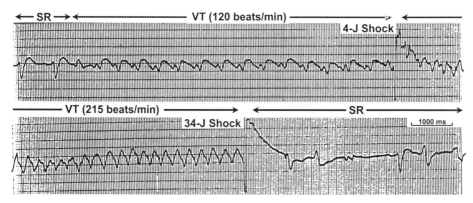

FIGURE 6-73. Example of ICD proarrhythmia with low energy cardioversion-induced acceleration of ventricular tachycardia from 120 beats/min to 215 beats/min after delivery of a 4-J shock. The patient was subsequently rescued after re-detection by the ICD and delivery of a maximum 34-J shock. SR, sinus rhythm; VT, ventricular tachycardia.

6.5.6 HIGH ENERGY DEFIBRILLATION

The original, and most critical, function of an ICD system is termination of ventricular fibrillation using a high energy defibrillation shock (Figure 6-74). ICD programming must always include a therapy zone to provide high energy shock of fast, hemodynamically-unstable ventricular tachycardia or ventricular fibrillation.

6.6   Bradyarrhythmia Therapy

The operation and programmability of the single chamber and dual chamber pacing systems included in ICD systems are largely identical to those already discussed for standalone permanent pacemaker systems (see "Pacemaker Operation, Programmability & Timing Cycles" on page 211). In general, the antibradycardia pacing output, sensitivity, and other features are separately programmable from the operation of the antitachycardia pacing circuit.

6.7   ICD System Implantation

As with pacemaker systems, it is popular to implant the newest ICD device with the most "bells and whistles", regardless of the immediate need for all these features by the patient. The available features and options increase with each new generation of devices. However, these "advances" come at a cost that includes: 1) increased risk of lead-related problems associated with the implantation of multiple leads, 2) accelerated battery drainage, particularly when the myriad of features and options are activated, and 3) more complex (time-consuming) follow-up and troubleshooting, especially when multiple detection schemes and therapy protocols are activated in devices with dual chamber therapy capabilities. The significance of these factors cannot be underestimated and should be carefully considered before automatically committing a patient to the "latest and greatest" system.

6.7.1 DEFIBRILLATION PATHWAYS

Electrical termination of ventricular fibrillation is accomplished by the passage of current between two or more electrodes. Each electrode pair defines a pathway for current. When initially developed, ICD systems required a thoracotomy procedure with epicardial placement of two or three patch electrodes around the heart. Since the introduction of the transvenous lead system and the biphasic shock waveform, the thoracotomy procedure has been abandoned accept in extreme cases. According to the common theories of ventricular defibrillation (see "Theories of Defibrillation" on page 292), either a critical mass of myocardium must be depolarized by the shock wave, or the shock must generate a critical current density throughout the entirety of the ventricular myocardium. There-

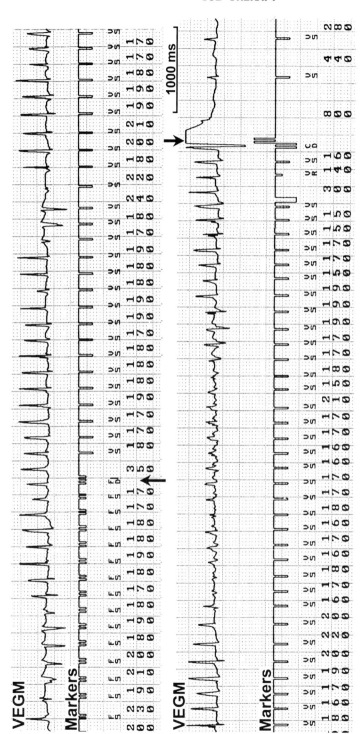

FIGURE 6-74. Stored continuous strip recording showing termination of spontaneously occurring ventricular fibrillation (VF) by a high energy shock. Detection of VF (upward arrow) is followed by charging of the ICD capacitor, after which the shock is delivered to the heart (downward arrow) followed by termination of the arrhythmia. CD, charge delivery; FD, fibrillation detection; FS, fibrillation sense; VEGM, ventricular electrogram; VS, ventricular sense.

fore, the number, size, and location of the defibrillating electrodes are critical to defining the current pathways and may significantly impact defibrillation efficacy.

The most commonly utilized electrode configurations include a 2-electrode system (Figure 6-75) or a 3-electrode system (Figure 6-76). With the 2-electrode configuration there is a single current pathway, while a 3-electrode configuration provides two current pathways. Both these configurations have been used extensively and both deliver clinically-acceptable DFTs ($\leq$ 15-J). Using a 2-electrode configuration, defibrillation electrodes may be placed in the superior vena cava/high right atrium, coronary sinus, right ventricular apex, or subcutaneously in the left lateral chest wall. In addition, modern ICD pulse generators, also can function as an electrode in a fashion similar to a unipolar pacing system. A 3-electrode system will consist of a combination electrodes positioned in the superior vena cava, coronary sinus, right ventricular apex, subcutaneous patch, and pulse generator. There is no optimum electrode configuration for all patients and, therefore, it is impossible to determine a priori which configuration is the best for any particular patient. Defibrillation energy is not clearly related to the type or extent of cardiac disease, infarction, heart size, ejection fraction, or body size. Theoretically, however, the 3-electrode system should better distribute the defibrillation current, resulting in lower DFTs. A clinically popular system utilizes a 3-electrode system with a single transvenous lead incorporating two defibrillation electrodes in conjunction with a defibrillation electrode integrated within the pulse generator (see panel E in Figure 6-76).

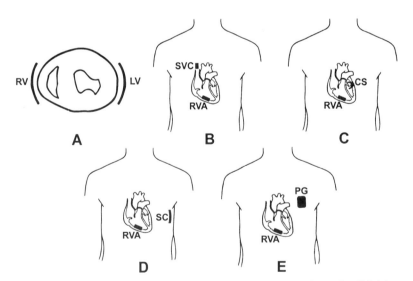

FIGURE 6-75. Most commonly used 2-electrode defibrillation pathways. Panel A: epicardial right ventricular (RV) and left ventricular (LV) electrode patches. Panel B: transvenous defibrillation electrodes at right ventricular apex (RVA) and within superior vena cava (SVC). Panel C: transvenous defibrillation electrodes at RVA and within coronary sinus (CS). Panel D: transvenous defibrillation electrode at RVA and subcutaneous (SC) patch/array electrode in left lateral chest wall. Panel E: transvenous defibrillation electrode at RVA and as part of the ICD pulse generator (PG) housing ("can"). Adapted from [145].

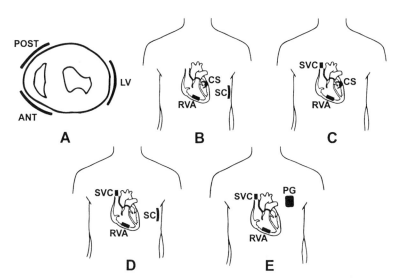

FIGURE 6-76. Most commonly used 3-electrode defibrillation pathways. Panel A: epicardial patch electrodes located over posterior (POST) and anterior (ANT) right ventricle, and lateral left ventricle (LV). Panel B: transvenous defibrillation electrodes at right ventricular apex (RVA), within the coronary sinus (CS), and a subcutaneous (SC) patch/array electrode in left lateral chest wall. Panel C: transvenous defibrillation electrodes at RVA, and within the CS and superior vena cava (SVC). Panel D: transvenous defibrillation electrodes at right ventricular apex (RVA), within SVC, and a subcutaneous (SC) patch/array electrode in left lateral chest wall. Panel E: transvenous defibrillation electrode at RVA, in SVC, and as part of the ICD pulse generator (PG) housing ("can"). Adapted from [145].

6.7.2 OVERVIEW OF IMPLANTATION PROCEDURE

Surgical implantation of an ICD system involves seven basic steps: 1) creation of the pocket for the pulse generator, 2) insertion and positioning of the lead(s), 3) testing the pacing and sensing functions of the lead(s), 4) connecting the lead(s) to the pulse generator, 5) defibrillation testing for adequate energy safety margin, 6) final evaluation of system function and system modification, if necessary (e.g., enlarge pocket, changes in shocking polarity, additional leads, etc.), and 7) wound closure. Implantation of an ICD must be performed in such a fashion to ensure successful functioning during the worst case scenario, i.e., in the event of a cardiac arrest due to ventricular fibrillation. Therefore, for successful implantation all components (sensing, pacing, shocking, and lead performance) must meet certain minimal levels of function.

The optimum location of ICD generator implantation using current devices is the left or right pectoral region. The left side is preferred because it allows for somewhat easier lead insertion/positioning and creates an optimal defibrillation shock vector when the ICD housing acts as an electrode (enhances current flow through left ventricle and especially interventricular septum). Most operators prefer placement of the pulse generator in a subcutaneous pocket (particularly as devices decrease in size), while some physicians continue to routinely use a submuscular approach. Care should be used to create a pocket of sufficient size to allow adequate room for the ICD generator. Too tight a fit, especially in thin patients with less overlying subcutaneous tissue, may predispose to erosion of the generator through the skin. However, an excessively large pocket may allow migration of the device, particularly if the connector block is not secured with suture to a muscle or facial layer. Migration, especially into the axillae, may lead to unnecessary patient discomfort and require a pocket revision.

Inserting, positioning, and securing the lead(s) is the most crucial aspect of the implantation procedure. In all transvenous ICD implantation procedures, a lead incorporating pace/sense and defibrillation electrodes must be positioned at the right ventricular apex (Figure 6-77). In general, to minimize the chance for post-implant disruption of the lead insulation or conductor, the transvenous lead(s) should be inserted through the cephalic or axillary veins. The subclavian approach should be avoided if possible to prevent "crush" damage as the lead passes between the clavicle and first rib (see "Pacemaker Implantation" on page 245). Lead dislodgment, if it occurs, it most common in the early post-implant period. To help

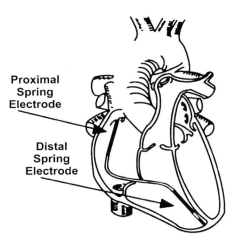

Proximal Spring Electrode

Distal Spring Electrode

FIGURE 6-77. Typical position of transvenous defibrillation lead with proximal and distal shocking electrodes and tip (with pace/sense electrode) at the right ventricular apex.

prevent this possibility, the lead body must be secured to a muscle layer within the subcutaneous or submuscular pocket. However, to avoid lead insulation damage secondary to applying a suture tie directly to the lead body, care should be taken to secure the lead using the anchoring sleeve (Figure 6-78).

Testing the pacing and sensing function of the leads is mandatory prior to continuation with the implantation procedure (Table 6-9.) Suboptimal positioning, antiarrhyth-

FIGURE 6-78. Anchoring the lead body to the fascia/muscle tissue is crucial for successful implantation. Top panel: triple groove anchoring sleeve. Middle panel: care should be taken to avoid suturing directly to the lead body, which can result in insulation or conductor damage. Bottom panel: suturing the anchoring sleeve to the fascia/muscle tissue is the preferred technique. Courtesy of Medtronic.

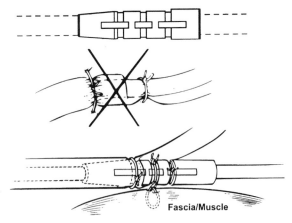

Fascia/Muscle

mic drugs, previous myocardial infarction, or myocardial scar may compromise implantation parameters, including the R- or P-wave amplitudes, slew rate, or pacing threshold. Several attempts at repositioning of the lead tip may be necessary. In most cases, passive fixation leads can be used, particularly for positioning at the right ventricular apex. However, secure positioning and fixation of the tip of a pace/sense lead outside the right ventricular apex or right atrial appendage may require the use of an activation fixation lead (see "Pacemaker Implantation" on page 245).

TABLE 6-9. Recommended lead measurements during ICD implantation

Parameter	Acute Lead System	Chronic Lead System
Ventricular capture threshold	≤ 1.0-V (@ 0.5-msec pulse width)	≤ 3.0-V (@ 0.5-msec pulse width)
Pacing impedance	$200 - 1000$-Ω	$200 - 1000$-Ω
Defibrillation impedance	≤ 80-Ω	≤ 80-Ω
Filtered R-wave amplitude	≥ 5-mV (during sinus rhythm)	≥ 3-mV (during sinus rhythm)
Slew rate	≥ 0.75-V/sec	≥ 0.45-V/sec

The connector pins from the lead(s) must be secured to the connector block of the ICD generator (Figure 6-79). It is important to ensure that: 1) tissue, blood or fluids are not deposited inside the lead connector ports, 2) the pins are inserted into the correct lead connector ports, 3) each lead pin is advanced past its set crew, 4) the set screws are not over-tightened (use manufacturer supplied "torque wrench"), and 5) the tip of the tightening wrench does not break-off in the head of the set screw, making removal impossible at the time of generator replacement. After securing the lead pins into their respective connector ports, the pulse generator should be inserted into the subcutaneous or submuscular pocket. Care should be used to ensure that any excess length of lead(s) resides comfortably within the pocket, avoiding coiling of the lead(s) or creation of acute angles to the lead body, especially where the lead(s) exit the connector block (Figure 6-80). If necessary, the pocket should be enlarged to comfortably accommodate the excess lead

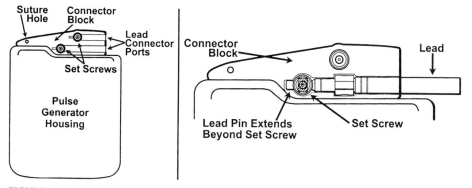

FIGURE 6-79. Schematic diagram illustrating typical features of a ICD pulse generator (left) and detailed view of connector block showing lead pin in connector port extending beyond the set screw (right).

body and the generator. Securing the pulse generator to a muscle or facial layer using the suture hole in the connector block is helpful in selected patients to prevent migration of the device (Figure 6-79).

Verification of reliable termination of ventricular fibrillation with an adequate energy safety margin is goal of DFT testing. The physician must demonstrate that ventricular fibrillation can be reproducibly terminated using the implanted lead configuration and energy capabilities of the device. Device-based DFT testing can be performed using the pacing, programmed stimulation, and shocking capabilities of the device. Typically, ventricular fibrillation can be induced using the programmable automatic *shock on T-wave* protocol included in the device (Figure 6-81). After fibrillation induction, the efficacy of a programmed energy to terminate ventricular fibrillation can be

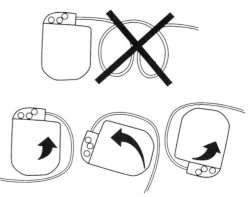

FIGURE 6-80. Proper positioning of excess lead length within the pocket. Top panel: when placing the device and leads in the pocket, do not coil the lead, which may increase the risk of lead dislodgment. Lower panel: to prevent undesirable twisting of the lead body, wrap the excess lead length loosely around the device and place both in the pocket. Extra care should be taken to ensure that the lead body lacks any acute angles that could be stress on the insulation or the conductors. Courtesy of Medtronic.

tested. This procedure is sequentially repeated to determine the estimated DFT (Figure 6-82). The details of DFT testing are discussed in the next section.

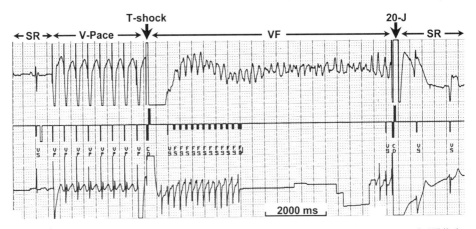

FIGURE 6-81. Example of device-based defibrillation testing using the shock on T-wave protocol. While in sinus rhythm (SR), a train of eight pacing stimuli are delivered at a cycle length of 400-msec (V-pace), after which a low energy shock (1.2-J) is delivered at a coupling interval of 300-msec. The T-shock induces ventricular fibrillation (VF) that is promptly detected and terminated by a 20-J shock, restoring sinus rhythm. As is discussed below (see "Defibrillation Threshold Testing" on page 373), this process can be repeated to determine the energy safety margin for reliable defibrillation. CD; shock (charge) delivered; FD, ventricular fibrillation detected; FS, ventricular fibrillation sense; VP, ventricular pace; VS, ventricular sense.

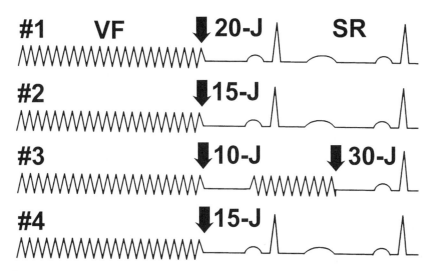

FIGURE 6-82. Example of intraoperative DFT testing. Confirmation of VF termination with 15-J (episode #4) may be taken as providing an adequate defibrillation safety margin when using an ICD with maximum output energy of 30-J. SR, sinus rhythm; VF, ventricular fibrillation. See "Defibrillation Threshold Testing" on page 373 for further details.

Many of the principles guiding initial ICD implantation are equally applicable at the time of generator replacement, including the evaluation of the pacing and sensing functions of the pre-existing ICD leads and documentation of appropriate sensing and conversion of induced ventricular fibrillation. In particular, visual inspection and electrical analysis should be performed to rule out a breach of the insulation. Typically, to evaluate the impedance, pacing, and sensing functions of the lead requires disconnecting the lead pins from the connector block ports of the ICD that is to be explanted, testing electrical functioning, and reconnecting to the connector ports of the new ICD generator. Some manufacturers offer generators with removable interchangeable connector blocks, obviating the need to disconnect the lead pins from the old connector block. Testing the impedance, sensing, and pacing function is then performed through the new generator after connecting the old connector block to the new generator (Figure 6-83). However, the disadvantage of this system is that the interchangeable connector block only fits generators from the original manufacturer. Should evaluation indicate that the sensing, pacing, or defibrillating capabilities of the lead(s) are inadequate, it may be necessary to replace and revise the chronic leads. Testing to establish the presence of an adequate energy safety margin for defibrillation is most critical for patients with a known pre-existing borderline safety margin.

Surgical complications associated with ICD implantation [58] include death resulting from unsuccessful rescue after induction of ventricular fibrillation, cardiac perforation and tamponade during implantation of the transvenous endocardial lead, infection

FIGURE 6-83. Schematic diagram illustrating features of ICD pulse generator with interchangeable connector block. The connector block can slide on and off the pulse generator. At the time of generator replacement, the depleted pulse generator can be removed from the connector block and a new ICD generator can be reattached to the same connector block. Therefore, the lead pins can remain attached to the original connector block. Courtesy of Medtronic.

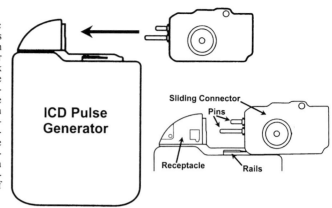

due to implantation of a foreign body, and post-operative hemorrhage within the newly formed ICD generator pocket (Table 6-10.) Lead dislodgment, if it occurs, is noted usually within the first few days following implantation. Since patients often go home the day following implantation of the device, it is critical the see the patient within one week of discharge to assess the healing wound and rule out lead dislodgment, usually by measuring the R-wave and evaluate pacing and sensing function. A chest x-ray is obtained

TABLE 6-10. Potential acute and chronic adverse effects of ICD implantation

Air embolism	Lead fracture
Allergic reaction	Lead insulation break
Bleeding	Lead tip deformation &/or breakage
Cardiac perforation ± effusion/tamponade	Local tissue reaction
Chronic nerve damage	Low amplitude signals during arrhythmia
Death	Myocardial injury
Lead displacement/dislodgment	Myocardial irritability
Lead/generator erosion/extrusion	Pneumothorax/hemothorax
Hematoma	Post-shock rhythm disturbance
Inappropriate therapies	Excessive appropriate therapies
Loose lead pin connection	Lead-related thrombosis/thromboembolism
Infection/sepsis	Pacing/defibrillation threshold elevation
Keloid formation	Pacemaker syndrome
"Frozen" shoulder/reduced mobility	Twiddler's syndrome
Pulse generator migration	Random component failure
Lead abrasion	Venous perforation
Arterio-venous fistula	Nerve/muscle stimulation (e.g., diaphragmatic pacing)
Pericarditis	Chronic pain
Psychological difficulties	Interpersonal & family problems

prior to discharge home and compared to the immediate post-operative film to rule-out early lead dislodgment. Either at the time of implant, or prior to discharge, a number of ICD parameters must be assessed in order to ensure that the ICD system will deliver safe and effective therapy for the patient's clinical arrhythmias and any worst case scenarios such as ventricular fibrillation (Table 6-11.)

TABLE 6-11. ICD Pre-Discharge Checklist

Document transvenous lead position by chest x-ray
Assess sensing and evaluate R-wave (and P-wave) amplitude(s)
Test efficacy and program VT therapies: ATP & LEC
Test and program VF therapy
Ensure that detection and therapies are activated
Assess pacing thresholds and program pacemaker options (mode, outputs, sensitivity, special features, etc.)
Provide patient and family education
Plan outpatient follow-up

*Some physicians empirically program antitachycardia pacing (ATP) and low energy cardioversion (LEC). VF, ventricular fibrillation; VT, ventricular tachycardia

6.7.3 DEFIBRILLATION THRESHOLD TESTING

Despite the pitfalls associated with the use of energy as a defibrillation dosage parameter, it is nevertheless widely used by device manufacturers as well as the clinical electrophysiologists. This is primarily because it is easy to calculate (see Equations 14 & 15), is a programmable option on ICD programmers, and has been widely used by clinical researchers for over the 30 years. In addition, while energy is meaningful only when capacitance, resistance, or pulse duration (or tilt) are all fixed, this condition is generally satisfied in most clinical situations. However, it is important to understand the limitations of energy as a defibrillation dosage parameter (see "Basic Concepts of Defibrillation" on page 291). During the implantation procedure, the electrophysiologist must determine that the energy required to assure termination of ventricular fibrillation is well within the output capabilities of the ICD generator, given the lead system, waveform, resistance, and clinical characteristics of the patient. To evaluate the energy safety margins for defibrillation it is crucial to appreciate the defibrillation success curve, discussed immediately below.

Defibrillation success curve and defibrillation threshold
A patient's defibrillation requirement, whether expressed in terms of energy, voltage, or current, is best described by a dose response relationship, termed the *defibrillation success curve* (Figure 6-84). The statistical character of defibrillation efficacy implied by this curve may be due to moment-to-moment variations in a variety of physiologic and non-physiologic factors that are neither known, nor controllable. In order to construct a defibrillation dose-response curve for each patient repeated defibrillation attempts at dif-

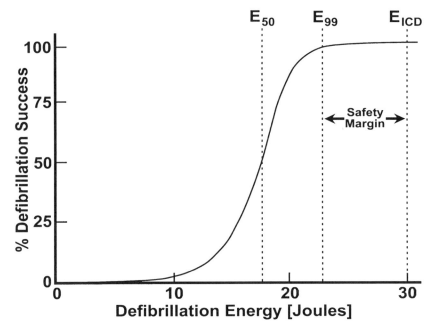

FIGURE 6-84. Example of defibrillation success curve showing probability of defibrillation success versus ICD output energy (stored energy). The shape of the curve implies a dose-response relationship in which increased doses of delivered energy are associated with an increased success rate of defibrillation. The true safety margin for the ICD system is defined as the difference between the maximum defibrillation output (E_{ICD}) and the upper shoulder of the defibrillation success curve corresponding to energy required to guarantee 99% defibrillation efficacy (E_{99}). The energy resulting in a 50% chance of defibrillation success is denoted by E_{50}. See text for additional discussion.

ferent energy levels would be required. In practice, however, this is impractical and potentially dangerous. Therefore, alternative means must be used to determine the defibrillation requirement for any particular patient. Note in Figure 6-84 that at very low or very high shock energies, there is very little increase in defibrillation success even with relatively large increases in delivered energy (flat portions of the curve). On the other hand, at energy levels producing 50% defibrillation success, even small increases in the energy dose results in a large increase in the success rate (steep portion of curve). Implantation requirements dictate that the patient must have an adequate safety margin between the defibrillation success curve and the output capabilities of the device. The key reason for this requirement is to ensure successful termination of ventricular fibrillation in spite of a temporary of chronic increase in the defibrillation threshold (rightward shift of the defibrillation success curve). Shifts in the defibrillation success curve to higher defibrillation energies may result from progression of underlying heart disease, changes in antiarrhythmic drug therapy, dislodgments of an endocardial defibrillation lead, or prolonged episodes of ventricular fibrillation, among other possibilities.

The relative position of the defibrillation success curve along the X-axis is typically denoted by certain points, such as the energy required for 99% (E_{99}) or 50% (E_{50}) defibrillation success. The *defibrillation threshold,* or *DFT*, expressed in terms of energy, refers to the minimum energy that terminates ventricular fibrillation 99% of the time (E_{99}). The energy *safety margin* is defined as the difference between the maximum energy output of the ICD (E_{ICD}) and the DFT. The safety margin should be wide enough to accommodate rightward (i.e., less favorable) shifts in the defibrillation success curve to higher energies that may result from progression of underlying heart disease, ischemia, changes in antiarrhythmic drugs, electrolyte or acid-base disturbances, prolonged fibrillation, or other unknowable and uncontrollable factors. The *actual* or *true DFT (DFT_{ACT})* and safety margin cannot be precisely defined, given practical and patient safety considerations. Therefore, it is expected that the *estimated defibrillation threshold (DFT_{EST})* will be less than the true DFT (E_{99}), because only a small, clinically-acceptable, number of inductions of ventricular fibrillation can be performed. As a consequence, the difference between the maximum energy output of the defibrillator, E_{ICD}, and DFT_{EST} – a difference that is best termed the *estimated safety margin* – is expected to be greater than the unknowable actual safety margin as defined above. Consequently, the electrophysiologist must assess at the time of implantation whether the estimated safety margin is "large enough" to protect the patient should a rightward shift occur in the defibrillation success curve. If not, the operator may need to modify or enhance the lead system, or implant an ICD generator with a higher output, assuming such a device is available. *Therefore, the critical feature of any ICD implantation procedure is to assess the adequacy of the estimated safety margin.*

Methods for evaluating safety margin
Methods for assessing the energy safety margin can be classified into two general categories: *threshold* techniques and *verification* techniques. Threshold methods are more rigorous and involve a sequence of repeated episodes of fibrillation and defibrillation attempts using various shock energies until an energy that succeeds at defibrillation with nearby slightly lower energies failing to terminate fibrillation is encountered. The purpose of these techniques is to determine the general location of the defibrillation success curve so as to ensure that an adequate energy margin can be provided. On the other hand, verification techniques are more abbreviated techniques that determine safe energy margins but do not require that the patient be tested using energies that fail to terminate ventricular fibrillation. Verification techniques are even less successful at precisely defining the defibrillation success curve than the threshold techniques.

   Determination of energy safety margins using threshold techniques. The *standard DFT protocol* involves a test sequence of consecutive fibrillation/defibrillation trials using declining shock energies until a defibrillation attempt fails (after which a high energy rescue shock is delivered) (Figure 6-85). The DFT_{EST} is defined as the lowest energy that successfully terminates ventricular fibrillation (Figure 6-86). Remember that the actual DFT ($DFT_{ACT} = E_{99}$) can only be determined by verifying that the "lowest successful energy" repeatedly terminates ventricular fibrillation in the patient. Therefore, a single success at an energy level immediately above an unsuccessful energy level only identifies the estimated DFT, DFT_{EST}. As a result, many electrophysiologists use an *enhanced DFT protocol* in which one or two additional fibrillation/defibrillation trials are performed at the lowest successful energy level [59]. For example, if 10-J is successful at terminating ventricular fibrillation, this energy could be retested additional times to confirm that this energy is reliably successful. The enhanced *DFT+ protocol* requires two of two successes at the lowest energy, while the *DFT++ protocol* demands three of three success at this energy [60-62]. If any of these additional repeat attempts are unsuccessful, the electrophysiologist may choose to test a nearby higher energy for defibrillation efficacy using one of the enhanced protocols. Data from experimental studies, as well as probability analysis, indicates that the DFT_{EST} will more closely approximate DFT_{ACT} as the number of consecutive successes (without intervening failures) increases.

Due to the probabilistic nature of defibrillation, the bulk of defibrillation successes will be distributed along the steep portion of the defibrillation success curve [63]. The accuracy of threshold techniques to establish the energy margin will depend upon the variability of threshold measurements. Animal studies as well as analysis of defibrillation probability indicates that DFTs obtained using a decreasing step protocol as described above (Figure 6-85) are distributed in an asymmetrical fashion toward the upper portion of the defibrillation success curve, with the average location at the energy that yields 71% success (E_{71}, range E_{25} to E_{100}) [59-64]. Thus, DFT_{EST} determined using the step-down to failure approach is usually located along the top three-fourths of the success curve with the statistically most common position being at approximately 70% success, while the true DFT (DFT_{ACT}) lies at the 99% success point.

The location of the DFT_{EST} along the success curve has an important bearing on adequacy of the safety margin for the patient. If DFT_{EST} is located near DFT_{ACT} (at E_{99} on the defibrillation success curve), the estimated safety margin (E_{ICD} – DFT_{EST}) will closely approximate the actual safety margin (E_{ICD} – E_{99}). If, however, DFT_{EST} is located low on the defibrillation success curve, the measured energy safety margin (E_{ICD} – DFT_{EST}) will be greater than the actual safety margin (E_{ICD} – E_{99}) (Figure 6-87). Therefore, the unsuspecting clinician may mistakenly assume a greater safety margin than is really available.

Because the standard DFT protocol does not establish the location of the DFT_{EST} along the defibrillation success curve there is uncertainty as

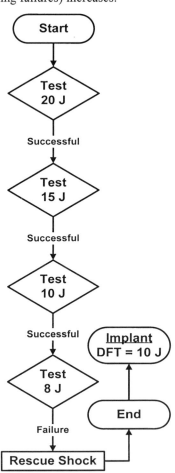

FIGURE 6-85. Determination of the estimated defibrillation threshold (DFT_{EST}) using standard step-down approach. Ventricular fibrillation is successfully terminated during consecutive fibrillation/defibrillation trials using 20 J, 15 J, and 10 J. However, an 8 J shock fails to terminate ventricular fibrillation. After a high energy rescue shock the procedure ends and the DFT is estimated to be 10 J.

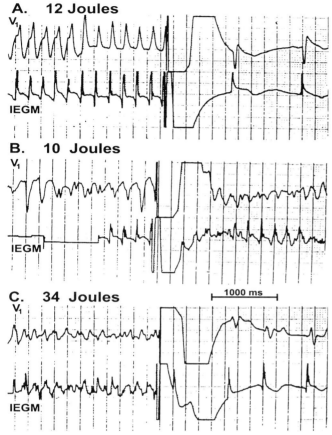

A. 12 Joules

V₁

IEGM

B. 10 Joules

V₁

IEGM

C. 34 Joules

V₁

IEGM

1000 ms

FIGURE 6-86. Determination of ventricular defibrillation threshold using DFT+ protocol. In each panel, ECG lead V₁ and right ventricular endocardial electrogram (IEGM) are displayed. Panel A: A biphasic shock of 12 joules converts ventricular fibrillation to sinus rhythm. Panel B: A biphasic shock of 10 joules fails to terminate ventricular fibrillation, which is subsequently converted to sinus rhythm with a rescue shock of 34 joules. After verifying a second time that this energy successfully converts ventricular fibrillation to sinus rhythm, 12 joules is defined as the estimated DFT.

to whether the estimated safety margin ($E_{ICD} - DFT_{EST}$) truly reflects the actual safety margin ($E_{ICD} - E_{99}$) for the patient. As mentioned, using the standard step-down to failure approach to determine the DFT, it is possible that DFT_{EST} may be localized at the lower extreme (E_{25}) of the probabilistic range (E_{25} to E_{100}) (curve D on Figure 6-87). Thus, it is essential to program the ICD shock energy for ventricular fibrillation high enough above DFT_{EST} in order to guarantee an adequate safety margin even for those patients in which $DFT_{EST} = E_{25}$. Experimental and theoretical studies indicate that if $DFT_{EST} = E_{25}$, the minimum output energy of the ICD device to ensure 99% defibrillation success is 1.7 – 2.0 x DFT_{EST} [60-62,64,65] (Table 6-12.) Consequently, patients with $DFT_{EST} = 15$-J (determined using the step-down protocol) can be safely implanted with an ICD device having a maximum output energy of at least 30-J. As note above, an enhanced DFT protocol (e.g., DFT+ or DFT+) may needed to confirm the DFT_{EST} in cases where the standard DFT protocol using the step-down approach suggests a high DFT and inadequate estimated safety margin using a standard 30–35-J device. Use of the enhanced protocols increases the likelihood that the DFT_{EST} that is finally measured is located high on the defibrillation success curve. This means that the safe energy margins for device implant

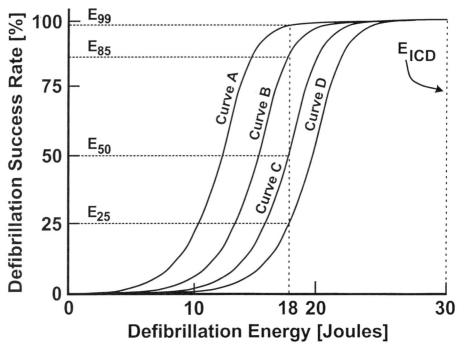

FIGURE 6-87. Hypothetical example illustrating variable location of four defibrillation success curves in four patients all of whom had a DFT_{EST} of 18 J. DFT_{EST} determined using standard step-down defibrillation protocol. Curve A represents a patient where DFT_{EST} is located at E_{99} (the true DFT). However, depending upon the actual position of the defibrillation success curve, the measured DFT_{EST} may be positioned at E_{85} (curve B), E_{50} (curve C), or in the worst case scenario, E_{25} (curve D). The likelihood that DFT_{EST} is near E_{99} increases as the number of successful shocks at this energy also increases (after determining the step-down energy that fails to successfully defibrillate). In order to avoid the necessity of doing repeat fibrillation/defibrillation trials, the DFT_{EST} must be multiplied by a "probability factor" to determine the E_{ICD} necessary to assure an adequate energy safety margin (see Table 6-12.) See text for an additional discussion.

can be smaller: 1.5 x DFT_{EST} using the DFT+ protocol and 1.2 x DFT_{EST} using the DFT++ protocol [61]. Therefore, for a 30-J device, these smaller energy margins would permit successful ICD implantation for patients with DFT_{EST} of 20-J (DFT+ protocol) or DFT_{EST} of 25-J (DFT++ protocol).

Determination of energy safety margins using verification techniques. Verification protocols minimize the number of fibrillation and defibrillation attempts, and consequently, are viewed as more clinically-acceptable than threshold techniques to determine ICD safety margins. During a verification protocol, termination of ventricular fibrillation is attempted with an intermediate energy which, if successful, would provide an adequate safety margin for the patient (given the energy output capabilities of the ICD generator). The most commonly used verification protocols include the *single energy success protocols* (3-shock, 2-shock, and 1-shock protocols), as well as the *step-down success protocol.*

The step-down success (SDS) protocol is very similar to the standard step-down DFT protocol except that by design the fibrillation/defibrillation trials do not continue until a defibrillation attempt is unsuccessful (i.e., there is no intention to determine DFT_{EST}). For example, as seen in Figure 6-85, if further fibrillation/defibrillation attempts are halted after the successful 10-J shock, the 10-J point would provide an estimate of the upper limit of the actual DFT. Therefore, the worst case scenario for the SDS protocol is that the final successful energy level (E_{SDS}) will equal DFT_{EST}. This similarity between the standard DFT protocol and the SDS protocol means that the E_{SDS} has all the characteristics of the DFT_{EST} determined by the standard DFT protocol using decreasing energy steps. Therefore the average location of E_{SDS} on the defibrillation success curve is $\geq E_{71}$ with the worst case position for $E_{SDS} = E_{25}$. Because of these similarities, the energy margins for the SDS protocol are identical those for the standard DFT protocol using decreasing energy steps, i.e., implant if $E_{ICD} \geq 2.0$ x E_{SDS}. To satisfy this implant criterion for a 30-J device, the highest energy for E_{SDS} is 15, with the initial starting energy usually 18–20-J. For a 20-J device, the maximum E_{SDS} should be 10-J with the initial energy one step higher at 13–15-J.

TABLE 6-12. ICD energy margins for commonly used threshold and verification protocols.

Test Protocol	Worst Case Location on Defibrillation Success Curve	Implant if $E_{ICD} \geq$	Maximal Implant Energy with 30-J Device
Standard Step-Down DFT	E_{25}	2.0 x DFT_{EST}	15-J
DFT+	E_{50}	1.5 x DFT_{EST}	20-J
DFT++	E_{75}	1.2 x DFT_{EST}	25-J
Step-Down Success	E_{25}	2.0 x E_{SDS}	15-J
Single Energy 1-Shock	E_5	2.7 x E_{1S}	11-J
Single Energy 2-Shock	E_{40}	2.0 x E_{2S}	15-J
Single Energy 3-Shock	E_{25}	1.7 x E_{3S}	17-J

DFT, defibrillation threshold; E, shock energy; EST, estimated; ICD, implantable cardioverter-defibrillator; S, shock; SDS, step-down success. Adapted from [61,62,66].

The single energy success (SES) protocol is the alternative to the SDS protocol. With an SES protocol, a shock energy is selected and one (1-shock protocol), two (2-shock protocol), or three (3-shock protocol) fibrillation/defibrillation trials are performed. The worst case locations on the defibrillation success curve, and the energy margins required for implant, are summarized in Table 6-12. In each case, all shocks (one, two, or three) at a selected energy must be successful to utilize these protocols. As with any verification protocol, the SES protocols do not localize the defibrillation success curve, but rather merely estimate its upper boundary. The 3-shock SES protocol establishes the upper limit of the DFT with greatest accuracy, while the 1-shock protocol is least accurate, and therefore requires the greatest energy margin ($E_{ICD} - E_{1\text{-Shock}}$) of any threshold or verification protocol (Table 6-12.) For example, for a 30-J device, a single

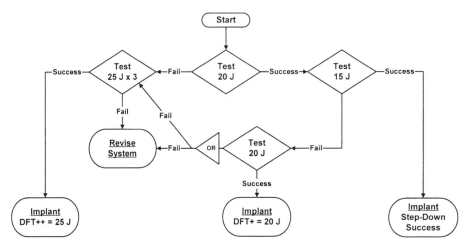

FIGURE 6-88. Flowchart summarizing commonly used defibrillation testing regimen used to evaluate energy margins during ICD implantation procedure. Shown here are both threshold techniques (DFT+ and DFT++) and a step-down success verification protocol. Energies used here are for a device with energy output of at least 30 J. For lower energy devices, testing using the SDS protocol would begin with an energy level one step higher than that equal to 50% of the maximum output. See text for additional discussion. Adapted from [61].

shock of 11-J (2.7 x 11-J = 30-J) must be successful to ensure an adequate safety margin for the patient after implantation.

During an implantation procedure it is often necessary to be flexible and be prepared to use a combination of verification and threshold protocols, although an SDS verification protocol is the first choice of most electrophysiologists. For example, Figure 6-88 summarizes a commonly used defibrillation testing regimen used for ICD devices with a 30–35-J output energy. As seen in this figure, the testing protocol begins with a defibrillation attempt at 20-J. If there is a step-down success with a E_{SDS} of 15-J, implantation can proceed without further testing. If first SDS test at 20-J is successful, but the second test at 15-J fails, then the SDS test becomes equivalent to a standard step-down DFT test with the $DFT_{EST} = 20$-J. Therefore, a repeat defibrillation attempt should be performed at 20-J, and if successful, implant can proceed based upon the DFT+ protocol criterion (Table 6-12.) Finally, if a 20-J shock fails, either initially or as part of a SDS or DFT+ protocol, implantation of a 30-J device can still be accomplished according to the DFT++ protocol if three of three 25-J shocks are successful. If any of the 25-J shocks are unsuccessful (or possibly if the second 20-J shock of the DFT+ protocol fails) the lead system may have to be revised and/or consideration be given to implanting a higher energy device, if available.

Some electrophysiologists have traditionally recommended the "10-J Rule", meaning that two successful shocks at 20-J provides an adequate energy margin for implantation of an ICD with a maximum output of 30-J. However, the above analysis makes clear that there is no experimental or theoretical support for this recommendation (Table 6-12.) An SES protocol performed with a 30-J device would require two successes at 15-J, not 20-J, to provide an adequate safety margin. Two successes at 20-J only meets implant criterion if it is part of a DFT+ protocol (i.e., 20-J success, 15-J failure, 20-J success).

Upper limit of vulnerability and defibrillation threshold
Determination of the upper limit of ventricular vulnerability has been proposed as another method to estimate the DFT using only a small number of fibrillation episodes (possibly one). To fully appreciate this concept it is helpful to understand the phenomenon of the *ventricular vulnerability zone* [67]. The ventricular vulnerability zone corresponds to a portion of ventricular repolarization (T-wave) during which administration of a shock of sufficient magnitude provokes ventricular fibrillation. The ventricular vulnerability zone generally extends from approximately 60 – 80-msec before the peak of the T-wave to approximately 20–30-msec after the T-wave peak. In addition to a time-dependence, the ventricular vulnerability zone also exhibits a shock energy-dependence. If the shock energy is too low or too high, ventricular fibrillation cannot be provoked, even though the shock is delivered well within the time borders of the ventricular vulnerability zone. The time- and voltage-dependence of ventricular vulnerability is best viewed by overlaying it on the ventricular strength-interval curve (Figure 6-89). Delineation of the

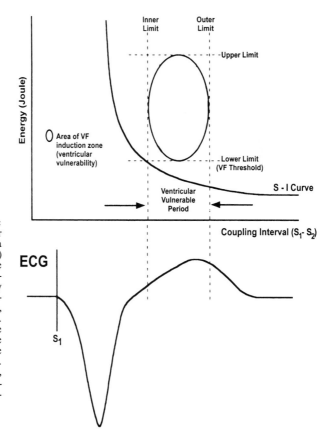

FIGURE 6-89. Schematic illustration of the ventricular vulnerable period and the area of ventricular fibrillation (VF) induction zone. Shown in the upper panel is the strength-interval (S-I) curve overlaid by the zone of ventricular vulnerability defined by the upper, lower, inner, and outer limits. The approximate region of the T-wave that corresponds to the ventricular vulnerability zone is shown in the lower panel. S_1, basic drive stimulus; S_2, premature ventricular stimulus. See text for complete discussion. Adapted from [67].

FIGURE 6-90. Determination of outer limit of ventricular vulnerability. In each panel, ECG lead V_1 and right ventricular endocardial electrogram (IEGM) are displayed. Panel A: Right ventricular fixed rate pacing is performed at a cycle length of 400-msec followed by delivery of a low energy shock (0.8-J) at a coupling interval of 320-msec after the last paced stimulus (shock on T-wave), eliciting two repetitive ventricular depolarizations. Panel B: Same protocol as in panel A, except that the low energy shock coupling interval is reduced from 320-msec to 310-msec, resulting in a non-sustained episode of ventricular fibrillation. Panel C: Same protocol as panels A and B, but shock coupling interval is further reduced to 300-msec, resulting in a sustained episode of ventricular fibrillation. The coupling interval of 300-msec at a pacing cycle length of 400-msec is the outer limit of ventricular vulnerability.

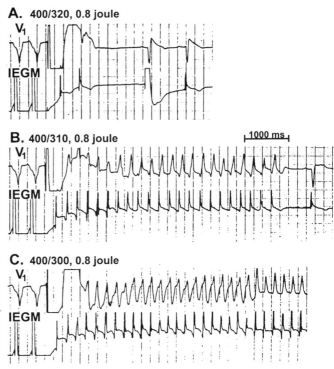

ventricular vulnerability zone requires delivering a series of shocks of different energies at precisely timed intervals during ventricular repolarization. The first stage involves determining the outer and inner borders of the ventricular vulnerable period. Typically, a shock is delivered into the T-wave after a fixed ventricular pacing train of 8–10 stimuli to stabilize the QT interval. The coupling interval between the lasted paced stimulus (S_1) and the ventricular shock (S_2) is sequentially reduced. Using an arbitrary fixed low energy for S_2 (e.g., 0.8-J), as S_1-S_2 is reduced, a critical coupling interval is eventually reached at which ventricular fibrillation is induced (Figure 6-90). With further reductions in the S_1-S_2 coupling interval, fibrillation continues to be provoked until, finally, a coupling interval is reached at which the fixed energy shock fails to provoke fibrillation (Figure 6-91). These outer and inner boundaries for induction of ventricular fibrillation are termed the *outer* and *inner limits of ventricular vulnerable period* (Figure 6-89). This process could be repeated using a higher shock energy to more precisely define the inner and outer limits.

In a similar fashion, the upper and lower boundaries of the ventricular vulnerability zone period also defined. In this case, one can choose a fixed coupling interval (usually a point midway between the inner and outer limits already determined) and then, starting from a high shock energy, deliver shocks of progressively decreasing energy. As the shock energy is reduced, an energy will be reached which provokes ventricular fibrillation (*upper limit of ventricular vulnerability*). As the shock energy is further reduced, fi-

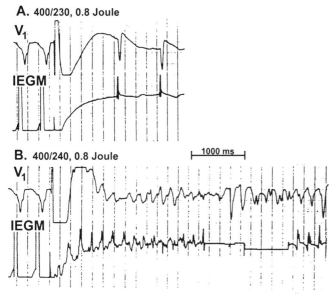

A. 400/230, 0.8 Joule

V_1

IEGM

B. 400/240, 0.8 Joule |⊢ **1000 ms** ⊣|

V_1

IEGM

FIGURE 6-91. Determination of the inner limit of ventricular vulnerability. In each panel, ECG lead V_1 and right ventricular endocardial electrogram (IEGM) are displayed. Panel A: Right ventricular fixed rate pacing is performed at a cycle length of 400-msec followed by delivery of a low energy shock (0.8-J) at a coupling interval of 230-msec after the last paced stimulus (shock on T-wave). This shock elicits no repetitive ventricular activity. Panel B: Same protocol as in panel A, except that the low energy shock coupling interval is increased from 230-msec to 240-msec, resulting in a sustained episode of ventricular fibrillation. The coupling interval of 240-msec at a pacing cycle length of 400-msec is the inner limit of ventricular vulnerability.

brillation will continue to be provoked until eventually a shock energy will be reached that is too small to induce ventricular fibrillation (*lower limit of ventricular vulnerability,* also referred to as the *ventricular fibrillation threshold*). This process could be repeated using different coupling intervals to more precisely define the upper and lower limits (see below).

Experimental studies indicate that there is a correlation between the DFT and the upper limit of ventricular vulnerability [31,32,68-70]. In order to estimate the upper limit of ventricular vulnerability at the time of ICD implantation, an intermediate energy shock (e.g., 10 – 12-J) must be delivered during cardiac repolarization at various coupling intervals (e.g., at the peak of the T-wave, 20-msec after the peak, and 20, 40, and 60-msec before the peak [68,69]. This process is sequentially performed at lower and lower shock energies until ventricular fibrillation is induced (Figure 6-92). The upper limit of ventricular vulnerability is the highest shock energy that triggers ventricular fibrillation. The DFT_{EST} and the upper limit of ventricular vulnerability appear to be well correlated in humans as long as the T-wave shocks are delivered with proper timing [70,71]. The value of the upper limit of ventricular vulnerability is sensitive to the exact placement of the shock on the T-wave [72-74]. Therefore, as with any measurement of DFT_{EST}, the upper limit of vulnerability determination is probabilistic: the shock energy at the upper limit of ventricular vulnerability plus 3-J appears to correspond to E_{90} on the defibrillation success curve, while the upper limit of ventricular vulnerability energy plus 5-J appears to closely approximate E_{99}, (i.e., DFT_{ACT}) [68,69]. Ideally, the DFT can be estimated with a single fibrillation induction, although multiple intermediate and low energy shocks must be delivered before the upper limit of ventricular vulnerability is determined.

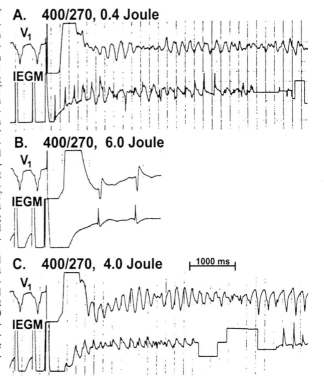

FIGURE 6-92. Determination of the lower and upper limits of ventricular vulnerability. In each panel, ECG lead V$_1$ and right ventricular endocardial electrogram (IEGM) are displayed. Panel A: Right ventricular fixed rate pacing is performed at a cycle length of 400-msec followed by delivery of a low energy shock at the lowest programmable energy (0.4 joule) at a coupling interval of 270-msec after the last paced stimulus (shock on T-wave). An episode of sustained ventricular fibrillation is provoked. Therefore, the lower limit of ventricular vulnerability is ≤ 0.4 joule. The coupling interval of 270-msec is chosen because it is mid-way between the coupling intervals that define the outer and inner limits of ventricular vulnerability (See Figures 6-90 & 6-91). Panel B: Same protocol as in panel A, except that the shock energy is increased to 6.0 joules. No ventricular fibrillation is induced. Panel C: Same protocol as panels B, but shock energy is reduced to 4.0 joules. Using this energy, a sustained episode of ventricular fibrillation is induced. Therefore, the upper limit of ventricular vulnerability is approximately 4.0 joules.

Effect of pulse waveform and polarity on defibrillation threshold

Damped sinusoidal waveforms, generated by capacitor discharge through a series inductor and the body's resistance, have become the waveform used by most portable external defibrillators. However, because of their size requirements, they cannot be used for implantable internal defibrillators. Initial work on implantable defibrillators focused on monophasic truncated pulses that avoided the re-fibrillating effects of a non-truncated capacitor discharge. Biphasic truncated exponential waveforms were introduced and found to defibrillate with lower energy requirements than monophasic pulses [75-78].

The traditional preferred polarity for endocardial lead systems had the right ventricular coil as the cathode (negative). This may have been based upon the early pacemaker experience which suggested that cathodal stimulation was less likely to trigger fibrillation. There is conflicting data concerning the effects of polarity on the DFT. Some investigators have found no statistical difference between DFTs obtained using the standard polarity (cathode at right ventricular apex) compared with the reverse polarity (anode at right ventricular apex) [78-81]. However, other researchers have shown that making the right ventricular coil as the anode actually reduces the DFT [82-84]. Regardless of the statistical validity, it is clear that in individual patients polarity changes may have a significant effect on the DFT.

Effects of antiarrhythmic drugs on defibrillation threshold

Since antiarrhythmic drugs are used as adjunctive therapy for patients with ICDs, especially to minimize therapeutic shocks or antitachycardia pacing (see "Drug Therapy in Patients with ICDs" on page 402), knowledge of their potential effects on the DFT and safety margin is important. In general, potent Na^+ channel blocking agents, such as class IC drugs, appear to increase the DFT [85-87], although propafenone in moderate doses appears to have little effect [88]. Less potent Na^+ channel blocking agents (class IA or IB), including procainamide, quinidine, lidocaine, and mexiletine, appear to have little or no effect on the ventricular threshold [89-96]. The class III agents sotalol and *N*-acetyl-procainamide (NAPA), which block membrane K^+ channels, appear to decrease the DFT [90,97,98]. The class III agent amiodarone, which is commonly used to control the frequency of tachyarrhythmia episodes in patients with ICDs, appears to decrease the DFT acutely [99-102], but increases the DFT after chronic administration [92,100,103]. It should be noted that most of the studies evaluating the effect of antiarrhythmic drugs on DFT were performed using monophasic shocks; it is likely that results will be quantitatively similar for biphasic waveforms.

Management of the patients with a high defibrillation threshold

The true incidence of high DFTs preventing implantation with an adequate (or any safety margin) is unknown but may range from 0.4–4.6% [102,104]. When confronted with a patient with an excessively high DFT, there are a number of maneuvers that may lower the threshold. The simplest options (if available) include: reversing the shock polarity, changing pulse duration or tilt (see "Defibrillation Parameters" on page 293), or switching from a monophasic to a biphasic pulse (or even *vice versa* [105]). While most devices provide the programmability to change polarity, the ability to alter the tilt or pulse duration is less common. Repositioning the endocardial lead deeper into the right ventricular apex so as to maximize the defibrillating electrical field to the cardiac mass also may lower the DFT. Beyond these maneuvers, further reductions in DFT may be achieved by adding an additional lead to the system, such as a subcutaneous patch or epicostal array lead. Switching to a pulse generator with a higher stored energy may also be an option. However, higher energy devices with larger capacitors and longer pulse durations (or different tilt) may actually deliver a lower effective defibrillating current (I_{EFF}) than the smaller, lower energy device, as already discussed (see "Defibrillation Parameters" on page 293). Finally, discontinue of antiarrhythmic drugs, such as class IC agents or amiodarone, may result in lower DFTs. Some patients with a a very high DFT may be candidates for thoracotomy and implantation of an ICD system using epicardial leads. Despite all attempts to optimize the DFT, there may still be a very few patients that continue to have inadequate energy safety margins. Even in those patients with $DFT_{EST} > 25$-J, implantation of ICD system is still supported by some data [102]. The rationale used to support this practice include the fact that some patients may present clinically with rapid, life-threatening monomorphic ventricular tachycardia, as opposed to ventricular fibrillation. Therefore, a shock that may not terminate ventricular fibrillation may nevertheless terminate monomorphic ventricular tachycardia, thereby preventing a sudden arrhythmic death resulting from the degradation of the ventricular tachycardia into ventricular fibrillation. In addition, even if DFT$_{EST}$ is > 25-J, this does not mean that defibrillation will fail 100% of the time even with an output of only 25-J. Finally, the ICD is capable of delivering multiple shocks (e.g., usually 4 or 5) during each episode of a ventricular fibrillation; subsequent shocks may terminate the arrhythmia even if the first shock is unsuccessful. Therefore, device implantation in these patients may provide better protection than would otherwise be predicted by standard DFT analysis.

6.8 Clinical Follow-up and Troubleshooting of ICD Systems

The implantation of an ICD is actually only the initial step in the management of the patient with medically-refractory ventricular tachyarrhythmias. The ICD fails to address the ongoing problems that face the patient, including new or progressive ischemia, worsening left ventricular function, electrolyte disorders, etc. All these, and other factors (Figure 6-93), may effect the patient's propensity to the development of recurrent ventricular tachycardia or ventricular fibrillation, frequency of shocks or hospitalizations, and can compromise quality of life.

In general, there are two types of clinical follow-up of patients with ICDs: 1) chronic surveillance to assess and document routine device operation, as well as the clinical progress of a largely asymptomatic patient, and 2) acute unexpected evaluations prompted by patient concerns, symptoms, delivery of ICD therapy, unsuccessful therapy, or presumed failure to deliver expected therapy. Chronic follow-up, usually performed in the office or clinic, is typically a stereotyped procedure that may often be performed by well-trained nursing personnel. On the other hand, acute evaluations may be performed in the office, emergency room, or inpatient setting. These evaluations are designed to answer two basic questions: *what did the device do and why did it do it?* Consequently, acute

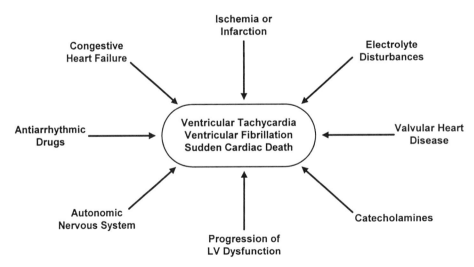

FIGURE 6-93. Clinical and physiological factors affecting the development, incidence, and frequency of ventricular tachyarrhythmias. LV, left ventricular.

evaluations often require detective work by the clinician in order to determine if device function was clinically appropriate or inappropriate and, if so, establish whether the device is malfunctioning and define the precise etiology. Troubleshooting suspicious device function has become immensely simpler thanks to the real-time and stored event, marker, and electrogram data available in modern devices. Unlike chronic follow-up visits, acute evaluations may often result in further diagnostic tests, or changes in therapy, including device reprogramming or alterations in the medical regimen.

6.8.1 ROUTINE CLINICAL FOLLOW-UP

A scheduled outpatient follow-up visit every three to four months provides the opportunity to assess the patient, the ICD device, the underlying cardiac disease, and patient-device, drug-device, and possible ICD-pacemaker interactions. The basic components of follow-up in patients with ICD systems are summarized in Table 6-13.

TABLE 6-13. Overview of ICD outpatient follow-up

Patient's clinical status and interval history of shocks/therapies/symptoms

    Cardiac review of systems

    Symptoms: e.g., palpitations, syncope, near-syncope

    Reports of shocks or episodes of antitachycardia pacing

Focused clinical exam (if indicated)

Device interrogation and analysis

    Document and review current programmed settings, including "on/off" status (mandatory)

    Evaluate sensing function with marker telemetry and document under- or oversensing (mandatory)

    Measure R-wave (and P-wave, if indicated) amplitude (mandatory)

    Document and review pace/sense & shocking (if available) impedances (mandatory)

    Document new tachyarrhythmia episodes/therapies; determine type & cause of arrhythmia (mandatory)

    Reform capacitor (mandatory if not done automatically)

    Determination of pacing threshold(s) (not mandatory at every visit)

    Generate final printout documenting interrogation results, stored & real-time data and programming changes (mandatory)

Formulate final assessment regarding patient's cardiac status, arrhythmia, and device function

Treatment plan &/or further evaluation

    ICD reprogramming (if indicated)

    Diagnostic interventions (Holter, ECG, echocardiogram, etc., if indicated)

    Changes/additions to general cardiac or non-cardiac medications (if indicated)

    Changes/additions to antiarrhythmic drug regimen

6.8.2 ACUTE PATIENT EVALUATION AND ICD TROUBLESHOOTING

Common clinical problems encountered in patients with ICD systems are summarized in Table 6-14.

TABLE 6-14. Classification of clinical problems encountered during ICD follow-up

---

ICD therapy (possibly "excessive") in asymptomatic or minimally symptomatic patients

Delayed or absent ICD therapy in patients with documented VT/VF

Unsuccessful ICD therapy in patients with documented VT/VF

Failure to deliver ICD therapy in patients with symptoms consistent with an episode of tachyarrhythmia

Psychological, interpersonal, or family problems related to ICD therapies (or risk for therapies)

VF, ventricular fibrillation; VT, ventricular tachycardia. Adapted from [106].

ICD therapy in asymptomatic or minimally symptomatic patients
Not uncommonly, ICD therapies may be delivered to asymptomatic, minimally symptomatic, and conscious patients. The development of frank syncope prior to an ICD shock occurs in less than 20% of patients [107,108]. As many as 40% of patients will be entirely symptom-free immediately prior to an ICD discharge [109,110]. Frequent shocks can be an especially bothersome problem in occasional patients. The definition of "frequent" is hard to define, with some patients bothered less by shocks than other patients. In addition, a sudden change in a patient's pattern of shocks, particularly a clustering of shocks in a short period of time, is of concern. For example, a patient who has had defibrillator for three years and never had any shocks but suddenly experiences three shocks over a 10 day period has clearly had a change in the therapy pattern and this change warrants investigation.

In general, the electrophysiologist should try to explain the reason for every shock received by a patient, especially since as many as 30% of ICD shocks may be unnecessary [111-116]. In particular, patients with "frequent" shocks should be evaluated to determine if the shocks are *clinically appropriate* or *inappropriate* (Table 6-15.) A clinically appropriate therapy is one delivered for the target arrhythmia after satisfaction of all programmed detection criteria (including rate, onset, stability, morphology, etc.). The major appropriate cause of ICD therapy in the conscious patient is hemodynamically tolerated ventricular tachycardia. Less frequently, fast ventricular tachycardia or even ventricular fibrillation may be detected and terminated by the device so quickly that the patient experiences minimal prodromal symptoms.

TABLE 6-15. Causes of ICD therapies in asymptomatic or minimally symptomatic patients

---

Clinically appropriate

    Hemodynamically tolerated, monomorphic sustained VT

    Rapidly detected and terminated fast VT or VF

Clinically inappropriate

    SVTs (AVNRT, AVRT, AF, AFL, AT)

    Nonsustained VT or SVT in patients with committed therapy

    Oversensing of non-R-wave signals

        T-wave or P-wave oversensing

        Lead or adapter conductor fractures ("make or break" potentials)

        Lead or adapter insulation failures

        Loose setscrew connections

        Sensing of pacemaker stimulus artifacts

        Oversensing due to automatic gain control [117]

    Oversensing of external signals (electrocautery, electromagnetic interference (EMI))

AF, atrial fibrillation; AFL, atrial flutter; AT, atrial tachycardia; AVNRT, atrioventricular nodal reentrant tachycardia; AVRT, atrioventricular reciprocating tachycardia; SVT, supraventricular tachycardia; VT, ventricular tachycardia; VF ventricular fibrillation. Adapted from [106].

However, the mere occurrence of a shock does not prove that the patient had an episode of ventricular tachycardia or ventricular fibrillation. The differential diagnosis of ICD therapy (that is not due to sustained ventricular tachycardia or fibrillation) in conscious or minimally symptomatic patients include: 1) non-sustained ventricular tachycardia, especially when using committed therapy zones; 2) supraventricular tachycardia that satisfies the programmed detection criteria, especially when employing a tachycardia zone with a low rate cut-off or if rate-only detection algorithms are utilized; 3) detection of unwanted cardiac signals, including T-waves (Figures 6-94 & 6-95), or possibly P-waves, by the ventricular channel resulting in "double counting"; 4) detection of signals from a separate permanent pacemaker system; and 5) detection of non-cardiac signals, including lead fractures (Figure 6-96), insulation breaks, myopotentials, loose connections within the connector block, or electromagnetic interference (Table 6-16.)

TABLE 6-16. Possible sources of interference or EMI that may affect ICD function

Medical

    Electrosurgical equipment

    Magnetic resonance imaging systems

    Therapeutic diathermy

    Pacemaker programming [118]

    Lithotripsy

Non-Medical

    Arc welding equipment

    Robotic jacks

    Strong electrical & magnetic fields (industrial transformers, motors) [119]

    Automobile alternators/magnetos

    Electrical smelting furnaces

    Large radiofrequency transmitters (e.g., radar)

    Large stereo speakers [120]

    Radiofrequency remote control devices [121]

    Slot machines [122]

    Cellular phones [123-127]

    Store security systems [128,129]

    Magnetic wands (e.g., "bingo wands") [130]

EMI, electromagnetic interference

In order to distinguish between appropriate and inappropriate shocks, as well as determine the precise cause of inappropriate shocks, the physician must perform a systematic evaluation, by obtaining a history, analyzing real-time and stored data from the device and, if necessary, pursuing additional diagnostic tests (Table 6-17.) The physician should determine if the therapy episodes are preceded by symptoms such as palpitations, dizziness, near-syncope, syncope, chest discomfort, or shortness breath. Prodromal symptoms strongly suggest that the shock is delivered in response to a tachyarrhythmia, although not necessarily for ventricular tachycardia. The absence of a prodrome, however, does not necessarily rule-out an appropriate shock.

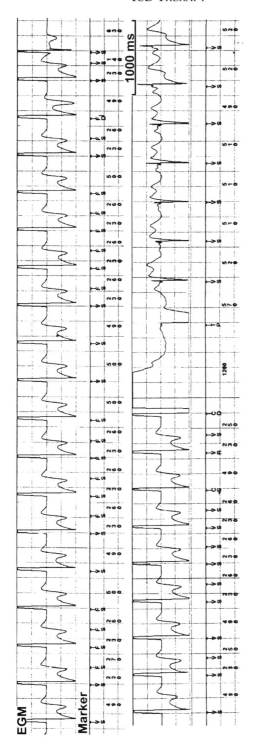

FIGURE 6-94. Oversensing of T-waves during slow ventricular tachycardia. Ventricular tachycardia develops at a rate of approximately 120 beats/min. However, this slow tachycardia is detected as ventricular fibrillation due to oversensing of T-waves ("double-counting"). Therefore, instead of antitachycardia pacing being delivered to treat the slow ventricular tachycardia, fibrillation therapy is delivered (25-J shock), terminating the ventricular tachyarrhythmia. T-wave oversensing can be eliminated by increasing the ventricular sensitivity setting from 0.3-msec to 0.45-msec. CE, end of charge; CD, delivery of cardioversion/defibrillation charge; FD, fibrillation detection; FS, fibrillation sense; TP, tachycardia pace; VR, ventricular sense during refractory period; VS, ventricular sense

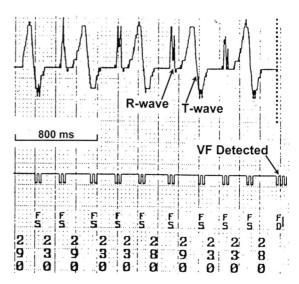

FIGURE 6-95. Stored episode record for an inappropriate Ventricular fibrillation (VF) detection due to T-wave oversensing. During sinus rhythm, R-wave amplitude was only 2-mV whereas T-wave amplitude are abnormally large with high slew rates. Courtesy of Medtronic.

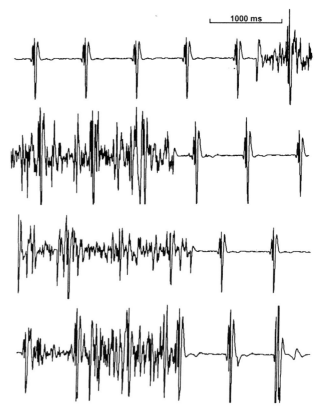

FIGURE 6-96. Real-time Intracardiac ventricular electrogram recording from a patient with an epicardial sensing lead and inappropriate ICD shocks. Not the prominent high frequency electrical noise detected by the sensing circuit consistent with an insulation break. Inspection of the sensing leads at the time of surgery showed cracked and missing insulation.

TABLE 6-17. Approach to the patient with possible ICD system malfunction

Chest x-ray

    Evaluate lead position and for possible signs of lead fracture

Device interrogation

    Real time measurements (battery status, pacing lead impedance, EGM amplitudes)

    Review of programmed ventricular (and atrial, if any) detection criteria

    Review of programmed ventricular (and atrial, if any) therapies

    Review of diagnostic data (events, delivered therapies, shocking lead impedance)

    Review of R-R interval and stored EGM data during tachycardia episodes, including comparison of EGM morphology during tachycardia compared with morphology during SR

When sensing or detection malfunction is suspected (causing inappropriate, delayed or no therapy delivery)

    Evaluate marker telemetry, "beep-o-gram", real-time EGM recordings

    Assess for sensing of T-waves or pacing stimuli

    Assess for under- or oversensing during device/lead manipulation (real-time markers, EGMs)

    Reassessment of sensing function after VT/VF induction

    Reassessment of programmed detection criteria for VT

    Evaluate possibly of device-device interactions in patients with separate pacemakers & ICDs

    Assess for undersensing of VT/VF re-detection after a failed high energy shock

When primary failure of delivered therapy is suspected

    If ATP programmed, revaluate pacing threshold

    If ATP or LEC programmed, reassess ATP, CER, and DFT during VT/VF

    Consider other contributing factors such as concomitant AAD therapy or change in cardiac substrate

AAD, antiarrhythmic drugs; ATP, antitachycardia pacing; CER, cardioversion energy requirement; DFT, defibrillation threshold; EGM, electrogram, LEC, low energy cardioversion; SR, sinus rhythm. Adapted from [106].

Devices capable of real-time telemetry should be fully interrogated to determine impedance of the rate sensing lead as a clue for a lead fracture (high impedance) or lead insulation failure (low impedance), either of which can cause oversensing of non-cardiac signals. The most common way to assess for the presence of oversensing is by evaluating marker telemetry data. The marker data indicates how the device interprets sensed events or intervals (Figures 6-19 & 6-20). To rule out spurious, non-tachycardia-related signals (e.g., myopotentials, T-waves, pacing stimulus artifacts) as the cause of unexpected therapies, it is helpful to record real-time marker data while the patient is performing activities or postural changes that provoke the therapy episodes. The provocation of over-sensing by the device while performing these maneuvers is diagnostic of a sensing lead malfunction, usually a failure of the insulation or "make-or-break" potentials associated with a conductor fracture. In some devices, sensing can also be evaluated by magnet application triggering audible beep tones every time an event is sensed. Correlation of these beeps with simultaneous ECG recording and provocative maneuvers may demonstrate oversensing. It is important to realize that lead problems may manifest themselves only sporadically. Therefore, a high degree of suspicion and investment of effort by the clinician may be necessary to document the specific malfunction. However, this effort must be made because most *lead malfunctions require an immediate remedy*. This may merely entail programming changes, such as changing sensitivity or refractory periods in the case of T-wave sensing, or surgical intervention in the case of loose setscrew connections or insulation/conductor failures. Without a functional lead system there is significant risk that the ICD will not perform as required at the time of a life-threatening ventricular tachyarrhythmia, or may deliver unnecessary and potentially proarrhythmic therapies.

TABLE 6-18. Causes of absent or delayed effective ICD therapy in patients with documented VT or VF

Inactivated ICD

Undersensing of ventricular EGMs

    Diminution of sensed ventricular EGM amplitude at lead-tissue interface

    Low amplitude ventricular EGM after a failed high energy discharge

    Marked fluctuation in EGM amplitude in ICD with automatic gain control

    Lead malfunction or displacement

    Generator malfunction

Underdetection

    Inappropriately high programmed rate cutoff for VT/VF

    Failure to satisfy multiple detection criteria

    Tachycardia rates at or near VT/VF detection interval in ICDs with multiple programmable tachycardia detection zones

Ineffective antitachycardia pacing algorithms or extremely low energy shocks for VT

Delayed VF or VT detection due to sensing of large amplitude pacing stimuli or noise reversion in patients with permanent pacing systems

---

EGM, electrogram; VF, ventricular fibrillation; VT, ventricular tachycardia. Adapted from [106].

Delayed or absent ICD therapy in patients with documented tachyarrhythmias
On occasion, patients with documented ventricular tachycardia or fibrillation will either have no therapy administered or there will be a delay in the delivery of therapy (Table 6-18.) The causes for this phenomenon include: 1) accidental failure to activate the device; 2) undersensing due to physiological and non-physiological causes (Figure 6-97); 3) underdetection (despite normal sensing) due to inappropriate programming relative to the patient's clinical arrhythmias; 4) programming initial ineffective therapies, delaying delivery of more effective therapies; and 5) ICD-pacemaker interactions with oversensing of pacemaker stimuli by the ICD. Undersensing by the ICD may be due to ICD failure or deterioration of the sensed signal at the interface of the rate sensing electrode and the cardiac tissue. When consecutive counting algorithms are utilized, transient undersensing of R-R intervals can result in resetting to zero a detection counter, thereby delaying

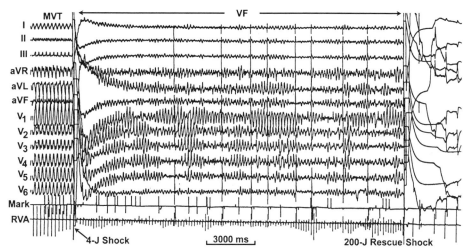

FIGURE 6-97. Example of ICD shock-related proarrhythmia and post-shock undersensing of shock-induced ventricular fibrillation (VF). Displayed from top-to-bottom is a a continuous 12-lead ECG, the ICD marker channel (Mark), and an endocardial electrogram recorded from the right ventricular apex RVA) using a separate temporary transvenous electrode catheter. Monomorphic ventricular tachycardia (MVT) is induced (far left side) at a cycle length of 225-msec. After satisfying detection criterion, a low energy shock (4-J) is delivered by the device. Instead of terminating the arrhythmia, the shock converts the MVT to VF. Note on the Mark recording that the device only sporadically senses the VF, resulting in the failure to meet detection criterion for delivery of tachyarrhythmia therapy. Consequently the device fails to deliver life-saving therapy. The patient is rescued with a external transthoracic shock (200-J). This scenario would likely have resulted in the death of the patient had it occurred clinically. Caution must be exercised in programming low energy cardioversion to avoid dangerous proarrhythmia.

(or preventing) the delivery of therapy. Conductor fracture or insulation break is a common cause of sensing failure.

Unsuccessful ICD therapy in patients with documented tachyarrhythmias
The most serious problem encountered during ICD follow-up is failure of the device to successfully terminate ventricular tachycardia or fibrillation, possibly necessitating emergency resuscitation measures or even leading to demise of the patient (Table 6-19.) Potential causes for this include: 1) battery depletion (usually due to inadequate clinical follow-up); 2) inadequate energy safety margins for defibrillation (high DFT); 3) programming ineffective antitachycardia pacing algorithms or low energy shock therapies; 4) failure or malfunction of a component of the ICD hardware or software.

The terminal events were analyzed in 51 patients with first-generation ICD systems who died suddenly (30 of the patients were monitored at the time of death) [131]. Two thirds of monitored episodes demonstrated ventricular tachycardia or fibrillation as the initial rhythm. Of the patients with documented or presumed death due to a tachyarrhythmia (based on witnessed shocks), 41% had active, non-depleted devices with DFTs ≤ 20-J (monophasic waveform), although possible contributory factors were noted in over half of these patients. Of note, battery depletion was present in 15% of the patients with documented or presumed death due to a tachyarrhythmia, confirming the importance of routine follow-up to assess battery reserve.

ICD therapy, which had previously been found to be effective, may lose its efficacy during long-term follow-up. Antitachycardia pacing may become ineffective due to increases in pacing threshold in the chronic setting [132] or lead fracture. Migration, wrinkling, or folding of epicardial or subcutaneous patch electrodes may significantly increase the DFT.

TABLE 6-19. Causes of failed ICD therapy in patients with documented VT or VF

Battery depletion
High defibrillation threshold
Dislodgment of transvenous defibrillator leads
Alteration of the contour of epicardial defibrillating patches
Drug-induced increase in defibrillation threshold
Spontaneous time-dependent change in defibrillation threshold
Ineffective antitachycardia pacing algorithms or extremely low energy shocks for VT
ICD component failure resulting in absent or inadequate pacing or shock therapy

VT, ventricular tachycardia; VF ventricular fibrillation. Adapted from [106].

Epicardial or extra-pericardial patches that come in contact with each other may cause current to be shunted away from the myocardium, leading to ineffective high energy discharges. Dislodgment or migration of transvenous defibrillating electrodes may also lead to ineffective defibrillation. With both epicardial and transvenous systems, defibrillating lead fracture can lead to unsuccessful cardioversion or defibrillation attempts [133].

Occasionally, antiarrhythmic drugs may result in the development of incessant ventricular tachycardia. Therefore, therapy may result only in transient termination of ventricular tachycardia with antitachycardia pacing. Although DFTs in epicardial systems have a tendency to remain stable [134], DFTs may rise during follow-up in transvenous systems [135]; this is not usually clinically significant, especially since the development and implementation of biphasic waveforms.

Antiarrhythmic medications such as amiodarone and class IA and IC agents may also raise the DFTs to unacceptable values [94,101,136,137]. Failure of initially effective programmed values for high energy shocks to treat ventricular fibrillation may also occur in patients with low safety margins [102,138]. The presence of concomitant conditions such as myocardial infarction or ischemia, drug-induced torsade de pointes, or electrolyte abnormalities, may produce ventricular arrhythmias refractory to therapy that had previously been shown to be effective.

Patients with documented failure of high energy shocks to terminate ventricular tachycardia or fibrillation will require re-evaluation of ICD function if battery depletion has been ruled-out. The shocking lead impedance registered at the time of the last shock should be carefully checked. Any increase in impedance should raise questions as to the integrity and position of the lead systems. A chest x-ray should be obtained to assess lead position and contour of epicardial patches. Ventricular tachycardia and ventricular fibrillation should be induced in the electrophysiology laboratory and the DFT reassessed. Impedance during shocks should be checked and compared to prior measurements, including those obtained at the time of implantation.

If the DFT is high, medications known to raise the threshold should be discontinued if possible. For patients with transvenous systems, an evaluation for possible lead dislodgment or migration should be performed, as even small changes in position may effect defibrillation efficacy. Occasionally, patients with marginal DFTs may benefit by programming the use of another current pathway, or changing polarity of the current vector. This may involve revision of the system, possibly with the addition of other leads or subcutaneous patch electrodes.

Symptoms of a tachyarrhythmia without delivery of ICD therapy
Patients with known ventricular tachycardia or ventricular fibrillation may develop symptoms (e.g. palpitations, near-syncope, or syncope) suggestive of arrhythmia, but without shock delivery (Table 6-20.) In most instances, this does not represent ICD malfunction. Such a phenomenon may result from supraventricular or ventricular arrhythmias with either too slow a rate or too short a duration to satisfy detection criteria. These occurrences are more likely with non-committed therapies (Figure 6-31) in which a "second look" is performed after capacitor charging to establish that the arrhythmia continues before committing to delivery of the charge. Hemodynamically tolerated ventricular tachycardia may initiate antitachycardia pacing and tachycardia termination with only a minimum of symptoms. Similarly, antitachycardia pacing may be successful in terminating ventricular tachycardia associated with syncope without obvious ICD function (i.e. high energy shock delivery) being evident to the patient or witnesses. Inappropriate antitachycardia pacing (e.g for a supraventricular tachycardia) also may mimic symptoms of a spontaneous tachyarrhythmia. Malfunction of the ICD system should also be considered in this setting. As previously discussed, undersensing or underdetection of a sustained ventricular tachycardia may cause the device to ignore a tachyarrhythmia that otherwise should have been detected and treated. ICD failure due to battery depletion or component failure may also cause the same phenomenon.

TABLE 6-20. Causes of symptoms suggesting VT or VF without noticed therapy

Non-sustained VT or SVT not satisfying detection criteria
Hemodynamically tolerated VT terminated with antitachycardia pacing
Undersensing of VT
Oversensing of non-R-wave signals or SVTs triggering symptomatic antitachycardia pacing

SVT, supraventricular tachycardia; VT, ventricular tachycardia; VF ventricular fibrillation. From [106].

Psychological, interpersonal, or family problems related to ICD therapy
A small minority of patients may have psychological, interpersonal, marital, or family problems develop after implantation of the ICD system. This is especially true if the patient has frequent shocks (appropriate or inappropriate), develops feelings that he/she has

lost independence secondary to the illness and cardiac condition, or resents the "hovering" or "mothering" coming from family members or loved ones. Sensitivity to these issues and early referral to social workers, counselors, support groups, psychologists, or psychiatrists is sometimes warranted.

6.8.3 SUDDEN ARRHYTHMIC DEATH DESPITE ICD THERAPY

Despite the best efforts of physicians and the engineering expertise of device manufacturers, patients with ICD systems may still die because of a ventricular tachyarrhythmia. In all these cases, exhaustive efforts must be made to identify the cause of the failure of ICD therapy so as to avoid future recurrences. Potential causes of tachyarrhythmic death in patients with ICD systems are summarized in Table 6-21.

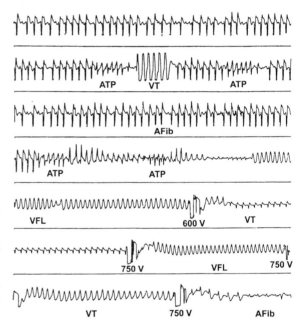

FIGURE 6-98. Clinically inappropriate delivery of ICD therapy during atrial fibrillation with a rapid ventricular response. Continuous ambulatory ECG recording (V_1) shows initiation of antitachycardia pacing (ATP) because the ventricular rate during the atrial fibrillation (AFib) is > the ventricular tachycardia (VT) detection rate. This results in one episode of nonsustained VT and then polymorphic VT degenerating into ventricular flutter (VFL). The VFL is terminated only after four ICD shocks. From [140] with permission.

6.8.4 ICD PROARRHYTHMIA

Potential causes of ICD-induced proarrhythmia are summarized in Table 6-22. Low or high energy shocks, antitachycardia pacing, or even antibradycardia pacing may rarely provoke tachyarrhythmias (Figures 6-73, 6-98, 6-99, 6-100 & 6-101). Most ominous is therapy-induced acceleration of ventricular tachyarrhythmias. Fortunately, this situation develops rarely.

TABLE 6-21. Summary of possible causes of sudden arrhythmic death in patients with ICD systems

Device inactivated

Intentionally (e.g., to avoid shocks)

Accidentally (e.g., strong magnetic field at home or work)

Erroneously

Sensing or detection failure

Low R-wave amplitude

Intrinsic from time of implant

Chronic attenuation

New local scar

Dynamic

Erroneous assumption of conversion to sinus rhythm (despite persistence of VT or VF) due to pseudo-long R-R intervals resulting from signal dropout or automatic gain control-related undersensing

Post shock, especially in ICD system with transvenous integrated sensing/defibrillation lead

Drug/electrolyte effect

Sensing lead dislodgment

Sensing lead fracture

Loose connection of sensing lead to ICD generator

Pacemaker stimulus artifact sensed during VF, and inhibiting tachyarrhythmia detection by ICD

Programming-related problem

Tachycardia rate cutoff zones set too high, resulting in under- or non-detection

Lower rate tachycardia zone set too close to VT rate, periodically resetting interval counter during VT thereby preventing attainment of minimum number of intervals for satisfying tachycardia detection

Fast VT with cycle length oscillating between VF and VT zones, markedly delaying declaration of tachyarrhythmia by certain algorithms*

Threshold voltage for sensing set higher than actual R-wave voltage (i.e., inappropriate sensitivity)

ICD sensing circuit (i.e., electronic) malfunction

VT or VF rates sensed, but ICD therapy not delivered

Battery depletion

Expected

Elective Replacement Indicator known to be attained, but generator not yet replaced

Not appreciated prior to death (e.g., patient lost to follow-up, excessive recent utilization secondary to SVT or VT/VF storm, etc.)

Premature (e.g., battery failure, excessive current leakage, etc.)

Programming-related problem (e.g., therapy delivery held back by erroneous assumption of SVT on the basis of enhancement criteria for tachycardia discrimination)

*Protracted time in VT or VF (due to prolonged detection time or delivery of initially ineffective therapies) may secondarily cause failure of otherwise effective electrical therapy or predispose to post-shock asystole or electromechanical dissociation, especially in patients with very poor left ventricular function. Abbreviations: ATP, antitachycardia pacing; DFT, defibrillation threshold; SVT, supraventricular tachycardia; VF, ventricular fibrillation; VT, ventricular tachycardia. Adapted from [139]

TABLE 6-21. Summary of possible causes of sudden arrhythmic death in patients with ICD systems

Failure to detect true conversion to normal rate rhythm between successive rapid VT or VF episodes which are reinitiated by recurring salvos of post-conversion non-sustained VT, with eventual automatic deactivation of VF therapy (ICD interprets independent VF episodes occurring in rapid succession as a "single event", with consecutive defibrillation failures leading to exhaustion of fixed allotment of (typically 4-6) shocks for such an "event")

ICD circuitry (i.e., electronic) malfunction

Loose connection between generator and antitachycardia pacing or defibrillation leads

Fracture of lead(s) for antitachycardia pacing or defibrillation

Dislodgment of antitachycardia pacing or defibrillation lead(s)

ICD therapy delivered, but patient not resuscitated

Antitachycardia pacing (ATP)

VT/VF "storm"

Incessant "pacing/shock resistant" VT (drug-related proarrhythmia)

Conversion to slower VT with reversion (in some devices) to the treatment algorithm of the low rate zone, thereby delaying prompt shock therapy*

Programming-related problem (i.e., inadequate or inappropriate type of ATP specified, or inappropriately high setting for upper limit of "low" rate ("VT") zone, leading to use of ineffective therapy for very fast, poorly-tolerated VT (or VF))*

Conversion of VT to VF in a patient with marginal DFT

Failure of pacing stimuli to capture

High pacing threshold

Since implantation

Subsequent to implantation (e.g., new scar, drugs, etc.)

Inappropriate programmed pacing stimulation parameters

Inappropriate type of ATP due to circuitry (i.e., electronic) malfunction

DC shock

VT/VF storm or incessant VT

Elevated DFT

Since implantation

Time dependent phenomenon (related to electrode-tissue interface)

Local anatomic resistive barrier (e.g., hematoma under epicardial patch electrode)

Transient (e.g., drug-related)

Subacute or chronic (adverse) change in underlying myocardial substrate

Shock-induced conversion of VT to VF in a patient with marginal or elevated DFT*

Inappropriately low shock energy*

Programming-related

ICD circuitry malfunction

Post-shock electromechanical dissociation or asystole (possibly with failure to capture during backup VVI pacing (due to shock itself or metabolically induced elevated pacing threshold))

*Protracted time in VT or VF (due to prolonged detection time or delivery of initially ineffective therapies) may secondarily cause failure of otherwise effective electrical therapy or predispose to post-shock asystole or electromechanical dissociation, especially in patients with very poor left ventricular function. Abbreviations: ATP, antitachycardia pacing; DFT, defibrillation threshold; SVT, supraventricular tachycardia; VF, ventricular fibrillation; VT, ventricular tachycardia. Adapted from [139]

TABLE 6-22.   Potential ICD-induced proarrhythmia

ICD-induced Tachyarrhythmias

   Clinically appropriate therapies

      Acceleration or degeneration of ventricular tachycardia

         Antitachycardia pacing

         Cardioversion shocks

      Deceleration of ventricular tachycardia

         Antitachycardia pacing

         Cardioversion shocks

      Induction of supraventricular tachyarrhythmias

         Cardioversion or defibrillation shocks

   Clinically inappropriate therapies

      Antitachycardia therapies (antitachycardia pacing, cardioversion or defibrillation shocks)

         Failure to discriminate between supraventricular and ventricular tachyarrhythmias

         Committed behavior for non-sustained ventricular arrhythmias

         Signal oversensing

            Electronic noise

            T waves

            Pacing stimulation artifacts

            Electromagnetic interference

         Antibradycardia pacing

         Undersensing of spontaneous beats

ICD-induced Bradyarrhythmias

   Post-shock bradyarrhythmias

   Post-shock increase in pacing threshold leading to non-capture

   Post-shock reset of a separate pacemaker

   Inhibition of antibradycardia pacing due to T wave oversensing

---

Adapted from Pinski, 1995 #5106]

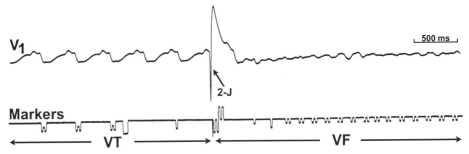

FIGURE 6-99. Degeneration of monomorphic ventricular tachycardia (VT) to ventricular fibrillation (VF) by a low energy (2-J) shock.

6.8.5 Drug Therapy in Patients with ICDs

Currently, when a patient receives an ICD for treatment of a ventricular tachycardia or fibrillation, it is the general intent and hope of the electrophysiologist that the device will provide all the necessary antiarrhythmic therapies the patient may need. In most cases, patients are implanted with an ICD in lieu of receiving antiarrhythmic drug therapy be-

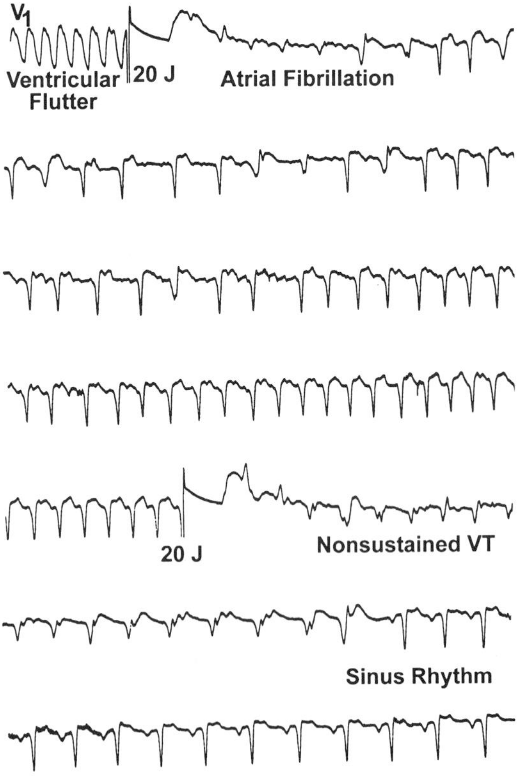

FIGURE 6-100. Initiation of atrial fibrillation by an ICD shock. Continuous ECG recording in a patient with an ICD system with epicardial patch electrodes. Ventricular flutter is terminated by a 20-J shock, but the shock triggers atrial fibrillation with a rapid ventricular response greater than the ventricular detection rate. The ICD responds with a clinically inappropriate second shock that induces nonsustained ventricular tachycardia (VT), eventually converting to sinus rhythm. With permission from [140].

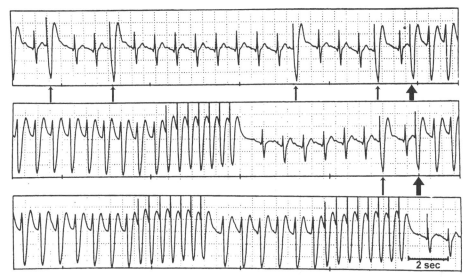

FIGURE 6-101. Inappropriate bradycardia pacing initiating ventricular tachycardia (VT). Continuous ambulatory ECG recording from a patient with an ICD device demonstrating intermittent undersensing in the bradycardia channel with delivery of asynchronous pacing pulses (small arrows). VT is initiated by a long-short pacing sequence on two occasions (large arrows) and terminated each time by antitachycardia pacing. From [140] with permission.

cause the latter is deemed to provide either insufficient or otherwise inadequate therapy for the patient's life-threatening cardiac arrhythmia. Why receive both an ICD and antiarrhythmic drug therapies if one can be avoided? A single therapeutic modality is generally less expensive than multiple therapies, as it exposes the patient to only one set of complications and side effects as opposed to multiple sets, and reduces the risk of adverse interactions between the multiple therapies. However, there clearly are clinical situations in which antiarrhythmic drug therapy can further reduce the risk to the patient from their ventricular tachyarrhythmia, as well as significantly improve their quality of life and acceptance of their device.

Indications for adjuvant use of antiarrhythmic drug therapy
In certain circumstances, patients with sustained ventricular tachycardia, ventricular fibrillation, or supraventricular tachyarrhythmias — especially atrial fibrillation/flutter with a ventricular response greater than the rate cut-off of the ICD — may require adjuvant medical therapy, even if advanced discrimination functions of the ICD are activated (see "Detection enhancements & tachycardia discrimination" on page 327). Patients with ICD systems who may require concomitant antiarrhythmic drug therapy generally fall into three groups:

1. Patients with frequent sustained ventricular fibrillation or fast ventricular tachycardia, not amenable to catheter-based treatments (i.e., radiofrequency catheter ablation), leading to syncope or complete hemodynamic collapse before arrhythmia termination by the delivery of effective ICD

therapy. This group of patients corresponds to those individuals with frequently recurrent, very dangerous, ventricular tachyarrhythmias that are extremely life-risking every time they occur, even in the presence of a functional ICD system. Slowing of the malignant tachyarrhythmia in these patients may reduce its risk by preventing hemodynamic collapse, obviate the need for any ICD-based therapy by suppressing the arrhythmia entirely, or allow the successful and reliable use of a less aggressive therapy modalities such as antitachycardia pacing if, for example, a very fast ventricular tachycardia is converted to a slow ventricular tachycardia.

2. Patients with frequent sustained ventricular tachycardia, regardless of its hemodynamic tolerability, not amenable to catheter-based treatments, and not reliably terminated by antitachycardia pacing, but instead requiring the delivery of an ICD shock, especially if the patient finds the shocks (regardless of their magnitude) intolerable. This group of patients corresponds to those with low risk ventricular tachycardia that cannot be treated by any other means except frequent ICD shocks. In these patients antiarrhythmic drug therapy may suppress the arrhythmia, negating the need for any ICD-based therapy, or make successful termination by antitachycardia pacing more reliable.

3. Patients with paroxysmal supraventricular tachyarrhythmias with ventricular rates greater than the mandated ICD rate cut-off (based upon the rate of the patient's clinical ventricular tachycardia), that lead to ICD therapy directed against a presumed ventricular tachyarrhythmia, and that cannot be managed by reprogramming the device or any available catheter-based or device-based treatment of supraventricular tachyarrhythmias. This group of patients corresponds to those who are receiving ICD therapies in their ventricles for arrhythmias occurring above the His bundle and which cannot be treated by any other means except suppression by drug therapy.

Some aspects of these specific indications need further discussion. Firstly, clinicians should *always* be alert that the development of new ventricular arrhythmias, particularly polymorphic ventricular tachycardia, fast monomorphic ventricular tachycardia, or cardiac arrest, may signify new or worsening myocardial ischemia, myocarditis, or congestive heart failure. Therefore, physicians should at least consider the necessity to pursue diagnostic or therapeutic interventions for these conditions if the frequency, pattern, or type of tachyarrhythmia changes. Treatment of these underlying triggering conditions may negate the need to institute antiarrhythmic drug therapy in these patients.

Secondly, patients implanted with a dual-chamber ICD device with an atrial sensing lead may have their supraventricular arrhythmias managed with specialized programming of devices, as previously discussed. In the case of a rapid paroxysmal supraventricular tachyarrhythmia, therapy that would normally be directed against a presumed, but non-existent, ventricular arrhythmia could be avoided by recognition that the rapid ventricular rate is the result of a supraventricular, as opposed to ventricular, tachycardia.

Thirdly, the word "frequent" is somewhat patient-dependent. From a psychological standpoint, some patients respond very poorly even to very rare and very low energy shocks delivered entirely appropriately for ventricular arrhythmias. At the other extreme, recurrent episodes of ventricular fibrillation or fast ventricular tachycardia occurring perhaps weekly (or even less commonly) and leading to rapid hemodynamic collapse may be "too frequent" for a particular patient given the malignant nature of this arrhythmia and the increased risk to which it exposes the patient. In this case, even if the patient "doesn't mind" these monthly or more frequent shocks, permitting this tachyarrhythmia to occur at such high rate poses an unacceptable life-threatening risk to the patient. Similarly, slower, less dangerous ventricular tachycardias, may need suppression by an antiarrhythmic drug if they cannot be terminated by overdrive ventricular pacing with a high success rate, resulting in bothersome pacing or shock therapies and more rapid rates of battery-depletion.

Fourthly, many supraventricular tachyarrhythmias, such as atrioventricular (AV) nodal reentrant tachycardia, AV reciprocating tachycardia utilizing a manifest or concealed accessory connection, atrial flutter, and many types of atrial tachycardia, are now generally curable using the technique of radiofrequency catheter ablation. In addition, scar-related reentrant monomorphic ventricular tachycardia and bundle branch reentrant ventricular tachycardia that may be causing unnecessary shocks also may be ablatable. For many of these patients with supraventricular and ventricular tachyarrhythmias leading to ICD therapies directed to the ventricles, the first line therapy may be an attempt at cure the arrhythmia using catheter ablation. Only if this option fails should the patient receive antiarrhythmic drugs.

Finally, the spectrum of atrial fibrillation creates some special circumstances that may negate the need to use antiarrhythmic drugs in all cases. Currently, patients receiving ICD shocks due to atrial fibrillation (usually paroxysmal) with rapid ventricular response refractory to medical therapy may be managed by total ablation of the AV junction with provision for backup bradycardia pacing either using the ICD device itself or implantation of a separate pacemaker. In addition, in some of these patients, moderation of the ventricular rates during atrial fibrillation may be achieved by "modifying" atrioventricular conduction.

Choice of the adjuvant antiarrhythmic drug
In patients with atrial fibrillation (generally paroxysmal) needing ventricular rate control, the first line therapy is generally digoxin, or AV nodal blocking drugs, such as Class II (β-adrenergic blockers) or Class IV (Ca^{2+} channel blockers). The negative inotropic effects of Class II and Class IV agents may pose a potential problem, but these are generally more effective than digoxin in controlling ventricular rate, especially in paroxysmal atrial fibrillation. In particular, β-adrenergic blockers may play an important role in situations associated with high sympathetic tone. In some refractory cases, clinicians have opted to use powerful agents such as amiodarone to control the ventricular response, but long-term use of this agent to merely control ventricular rate in atrial fibrillation may not be indicated in the majority of these patients. In many of these patients, complete AV

node ablation and institution of permanent pacing may be a better choice (either VVI(R) if chronic atrial fibrillation is present, or DDD(R) pacing with mode switching in patients with paroxysmal atrial fibrillation).

For suppression of non-ablatable supraventricular tachyarrhythmias, Ca^{2+} channel and β-adrenergic blockers can be tried, but true Na^+ channel or K^+ channel blocking agents may be necessary. In general, one would not use Class IA drugs in patients with the risk for ventricular tachyarrhythmias because they are often ineffective or may be frankly proarrhythmic. In patients under the protection of an ICD, the clinician has a bit more freedom to use these agents. Most electrophysiologists will not use Class IC agents in these patients, especially if they have significant left ventricular dysfunction.

For patients requiring suppression or slowing of monomorphic ventricular tachycardia or suppression of frequent fast ventricular tachycardia or ventricular fibrillation (not due to new or worsening myocardial ischemia, myocarditis, congestive heart failure, proarrhythmia, etc.) class IA, IB and III have been widely used. Class IA agents alone (especially quinidine or procainamide), occasionally in combination with a class IB agent (e.g., quinidine/mexiletine) are sometimes used and can be quite useful. In addition, for patients with renal failure, the N-acetylprocainamide (NAPA) metabolite of procainamide may reach toxic levels. In most cases, patients in this group are best treated with a class III agent, either racemic sotalol, dofetilide, or amiodarone. Sotalol, of course, also has β-adrenergic blocking effects which may be beneficial in some of these patients (if they can tolerate the negative inotropic and chronotropic effects), while amiodarone also has Na^+ and Ca^{2+} channel blocking effects. The use of sotalol must be monitored closely, especially in patients with renal insufficiency where drug accumulation could lead to dangerous QT prolongation and torsade de pointes. Amiodarone, which appears to have the least proarrhythmic risk of any of the antiarrhythmic agents (other than the β-adrenergic or Ca^{2+} channel blockers), nevertheless does have other problems including the potential for causing pulmonary fibrosis, hypothyroidism, hyperthyroidism, hepatitis, and even significant visual disturbances.

Antiarrhythmic drug-device interactions
Antiarrhythmic drugs can have both adverse and beneficial effects in patients with ICD devices. These effects are collectively referred to as *drug-device interactions*. A number of them have already been discussed above and these and others are summarized in Table 6-23. The worst adverse drug-device interactions include; 1) a drug-induced increase in the DFT [88,92,101,141], 2) drug-induced proarrhythmia that results in an increase in administered therapies, possibly with therapy-induced acceleration of ventricular tachycardia (Figure 6-73) or even induction of ventricular fibrillation [57]; and 3) drug-induced slowing of ventricular tachycardia below the programmed rate cut-off resulting in failure to deliver therapy. Patients with borderline DFTs or clinical monomorphic ventricular tachycardia may require re-testing of their DFT and the reassessment of the rates of their inducible ventricular tachycardias if they are placed on antiarrhythmic medications, especially amiodarone. Reprogramming of maximum shock energies, a new rate cut-off for ventricular tachycardia and ventricular fibrillation zones, and modification of ventricular tachycardia therapies may be necessary as well. Similarly, patients with antitachycardia pacing programmed for management of slow ventricular

tachycardia may need reevaluation of the rate cut-off and pacing protocol when a new antiarrhythmic therapy is initiated so as to avoid failure to treat or antitachycardia pacing-induced aggravation of a benign ventricular tachycardia into a more lethal form.

TABLE 6-23. Potential interactions of antiarrhythmic drug therapy and ICD devices

Increase in defibrillation threshold and/or cardioversion energy requirement [88,92,101,141].
Slowing of VT which may result in non-detection of the VT by the ICD, a more hemodynamically stable VT before termination, or easier (or more difficult) termination with low energy shocks or overdrive ventricular pacing.
Potentially decrease the frequency (antiarrhythmic effect) or increase the frequency (proarrhythmic effect) of the VT, requiring less or more therapies. This proarrhythmic potential could lead to many more therapies for non-sustained arrhythmias (especially in older model committed ICD devices), enhanced battery depletion, or risk of therapy-induced provocation or aggravation of ventricular arrhythmias [57,142].
Potentially decrease the frequency (antiarrhythmic effect) or increase the frequency (proarrhythmic effect) of atrial arrhythmias, leading to less or possibly more inappropriate therapies directed at the ventricle, and possible device-induced (by shock or antitachycardia pacing) lethal ventricular arrhythmias [57,140,142].
Any increase in frequency of the clinical arrhythmia (a type of proarrhythmia) from antiarrhythmic drug use risks an increase in device-induced aggravation of the arrhythmia, including antitachycardia pacing or shock-induced acceleration of VT or induction of VF from VT [57,140].
Induction of incessant ventricular arrhythmias, or ventricular arrhythmias exhibiting no excitable gap, making termination by antitachycardia pacing or low energy cardioversion difficult, risking device-induced proarrhythmia.

Adapted from [143].

6.8.6 PACEMAKER & ICD INTERACTIONS

In general, the safe coexistence of a separate pacemaker and ICD system requires that the pacemaker system be implanted with bipolar leads, employ bipolar pacing, and be resistant to reprogramming to unipolar pacing by a defibrillator shock. A pacemaker can interact with a defibrillator in a number of ways. During a ventricular tachyarrhythmia a potentially fatal interaction may occur if the pacemaker is not inhibited, but instead continues to deliver pacing stimuli despite the underlying tachyarrhythmia. If the local amplitude of the pacing pulses is greater than the local amplitude of the ventricular electrograms (as may be the case with unipolar pacing), the ICD system may only sense the regular slow rate of the pacing pulses and fail to sense the rapid activity of the underlying ventricular arrhythmia, resulting in failure to deliver life-saving shock therapy (Figure 6-102).

A second potential complication can occur if the pacemaker exhibits undersensing or failure to capture (due, for example, to lead dislodgment). In the former situation, failure to sense a spontaneous ventricular activation will result in inappropriate delivery of pacing stimuli. If this occurs frequently and repetitively, sensing of both the inappropriate pacing stimuli, as well as spontaneous ventricular depolarizations may result in satisfaction of the rate criterion, triggering the delivery of unnecessary anti-tachycardia therapy. Even if pacemaker sensing is appropriate, frequent and repetitive subthreshold

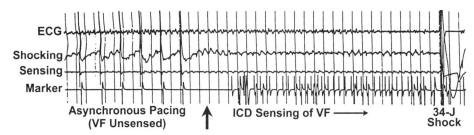

FIGURE 6-102. Example of ICD undersensing of ventricular fibrillation (VF) due to sensing of pacemaker stimuli in a patient implanted with an ICD system and a separate pacemaker. On the left side of the panel, VOO pacing is forced by magnet application over the pacemaker generator. The automatically adjusting gain control "sees" the pacemaker stimuli, but fails to detect the underlying low amplitude signals of the VF. Only after removing the magnet (with reversion to demand VVI pacing), does the pacing stop and the ICD sensing circuit is able to "find" and terminate the VF.

pacing stimuli that fail to produce a cardiac activation may result in fulfillment of the programmed rate criterion if the ICD senses both the pacing stimuli as well as spontaneous ventricular depolarizations. Finally, even if pacing stimuli capture the ventricle, in rare cases the ICD may count both the pacing stimuli and the resultant ventricular depolarization. This double counting may potentially lead to inappropriate delivery of ICD therapy if the rate criterion is met (Figure 6-103).

Some pacemaker systems have a STAT programming option that can be used in an emergency to rapidly program demand pacing. In many of these systems, STAT pacing results in unipolar pacing at very high current amplitudes. As mentioned above, development of a ventricular tachyarrhythmia during unipolar pacing may result in failure to detect the ventricular arrhythmia.

An ICD shock may damage the pacemaker pulse generator or alter the programmed settings (Figure 6-104). An external or an internal defibrillation shock (or any EMI, including electrocautery or radiofrequency ablation) may trigger a reset event in some vulnerable pacemaker pulse generators. During hardware reset, the pacemaker conducts a memory check to determine if the parameters essential for safe operation have been affected. If critical functions are nominal, the pacemaker will continue to operate as programmed. If essential parameters have been affected, the pacemaker will revert to a back-up mode, usually SSI or SOO, with sensing and pacing functions set at their default values. Should reversion to back-up mode occur, reprogramming to the original settings can ordinarily be accomplished without difficulty.

In order to minimize the potential for adverse interactions between a pacemaker and an ICD, the pacemaker and ICD leads should be positioned as far apart as possible from each other. This may entail using an active fixation bipolar ventricular pacemaker or ICD lead allowing implantation of the lead either at the ventricular septum or in the right ventricular outflow tract. To further minimize the potential for device-device interaction, certain additional precautions can be taken at the time of implantation. The electrophysiologist can use the ICD features, such as markers and real-time electrograms to help evaluate the potential for pacemaker interaction due to oversensing by the ICD. Ventricular fibrillation should be induced while the ICD is activated and the pacemaker is programmed to an asynchronous mode at maximum amplitude and pulse width. This

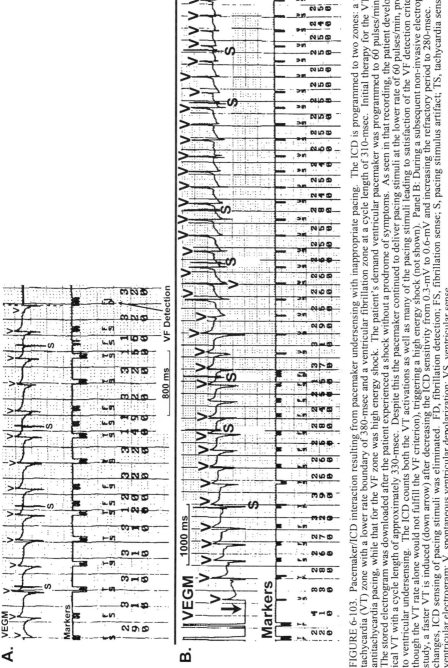

FIGURE 6-103. Pacemaker/ICD interaction resulting from pacemaker undersensing with inappropriate pacing. The ICD is programmed to two zones: a ventricular tachycardia (VT) zone with a lower rate boundary of 380-msec and a ventricular fibrillation zone at a cycle length of 310-msec. Initial therapy for the VT zone was antitachycardia pacing, while that for the VF zone was high energy shock. The patient's demand ventricular pacemaker was programmed to 60 pulses/min. Panel A: The stored electrogram was downloaded after the patient experienced a shock without a prodrome of symptoms. As seen in that recording, the patient developed a clinical VT with a cycle length of approximately 330-msec. Despite this the pacemaker continued to deliver pacing stimuli at the lower rate of 60 pulses/min, probably due to ventricular undersensing. The ICD counts both the VT activations as well as many of the pacing stimuli leading to satisfaction of the VF detection criterion (even though the VT rate alone would not fulfill the VF criterion), triggering a high energy shock (not shown). Panel B: During a subsequent non-invasive electrophysiology study, a faster VT is induced (down arrow) after decreasing the ICD sensitivity from 0.3-mV to 0.6-mV and increasing the refractory period to 280-msec. With these changes, ICD sensing of pacing stimuli was eliminated. FD, fibrillation detection; FS, fibrillation sense; S, pacing stimulus artifact; TS, tachycardia sense; VEGM, ventricular electrogram; V, spontaneous ventricular depolarization; VS, ventricular sense.

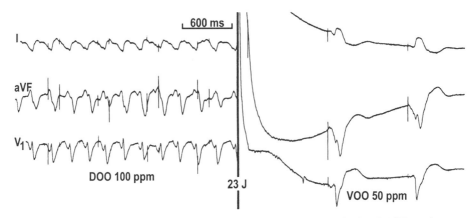

FIGURE 6-104. Resetting of pacemaker mode from DOO to VOO by an ICD shock. The ICD terminates an episode of induced ventricular tachycardia with a 23-J discharge. Following the shock the pacemaker reverts to its power-on-reset mode of VOO at 50 pulses/min (ppm). With permission from [140].

should provide the greatest opportunity for inhibition of arrhythmia detection due to detection of pacemaker pacing pulses. The pacemaker leads may have to be repositioned to eliminate detection of the pacing pulses by the ICD. Unfortunately, implantation of a ventricular defibrillation lead anywhere but the right ventricular apex may result in prohibitively high defibrillation energies required to terminate ventricular fibrillation. Consequently, some patients that require dual chamber pacing and an ICD may benefit by replacement of their existing system with a combined device equipped with both dual chamber pacing and the usual ICD functions.

References

1. Abilgard CP: Tentamina electrica in animalibus instituta. *Societatis Medicae Havniensis Collectanea* **2**:157, 1775.
2. Prevost JL, Battelli F: La mort par les courants electriques-courants alternatifs a haute tension. *J Physiol Path Gen* **1**:427, 1899.
3. Prevost JL, Batelli F: Sur quelques effets de decharges electriques sur le coeur des mammiferes. *Comptes Rendus Acad Sci* **129**:1267-68, 1899.
4. Wiggers CJ: The mechanism and nature of ventricular fibrillation. *Am Heart J* **20**:399-412, 1940.
5. Gurvich NL, Yuniev GS: Restoration of regular rhythm in the mammalian fibrillating heart. *Amer Rev Soviet Med* **3**:236-239, 1946.
6. Gurvich NL, Yuniev GS: Restoration of heart rhythm during fibrillation by a condenser discharge. *Amer Rev Soviet Med* **4**:252, 1947.
7. Zoll PM, Linenthal AJ, Gibson W, et al.: Termination of ventricular fibrillation in man by externally applied countershock. *N Engl J Med* **254**:727-732, 1956.
8. Lown B, Amarasingham R, Neuman J: New method for terminating cardiac arrhythmias: use of synchronized capacitor discharge. *JAMA* **182**:548-555, 1962.
9. Lown B, Axelrod P: Implanted standby defibrillators. *Circulation* **46**:637, 1972.
10. Mirowski M, Mower M, Staewen WS, et al.: Standby automatic defibrillator: An approach to prevention of sudden coronary death. *Arch Intern Med* **126**:158, 1970.

11. Mirowski M, Mower M, Staewen WS, et al.: Ventricular defibrillation through a single intravascular catheter electrode system (Abstract). *Clin Res* **19**:328, 1971.

12. Mirowski M, Mower M, Staewen WS, et al.: The development of the transvenous automatic defibrillator. *Arch Intern Med* **129**:773, 1972.

13. Mirowski M, Mower M, Gott VL, Brawley RK: Feasibility and effectiveness of low-energy catheter defibrillation in man. *Circulation* **47**:79, 1973.

14. Mirowski M, Mower MM, Langer A, et al.: A chronically implanted system for automatic defibrillation in active conscious dogs. Experimental model for treatment of sudden death from ventricular fibrillation. *Circulation* **58**:90-4, 1978.

15. Mirowski M, Mower MM, Reid PR: The automatic implantable defibrillator. *Am Heart J* **100**:1089-92, 1980.

16. Mirowski M, Reid PR, Mower MM, et al.: Termination of malignant ventricular arrhythmias with an implanted automatic defibrillator in human beings. *N Engl J Med* **303**:322-4, 1980.

17. Moss AJ, Hall WJ, Cannom DS, et al.: Improved survival with an implanted defibrillator in patients with coronary disease at high risk for ventricular arrhythmia. Multicenter Automatic Defibrillator Implantation Trial Investigators. *N Engl J Med* **335**:1933-40, 1996.

18. AVID Investigators: A comparison of antiarrhythmic drug therapy with implantable defibrillators in patients resuscitated from near-fatal ventricular arrhythmias. *New Engl J Med* **337**:1576-1583, 1997.

19. Bigger JT, Jr.: Prophylactic use of implanted cardiac defibrillators in patients at high risk for ventricular arrhythmias after coronary-artery bypass graft surgery. Coronary Artery Bypass Graft (CABG) Patch Trial Investigators. *N Engl J Med* **337**:1569-75, 1997.

20. Bigger JT, Jr., Whang W, Rottman JN, et al.: Mechanisms of death in the CABG Patch trial: a randomized trial of implantable cardiac defibrillator prophylaxis in patients at high risk of death after coronary artery bypass graft surgery. *Circulation* **99**:1416-21, 1999.

21. Gregoratos G, Cheitlin MD, Conill A, et al.: ACC/AHA guidelines for implantation of cardiac pacemakers and antiarrhythmia devices: a report of the American College of Cardiology/American Heart Association Task Force on Practice Guidelines. *J Am Coll Cardiol* **31**:1175-209, 1998.

22. Kroll MW, Lehmann MH, eds. *Implantable Cardioverter Defibrillator Therapy: The Engineering-Clinical Interface.* Norwell, MA: Kluwer Academic Publishers, 1996.

23. Block M, Breithardt G: Optimizing defibrillation through improved waveforms. *Pacing Clin Electrophys* **18**:526-538, 1995.

24. Zipes DP, Fischer J, King RM, et al.: Termination of ventricular fibrillation in dogs by depolarizing a critical amount of myocardium. *Am J Cardiol* **36**:37-44, 1975.

25. Witkowski FX, Penkoske PA: Epicardial activation times after defibrillation in open-chest dogs using unipolar DC-coupled activation recordings. *J Electrocardiol* **23 Suppl**:39-45, 1990.

26. Witkowski FX, Penkoske PA, Plonsey R: Mechanism of cardiac defibrillation in open-chest dogs with unipolar DC-coupled simultaneous activation and shock potential recordings. *Circulation* **82**:244-60, 1990.

27. Witkowski FX, Penkoske PA: Activation patterns during ventricular fibrillation. *Ann N Y Acad Sci* **591**:219-31, 1990.

28. Shibata N, Chen PS, Dixon EG, et al.: Epicardial activation after unsuccessful defibrillation shocks in dogs. *Am J Physiol* **255**:H902-9, 1988.

29. Shibata N, Chen PS, Dixon EG, et al.: Influence of shock strength and timing on induction of ventricular arrhythmias in dogs. *Am J Physiol* **255**:H891-901, 1988.

30. Witkowski FX, Kerber RE: Currently known mechanisms underlying direct current external and internal cardiac defibrillation. *J Cardiovasc Electrophysiol* **2**:562-572, 1991.

31. Chen PS, Wolf PD, Ideker RE: Mechanism of cardiac defibrillation: a different point of view. *Circulation* **84**:913-9, 1991.

32. Chen PS, Shibata N, Dixon EG, et al.: Comparison of the defibrillation threshold and the upper limit of ventricular vulnerability. *Circulation* **73**:1022-8, 1986.

33. Chen PS, Wolf PD, Melnick SD, et al.: Comparison of activation during ventricular fibrillation and following unsuccessful defibrillation shocks in open-chest dogs. *Circ Res* **66**:1544-60, 1990.

34. Sweeney RJ, Gill RM, Steinberg MI, Reid PR: Ventricular refractory period extension caused by defibrillation shocks. *Circulation* **82**:965-72, 1990.

35. Kroll MW: A minimal model of the monophasic defibrillation pulse. *Pacing Clin Electrophysiol* **16**:769-77, 1993.

36. Kroll MW, Lehmann MH, Tchou PJ. Defining the defibrillation dosage. In: Kroll MW, Lehmann MH, eds. *Implantable Cardioverter Defibrillator Therapy: The Engineering-Clinical Interface*. Norwell, MA: Kluwer Academic Publishers, 63-88: 1996.

37. Koning G, Schneider H, Hoelen AJ, et al.: Amplitude-duration relation for direct ventricular defibrillation with rectangular current pulses. *Med Biol Eng* **13**:388-95, 1975.

38. Bourland JD, Tacker WA, Geddes LA, et al.: Comparative efficacy of damped sine wave and square wave current for transchest ventricular defibrillation in animals. *Medical Instrum* **12**:38-41, 1978.

39. Hillsley RE, Walker RG, Swanson DK, et al.: Is the second phase of a biphasic defibrillation waveform the defibrillating phase? *Pacing Clin Electrophysiol* **16**:1401-11, 1993.

40. Feeser SA, Tang AS, Kavanagh KM, et al.: Strength-duration and probability of success curves for defibrillation with biphasic waveforms. *Circulation* **82**:2128-41, 1990.

41. Kroll MW: A minimal model of the single capacitor biphasic defibrillation waveform. *Pacing Clin Electrophysiol* **17**:1782-92, 1994.

42. Swartz JF, Fletcher RD, Karasik PE: Optimization of biphasic waveforms for human nonthoracotomy defibrillation. *Circulation* **88**:2646-2654, 1993.

43. Natale A, Sra J, Krum D, et al.: Relative efficacy of different tilts with biphasic defibrillation in humans. *Pacing Clin Electrophysiol* **19**:197-206, 1996.

44. Daubert JP, Frazier DW, Wolf PD, et al.: Response of relatively refractory canine myocardium to monophasic and biphasic shocks. *Circulation* **84**:2522-38, 1991.

45. Supino CG. The system. In: Kroll MW, Lehmann MH, eds. *Implantable Cardioverter Defibrillator Therapy: The Engineering-Clinical Interface*. Norwell, MA: Kluwer Academic Publishers, 163-172: 1996.

46. Holmes C. The battery. In: Kroll MW, Lehmann MH, eds. *Implantable Cardioverter Defibrillator Therapy: The Engineering-Clinical Interface*. Norwell, MA: Kluwer Academic Publishers, 205-221: 1996.

47. Higgins SL, Alexander DC, Kuypers CJ, et al.: The subcutaneous array - a new lead adjunct for the transvenous ICD to lower defibrillation thresholds. *Pacing Clin Electrophys* **19-8**:1540-48, 1995.

48. Bernstein AD, Camm AJ, Fisher JD, et al.: North American Society of Pacing and Electrophysiology policy statement. The NASPE/BPEG defibrillator code. *Pacing Clin Electrophysiol* **16**:1776-80, 1993.

49. Singer I, Adams L, Austin E: Potential hazards of fixed gain sensing and arrhythmia reconfirmation for implantable cardioverter defibrillators. *Pacing Clin Electrophys* **16**:1070-1079, 1993.

50. Ellenbogen KA, Wood MA, Stambler BS, et al.: Measurement of ventricular electrogram amplitude during intraoperative induction of ventricular tachyarrhythmias. *Am J Cardiol* **70**:1017-22, 1992.

51. Kaemmerer WF, Olson WH: Dual chamber tachyarrhythmia detection using syntactic pattern recognition and contextual timing rules for rhythm classification. *Pacing Clin Electrophys* **18(Pt II)**:872, 1995.

52. Jenkins J, Wu D, Arzbaecher RC: Computer diagnosis of supraventricular and ventricular arrhythmias. *Circulation* **60**:977-987, 1979.

53. Arzbaecher RC, Bump T, Jenkins J, et al.: Automatic tachycardia recognition. *Pacing Clin Electrophys* **7(Pt II)**:541-547, 1984.

54. Catanzariti D, Pennisi V, Pangallo A, et al.: Efficacy and safety of antitachycardia pacing in ICD patients: analysis of two-years follow-up. *Eur J Card Electrophys* **5**:248-252, 1995.

55. Nasir N, Jr., Pacifico A, Doyle TK, et al.: Spontaneous ventricular tachycardia treated by antitachycardia pacing. Cadence Investigators. *Am J Cardiol* **79**:820-2, 1997.

56. Connelly DT, Cardinal D, Foley L, et al.: Is routine pre-discharge testing necessary for patients with implantable cardioverter-defibrillators. *Pacing Clin Electrophysiol* **19**:614, 1996.

57. Lauer MR, Young C, Liem LB, et al.: Ventricular fibrillation induced by low-energy shocks from programmable implantable cardioverter-defibrillators in patients with coronary artery disease. *Am J Cardiol* **73**:559-63, 1994.

58. Grimm W, Flores BF, Marchlinski FE: Complications of implantable cardioverter defibrillator therapy: follow- up of 241 patients. *Pacing Clin Electrophysiol* **16**:218-22, 1993.

59. Lang DJ, Cato EL, Echt DS: Protocol for evaluation of internal defibrillation safety margins. *J Am Coll Cardiol* **13**:111A, 1989.

60. Singer I, Lang D: Defibrillation threshold, clinical utility and therapeutic implications. *Pacing Clin Electrophysiol* **15**:932-49, 1992.

61. Singer I, Lang D. The defibrillation threshold. In: Kroll MW, Lehmann MH, eds. *Implantable Cardioverter Defibrillator Therapy: The Engineering-Clinical Interface.* Norwell, MA: Kluwer Academic Publishers, 89-129: 1996.

62. Davy JM, Fain ES, Dorian P, Winkle RA: The relationship between successful defibrillation and delivered energy in open-chest dogs: reappraisal of the "defibrillation threshold" concept. *Am Heart J* **113**:77-84, 1987.

63. McDaniel WC, Schuder JC: The cardiac ventricular defibrillation threshold - inherent limitations in its application and interpretation. *Med Instrum* **21**:170-76, 1987.

64. Rattes MF, Jones DL, Sharma AD, Klein GJ: Defibrillation threshold: a simple and quantitative estimate of the ability to defibrillate. *Pacing Clin Electrophysiol* **10**:70-7, 1987.

65. Jones DL, Klein GJ, Guiraudon GM, Sharma AD, Yee R, Kallok MJ: Prediction of defibrillation success from a single defibrillation threshold measurement with sequential pulses and two current pathways in humans. *Circulation* **78**:1144-9, 1988.

66. Lang DJ, Swanson DK. Safety margin for defibrillation. In: Alt E, Klein H, Griffin JC, eds. *The Implantable Cardioverter/Defibrillator.* Berlin: Springer-Verlag, 272: 1992.

67. Hou CJ, Chang-Sing P, Flynn E, et al.: Determination of ventricular vulnerable period and ventricular fibrillation threshold by use of T-wave shocks in patients undergoing implantation of cardioverter/defibrillators. *Circulation* **92**:2558-64, 1995.

68. Swerdlow CD, Ahern T, Kass RM, et al.: Upper limit of vulnerability is a good estimator of shock strength associated with 90% probability of successful defibrillation in humans with transvenous implantable cardioverter-defibrillators. *J Am Coll Cardiol* **27**:1112-8, 1996.

69. Swerdlow CD, Davie S, Ahern T, Chen PS: Comparative reproducibility of defibrillation threshold and upper limit of vulnerability. *Pacing Clin Electrophysiol* **19**:2103-11, 1996.

70. Chen PS, Feld GK, Kriett JM, et al.: Relation between upper limit of vulnerability and defibrillation threshold in humans. *Circulation* **88**:186-92, 1993.

71. Hwang C, Swerdlow CD, Kass RM, et al.: Upper limit of vulnerability reliably predicts the defibrillation threshold in humans. *Circulation* **90**:2308-14, 1994.

72. Behrens S, Li C, Kirchhof P, et al.: Reduced arrhythmogenicity of biphasic versus monophasic T-wave shocks. Implications for defibrillation efficacy. *Circulation* **94**:1974-80, 1996.

73. Kirchhof PF, Fabritz CL, Zabel M, Franz MR: The vulnerable period for low and high energy T-wave shocks: role of dispersion of repolarisation and effect of d-sotalol. *Cardiovasc Res* **31**:953-62, 1996.

74. Fabritz CL, Kirchhof PF, Behrens S, et al.: Myocardial vulnerability to T wave shocks: relation to shock strength, shock coupling interval, and dispersion of ventricular repolarization. *J Cardiovasc Electrophysiol* **7**:231-42, 1996.

75. Bardy GH, Ivey TD, Allen MD, et al.: A prospective randomized evaluation of biphasic versus monophasic waveform pulses on defibrillation efficacy in humans. *J Am Coll Cardiol* **14**:728-33, 1989.

76. Saksena S, An H, Mehra R, et al.: Prospective comparison of biphasic and monophasic shocks for implantable cardioverter-defibrillators using endocardial leads. *Am J Cardiol* **70**:304-10, 1992.

77. Wyse DG, Kavanagh KM, Gillis AM, et al.: Comparison of biphasic and monophasic shocks for defibrillation using a nonthoracotomy system. *Am J Cardiol* **71**:197-202, 1993.

78. Block M, Hammel D, Bocker D, et al.: A prospective randomized cross-over comparison of mono- and biphasic defibrillation using nonthoracotomy lead configurations in humans. *J Cardiovasc Electrophys* **5**:581-590, 1994.

79. Strickberger SA, Man KC, Daoud E, et al.: Effect of first-phase polarity of biphasic shocks on defibrillation threshold with a single transvenous lead system. *J Am Coll Cardiol* **25**:1605-8, 1995.

80. Shorofsky SR, Gold MR: Effects of waveform and polarity on defibrillation thresholds in humans using a transvenous lead system. *Am J Cardiol* **78**:313-6, 1996.

81. Usui M, Walcott GP, Strickberger SA, et al.: Effects of polarity for monophasic and biphasic shocks on defibrillation efficacy with an endocardial system. *Pacing Clin Electrophysiol* **19**:65-71, 1996.

82. Strickberger SA, Hummel JD, Horwood LE, et al.: Effect of shock polarity on ventricular defibrillation threshold using a transvenous lead system. *J Am Coll Cardiol* **24**:1069-72, 1994.

83. Thakur RK, Souza JJ, Chapman PD, et al.: Electrode polarity is an important determinant of defibrillation efficacy using a nonthoracotomy system. *Pacing Clin Electrophysiol* **17**:919-23, 1994.

84. Natale A, Sra J, Axtell K, et al.: Preliminary experience with a hybrid nonthoracotomy defibrillating system that includes a biphasic device: comparison with a standard monophasic device using the same lead system. *J Am Coll Cardiol* **24**:406-12, 1994.

85. Reiffel JA, Coromilas J, Zimmerman JM, Spotnitz HM: Drug-device interactions: clinical considerations. *Pacing Clin Electrophysiol* **8**:369-73, 1985.

86. Fain ES, Dorian P, Davy JM, et al.: Effects of encainide and its metabolites on energy requirements for defibrillation. *Circulation* **73**:1334-41, 1986.

87. Hernandez R, Mann DE, Breckenridge S, et al.: Effects of flecainide on defibrillation thresholds in the anesthetized dog. *J Am Coll Cardiol* **14**:777-781, 1989.

88. Stevens SK, Haffajee CI, Naccarelli GV, et al.: Effects of oral propafenone on defibrillation and pacing thresholds in patients receiving implantable cardioverter-defibrillators. Propafenone Defibrillation Threshold Investigators. *J Am Coll Cardiol* **28**:418-22, 1996.

89. Echt DS, Gremillion ST, Lee JT: Effects of procainamide and lidocaine on defibrillation energy requirements in patients receiving implantable cardioverter defibrillator devices. *J Cardiovasc Electrophysiol* **5** 1994.

90. Echt DS, Black JN, Barbey JT, et al.: Evaluation of antiarrhythmic drugs on defibrillation energy requirements in dogs. Sodium channel block and action potential prolongation. *Circulation* **79**:1106-17, 1989.

91. Dorian P, Fain ES, Davy JM, Winkle RA: Lidocaine causes a reversible, concentration-dependent increase in defibrillation energy requirements. *J Am Coll Cardiol* **8**:327-32, 1986.

92. Jung W, Manz M, Pizzulli L, et al.: Effects of chronic amiodarone therapy on defibrillation threshold. *Am J Cardiol* **70**:1023-1027, 1992.

93. Ujhelyi MR, Schur M, Frede T, et al.: Differential effects of lidocaine on defibrillation threshold with monophasic versus biphasic shock waveforms. *Circulation* **92**:1644-1650, 1995.

94. Marinchak RA, Friehling TD, Line RA, et al.: Effect of antiarrhythmic drugs on defibrillation threshold: case report of an adverse effect of mexiletine and review of the literature. *Pacing Clin Electrophysiol* **11**:7-12, 1988.

95. Koo CC, Allen JD, Pantridge JF: Lack of effect of bretylium tosylate on electrical ventricular defibrillation in a controlled study. *Cardiovasc Res* **18**:762-767, 1984.

96. Kerber RE, Pandian NG, Jensen SR: Effect of lidocaine and bretylium on energy requirements for transthoracic defibrillation: experimental studies. *J Am Coll Cardiol* **7**:397-405, 1986.

97. Wang M, Dorian P: Defibrillation energy requirements differ between anesthetic agents. *J Electrophysiol* **3/2**:86-94, 1989.

98. Dawson AK, Steinberg MI, Shephard JE: Effects of class I and class III drugs on current and energy required for internal defibrillation. *Circulation* **72**:III-384, 1985.

99. Fain ES, Lee JT, Winkle RA: Effects of acute intravenous and chronic oral amiodarone on defibrillation energy requirements. *Am Heart J* **114**:8-17, 1987.

100. Fogoros RN: Amiodarone-induced refractoriness to cardioversion. *Ann Intern Med* **100**:699-700, 1984.

101. Guarnieri T, Levine JH, Veltri EP, et al.: Success of chronic defibrillation and the role of antiarrhythmic drugs with the automatic implantable cardioverter/defibrillator. *Am J Cardiol* **60**:1061-4, 1987.

102. Epstein AE, Ellenbogen KA, Kirk KA, et al.: Clinical characteristics and outcome of patients with high defibrillation thresholds. A multicenter study. *Circulation* **86**:1206-16, 1992.

103. Borbola J, Denes P, Ezri MD, et al.: The automatic implantable cardioverter-defibrillator: clinical experience, complications, and follow-up in 25 patients. *Arch Intern Med* **148**:70-76, 1988.

104. Troup PJ: Implantable cardioverters and defibrillators. *Curr Probl Cardiol* **14**:673-843, 1989.

105. Martin DT, John R, Venditti FJ: Increase in defibrillation threshold in non-thoracotomy implantable defibrillators using a biphasic waveform. *Am J Cardiol* **76**:263-66, 1995.

106. Rosenthal ME, Alderfer JT, Marchlinski FE. Troubleshooting suspected ICD malfunctions. In: Kroll MW, Lehmann MH, eds. *Implantable Cardioverter Defibrillator Therapy: The Engineering-Clinical Interface*. Norwell, MA: Kluwer Academic Publishers, 435-476: 1996.

107. Axtell KA, Akhtar M: Incidence of syncope prior to implantable cardioverter-defibrillator discharges. *Circulation* **82**:211A, 1990.

108. Kou WH, Calkins H, Lewis RR, et al.: Incidence of loss of consciousness during automatic implantable cardioverter-defibrillator shocks. *Ann Intern Med* **115**:942-5, 1991.

109. Grimm W, Flores BF, Marchlinski FE: Symptoms and electrocardiographically documented rhythm preceding spontaneous shocks in patients with implantable cardioverter- defibrillator. *Am J Cardiol* **71**:1415-8, 1993.

110. Marchlinski FE, Flores BT, Buxton AE, et al.: The automatic implantable cardioverter-defibrillator: efficacy, complications, and device failures. *Ann Intern Med* **104**:481-8, 1986.

111. Newman D, Dorian P, Downar E, et al.: Use of telemetry functions in the assessment of implanted antitachycardia device efficacy. *Am J Cardiol* **70**:616-21, 1992.

112. Grimm W, Flores BF, Marchlinski FE: Electrocardiographically documented unnecessary, spontaneous shocks in 241 patients with implantable cardioverter defibrillators. *Pacing Clin Electrophysiol* **15**:1667-73, 1992.

113. Grimm W, Flores BT, Marchlinski FE: Shock occurrence and survival in 241 patients with implantable cardioverter-defibrillator therapy. *Circulation* **87**:1880-8, 1993.

114. Grimm W, Marchlinski FE: Shock occurrence in patients with an implantable cardioverter- defibrillator without spontaneous shocks before first generator replacement for battery depletion. *Am J Cardiol* **73**:969-70, 1994.

115. Grimm W, Marchlinski FE: Shock occurrence and survival in 49 patients with idiopathic dilated cardiomyopathy and an implantable cardioverter-defibrillator. *Eur Heart J* **16**:218-22, 1995.

116. Fogoros RN, Elson JJ, Bonnet CA: Actuarial incidence and pattern of occurrence of shocks following implantation of the automatic implantable cardioverter defibrillator. *Pacing Clin Electrophysiol* **12**:1465-73, 1989.

117. Kelly PA, Mann DE, Damle RS, Reiter MJ: Oversensing during ventricular pacing in patients with a third-generation implantable cardioverter-defibrillator. *J Am Coll Cardiol* **23**:1531-4, 1994.

118. Gottlieb C, Miller JM, Rosenthal ME, Marchlinski FE: Automatic implantable defibrillator discharge resulting from routine pacemaker programming. *Pacing Clin Electrophysiol* **11**:336-8, 1988.

119. Fetter JG, Benditt DG, Stanton MS: Electromagnetic interference from welding and motors on implantable cardioverter-defibrillators as tested in the electrically hostile work site. *J Am Coll Cardiol* **28**:423-7, 1996.

120. Karson T, Grace K, Denes P: Stereo speaker silences automatic implantable cardioverter defibrillator. *N Engl J Med* **320**:1628-29, 1989.

121. Man KC, Davidson T, Langberg JJ, et al.: Interference from a hand held radiofrequency remote control causing discharge of an implantable defibrillator. *Pacing Clin Electrophysiol* **16**:1756-8, 1993.

122. Madrid A, Sanchez A, Bosch E, et al.: Dysfunction of implantable defibrillators caused by slot machines. *Pacing Clin Electrophysiol* **20**:212-4, 1997.

123. Fetter JG, Ivans V, Benditt DG, Collins J: Digital cellular telephone interaction with implantable cardioverter-defibrillators. *J Am Coll Cardiol* **31**:623-8, 1998.

124. Naegeli B, Osswald S, Deola M, et al.: Intermittent pacemaker dysfunction caused by digital mobile telephones. *J Am Coll Cardiol* **27**:1471-77, 1996.

125. Barbaro V, Bartolini P, Donato A, et al.: Do European GSM mobile cellular phones pose a potential risk for pacemaker patients? *Pacing Clin Electrophysiol* **18**:1218-24, 1995.

126. Ellenbogen KA, Wood MA: Cellular telephones and pacemakers: urgent call or wrong number? *J Am Coll Cardiol* **27**:1478-9, 1996.

127. Stanton MS, Grice S, Trusty J, et al.: Safety of various cellular phone technologies with implantable cardioverter defibrillators. *Pacing Clin Electrophysiol* **19**:583, 1996.

128. McIvor ME: Environmental electromagnetic interference from electronic article surveillance devices; interactions with an ICD. *Pacing Clin Electrophysiol* **18**:2229-30, 1995.

129. Mathew P, Lewis C, Neglia J, et al.: Interaction between electronic article surveillance systems and implantable defibrillators: insights from a fourth generation ICD. *Pacing Clin Electrophysiol* **20**:2857-9, 1997.

130. Ferrick KJ, Johnston D, Kim SG, et al.: Inadvertent AICD inactivation while playing bingo. *Am Heart J* **121**:206-7, 1991.

131. Lehmann MH, Thomas A, Nabih M: Sudden death in recipients of first generation implantable cardio-verter-defibrillators: analysis of terminal events. *J Intervent Cardiol* **7**:487-503, 1994.

132. Saksena S, Poczobutt-Johanos M, Castle LW, et al.: Long-term multicenter experience with a second-generation implantable pacemaker-defibrillator in patients with malignant ventricular tachyarrhythmias. The Guardian Multicenter Investigators Group. *J Am Coll Cardiol* **19**:490-9, 1992.

133. Jones GK, Bardy GH, Kudenchuk PJ, et al.: Mechanical complications after implantation of multiple-lead nonthoracotomy defibrillator systems: implications for management and future system design. *Am Heart J* **130**:327-33, 1995.

134. Frame R, Brodman R, Furman S, et al.: Long-term stability of defibrillation thresholds with intraperi-cardial defibrillator patches. *Pacing Clin Electrophysiol* **16**:208-12, 1993.

135. Venditti F, Martin DT, Vassolas G, Bowen S: Rise in chronic defibrillation thresholds in nonthoracoto-my implantable defibrillator. *Circulation* **89**:216-223, 1994.

136. Callans DJ, Hook BG, Marchlinski FE: Paced beats following single nonsense complexes in a "code-pendent" cardioverter defibrillator and bradycardia pacing system: potential for ventricular tachycardia induction. *Pacing Clin Electrophysiol* **14**:1281-7, 1991.

137. Haberman RJ, Veltri EP, Mower MM: The effect of amiodarone on defibrillation threshold. *J Electro-physiol* **5**:415-23, 1988.

138. Pinski SL, Vanerio G, Castle LW: Patients with a high defibrillation threshold: clinical characteristics, management, and outcome. *Am Heart J* **122**:89-95, 1991.

139. Lehmann MH, Pires LA, Olson WH, et al. Sudden death despite ICD therapy: why does it happen? In: Kroll MW, Lehmann MH, eds. *Implantable Cardioverter Defibrillator Therapy: The Engineering-Clinical Interface*. Norwell, MA: Kluwer Academic Publishers, 501-523: 1996.

140. Pinski SL, Fahy GJ: The proarrhythmic potential of implantable cardioverter-defibrillators. *Circulation* **92**:1651-1664, 1995.

141. Peters RW, Gilbert TB, Johns-Walton S, Gold MR: Lidocaine-related increase in defibrillation thresh-old. *Anesth Analg* **85**:299-300, 1997.

142. Vlay LC, Vlay SC: Pacing induced ventricular fibrillation in internal cardioverter defibrillator patients: a new form of proarrhythmia. *Pacing Clin Electrophysiol* **20**:132-3, 1997.

143. Gottlieb CD, Horowitz LN: Potential interactions between antiarrhythmic medication and the automatic implantable cardioverter defibrillator. *PACE* **14(Part II)**:898, 1991.

144. Bach SM, Lehmann MH, Kroll MW. Tachyarrhythmia detection. In: Kroll MW, Lehmann MH, eds. *Im-plantable Cardioverter Defibrillator Therapy: The Engineering-Clinical Interface*. Norwell, MA: Kluw-er Academic Publishers, 303-323: 1996.

145. Kallok MJ. Pathways for defibrillation. In: Kroll MW, Lehmann MH, eds. *Implantable Cardioverter Defibrillator Therapy: The Engineering-Clinical Interface*. Norwell, MA: Kluwer Academic Publishers, 131-146: 1996.

146. Brumwell DA, Kroll K, Lehmann MH. The amplifier: sensing and depolarization. In: Kroll MW, Leh-mann MH, eds. *Implantable Cardioverter Defibrillator Therapy: The Engineering-Clinical Interface*. Norwell, MA: Kluwer Academic Publishers, 275-302: 1996.

147. Nelson RS, Gilman BL, Shapland E, Lehmann MH. Leads for the ICD. In: Kroll MW, Lehmann MH, eds. *Implantable Cardioverter Defibrillator Therapy: The Engineering-Clinical Interface*. Norwell, MA: Kluwer Academic Publishers, 173-204: 1996.

148. Hardage ML, Sweeney MB. Anti-tachycardia pacing and cardioversion. In: Kroll MW, Lehmann MH, eds. *Implantable Cardioverter Defibrillator Therapy: The Engineering-Clinical Interface*. Norwell, MA: Kluwer Academic Publishers, 325-342: 1996.

CHAPTER 7

DIAGNOSIS AND ACUTE MANAGEMENT OF PATIENTS WITH SYMPTOMATIC BRADYARRHYTHMIAS

Bradyarrhythmias can occur secondary to a wide variety of normal physiological and abnormal pathological conditions, ranging from mild conditions such as vasovagal episodes or unintentional drug overdose, to more serious conditions such as severe sepsis, multiorgan failure, or intracranial catastrophe (Table 7-1.) In fact, the large majority of symptomatic bradyarrhythmias are due to causes *extrinsic* to the specialized cardiac conduction system (*secondary* or *functional* bradycardia). *Primary* bradyarrhythmias truly due to *intrinsic* disease of the sinoatrial node, atrioventricular node, or His-Purkinje system are relatively rare (Table 7-1.)

TABLE 7-1. General classification and causes of bradyarrhythmias seen in emergency department setting

Cause of bradycardia	Incidence
Intrinsic (Primary)	15%
Calcification and fibrotic degeneration of SA node and AV node, and their transitional zones and His-Purkinje system	
Extrinsic (Secondary)	85%
Acute myocardial ischemia	40%
Pharmacological/toxicological	20%
Metabolic	5%
Neurological	5%
Miscellaneous	15%
Adapted from [1]	

Consequently, optimum diagnosis and urgent management of patients with symptomatic bradyarrhythmias should include as complete an evaluation of the patient as necessary to establish the presence of extrinsic factors/agents or underlying acute/chronic medical conditions/diseases which may be responsible for the bradyarrhythmia. In this case, treating the underlying condition or withdrawing a potentially offending agent often is sufficient to reverse the bradycardia, whether it be at the level of the SA or AV node, or His-Purkinje system. Secondary or functional bradycardias also are more likely to respond to pharmacological interventions (see below), such as intravenous administration of atropine or β-adrenergic agonists, than primary bradyarrhythmias. A complete discussion of secondary causes of bradyarrhythmias is well beyond the scope of this book and the interested reader is referred to other sources [1].

The most common type of secondary bradycardia, *vasovagal* episodes, may merely be a normal variant of a healthy autonomic nervous system. Because of this and its general benign natural history (although see below under malignant vasovagal syncope), it is important to distinguish this cause of symptomatic bradycardia from those with pathological or drug-induced secondary causes, as well as from bradyarrhythmias resulting from intrinsic conduction system disease. Failure to do so may not only prevent correct treatment of the underlying pathological condition but may also result in unnecessary implantation of a permanent pacemaker in a patient with a normal conduction system.

Because primary bradyarrhythmias result from intrinsic conduction system disease, they generally are not reversible, often are progressive, and respond poorly to urgent pharmacological interventions such as intravenous atropine or β-adrenergic agonists. This is not to say these agents should not be tried, especially in emergency situations, because: 1) there may be a secondary (functional) component to the bradycardia and 2) agents such as isoproterenol may enhance the activity of subsidiary or ectopic pacemakers in the ventricles providing a life-saving ventricular rate with adequate organ perfusion until a temporary pacemaker can be placed. In general, most of these patients require implantation of a permanent pacemaker after stabilization with a temporary transcutaneous or transvenous pacemaker. Nevertheless, localization of the site of conduction block within the specialized conduction system may aid in both the acute management of these patients and suggest the optimum type of long-term pacing treatment.

7.1   Localization of Conduction Disturbance

7.1.1 SINOATRIAL NODE DYSFUNCTION AND EXIT BLOCK

This condition is discussed in detail in Chapter 8 "Disturbances of Sinoatrial Node Function" on page 453 (see especially section "Sinoatrial Node Dysfunction and Exit Block" on page 454). The "sinus node pauses" seen with this condition (see Figure 9-2 on page 454, Figure 9-3 on page 455 & Figure 9-5 on page 457) generally do not represent a failure of impulse generation within the SA node, but rather from conduction block of the impulse as it travels from the SA node proper through the border zone of transitional cells to the atrial muscle proper (SA node exit block). The widespread replacement of transitional border zone cells with non-excitable fibrocytes may explain the exit block seen with this condition. There is an increased incidence of this disorder in the elderly, but it can be congenital as well as familial, and therefore seen in young people.

Because this disorder usually results from a failure of impulse conduction through the border zone tissue at the sinoatrial junction and not action potential generation, drugs such as atropine or β-adrenergic agonists which exert their effects by enhancing the ionic currents responsible for the SA node action potential, have little or no effect in preventing the periods of asystole responsible for the symptoms in this condition. In fact, such agents may at least theoretically worsen this disorder by increasing the rate of action potential generation which may exacerbate any exit block which has a rate-related component.

7.1.2 CONDUCTION BLOCK WITHIN THE ATRIOVENTRICULAR NODE

Normal and AV nodal conduction is discussed in detail in Chapter 9 "Disturbances of Atrioventricular Conduction" on page 469 (see especially "Classification of Disturbances of AV Conduction" on page 472). Conduction block within the AV node proper (see Figure 10-5 on page 473) or its perinodal transitional cell regions is rare, but can occur secondary to fibrous or sclerotic replacement, as a complication following some types of cardiac surgery, or can be congenital. As such it may represent a manifestation of widespread conduction system involvement also affecting the SA nodal region and His-Purkinje system. Without a His bundle recording, certain localization of the conduction block to the AV node is impossible. Clinical factors supporting a diagnosis of AV block within the AV node include: 1) an escape rhythm exhibiting a narrow QRS complex morphology, 1) absence of surface ECG pattern showing fixed bundle branch block or intaventricular conduction delay (especially in association with first degree AV block) during sinus rhythm, and 3) reversal of the block by pharmacologic agents such as atropine or isoproterenol. With a His bundle recording, a diagnosis of site of block is generally easily made. Conduction block can be localized to the AV node if atrial activation occurs without subsequent His bundle activation (no His bundle electrogram observed), while intra- or infra-Hisian block is present if atrial activation is followed by His bundle depolarization without subsequent ventricular activation.

Functional block within the AV node due, for example, to hypervagotonia, could present identically but it should be easily distinguishable from intrinsic AV nodal disease by responding promptly to intravenous administration of atropine or β-adrenergic agonists. As with SA nodal exit block, intrinsic AV nodal disease generally does not represent a failure of conduction of ionic currents in viable electrically-excitable cells; therefore, these agents will provide little beneficial effects in primary AV node block.

7.1.3 CONDUCTION BLOCK WITHIN THE HIS-PURKINJE SYSTEM

Conduction block within the His-Purkinje system is discussed in more detail in Chapter 9 "Disturbances of Atrioventricular Conduction" on page 469 (see especially "Classification of Disturbances of AV Conduction" on page 472). Classically, *Lenegre's disease* describes a fibrotic and calcific degenerative disease of the His-Purkinje conduction system of unknown cause. *Lev's disease* presents similarly but traditionally has involved the spread of fibrotic and calcific changes from neighboring structures of the cardiac fibrotic skeleton. Both conditions can lead to bradycardia secondary to varying degrees of AV block (see Figure 10-14 on page 479). As with other intrinsic causes of bradycardia, AV block due to degenerative diseases of the His-Purkinje system respond poorly to pharmacologic interventions.

7.1.4 THE AUTONOMIC NERVOUS SYSTEM AND FUNCTIONAL CONDUCTION BLOCK

While not reflected in the statistics (Table 7-1.) because these patients generally are not hospitalized and may never seek emergency care, cardioinhibitory (vasovagal) or vasodepressor syncope are probably the most common cause of syncope when all episodes are counted, especially in patients with structurally normal hearts. Often, but not always, these episodes may have a demonstrable "trigger" such as pain, fear, excitement, or anger. Sometimes normal biological functions such as micturition or even swallowing can trigger this type of syncope. Although the mechanism is not completely clear, there is evidence that a common neurohumoral trigger for these forms of syncope is β-adrenergic- or sympathetic activation which results in a subsequent and abrupt inappropriate degree of sympathetic withdrawal and parasympathetic (vagal) activation. Not only can this produce inappropriate vasodilation and bradycardia due to asystole or AV block, but it can also induce diaphoresis, nausea, and vomiting. In fact a prodrome of dizziness, sweating, nausea and vomiting is the classic diagnostic prodrome of vasovagal or vasodepressor syncope.

Accurate and early diagnosis of this syndrome in patients can spare them an unnecessary expensive, uncomfortable, and possibly invasive work-up including computerized brain scans, magnetic resonance imaging, or even electrophysiology testing. At a maximum, diagnosis may require a tilt table test. However, in most cases the diagnosis is readily apparent from the patient history, especially in young individuals lacking structural heart disease. Furthermore, treatment in patients with recurrent episodes often may require nothing more than β-adrenergic blocking agents which have been shown to work well [2-5], possibly by preventing the triggering increase in sympathetic activity. Other treatments include support hose, mineralocorticoids (fludrocortisone acetate) [6-8], α-adrenergic agonists (midodrine) [9-12], inhibitors of serotonin re-uptake (sertraline, fluoxetine) [13-15], and anticholinergic agents (propantheline, disopyramide) [8,16-18], although scopolamine has been shown to be ineffective [19].

Patients with the "garden variety" cardioinhibitory (vasovagal) syncope rarely require implantation with permanent pacemakers. In fact, pacemaker implantation alone rarely relieves these patients of all their symptoms because they usually have a mixed syndrome of vasodilation (vasodepressor) and bradycardia (vasovagal), the former of which is unaffected by the pacemaker. In these typical cases, medical therapy alone with one or more of the above agents treats both the vasodepressor and vasovagal components. There is a small subgroup, however, of patients with "malignant" cardioinhibitory syncope who have recurrent episodes of syncope associated with very long periods of asystole, sometimes up to 45 sec or longer (for example see Figure 9-1 on page 453). These long pauses may trigger polymorphic ventricular tachycardia or ventricular fibrillation making permanent pacemaker implantation, in conjunction with medical therapy, a necessity in some of these patients.

The *hypersensitive carotid sinus syndrome* is a very rare cause of neurally-mediated syncope in which symptomatic asystolic episodes result from even mild stimulation of the carotid sinus baroreceptors. Patients may give a history of syncope when wearing tight shirt collars, when looking up at flying airplanes, or when turning/twisting their neck in certain directions. Confirmatory diagnosis is considered to be a 3 sec pause induced by up to a 5 sec massage of the right or left carotid sinus (see Figure 9-6 on page 459). In our personal experience, the sensitivity and specificity of this diagnostic maneuver is increased by noting a positive result with even low pressure massage of the carotid sinus region. These patients generally require treatment with a permanent AV sequential pacemaker.

7.2 Urgent Management of Conduction Failure

7.2.1 OVERVIEW

As mentioned above at the beginning of this chapter urgent management of patients with symptomatic bradyarrhythmias should include a complete evaluation of the patient to assess for the presence of *extrinsic* or *secondary* factors/agents or underlying acute/chronic medical conditions/diseases which may be responsible for the bradyarrhythmia. In these cases, directing treatment at the underlying condition or withdrawing the potentially offending agent often is sufficient at reversing the bradycardia, whether it be at the level of the SA or AV node, or His-Purkinje system. Symptomatic secondary or functional bradycardias also are more likely to respond to conservative measures, such as volume expansion and reverse Trendelenberg positioning or pharmacological interventions such as intravenous anti-cholinergic agents or β-adrenergic agonists (Table 7-2.) Primary bradyarrhythmias resulting from fixed intrinsic conduction system disease generally fail to respond to these pharmacological interventions and instead require temporary pacing until permanent pacemaker implantation can be arranged.

TABLE 7-2. Acute treatment options for symptomatic bradyarrhythmias

---

Reverse Trendelenberg position

Volume expansion

Pharmacological interventions

  Anticholinergic agents

    Atropine: 0.6 mg - 1.0 mg IV bolus every 5 min (maximum dosage of 0.04 mg/kg)

  β-adrenergic agonists and activators of adenylyl cyclase

    Isoproterenol: beginning dose 0.5 - 1.0 μg/min continuous IV infusion; titrate up for heart rate effect

    Glucagon: 0.05 - 0.15 mg/kg IV bolus; repeat boluses as needed or continuous IV infusion (2 - 5 mg/hr)

  Anti-purinergic agents (methylxanthines)

    Aminophylline: 5 - 15 mg/kg IV infused over 5 min

  Digoxin toxicity

    Digoxin-specific antibody Fab fragments (Digibind)

Temporary pacing

  Temporary transcutaneous pacing

  Temporary transvenous pacing

7.2.2 PHARMACOLOGIC OPTIONS

Anti-cholinergic agents

Atropine exerts its effects on the SA and AV node by enhancing the rate of impulse formation in the SA node and transnodal conduction in the AV node (See "Neurohumoral Regulators of Ionic Currents" on page 109.) The initial dose of atropine is 0.6 to 1.0 mg [1]. This dose can be repeated until a satisfactory rate response is achieved. The maximal dose is generally 0.04 mg/kg. Generally speaking, if the initial dose does not relieve the reverse the bradycardia, whether due to problems with the SA node or AV conduction, subsequent doses are unlikely to work any better. In some patients with AV block, especially if the block is at the level of the His-Purkinje system, administration of atropine may significantly further slow the heart rate. This paradoxical response may result because while atropine may enhance AV nodal conduction of the sinus or atrial impulses, it does not relieve the His-Purkinje block. In fact, enhanced conduction of supraventricular impulses into the His-Purkinje system can worsen the block (concealed conduction) resulting in further slowing of the ventricular response. Patients who receive atropine should also be monitored for systemic anti-cholinergic effects of this drug. In addition, individuals with acute ischemia may potentially have a worsening of their symptoms due to an increase in ventricular rate.

β-adrenergic agonists

As with atropine, β-adrenergic agonists exert their effects on the SA and AV node by enhancing the rate of impulse formation in the SA node and transnodal conduction in the AV node (See "Neurohumoral Regulators of Ionic Currents" on page 109.) The starting dose of isoproterenol is 0.5 - 1.0 μg/min [1]. Generally speaking, if there is going to be a response it is apparent at a dose of 1 - 3 μg/min (Table 7-2.) Higher doses, even greater than 10 μg/min are required in patients on high dose β-adrenergic blocker therapy. Limiting side effects may include tachyarrhythmias, angina, anxiety, uncontrollable tremor, and paradoxical vagal activation with nausea, enhancement of the bradycardia along with a vasodepressor response with vasodilation, flushing, and worsening of hypotension.

Glucagon, which activates adenylyl cyclase, may be useful in patients who have bradycardia secondary to an overdose of β-adrenergic antagonists and Ca^{2+} channel blocking agents [1]. It may enhance sinus rhythm and junctional escape rhythms in these patients. Initial dose is 0.05 - 0.15 mg/kg intravenous bolus with repeat boluses as needed or continuous IV infusion up to 2 - 5 mg/hr [1]. Side effects, including nausea and vomiting, hyperglycemia, hypokalemia, and excessive respiratory secretions may limit re-boluses and the continuous intravenous infusion.

Anti-purinergic agents

Some secondary forms of AV nodal conduction block or sinus asystole, for example during acute myocardial ischemia, may result from release of endogenous stores of adenosine. Adenosine is a potent inhibitor of AV nodal conduction and can also completely suppress SA nodal activity by modulation of ionic currents (See "Neurohumoral Regulators of Ionic Currents" on page 109.) Aminophylline is a methylxanthine which can competitively inhibit adenosine at the receptor site and thereby reverse the bradycardia induced by adenosine (Table 7-2.) The dose is 5 - 15 mg/kg infused over 5 min [1].

Digoxin intoxication prevents a special challenge. Life-threatening hyperkalemia may occur secondary to severe digoxin toxicity. This hyperkalemia, along with the digoxin elevation, *per se*, may produce profound bradycardia (Figure 7-1) (and also possibly ventricular tachyarrhythmias). Acute management includes the administration of sodium bicarbonate, glucose, and insulin, sodium polystyrene sulfonate (Kayexalate), to quickly reduce the serum K^+ level., and digoxin-specific antibody Fab fragments (Digibind) to bind digoxin molecules. The bound digoxin and Fab fragments are excreted in the urine by the kidneys. The effects of treatment with digoxin-specific antibody Fab fragments is generally evident within 1-2 hours. The reader is referred to the package insert for dosing regimens for Digibind.

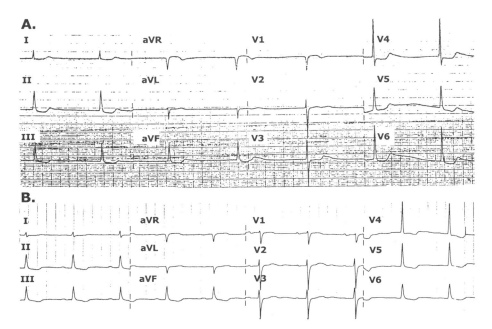

FIGURE 7-1. Digitalis-toxicity-induced sinus arrest or sinoatrial exit block. Panel A: 12-lead ECG taken from 84-year-old woman with a near-syncopal episode associated with a serum digoxin level of 4.9 nmol/L. The ECG shows an AV junctional rhythm at a rate of 39/min without any identifiable P wave activity. Panel B: Within 2 hours of administering digoxin-specific antibody Fab fragments (Digibind), sinus rhythm is restored at a rate of 60/min with a PR interval of 0.22 sec. Paper speed 25 mm/sec.

7.2.3 TEMPORARY PACING

Transcutaneous ventricular pacing

Transcutaneous pacing [20] is initiated by applying adhesive patch electrodes to the skin of the anterior and posterior chest walls (Figure 7-2). Standard ECG electrodes must also be applied for continuous ECG monitoring. The pacing electrodes, which have an

8-cm diameter conducting surface, are applied over the left anterior and posterior chest with the anterior (positive) patch placed over the point of maximal cardiac impulse. The electrodes are connected to a pacing pulse generator which is often incorporated into an external cardioverter-defibrillator unit. After application of the pacing and recording electrodes, the pulse generator should be activated and the current slowly increased until electrical capture of the ventricles occurs as assessed both from the filtered ECG and simultaneous palpation of a pulse wave directly related to the discharge of the pulse generator. The current output and pacing rate should be maintained as low as possible to maintain stable capture with acceptable blood pressure with minimization of patient discomfort. Sedation is often necessary to minimize patient anxiety and pain.

Transcutaneous pacing has been shown to be useful in patients with symptomatic bradycardias which fail to respond to atropine [20]. Complications of transcutaneous pacing include pain, induction of cardiac arrhythmias, tissue damage, failure to recognize underlying dangerous arrhythmias, such as ventricular fibrillation. Chest compressions over pacing patches can be performed without risk of electrical shock to health care personnel. Because of the potential complications and risk of loss of capture, transcutaneous pacing is strictly temporary and should be replaced with

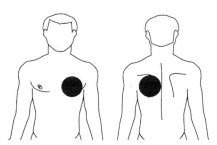

FIGURE 7-2. Proper Positioning of anterior (left) and posterior (right) transcutaneous adhesive pacing electrodes.

transvenous pacing, whether temporary or permanent, as soon as is feasible, but preferably within one hour [20].

Transvenous ventricular pacing

Patients who fail to respond to pharmacologic interventions, those who do respond but are deemed to be at recurrent risk of further episodes of symptomatic bradycardia, or those who have been temporarily stabilized with transcutaneous pacing, temporary placement of a transvenous pacing wire is usually the next step. The equipment needed for insertion of a temporary transvenous pacemaker is listed in Table 7-3.

TABLE 7-3. Equipment needed for temporary transvenous pacemaker insertion

Central venous introducer kit with intravenous 6-7 Fr cannula (sheath) and side-port

Fluoroscopy C-arm (optimum) or ECG machine (less optimum)

Portable constant current bipolar pulse generator

Bipolar 5-6 Fr balloon-tipped electrode catheter or balloon-tipped, flotation-directed pulmonary artery catheter with pace-port and pacing wire

Cabling to connect pacing wires to V lead of ECG machine and pulse generator

Intravenous access is obtained and placement of an introducer cannula (sheath) is accomplished using the modified Seldinger technique (Figure 2-9 on page 36). Access for transvenous pacing is usually achieved through the right internal jugular, left or right subclavian, or right or left femoral veins. Since many of these patients go on to receive a permanent pacemaker, the left subclavian vein is usually the least desirable site for the temporary pacing wire.

The pulse generator has indicator lights indicating when it paces and when it senses a ventricular depolarization. In addition, it should allow bipolar asynchronous and synchronous pacing with variably adjustable rate, current and sensitivity settings (Figure 7-3).

Placement of a transvenous pacing wire is most expeditiously accomplished using fluoroscopic guidance. In many cases, unfortunately, urgent transvenous pacemaker placement precludes the use of fluoroscopy. In these cases, a balloon-tipped, flow directed bipolar electrode catheter or a balloon-tipped, flow directed pulmonary artery catheter with a right ventricular port for a pacing wire are the preferred alternatives. Placement of the electrode catheter tip in the right ventricle is then accomplished either blindly or using electro-cardiographic guidance.

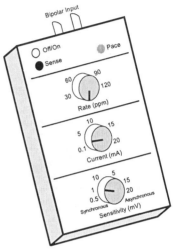

FIGURE 7-3. Example of constant current pulse generator with input for bipolar pacing leads and variably adjustable rate, sensitivity, and current settings.

For blind placement, the wire is connected to the pulse generator and the generator is turned on and adjusted to the maximum sensitivity. Pacing amperage should be set very low (<0.5 mA). The balloon should be inflated and the pacing wire advanced. Assuming there is blood flow across the tricuspid valve, the balloon should easily enter the right ventricle. Upon entering the ventricle, sensing of the right ventricle activation by the pulse generator should be evident (usually by a blinking light corresponding to every ventricular activation). At this point, the amperage should be increased to 5 mA and the lower rate increased to a rate above the patients intrinsic ventricular rate. The balloon should be deflated and the pacing lead slowly advanced further until pacing capture is achieved, documented by electrocardiographic recording and/or palpable pulse increase to the pacing rate. If there is failure to achieve capture after advancing the pacing lead 4-8 cm after entering the right ventricle, the operator should pull back the pacing lead to the original site of sensing of right ventricular activation, torque the lead slightly clockwise or counterclockwise, and re-advance the lead until capture is obtained. At this point the current should be reduced to determine the lowest amperage necessary to activate the ventricle. The final setting should be 2-3 times the minimal current require to pace the ventricle. In extremely urgent situations with asystole, advancing the wire with the pulse generator programmed to the asynchronous mode with the current output set to the maximum.

For placement using ECG guidance, the patient should be connected to the limb leads of an ECG machine. The distal electrode of the pacing wire is then connected to a V lead of the ECG machine and advanced as above. As the distal electrode travels through the superior vena cava to right atrium and into the right ventricle, the inscribed P wave will change from being negative and larger than the QRS complex (upper right atrium) to become positive and smaller than QRS complex as it finally arrives in the right ventricle. Once in the right ventricle, the balloon should be deflated and the lead advanced further. Upon contact with the ventricular endocardium, marked ST-elevation should be noted and synchronous sensing and pacing possible. As above, re-attempts with partial removal and torquing of the catheter may be necessary for eventual stable positioning with achievement of an acceptable pacing threshold.

Using the pace-port pulmonary artery flotation catheter is often the easiest. After floating the catheter into the pulmonary artery and localizing the "wedge" position, the RV port is used for easy placement of the small gauge pacing wire. This wire, furnished with the pulmonary artery catheter kit, can be advanced through the pacing port and connected to the pulse generator. After advancement beyond the opening in the right ventricle, the wire can be further advanced a few centimeters with the pulse generator set to the synchronous mode, with the current set at 5 mA, and the rate above the patient's intrinsic ventricular rate. For patients with very slow ventricular rates or asystole, the pulse generator should be set to the asynchronous mode.

Following insertion, by whichever technique, an anterior-posterior or posterior-anterior chest radiograph (and if possible, a lateral view as well) should be obtained to verify correct positioning near the right ventricular apex (Figure 7-4). A common problem is placement of the lead in the coronary sinus. In this case, pacing of the atria, and not the ventricle results.

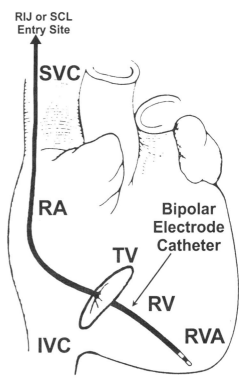

FIGURE 7-4. Schematic diagram illustrating optimum position of temporary pacing wire at right ventricular apex (RVA). Equivalent of radiograph AP view. IVC, inferior vena cava; RA, right atrium; RIJ, right internal jugular vein; RV, right ventricle; RVA, right ventricular apex; SCL, subclavian vein; SVC, superior vena cava; TV, tricuspid valve

However, ventricular pacing may be possible from the coronary sinus but in this case ECG during pacing will show a RBBB pattern in lead V_1 (left ventricular pacing), as opposed to the normal LBBB pattern in lead V_1 with pacing from the right ventricle. In addition, a lateral radiograph would show the pacemaker lead projecting along the posterior aspect of the heart in the great cardiac vein instead of anteriorly, where the right ventricular apex is located.

In addition, the final pacing threshold and sensing parameters should be assessed. The pacing threshold is tested by increasing the lower rate to 10-20/min greater than the patients intrinsic ventricular rate and decrease the current until capture is lost. This setting measures, in mA, the minimum current that must be applied from the constant current pulse generator to fully activate the cardiac tissue in contact with the distal bipolar pair of the pacing catheter. The final current setting should be set at 2-3 times the threshold level. Ideally, the pacing threshold should be less than 1 mA, but higher levels (<3 mA) are acceptable when blind, non-fluoroscopic placement is performed.

To assess the sensing function of the pacing system, the pulse generator should be adjusted to maximum sensitivity ("synchronous" mode) the rate should be set 10-20/min less than the patient's intrinsic ventricular rate (if possible) so that the patient's heart is not being paced, but is instead is beating spontaneously. Then, the sensitivity is decreased (turn the control knob slowly away from the synchronous mode toward the "asynchronous" mode) until pacing spikes appear and pacing resumes. At this point the pulse generator sensitivity has been decreased just to the point where the circuitry is no longer "seeing" the wavefront of ventricular activation and therefore the device has begun pacing the ventricle again. This setting measures the maximum amplitude of the ventricular systolic depolarization that can be sensed by the bipolar electrode pair in its current position within the heart. The higher the number (greater sensitivity), in mV, as read off the pulse generator sensitivity scale, the larger the voltage amplitude of the sensed ventricular systolic wavefront. Ordinarily, the final sensitivity setting should be set to a voltage at least one-half of the sensed voltage, but many operators just routinely set the sensitivity at its most sensitive position, ensuring pacing when needed and avoiding any competing asynchronous pacing with the patients own spontaneous ventricular rate, thereby reducing the risk of inducing ventricular tachyarrhythmias.

References

1. Brady WJ, Harrigan RA: Evaluation and management of bradyarrhythmias in the emergency department. *Emerg Med Clin NA* **16**:361-388, 1998.
2. Benditt DG, Erickson M, Gammage MD, et al.: A synopsis: neurocardiogenic syncope, an international symposium, 1996. *Pacing Clin Electrophysiol* **20**:851-60, 1997.
3. Cox MM, Perlman BA, Mayor MR, et al.: Acute and long-term beta-adrenergic blockade for patients with neurocardiogenic syncope. *J Am Coll Cardiol* **26**:1293-8, 1995.
4. Natale A, Newby KH, Dhala A, et al.: Response to beta blockers in patients with neurocardiogenic syncope: how to predict beneficial effects. *J Cardiovasc Electrophysiol* **7**:1154-8, 1996.
5. Sra JS, Jazayeri MR, Dhala A, et al.: Neurocardiogenic syncope. Diagnosis, mechanisms, and treatment. *Cardiol Clin* **11**:183-91, 1993.
6. Scott WA, Pongiglione G, Bromberg BI, et al.: Randomized comparison of atenolol and fludrocortisone acetate in the treatment of pediatric neurally mediated syncope. *Am J Cardiol* **76**:400-2, 1995.
7. Lazarus JC, Mauro VF: Syncope: pathophysiology, diagnosis, and pharmacotherapy. *Ann Pharmacother* **30**:994-1005, 1996.
8. Wolff GS: Unexplained syncope: clinical management. *Pacing Clin Electrophysiol* **20**:2043-7, 1997.

9.   Sra J, Maglio C, Biehl M, et al.: Efficacy of midodrine hydrochloride in neurocardiogenic syncope re-
      fractory to standard therapy. *J Cardiovasc Electrophysiol* **8**:42-6, 1997.

10.   Low PA, Gilden JL, Freeman R, et al.: Efficacy of midodrine vs. placebo in neurogenic orthostatic hy-
      potension. A randomized, double-blind multicenter study. Midodrine Study Group. *JAMA* **277**:1046-
      51, 1997.

11.   Ward C, Kenny RA: Observations on midodrine in a case of vasodepressor neurogenic syncope. *Clin
      Auton Res* **5**:257-60, 1995.

12.   Ward CR, Gray JC, Gilroy JJ, Kenny RA: Midodrine: a role in the management of neurocardiogenic
      syncope. *Heart* **79**:45-9, 1998.

13.   Grubb BP, Wolfe DA, Samoil D, et al.: Usefulness of fluoxetine hydrochloride for prevention of resis-
      tant upright tilt induced syncope. *Pacing Clin Electrophysiol* **16**:458-64, 1993.

14.   Grubb BP, Samoil D, Kosinski D, et al.: Use of sertraline hydrochloride in the treatment of refractory
      neurocardiogenic syncope in children and adolescents. *J Am Coll Cardiol* **24**:490-4, 1994.

15.   Tandan T, Giuffre M, Sheldon R: Exacerbations of neurally mediated syncope associated with sertra-
      line. *Lancet* **349**:1145-6, 1997.

16.   Yu JC, Sung RJ: Clinical efficacy of propantheline bromide in neurocardiogenic syncope: pharmacody-
      namic implications. *Cardiovasc Drugs Ther* **10**:687-92, 1997.

17.   Grubb BP, Temesy-Armos P, Moore J, et al.: The use of head-upright tilt table testing in the evaluation
      and management of syncope in children and adolescents. *Pacing Clin Electrophysiol* **15**:742-8, 1992.

18.   Grubb BP, Kosinski D, Mouhaffel A, Pothoulakis A: The use of methylphenidate in the treatment of re-
      fractory neurocardiogenic syncope. *Pacing Clin Electrophysiol* **19**:836-40, 1996.

19.   Lee TM, Su SF, Chen MF, et al.: Usefulness of transdermal scopolamine for vasovagal syncope. *Am J
      Cardiol* **78**:480-2, 1996.

20.   Barthell E, Troiano P, Olson D, et al.: Prehospital external cardiac pacing: a prospective, controlled
      clinical trial. *Ann Emerg Med* **17**:1221-6, 1988.

CHAPTER 8

DIAGNOSIS AND ACUTE MANAGEMENT OF PATIENTS WITH SYMPTOMATIC TACHYARRHYTHMIAS

The acute management of patients with symptomatic tachyarrhythmias is complicated by the fact that the mechanism of the tachycardia is often difficult to quickly determine. The familiar classification of supraventricular tachycardias displaying a narrow QRS complex while ventricular tachycardias exhibit a wide QRS complex is a potentially dangerous oversimplification. Likewise, the common assumption that a patient with a hemodynamically stable tachycardia — narrow or wide QRS complex — must be having a supraventricular tachycardia can lead to disastrous results if treated inappropriately. Patients with hemodynamically unstable tachycardias should always be treated emergently with electrical shock according to the guidelines of the American Heart Association presented in their Advanced Cardiac Life Support course. All patients with a hemodynamically stable tachycardia should be approached and managed systematically. In particular, the tachycardia should be safely terminated so as to avoid converting a hemodynamically stable tachyarrhythmia into an unstable one. Also, without compromising the acute management of the patient, the physician should make an effort establish the mechanism of the tachycardia.

8.1 Supraventricular Tachyarrhythmias

The term "supraventricular tachyarrhythmias" refers to abnormally rapid rhythms originating above the bifurcation of the His bundle of the AV conduction system. These arrhythmias include sinus tachycardia, high cristal atrial (sinoatrial reentrant) tachycardia, inappropriate sinus tachycardia, focal and reentrant atrial tachycardias, multifocal atrial tachycardia, atrial flutter, atrial fibrillation, accelerated AV junctional rhythm (tachycardia), AV nodal reentrant tachycardia, and AV reciprocating tachycardia involving an accessory AV connection. Because the process of ventricular depolarization remains normal, the QRS complex during these arrhythmias is identical to that seen in sinus rhythm unless there is a development of functional (rate-dependent) bundle branch block (aberrant conduction), or ventricular preexcitation due to the presence of an accessory AV connection.

8.1.1 HEMODYNAMIC CONSEQUENCES OF SUPRAVENTRICULAR TACHYARRHYTHMIAS

The AV node possesses decremental conduction properties and functions as a protective barrier by limiting the rate of ventricular response during supraventricular tachyarrhyth-

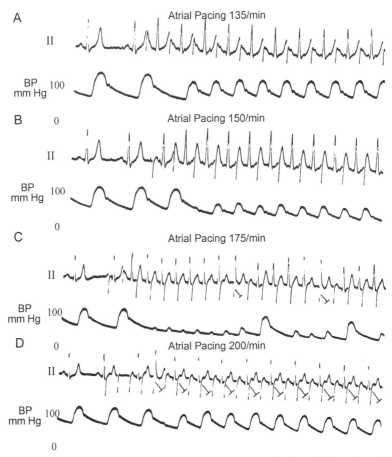

FIGURE 8-1. AV node functioning as a protective barrier. ECG lead II and femoral arterial blood pressure are simultaneously recorded. Panel A, With atrial pacing at 135/min, there is 1:1 AV conduction. The corresponding blood pressure is slightly decreased from a control of 125/65 to 115/65 mm Hg. Panel B, With atrial pacing at 150/min, 1:1 AV conduction results in a decrease of blood pressure to 95/60 mm Hg. Panel C, With atrial pacing at 175/min, there is development of an AV Wenckebach phenomenon. Preceding the appearance of the AV Wenckebach phenomenon, the 1:1 AV conduction resulted in a significant fall of blood pressure to 70/55 mm Hg. Note the restoration of blood pressure after the appearance AV Wenckebach block. Panel D, With atrial pacing at 200/min, development of 2:1 AV Wenckebach phenomenon (ventricular rate 100 per minute) prevents development of hypotension.

mias (Figure 8-1). However, during a sustained episode of tachycardia, loss of synchronized atrial contraction can reduce resting cardiac output by 5 to 15% in patients without structural heart disease, and by as much as 20 to 45% in patients with structural heart disease [1-4]. A rapid ventricular rate shortens ventricular diastole and compromises ventricular filling, thereby decreasing cardiac output and blood pressure.

Blood pressure falls dramatically with the onset of tachycardia. After 20 or 30 seconds, blood pressure is partially restored by reflex mechanisms that increase systemic arterial resistance and slow the rate of tachycardia. If reflex mechanisms fail to rescue blood pressure, symptoms may then develop in the patient. The severity of the hemodynamic instability depends on the ventricular rate, duration of tachycardia, and left ventricular function.

Patients with structurally normal hearts may experience no initial symptoms during tachycardia other than an awareness of palpitation. As the tachycardia continues for hours to days, cardiac output and blood pressure may further decline. Even patients without structural heart disease may develop symptoms of dizziness, chest pain, shortness of breath, and syncope [5].

The presence of structural heart disease will alter hemodynamic tolerance of rapid heart rate when there is interference with left ventricular function. Left atrial thrombus or tumor and mitral valvular stenosis may severely limit left ventricular filling during tachycardia resulting in pulmonary venous congestion. Ventricular distortion with concentric or asymmetric hypertrophy [6-8] is accompanied by sluggish relaxation and poor diastolic compliance which may impede ventricular filling, reduce cardiac output, and lead to hypotension and syncope during tachycardia. Loss of atrial contraction may further aggravate these symptoms. Increased resistance to coronary blood flow has been demonstrated in hypertrophic ventricles [9]. This may limit subendocardial blood flow during tachycardia. In patients with congestive cardiomyopathy and with impairment of ventricular emptying as in aortic stenosis or severe ventricular hypertrophy, cardiac output and coronary perfusion may be compromised during tachycardia. Finally, reduction of blood flow to vital organs such as cerebral, renovascular, or peripheral vascular systems may be unmasked or worsened by supraventricular tachyarrhythmias [5].

8.1.2 ACUTE MANAGEMENT OF SUPRAVENTRICULAR TACHYARRHYTHMIAS

Vagal maneuvers
The sinus and AV nodal tissues have abundant autonomic innervation. Arrhythmias that depend on conduction at these two sites may respond to maneuvers that increase vagal tone. Recommended vagal maneuvers include: carotid sinus massage [10], gag reflex, Valsalva maneuver, eyeball compression, facial immersion in cold water, and the use of pharmacologic agents such as edrophonium [11,12] and α-adrenergic agonists (phenylephrine and metaraminol). These manipulations or pharmacologic agents (seldom used today) are effective in patients with normal reflex autonomic sensitivity. Baroreceptor sensitivity is diminished with age, chronic hypertension and congestive heart failure [13,14]. The use of α-adrenergic drugs is not without risks in patients with hypertension or depressed left ventricular function.

Vagal maneuvers can be applied to terminate reentrant supraventricular tachycardias such as sinoatrial reentrant tachycardia, AV nodal reentrant tachycardia, and AV reciprocating tachycardia involving the AV node as a part of the reentrant circuit. Vagal maneuvers can only temporarily slow the rate of ventricular response during atrial tachycardia, atrial flutter, and atrial fibrillation (Figure 8-2). In applying carotid sinus massage, the carotid arteries should never be manipulated simultaneously and the duration of massage should not exceed five seconds. Carotid sinus massage is immediately discontinued on termination of supraventricular tachycardia or with the appearance of ventricu-

Baseline

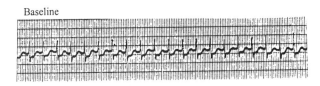

Carotid Sinus Pressure   Cessation of Carotid Sinus Pressure

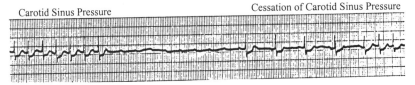

FIGURE 8-2. Carotid sinus pressure during atrial tachycardia fails to terminate the atrial tach-yarrhythmia, but does block AV conduction, revealing the P waves continuing at 150/min. Fol-lowing cessation of carotid sinus massage, the transient AV block resolves, and 1:1 AV conduction resumes. Continuous recording of ECG lead II is shown. Paper speed 25 mm/sec.

lar ectopy to avoid initiation of ventricular fibrillation (Figure 8-3) and post-conversion bradyarrhythmias. Ipsilateral cerebral infarction with contralateral hemiplegia can rarely occur following carotid sinus massage. Auscultation for carotid bruits and avoidance of carotid sinus massage in patients with known cerebrovascular disease or occlusive carot-id artery disease may reduce the risk of this catastrophic complication particularly in eld-erly patients. Carotid sinus massage should be avoided in patients with known carotid sinus hypersensitivity unless it is performed for diagnostic purposes, and it is contraindi-

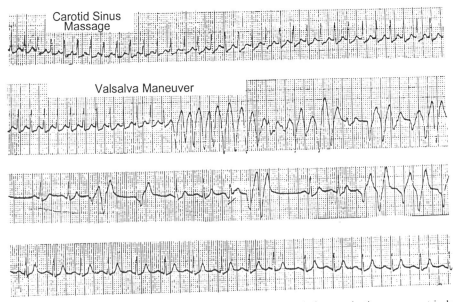

FIGURE 8-3. Transient ventricular arrhythmia during vagal maneuvers before terminating a supraventricular tachycardia. Continuous recording of ECG lead II is shown. Carotid sinus massage fails to terminate the arrhythmia (top tracing). Valsalva maneuver induces transient ventricular tachyarrhythmia (two middle trac-ings) but also terminates the supraventricular tachycardia. Paper speed 25 mm/sec.

Adenosine, 6 mg, IV bolus

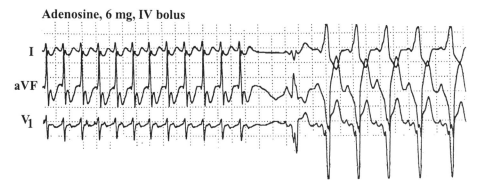

FIGURE 8-4. Termination of supraventricular tachycardia by adenosine. Rapid intravenous bolus infusion of 6 mg of adenosine terminates the tachycardia within 10 sec. Note the appearance of a delta wave during sinus rhythm after conversion of the arrhythmia, suggesting that atrioventricular reciprocating tachycardia is the mechanism of preceding supraventricular tachycardia. ECG leads I, aVF, and V_1 are simultaneously recorded. Paper speed 25 mm//sec.

cated in patients with suspected digitalis intoxication as it may provoke fatal ventricular fibrillation.

Antiarrhythmic agents

For acute termination of reentrant supraventricular tachycardias, intravenous verapamil (5-10 mg/3min) [15], diltiazem (15-20 mg/5min) [16], digoxin, and β-adrenergic blocking agents such as metoprolol and propranolol are effective as theses agents depress conduction and increase refractoriness of the sinoatrial and AV nodes. Clinically, adenosine given as an intravenous bolus (6 or 12 mg) is most often used because of its having a very short half-life of 5-9 seconds (Figure 8-4) [17-19]. Adenosine exerts its electrophysiologic effects (through A_1 receptors) either by directly increasing the intracellular guanosine triphosphate-binding protein G_i or by indirectly inhibiting the G_s/adenylyl cyclase/cyclic adenosine monophosphate (cAMP) system. The precise mechanism by which these adenosine-induced alterations depress sinoatrial and AV node conduction remains to be defined. It is proposed that G_i directly activates adenosine-sensitive potassium channels, thereby increasing an outward potassium current, $I_{K(Ado)}$ and driving the cellular resting potential more negatively toward the potassium equilibrium potential (hyperpolarization) [17,20]. An alternative possibility is that the increase in G_i antagonizes the intracellular effects of G_s, thereby antagonizing the β-adrenergic-mediated increase in L-type Ca^{++} current (I_{Ca}), and also possibly the pacemaker current (I_f) [21].

Intravenous verapamil, diltiazem and β-adrenergic blocking agents may also be used to slow the ventricular rate of atrial tachycardia, atrial flutter, and atrial fibrillation [22]. In clinical settings in which a brief duration of β-adrenergic blockade is needed, intravenous esmolol (500 µg/kg in one minute followed by 100-200 µg/kg/min infusion) can be used as it has a short half life of 9 minutes [23]. Although various antiarrhythmic agents can be tried to terminate atrial flutter and atrial fibrillation [24-30], a new class III antiarrhythmic agent, ibutilide (0.5–1.0 mg/10 min intravenous infusion x 2, 10 min

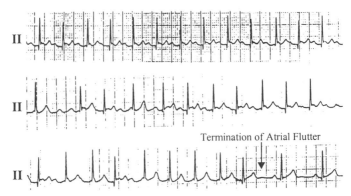

FIGURE 8-5. Termination of atrial flutter with ibutilide. After two intravenous bolus infusions of ibutilide, each 1 mg, administered 10 min apart, atrial flutter is converted to sinus rhythm. Top tracing: Baseline rhythm showing atrial flutter with 2:1 atrioventricular block. Middle tracing: Development of varying degrees of atrioventricular block after ibutilide infusions. Bottom tracing: Conversion of atrial flutter to sinus rhythm. ECG lead II recorded at a paper speed of 25 mm/sec.

apart), appears to have a greater efficacy in converting atrial flutter (50-70%) and atrial fibrillation (30-50%) to sinus rhythm (Figure 8-5) [31,32]. Ibutilide activates a slow inward Na^+ current and also blocks the rapidly-activating delayed rectifier K^+ current (I_{Kr}) thereby prolonging the duration of action potential [33-35]. The resultant increase in atrial refractoriness is believed to be the mechanism by which ibutilide terminates atrial flutter and atrial fibrillation.

Class I antiarrhythmic agents depress conduction and increase refractoriness of the atrium, His-Purkinje system, ventricle, and accessory AV connection [36,37]. Intravenous procainamide can be used for terminating AV reciprocity tachycardia by its action on accessory AV connection (Figure 8-6). Procainamide, quinidine, and disopyramide

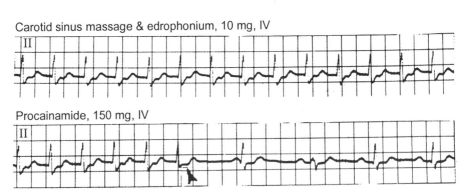

FIGURE 8-6. Termination of supraventricular tachycardia with intravenous procainamide. Panel A, Carotid sinus massage and edrophonium, 10 mg, IV, fail to terminate the tachycardia. Panel B, Within 2 minutes after infusion of procainamide, 150 mg, IV, the tachycardia is converted to sinus rhythm. The sudden disappearance of retrograde P wave (arrow) before termination of tachycardia suggests development of retrograde conduction block in an accessory AV connection or a fast AV nodal pathway induced by procainamide. Paper speed 25 mm/sec.

have also been demonstrated to be effective in suppressing retrograde fast AV nodal pathway conduction. Thus, intravenous procainamide may also be used for terminating the slow-fast form of AV nodal reentrant tachycardia [38]. Furthermore, intravenous procainamide (or lidocaine) is useful for slowing the rate of ventricular response during atrial flutter or fibrillation with ventricular preexcitation by virtue of its depressive action on accessory AV connection (Figure 8-7). In patients with rapid ventricular rate with ventricular preexcitation, the use of intravenous digitalis or verapamil is considered to be contraindicated. Digitalis may shorten the refractory period of the accessory AV connection and increase ventricular vulnerability to ventricular fibrillation [39]. Verapamil depresses AV nodal conduction and may thus enhance conduction of accessory AV connection [15]. Moreover, verapamil induces vasodilation which, in turn, decreases systemic vascular resistance and stimulates sympathetic reflex. Consequently, it may thereby shorten the refractory period of the accessory AV connection and increase the ventricular response leading to an onset of ventricular fibrillation (Figure 8-8).

Intravenous d,l-sotalol and amiodarone may not be effective in terminating reentrant supraventricular tachycardias, atrial flutter, and atrial fibrillation [28,29]. However, these two agents may be effective at maintaining sinus rhythm [40]. In acute clinical settings in which maintenance of sinus rhythm is critical, intravenous sotalol or amiodarone may be used before and after electrical conversion of supraventricular tachyarrhythmias. d,l-sotalol possesses both class III antiarrhythmic activity and beta-adrenergic blocking effects, while amiodarone affects Na^+, Ca^{++}, and K^+ channels and β-adrenergic receptors.

Atrial fibrillation with rapid ventricular response

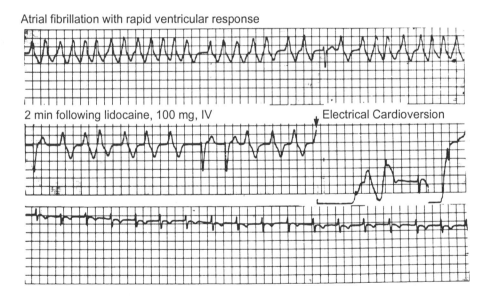

FIGURE 8-7. Slowing of rapid ventricular response with intravenous lidocaine during atrial fibrillation in a patient with the Wolff-Parkinson-White syndrome. Top panel, transvenous infusion of lidocaine, 100 mg, IV slows the rate of ventricular response. Middle panel, synchronized DC electrical cardioversion (down arrow) subsequently converts atrial fibrillation to sinus rhythm (bottom panel). Paper speed 25 mm/sec.

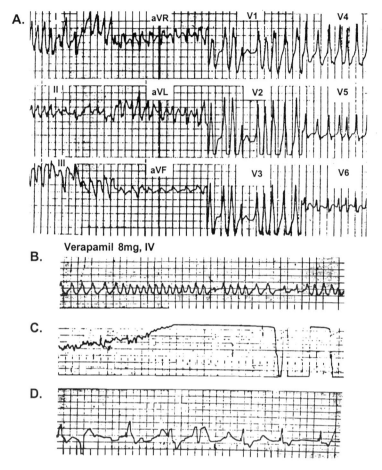

FIGURE 8-8. .Adverse effects of intravenous verapamil on atrial fibrillation with ventricular preexcitation. Panel A: Atrial fibrillation with ventricular preexcitation (Wolff-Parkinson-White syndrome) in 19 year old man. The 12-lead ECG shows findings indicating
the presence of a left-sided (posterolateral) accessory atrioventricular connection. Panel
B: The ventricular response of atrial fibrillation accelerates from 200/min to 300/min. after
infusion of verapamil, 8 mg. Panel C: The rhythm then degenerates into ventricular fibrillation. Panel D: delayed resuscitation results in idioventricular rhythm and demise of the
patient. Recordings in panels B, C, and D are not continuous. Paper speed 25 mm/sec.

Both agents prolong refractoriness of the atrium, AV node, ventricle, and accessory AV
connection.

Cardiac pacing
The techniques of cardiac pacing are particularly useful when a reentrant supraventricular tachycardia is resistant to pharmacological termination and repeated electrical cardioversion is impractical. The atrial pacing technique is an effective means of terminating
reentrant supraventricular tachycardia and atrial flutter [41]. The ventricular pacing

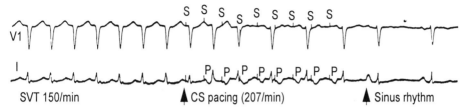

FIGURE 8-9. Termination of supraventricular tachycardia (SVT) with overdrive atrial pacing. ECG leads V1 and I are simultaneously recorded. Coronary sinus (CS) pacing at a rate of 207 per minute converts the tachycardia at a rate of 150 beats per minute to sinus rhythm. P = P wave. S = stimulus artifact. Paper speed 25 mm/sec

technique may be applied for terminating AV nodal reentrant tachycardia and AV reciprocating tachycardia.

For acute termination of a reentrant supraventricular tachycardia, the mode of pacing can be either overdrive or underdrive pacing. Overdrive pacing is to pace at a rate in excess of the rate of the arrhythmia (Figure 8-9), and underdrive pacing is to pace at a rate slower than the rate of the arrhythmia (Figure 8-10).

While overdrive atrial pacing is not expected to be effective in terminating automatic (ectopic) atrial tachycardia or atypical atrial flutter, atrial overdrive pacing will increase impulse bombardment at the AV node (concealed AV nodal conduction) thereby slowing the rate of ventricular response. This may yield beneficial hemodynamic effects in patients with symptomatic hypotension in an acute setting (Figure 8-1). Overdrive atrial pacing, however, may provoke atrial flutter or fibrillation. Thus, it may be hazardous in patients with ventricular preexcitation (Wolff-Parkinson-White syndrome).

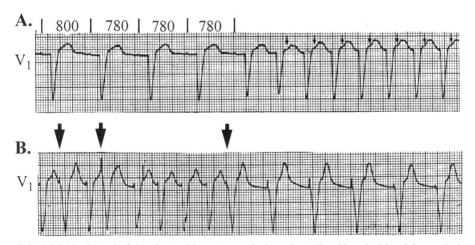

FIGURE 8-10. Control of chronic repetitive supraventricular tachycardia with underdrive right ventricular pacing. Panel A: Spontaneous initiation of supraventricular tachycardia after the sinus rate accelerated (shortening of the sinus cycle length from 800 to 780 msec). During tachycardia, there is complete left bundle branch block with a retrograde P wave inscribed immediately after the QRS complex (small arrows), suggestive of an AV reciprocating tachycardia (confirmed by electrophysiology study). Panel B: Underdrive right ventricular pacing at a rate of 88/min terminates the tachycardia at a rate of 136/min. Capture and fusion beats are denoted with the large arrows. Paper speed 25 mm/sec.

Electrical cardioversion

Emergency cardioversion is the treatment of choice for patients with severe hypotension and inadequate perfusion to vital organs during supraventricular tachyarrhythmias. This occurs more frequently in patients with a rapid ventricular rate, particularly atrial flutter with 1:1 AV conduction or atrial fibrillation with ventricular preexcitation. These patients may clinically manifest dizziness, syncope, angina, and congestive heart failure resulting from hemodynamic instability. The objective of direct current (DC) cardioversion is to drive electrical current across the heart to depolarize the entire or a portion of the entire heart, after which sinus rhythm may ensue [42].

DC cardioversion is applied under continuous ECG monitoring. The electrical discharge should be QRS synchronized to avoid current delivery during the ventricular vulnerable period [43]. Once the patient is anesthetized and electrically isolated, R-wave synchronized energy adequate to terminate a specific supraventricular tachyarrhythmia (usually less than 100 joules except for atrial fibrillation) is applied. In attempting to convert atrial fibrillation, initial management should include slowing of the ventricular rate, after which electrical cardioversion can be attempted. Direct current countershocks with energies up to 360 joules (monophasic waveform) or 200 joules (biphasic waveform) may be required. To ensure delivery of current through both atria, placement of the electrode pads at the right parasternal and left posterior infrascapular positions may provide the optimum current vector (Figure 8-11). Failure to terminate the arrhythmia should prompt reevaluation of the technique, equipment, and the patient's clinical status. A change of electrode pad placement from an anterior-posterior location to a apical-right subclavicular position, or vice-versa, may be required. Alternative methods for arrhythmia termination should be considered. These include addition of an antiarrhythmic agent before DC cardioversion such as intravenous procainamide or ibutilide for atrial flutter and fibrillation. In patients with atrial tachycardia with AV block due to digitalis intoxication, electrical countershock is contraindicated as it may expose serious ventricular tachyarrhythmias [44].

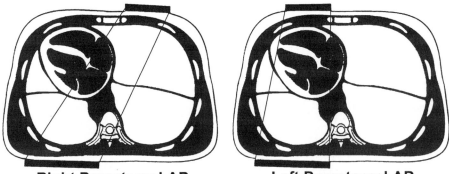

Right Parasternal AP   **Left Parasternal AP**

FIGURE 8-11. Options for electrode pad position for transthoracic cardioversion of atrial fibrillation. The right parasternal anterior-posterior (AP) position has the advantage of directing a current vector through both atria. However, the electrode distance is long and a the current pathway necessarily involves a significant amount of lung tissue. In contrast, the left parasternal AP position results in a shorter current pathway, although the current vector fails to completely encompass both atria.

Electrophysiology study and catheter ablation

In patients with recurrent supraventricular tachyarrhythmias refractory to pharmacologic therapy, precise diagnoses and characterization of the arrhythmias are required. Specifically, many supraventricular tachyarrhythmias are potentially curable with the technique of radiofrequency catheter ablation. These supraventricular tachyarrhythmias include AV reciprocating tachycardia, AV node reentrant tachycardia, atrial tachycardia, and atrial flutter [45]. The success rates of catheter ablation in these arrhythmias are very high and risks are relatively low and manageable.

8.1.3 SUPRAVENTRICULAR TACHYARRHYTHMIAS DURING THE POSTOPERATIVE PERIOD

Supraventricular tachyarrhythmias, particularly atrial flutter and atrial fibrillation, may occur in as high as 30% of patients undergoing cardiac surgery (e.g., aortocoronary bypass grafting and valvular replacement) during the postoperative period. The onset of these arrhythmias is usually triggered by a high catecholamine state (i.e., incision pain, intubation, vasopressor agents, etc.) with or without associated pericarditis. If there are no clinical contraindications, β-adrenergic blocking agents are the drugs of choice not only for slowing the ventricular response, but also for termination of the arrhythmia. Intravenous ibutilide may also be effective for terminating atrial flutter and atrial fibrillation in acute clinical settings [46], and intravenous or oral amiodarone may be needed for short-term maintenance of sinus rhythm.

8.2 Ventricular Tachyarrhythmias

Ventricular tachyarrhythmias are abnormally rapid rhythms originating at or below the bifurcation of the His bundle of the AV conduction system. These arrhythmias include ventricular tachycardia and ventricular fibrillation. Because of having abnormal process of ventricular depolarization, the QRS complexes of both ventricular tachycardia and ventricular fibrillation are broad ($\geq$ 120 ms) and bizarre (Figure 8-12). However, fascicular tachycardia, a form of ventricular tachycardia with an origin located at one of the fascicles of bundle branches, can manifest a relatively narrow (<120 ms) QRS complex particularly when it is arising at the proximal portion of a fascicle close to the His bundle proper (Figure 8-13) [47,48]. Fascicular tachycardia is often mistaken for supraventricular tachycardia.

8.2.1 HEMODYNAMIC CONSEQUENCES OF VENTRICULAR TACHYCARDIA

Ventricular tachycardia generally connotes a much worse clinical outcome than supraventricular tachyarrhythmias. This is because of its frequent association with structural heart disease such as atherosclerotic coronary heart disease and primary or secondary cardiomyopathy [49], and its lack of a protective barrier (e.g., the AV node in supraventricular tachycardia) to modulate the ventricular rate. Furthermore, loss of atrial

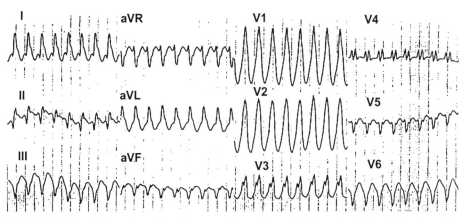

FIGURE 8-12. Ventricular tachycardia with a very wide and bizarre QRS complex. Note the duration of the QRS complex is 200 ms, the marked left axis deviation, and the monophasic QS in lead V6, all findings highly suggestive that the tachyarrhythmia is ventricular tachycardia and not supraventricular tachycardia with aberrancy. Paper speed 25 mm/sec.

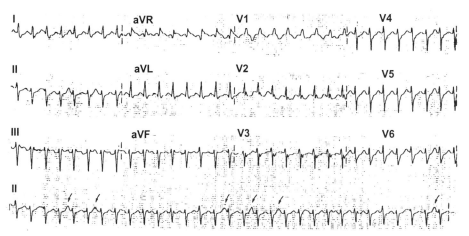

FIGURE 8-13. Surface 12-lead ECG from a 42 year-old man with a structurally normal heart and ventricular tachycardia with its origin in a fascicle of the left bundle branch. Intracardiac electrophysiologic evaluation confirmed this rhythm to be ventricular tachycardia. Note the relatively narrow duration of the QRS complex (100 ms), making this tachycardia often mistaken for supraventricular in origin. During electrophysiology study this tachycardia was mapped to the proximal portion of the left posterior fascicle of the left bundle branch where it was successfully ablated with radiofrequency energy (not shown). The downward arrows point to sinus P wave activity dissociated from the ventricular rhythm, an important finding which suggested the ultimate electrophysiologic diagnosis of ventricular tachycardia as opposed to supraventricular tachycardia. Paper speed 25 mm/sec.

contribution and the altered process of ventricular depolarization all contribute to reduction of cardiac output, blood pressure, and coronary perfusion. Consequently, ventricular tachycardia can easily produce symptoms of dizziness, syncope, angina, and congestive heart failure, and can rapidly degenerate into ventricular fibrillation causing cardiac arrest (sudden cardiac death syndrome).

8.2.2 DIFFERENTIAL DIAGNOSIS OF A WIDE QRS COMPLEX TACHYCARDIA

Although ventricular tachycardia usually manifests as a wide QRS complex tachycardia, supraventricular tachyarrhythmias with aberrant conduction (functional or preexisting bundle branch block) or with ventricular preexcitation can also present with wide QRS complexes. The clinical clues that are useful in distinguishing between SVT and VT are summarized below (Table 8-1.) and some of the critical ECG findings suggestive of VT are illustrated in Figures 8-12 through 8-14.

It should not be overemphasized that exceptions to the rules do exist. For instance, idiopathic ventricular tachycardia is often found in patients without clinical evidence of structural heart disease and may be responsive to adenosine and verapamil [50-52]; patients with ventricular tachycardia may manifest stable hemodynamics and supraventricular tachycardia with fast ventricular rate may cause syncope, angina and congestive heart failure, particularly in the presence of structural heart disease. In some cases, electrophysiology study is required for differential diagnosis (Figure 8-15 & Figure 8-16).

8.2.3 ACUTE MANAGEMENT OF VENTRICULAR TACHYARRHYTHMIAS

Cardioversion and ventricular defibrillation
Ventricular fibrillation usually causes cardiac arrest. Immediate defibrillation (without QRS synchronization) using a direct current countershock of ≥ 200 joules is recommended to restore sinus rhythm to minimize hypoperfusion to other vital organs such as the

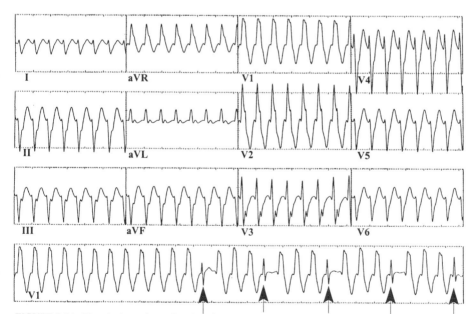

FIGURE 8-14. Ventricular tachycardia with bizarre QRS complex. The duration of the QRS complexes is 180 ms and there is marked left axis deviation. Note the intermittent sinus capture beats (upward arrows) in the rhythm strip at the bottom of the figure (ECG lead V1). Paper speed 25 mm/sec.

TABLE 8-1. Factors useful in the differentiation of wide QRS complex tachycardias: VT versus SVT.

Clinical Factors

Patients with structural heart disease, especially with prior MI, and recent onset of arrhythmia are more likely to have VT or, AFL with functional or preexisting bundle branch block. Patients with a structurally normal heart and a long history of arrhythmia are more likely to have an SVT with aberrant conduction.

Patients who present with serious symptoms such as angina, syncope, congestive heart failure and cardiac arrest are more likely to have ventricular tachycardia.

Termination of tachycardia by vagal maneuvers, and/or adenosine, favors reentrant SVT with aberrant conduction. Adenosine or vagal-induced transient AV nodal block without interruption of atrial activity indicates atrial tachycardia and atrial flutter with aberrant conduction [18,53-58].

Electrocardiographic Features [59-63].

QRS complex

RBBB pattern

Monophasic R in V_1 favors VT

Amplitude of left "rabbit ear" > right "rabbit ear" in V_1 Rsr' favors VT

RS pattern in V_1 favors VT

Monophasic Q or Qr' pattern in V_6 favors VT

LBBB pattern

qR or qS pattern in V_6 favors VT

R wave in V_1 or V_2 > 30 ms duration favors VT

Any Q wave in V6 favors VT

Time from onset of QRS to nadir of S wave in V_1 or V_2 > 60 ms favors VT

Notching on the downstroke of the S wave in V_1 or V_2 favors VT

QRS duration

≥ 0.14 sec favors VT (assuming no pre-existing BBB or use AAD)

QRS axis

LAD (<-30°) favors VT

RAD in association with LBBB pattern favors VT

QRS concordance in precordial leads

Positive concordance (in absence of RVH) favors VT; negative concordance less strongly favors VT

QRS capture/fusion complexes

Capture/fusion complexes strongly favors VT

AV relationship

AV dissociation strongly favors VT

Rhythm

Irregular rhythm is evidence against VT and instead favors AF with aberrant conduction or anterograde conduction over an accessory AV connection

AAD, antiarrhythmic drug; AF, atrial fibrillation; AFL, atrial flutter; BBB, bundle branch block; LAD, left axis deviation; LBBB, left bundle branch block; MI, myocardial infarction; RAD, right axis deviation; RBBB, right bundle branch block; RVH, right ventricular hypertrophy; SVT, supraventricular tachycardia; VT, ventricular tachycardia

brain, liver, and kidneys. Ventricular tachycardia also needs immediate cardioversion (with QRS synchronization) if it causes unstable hemodynamics, e.g., dizziness, syncope, angina, and congestive heart failure. The electrical energy required for converting ventricular tachycardia is relatively low as 20 to 50 joules is usually sufficient.

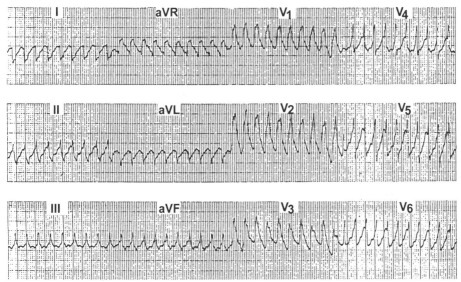

FIGURE 8-15. Surface 12-lead ECG from a 23-year-old woman without structural heart disease suffering from an episode of palpitation with near-syncope. The ECG shows wide bizarre QRS complexes with a right bundle branch block morphology with a right inferior frontal plane axis at a rate of 240/min. Note alternating QRS morphology in V_2 through V_6 (QRS duration 160 ms and 140 ms, respectively). Also note rS and QS patterns in leads I and aVL, respectively, suggestive of ventricular tachycardia. The electrophysiology study (Figure 8-16), however, shows that this is an AV nodal reentrant tachycardia with aberrant conduction (right bundle branch block and left posterior hemiblock). Paper speed 25 mm/sec.

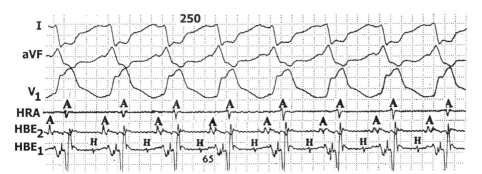

FIGURE 8-16. Intracardiac recordings obtained during electrophysiology study in the patient exhibiting the tachycardia shown in Figure 8-15. The study shows that the tachycardia is the slow-fast form of AV nodal reentrant tachycardia with aberrant ventricular conduction (right bundle branch block and left posterior hemiblock). The tachycardia cycle length is 250 ms and the H-V interval is 65 ms. HRA, high right atrium; HBE_{1-2}, distal to proximal His bundle electrographic lead. Paper speed 100 ms.

Pharmacotherapy

In patients who are successfully cardioverted for ventricular tachycardia or defibrillated for ventricular fibrillation, intravenous infusion of lidocaine (100 mg and 50 mg boluses 10 min apart followed by 1-4 mg/min maintenance drip) should be initiated. If lidocaine fails, intravenous procainamide (10-15 mg/kg infused at 50 mg/min followed by 1-4 mg/ min maintenance drip) may be used. If neither intravenous lidocaine nor intravenous procainamide is effective in preventing the arrhythmia from recurrence, then intravenous amiodarone therapy should be considered [40]. Clinical studies have shown that the efficacy of intravenous amiodarone ranges from 51 to 100% in suppressing ventricular tachycardia and ventricular fibrillation [64-71]. Intravenous amiodarone is administered at 150 mg bolus/20 min x 2, 30 min apart followed by 0.5-1.0 mg/min maintenance drip. If it is shown to be effective, oral amiodarone can be started with a loading of 800-1600 mg/day until a total of 10 grams (both IV and oral) has been given.

TABLE 8-2. Electropharmacologic effects of oral and intravenous amiodarone.

Variable	Oral amiodarone	Intravenous amiodarone
Prolongation of APD in atria and ventricles	+++	+
Na$^+$ channel blockade with decrease in AP upstroke	+++	++
Decrease in rate of phase 4 depolarization in SA node	+++	+
Ca^{++} channel blockade	+++	+++
AV node ERP	↑↑↑	↑↑↑
Atrial ERP	↑↑↑	↑
Ventricular ERP	↑↑↑	↑
QRS interval	↑↑	↑
QT$_C$ duration	↑↑↑	–/↑
A-H interval*	↑↑	↑↑↑
H-V interval*	↑	–
Non-competitive blockade of α- & β-adrenoreceptors	+	+ (faster)
Block conversion of thyroxine to triodothyronine	+++	–
Heart rate	↓↓	–/↓

AP, action potential; APD, action potential duration; AV, atrioventricular; ERP, effective refractory period. *A-H interval = time from initial rapid deflection of the atrial wave to the initial rapid deflection of His bundle potential; H-V interval = time from initial deflection of the His bundle potential to the onset of ventricular activity. + = yes or present; - = no or absent; ↑ = increase; ↓ = decrease. Adapted from [40].

The antiarrhythmic properties of intravenous amiodarone are potentiated by its ability to exert electrophysiologic actions faster than oral amiodarone (Table 8-2.) First, intravenous amiodarone substantially inhibits inactivated sodium channels, especially at shorter cycle lengths (use-dependency phenomenon) [72-76]. Thus, the short-term antiarrhythmic action of intravenous amiodarone is expected to be greater during rapid tachyarrhythmias. This action on the sodium channel has been shown to be more pronounced in ischemic myocardial tissues than in normal tissues [75].

Second, experimental studies have shown that intravenous amiodarone significantly decreases the frequency of ventricular fibrillation associated with a substantial reduction in intracellular calcium concentration. This finding suggests that the effect of intravenous amiodarone on cellular calcium homeostasis plays an important role in its antiarrhythmic action [77]. Third, intravenous amiodarone has also been shown to exert a more potent and faster anti-adrenergic action than does oral amiodarone [78].

Intravenous amiodarone has several favorable electropharmacologic properties that can theoretically help terminate ventricular arrhythmias related to myocardial infarction and improve the overall survival rate. If a ventricular arrhythmia is induced by acute myocardial ischemia, intravenous amiodarone may help relieve ischemia and thereby control the arrhythmia.

Several clinical trials have shown that short-term treatment with a β-adrenergic blocking agent improves the survival rate and reduces infarction size and reinfarction rate in acute myocardial infarction [79-81]. Intravenous amiodarone exerts the same anti-adrenergic effect and probably provides a benefit similar to that of β-adrenergic blocking agents [82].

Intravenous amiodarone may be particularly useful in patients who have had myocardial infarction and have a compromised hemodynamic status. Although it generates a negative inotropic effect, this action is counterbalanced by an afterload reduction and improvement in coronary blood flow, thereby increasing overall cardiac output with minimal or no decrease in blood pressure [82-84]. Therefore, intravenous amiodarone can often be used safely in patients with left ventricular systolic dysfunction with or without associated hypotension.

Advanced cardiac life support
Both clinical and experimental data support the use of intravenous amiodarone in protocols of advanced cardiac life support [70,71]. Intravenous bretylium is currently the only approved class III agent in this setting. However, clinical investigations have shown that one gram of intravenous amiodarone infused over 24 hours is as effective as intravenous bretylium in preventing recurrence of highly malignant ventricular arrhythmias. In fact, within the first six hours of monitoring, intravenous amiodarone is more effective than intravenous bretylium in preventing arrhythmia recurrence, and besides, intravenous bretylium is associated with a higher incidence of hypotension.

Ventricular overdrive pacing
If ventricular tachycardia recurs frequently, an electrode catheter may be inserted intravenously and placed in the right ventricular apex for delivering bursts of overdrive pacing to terminate ventricular tachycardia before and during antiarrhythmic therapy (Figure 8-17). However, the technique of ventricular overdrive pacing potentially may induce another form of ventricular tachycardia (Figure 8-18), accelerate the ventricular tachycardia rate and provoke ventricular fibrillation. Therefore, the technique should

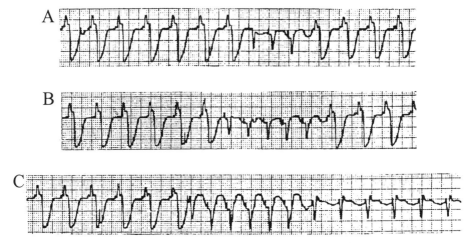

FIGURE 8-17. Should ventricular tachycardia recur during the course of antiarrhythmic therapy, a temporary pacing wire in the right ventricle can be used to deliver a single stimulus or a train of stimuli to terminate ventricular tachycardia. Ventricular tachycardia recurs at a rate of 120 beats per minute while on oral procainamide therapy. Short bursts of 3 (Panel A), 5 (Panel B), and 6 (Panel C) ventricular stimuli at a rate of 150/min are delivered during the ventricular tachycardia, the latter of which finally interrupts the tachycardia circuit (Panel C). This technique can be safely performed in an intensive care unit to avoid multiple DC countershocks. ECG lead V$_1$ shown. Paper speed 25 mm/sec.

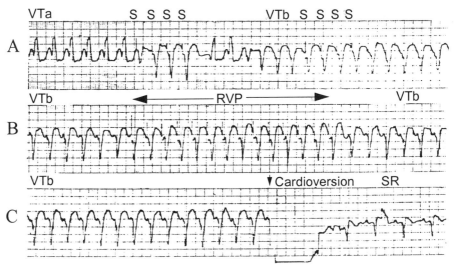

FIGURE 8-18. Provocation of another form of ventricular tachycardia while attempting overdrive ventricular pacing to terminate ventricular tachycardia. Panel A, Short burst of ventricular stimulation(S) (170/min) not only fails to terminate a sustained ventricular tachycardia (VTa, 150/min) but instead converts it to another form of ventricular tachycardia (VTb, 160/min) with a different QRS morphology. Panel B, Repeated bursts of rapid ventricular pacing (RVP) at 180/min fails to terminate VTb. Panel C, Finally, an electrical countershock of 50 watt-sec terminates VTb, resulting in resumption of sinus rhythm (SR). Paper speed 25 mm/sec.

only be performed under the supervision of a team consisting of an experienced cardiac electrophysiologist, nurses and/or technicians.

8.2.4 DIAGNOSTIC WORK-UP FOR PATIENTS WITH VENTRICULAR TACHYARRHYTHMIAS

After stabilization of the patient, they should be monitored closely, and further dianostic testing and additional treatment performed. Specifically, the following acute conditions should be considered and treated once the diagnosis is made (Table 8-3.)

TABLE 8-3. Acute causes of ventricular tachyarrhythmias requiring further urgent evaluation and treatment.

Acute myocardial ischemia/infarction

Congestive heart failure

Electrolyte imbalance

Hypoxia

Proarrhythmia effects of drugs

Long QT syndrome (congenital & acquired)

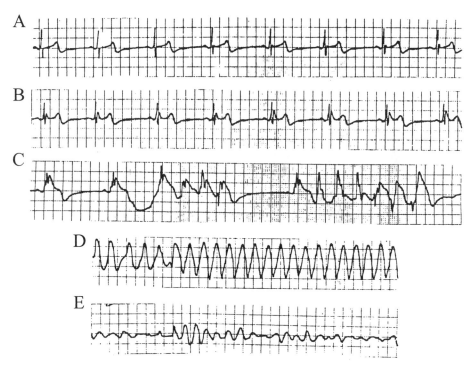

FIGURE 8-19. Recurrent cardiac arrest caused by coronary artery spasm with silent myocardial ischemia in a 58 year old man who has never experienced chest pain. ECG lead V_3 shown. Panel A: Baseline control recording. Panels B & C: Gradual development of ST-segment elevation and short bursts of non-sustained ventricular tachycardia. Panels D & E: Degeneration of ventricular tachycardia to ventricular flutter and fibrillation, resulting in a cardiac arrest. The patient was successfully resuscitated with external counter-shock. The ECG returned to the baseline control with isoelectric ST-segment. Paper speed 25 mm/sec.

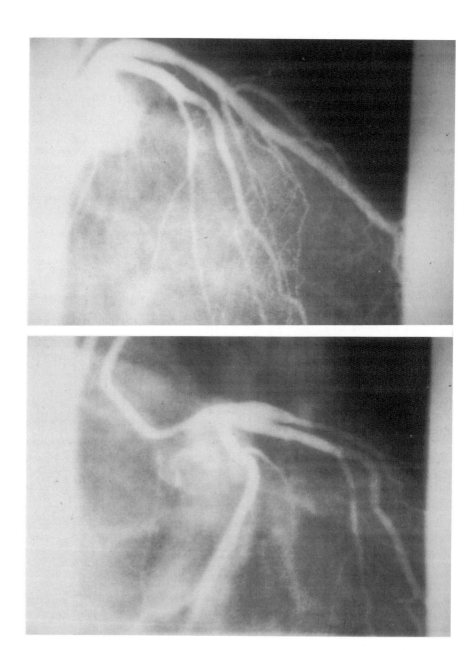

FIGURE 8-20. Induction of a silent coronary artery spasm in the patient presented in Figure 8-19. Upper panel: Coronary arteriography revealed a less than 30% occlusive lesion at the proximal portion of the left anterior descending artery. Lower panel: Ergonovine infusion provoked no symptom of chest pain but induced segmental spasm of the left anterior descending artery distal to the occlusive lesion. This was followed by development of ST-segment elevation and an onset of ventricular tachycardia and ventricular fibrillation similar to what had been observed spontaneously (tracings D and E of Figure 8-19).

Acute myocardial ischemia and infarction must be ruled out, especially in patients presenting with ventricular fibrillation or polymorphic VT and normal left ventricular function (Figure 8-19 & Figure 8-20).

Long-term antiarrhythmic therapy is not indicated for ventricular tachyarrhythmias due to reversible clinical conditions including those listed above except for the congenital long QT syndromes. Ventricular tachyarrhythmias related to structural heart disease, such as atherosclerotic heart disease with prior myocardial infarction or primary or secondary cardiomyopathy, may require an electrophysiology study to define the nature, characteristics, and optional treatment for the arrhythmia. Implantation of a cardioverter-defibrillator and/or long-term antiarrhythmic therapy, and radiofrequency catheter ablation may be indicated in selected patients.

References

1.	Benchimol A: Significance of the contribution of atrial systole to cardiac function in man. *Am J Cardiol* **23**:568-71, 1969.
2.	Curry PVL. The hemodynamic and electrophysiological effects of paroxysmal tachycardia. In: Narula OS, ed. *Cardiac Arrhythmias: Electrophysiology, Diagnosis and Management.* Baltimore: Williams and Wilkins, 364-381: 1979.
3.	Goldreyer BN, Kastor JA, Kershbaum KL: The hemodynamic effects of induced supraventricular tachycardia in man. *Circulation* **54**:783, 1976.
4.	Mitchell JH, Shapiro, W.: Atrial function and the hemodynamic consequences of atrial fibrillation in man. *Am J Cardiol* **23**:556, 1969.
5.	McIntosh HD, Morris JJ: The hemodynamic consequences of arrhythmias. *Progress in Cardiovascular Disease* **8**:330, 1966.
6.	Falicov RE, Resnekov L: Midventricular obstruction in hypertrophic obstructive cardiomyopathy. *Br Heart J* **39**:701, 1977.
7.	Sanderson JE, Gibson DG, Brown DJ, Goodwin JF: Left ventricular filling in hypertrophic cardiomyopathy. An angiographic study. *Br Heart J* **39**:661-70, 1977.
8.	Walston A, Behar VS: Spectrum of coronary artery disease in idiopathic hypertrophic subaortic stenosis. *Am J Cardiol* **38**:12, 1976.
9.	Eckberg DL, Drabinsky M, Braunwald E: Defective cardiac parasympathetic control in patients with heart disease. *N Engl J Med* **285**:877-83, 1971.
10.	Josephson ME, Seides SE, Batsford WB, et al.: The effects of carotid sinus pressure in re-entrant paroxysmal supraventricular tachycardia. *Am Heart J* **88**:694-7, 1974.
11.	Cantwell JD, Dawson JE, Fletcher GF: Supraventricular tachyarrhythmias: Treatment with edrophonium. *Arch Intern Med* **130**:221, 1972.
12.	Waxman MB, Wald RW, Sharma AD, et al.: Vagal techniques for termination of paroxysmal supraventricular tachycardia. *Am J Cardiol* **46**:655-64, 1980.
13.	Gribbin B, Pickering TG, Sleight P, Peto R: Effect of age and high blood pressure on baroreflex sensitivity in man. *Circ Res* **29**:424-31, 1971.
14.	O'Keefe DD, Hoffman JI, Cheitlin R, et al.: Coronary blood flow in experimental canine left ventricular hypertrophy. *Circ Res* **43**:43-51, 1978.
15.	Sung RJ, Elser B, McAllister RG, Jr.: Intravenous verapamil for termination of re-entrant supraventricular tachycardias: intracardiac studies correlated with plasma verapamil concentrations. *Ann Intern Med* **93**:682-9, 1980.
16.	Huycke EC, Sung RJ, Dias VC, et al.: Intravenous diltiazem for termination of reentrant supraventricular tachycardia: a placebo-controlled, randomized, double-blind, multicenter study. *J Am Coll Cardiol* **13**:538-44, 1989.

17. Lauer MR, Young C, Liem LB, Sung RJ: Efficacy of adenosine in terminating catecholamine-dependent supraventricular tachycardia. *Am J Cardiol* **73**:38-42, 1994.

18. DiMarco JP, Sellers TD, Berne RM, et al.: Adenosine: electrophysiologic effects and therapeutic use for terminating paroxysmal supraventricular tachycardia. *Circulation* **68**:1254-63, 1983.

19. DiMarco JP, Miles W, Akhtar M, et al.: Adenosine for paroxysmal supraventricular tachycardia: dose ranging and comparison with verapamil. Assessment in placebo-controlled, multicenter trials. The Adenosine for PSVT Study Group. *Ann Intern Med* **113**:104-10, 1990.

20. Lai WT, Wu SN, Sung RJ: Negative dromotropism of adenosine under beta-adrenergic stimulation with isoproterenol. *Am J Cardiol* **70**:1427-31, 1992.

21. Lerman BB, Belardinelli L: Cardiac electrophysiology of adenosine. Basic and clinical concepts. *Circulation* **83**:1499-509, 1991.

22. Salerno DM, Dias VC, Kleiger RE, et al.: Efficacy and safety of intravenous diltiazem for treatment of atrial fibrillation and atrial flutter. The Diltiazem-Atrial Fibrillation/Flutter Study Group. *Am J Cardiol* **63**:1046-51, 1989.

23. Byrd RC, Sung RJ, Marks J, Parmley WW: Safety and efficacy of esmolol (ASL-8052: an ultrashort-acting beta-adrenergic blocking agent) for control of ventricular rate in supraventricular tachycardias. *J Am Coll Cardiol* **3**:394-9, 1984.

24. Fenster PE, Comess KA, Marsh R, et al.: Conversion of atrial fibrillation to sinus rhythm by acute intravenous procainamide infusion. *Am Heart J* **106**:501-504, 1983.

25. Borgeat A, Goy JJ, Maendly R, et al.: Flecainide versus quinidine for conversion of atrial fibrillation to sinus rhythm. *Am J Cardiol* **58**:496-498, 1986.

26. Vita JA, Friedman PL, Cantillon C, Antman EM: Efficacy of intravenous propafenone for the acute management of atrial fibrillation. *Am J Cardiol* **63**:1275-1278, 1989.

27. Boahene KA, Klein GJ, Yee R, et al.: Termination of acute atrial fibrillation in the Wolff-Parkinson-White syndrome by procainamide and propafenone: importance of atrial fibrillatory cycle length. *J Am Coll Cardiol* **16**:1408-14, 1990.

28. Donovan KD, Power BM, Hockings BE, et al.: Intravenous flecainide versus amiodarone for recent-onset atrial fibrillation. *Am J Cardiol* **75**:693-697, 1995.

29. Sung RJ, Tan HL, Karagounis L, et al.: Intravenous sotalol for the termination of supraventricular tachycardia and atrial fibrillation and flutter: a multicenter, randomized, double-blind, placebo-controlled study. Sotalol Multicenter Study Group. *Am Heart J* **129**:739-48, 1995.

30. Suttorp MJ, Kingma JH, et al.: The value of class IC antiarrhythmic drugs for acute conversion of paroxysmal atrial fibrillation or flutter to sinus rhythm. *J Am Coll Cardiol* **16**:1722-1727, 1990.

31. Stambler BS, Wood MA, Ellenbogen KA, et al.: Efficacy and safety of repeated intravenous doses of ibutilide for rapid conversion of atrial flutter or fibrillation. Ibutilide Repeat Dose Study Investigators. *Circulation* **94**:1613-21, 1996.

32. Ellenbogen KA, Stambler BS, Wood MA, et al.: Efficacy of intravenous ibutilide for rapid termination of atrial fibrillation and atrial flutter: a dose-response study. *J Am Coll Cardiol* **28**:130-6, 1996.

33. Lee KS, Tsai TD, Lee EW: Membrane activity of class III antiarrhythmic compounds; a comparison between ibutilide, d-sotalol, E-4031, sematilide, and dofetilide. *Eur J Pharmacol* **234**:43-53, 1994.

34. Lee KS: Ibutilide, a new compound with potent class III antiarrhythmic activity, activates a slow inward Na current in guinea pig ventricular cells. *J Pharmacol Exp Ther* **262**:99-108, 1992.

35. Yang T, Snyders DJ, Roden DM: Ibutilide, a methanesulfonamide antiarrhythmic, is a potent blocker of the rapidly-activating delayed rectifier K+ current (Ikr) in AT-1 cells: concentration, time-, voltage-, and use dependent effects. *Circulation* **91**:1799-1806, 1995.

36. Wellens HJ, Bar FW, et al.: Effect of drugs in the Wolff-Parkinson-White syndrome. Importance of initial length of effective refractory period of the accessory pathway. *Am J Cardiol* **46**:665-9, 1980.

37. Shen EN, Keung E, Huycke E, et al.: Intravenous propafenone for termination of reentrant supraventricular tachycardia. A placebo-controlled, randomized, double-blind, crossover study. *Ann Intern Med* **105**:655-61, 1986.

38. Wu D, Denes P, Bauernfeind R, et al.: Effects of procainamide on atrioventricular nodal re-entrant paroxysmal tachycardia. *Circulation* **57**:1171-9, 1978.

39. Sellers TD, Jr., Bashore TM, Gallagher JJ: Digitalis in the pre-excitation syndrome. Analysis during atrial fibrillation. *Circulation* **56**:260-7, 1977.

40.   Desai AD, Chun S, Sung RJ: The role of intravenous amiodarone in the management of cardiac arrhythmias. *Ann Intern Med* **127**:294-303, 1997.
41.   Waldo AL, MacLean WA, Karp RB, et al.: Entrainment and interruption of atrial flutter with atrial pacing: studies in man following open heart surgery. *Circulation* **56**:737-45, 1977.
42.   Resnekov L: Present status of electroversion in the management of cardiac dysrhythmias. *Circulation* **47**:1356, 1973.
43.   Hou CJ, Chang-Sing P, Flynn E, et al.: Determination of ventricular vulnerable period and ventricular fibrillation threshold by use of T-wave shocks in patients undergoing implantation of cardioverter/defibrillators. *Circulation* **92**:2558-64, 1995.
44.   Castellanos A, Sung RJ..Ventricular arrhythmias and digitalis-induced arrhythmias. In: Sanders J, Gardner L, eds. *Handbook of Medical Emergencies*. 2nd ed. Garden City, New York: Medical Examination Publishing Co., 32-54: 1978.
45.   Chun HM, Sung RJ: Supraventricular tachyarrhythmias. Pharmacologic versus nonpharmacologic approaches. *Med Clin North Am* **79**:1121-34, 1995.
46.   Mattioni T, Denker S, Riggio D, et al.: Efficacy and safety of intravenous ibutilide in the treatment of atrial flutter and atrial fibrillation following valvular or coronary artery bypass surgery (abstract). *PACE Pacing and Clinical Electrophysiology* **20**:1059, 1997.
47.   Gonzalez RP, Scheinman MM, Lesh MD, et al.: Clinical and electrophysiologic spectrum of fascicular tachycardias. *Am Heart J* **128**:147-56, 1994.
48.   Bar FW, Brugada P, Dassen WR, Wellens HJ: Differential diagnosis of tachycardia with narrow QRS complex (shorter than 0.12 second). *Am J Cardiol* **54**:555-60, 1984.
49.   Moss AJ: Clinical significance of ventricular arrhythmias in patients with and without coronary artery disease. *Prog Cardiovasc Dis* **23**:33-52, 1980.
50.   Lee KL, Lauer MR, Young C, et al.: Spectrum of electrophysiologic and electropharmacologic characteristics of verapamil-sensitive ventricular tachycardia in patients without structural heart disease. *Am J Cardiol* **77**:967-73, 1996.
51.   Sung RJ, Keung EC, Nguyen NX, Huycke EC: Effects of beta-adrenergic blockade on verapamil-responsive and verapamil-irresponsive sustained ventricular tachycardias. *J Clin Invest* **81**:688-99, 1988.
52.   Sung RJ, Shapiro WA, Shen EN, et al.: Effects of verapamil on ventricular tachycardias possibly caused by reentry, automaticity, and triggered activity. *J Clin Invest* **72**:350-60, 1983.
53.   DiMarco JP, Sellers TD, Lerman BB, et al.: Diagnostic and therapeutic use of adenosine in patients with supraventricular tachyarrhythmias. *J Am Coll Cardiol* **6**:417-25, 1985.
54.   Camm AJ, Garratt CJ: Adenosine and supraventricular tachycardia. *N Engl J Med* **325**:1621-9, 1991.
55.   Garratt CJ, Griffith MJ, O'Nunain S, et al.: Effects of intravenous adenosine on antegrade refractoriness of accessory atrioventricular connections. *Circulation* **84**:1962-8, 1991.
56.   Griffith MJ, Linker NJ, Ward DE, Camm AJ: Adenosine in the diagnosis of broad complex tachycardia. *Lancet* **1**:672-5, 1988.
57.   Mehta D, Wafa S, Ward DE, Camm AJ: Relative efficacy of various physical manoeuvres in the termination of junctional tachycardia. *Lancet* **1**:1181-5, 1988.
58.   Rankin AC, Oldroyd KG, Chung E, et al.: Value and limitations of adenosine in the diagnosis and treatment of narrow and broad complex tachycardias. *Br Heart J* **62**:195-203, 1989.
59.   Brugada P, Brugada J, Mont L, et al.: A new approach to the differential diagnosis of a regular tachycardia with a wide QRS complex. *Circulation* **83**:1649-1659, 1991.
60.   Josephson ME, Horowitz LN, Waxman HL, et al.: Sustained ventricular tachycardia: role of the 12-lead electrocardiogram in localizing site of origin. *Circulation* **64**:257-72, 1981.
61.   Kindwall KE, Brown J, Josephson ME: Electrocardiographic criteria for ventricular tachycardia in wide complex left bundle branch block morphology tachycardias. *Am J Cardiol* **61**:1279-83, 1988.
62.   Sandler IA, Marriott HJL: The differential morphology of anomalous ventricular complexes of RBBB-type in lead V1. *Circulation* **31**:551-556, 1966.
63.   Wellens HJ, Bar FW, Lie KI: The value of the electrocardiogram in the differential diagnosis of a tachycardia with a widened QRS complex. *Am J Med* **64**:27-33, 1978.
64.   Morady F, Scheinman MM, Hess DS: Amiodarone in the management of patients with ventricular tachycardia and ventricular fibrillation. *Pacing Clin Electrophysiol* **6**:609-15, 1983.

65. Morady F, Scheinman MM, Shen E, et al.: Intravenous amiodarone in the acute treatment of recurrent symptomatic ventricular tachycardia. *Am J Cardiol* **51**:156-9, 1983.

66. Ochi RP, Goldenberg IF, Almquist A, et al.: Intravenous amiodarone for the rapid treatment of life-threatening ventricular arrhythmias in critically ill patients with coronary artery disease. *Am J Cardiol* **64**:599-603, 1989.

67. Saksena S, Rothbart ST, Shah Y, Cappello G: Clinical efficacy and electropharmacology of continuous intravenous amiodarone infusion and chronic oral amiodarone in refractory ventricular tachycardia. *Am J Cardiol* **54**:347-352, 1984.

68. Scheinman MM: Parenteral antiarrhythmic drug therapy in ventricular tachycardia/ventricular fibrillation: evolving role of class III agents-focus on amiodarone. *J Cardiovasc Electrophysiol* **6**:914-9, 1995.

69. Levine JH, Massumi A, Scheinman MM, et al.: Intravenous amiodarone for recurrent sustained hypotensive ventricular tachyarrhythmias. Intravenous Amiodarone Multicenter Trial Group. *J Am Coll Cardiol* **27**:67-75, 1996.

70. Kowey PR, Levine JH, Herre JM, et al.: Randomized, double-blind comparison of intravenous amiodarone and bretylium in the treatment of patients with recurrent, hemodynamically destabilizing ventricular tachycardia or fibrillation. The Intravenous Amiodarone Multicenter Investigators Group. *Circulation* **92**:3255-63, 1995.

71. Kowey PR, Marinchak RA, Rials SJ, Filart RA: Intravenous amiodarone. *J Am Coll Cardiol* **29**:1190-8, 1997.

72. Morady F, DiCarlo LA, Jr., Krol RB, et al.: Acute and chronic effects of amiodarone on ventricular refractoriness, intraventricular conduction and ventricular tachycardia induction. *J Am Coll Cardiol* **7**:148-57, 1986.

73. Mason JW, Hondeghem LM, Katzung BG: Amiodarone blocks inactivated cardiac sodium channels. *Pflugers Arch* **396**:79-81, 1983.

74. Mason JW, Hondeghem LM, Katzung BG: Block of inactivated sodium channels and of depolarization-induced automaticity in guinea pig papillary muscle by amiodarone. *Circ Res* **55**:278-85, 1984.

75. Mayuga RD, Singer DH: Effects of intravenous amiodarone on electrical dispersion in normal and ischaemic tissues and on arrhythmia inducibility: monophasic action potential studies. *Cardiovasc Res* **20**:571-579, 1992.

76. Yabek SM, Kato R, Singh BN: Effects of amiodarone and its metabolite, desethylamiodarone, on the electrophysiologic properties of isolated cardiac muscle. *J Cardiovasc Pharmacol* **8**:197-207, 1986.

77. Kojima S, Wu ST, Wikman-Coffeit J, Parmley WW: Acute amiodarone terminates ventricular fibrillation by modifying cellular Ca^{++} homeostasis in isolated perfused rat hearts. *J Pharmacol Exp Ther* **275**:254-262, 1995.

78. Du XJ, Elser MD, Dart AM: Sympatholytic action of intravenous amiodarone in the rat heart. *Circulation* **91**:462-470, 1995.

79. Norris RM, Barnaby PF, Brown MA, et al.: Prevention of ventricular fibrillation during acute myocardial infarction by intravenous propranolol. *Lancet* **2**:883-6, 1984.

80. Roberts R, Rogers WJ, Mueller HS, et al.: Immediate versus deferred beta-blockade following thrombolytic therapy in patients with acute myocardial infarction. Results of the Thrombolysis in Myocardial Infarction (TIMI) II-B Study. *Circulation* **83**:422-37, 1991.

81. Yusuf S, Peto R, Lewis J, et al.: Beta blockade during and after myocardial infarction: an overview of the randomized trials. *Prog Cardiovasc Dis* **27**:335-371, 1985.

82. Hohnloser SH, Meinertz T, et al.: Electrocardiographic and antiarrhythmic effects of intravenous amiodarone: results of a prospective, placebo-controlled study. *Am Heart J* **121**:89-95, 1991.

83. Remme WJ, Kruyssen HA, Look MP, et al.: Hemodynamic effects and tolerability of intravenous amiodarone in patients with impaired left ventricular function. *Am Heart J* **122**:96-103, 1991.

84. Twidale N, Roberts-Thomson P, McRitchie RJ: Comparative hemodynamics effects of amiodarone, sotalol, and d-sotalol. *Am Heart J* **126**:122-129, 1992.

CHAPTER 9

DISTURBANCES OF SINOATRIAL NODE FUNCTION

The spectrum of human cardiac performance is amazingly broad with cardiac output varying 10-20-fold between that measured during the deepest of sleep to that seen at peak of exercise. In large part this tremendous cardiac reserve is modulated both by cardiac contractility as well as the heart rate itself. While many factors can affect contractility, heart rate as almost entirely regulated by the autonomic mediation of the sinoatrial (SA) node pacemaker. While uninhibited enhancement of sympathetic tone can result in normal sinus rates over 200/min in many young health individuals, uninhibited and unhindered parasympathetic (vagal) tone can completely suppress all SA nodal activity, even when there is no intrinsic abnormality of the node itself. Consequently, "SA node dysfunction," manifested as symptomatic sinus pauses or SA nodal exit block, may not represent true *intrinsic* SA node disease, but instead, could merely result from dramatic neurogenic influences exerted by the autonomic nervous system (Figure 9-1). Therefore, one of the challenges facing the electrophysiologist in evaluating assumed abnormalities

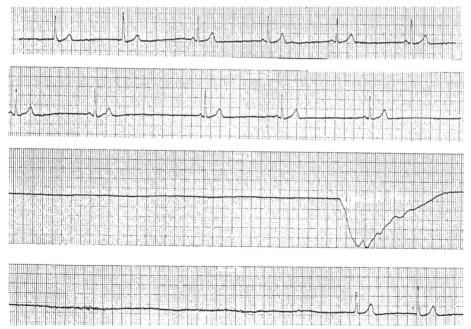

FIGURE 9-1. Long sinus pause induced by hypervagotonia during head-up tilt table test in 25-year-old woman with vasovagal syncope. Recurrent episodes successfully treated with β-adrenergic blocking agent alone. Paper speed 25 mm/sec.

of the SA node is distinguishing between *intrinsic* SA node disease and *functional* (physiological) disturbances of SA node function related to *extrinsic* influences such as the autonomic nervous system.

TABLE 9-1. Clinical manifestations of sinoatrial node dysfunction

---

Sinus bradycardia (chronically < 40/min resting while awake except in well-conditioned athletes), especially if symptomatic

"Pronounced" or "dramatic" sinus arrhythmia (lower sinus rate consistently below 40/min during daytime while awake or sinus pauses ≥ 2.5 to 3.0 sec while awake; beat-to-beat P-P interval variations >160 ms)

Exercise-induced chronotropic incompetence, especially if patient complains of symptoms of exercise intolerance

Sinus pauses (≥ 2.5 to 3.0 sec during daytime while awake), especially if associated with symptoms

Episodes of bradycardia or sinus pauses (as described above) following termination of and/or interspersed with episodes of paroxysmal atrial tachycardia, flutter, or fibrillation.

Chronic atrial tachycardia, flutter, or fibrillation

9.1   Sinoatrial Node Dysfunction and Exit Block

The so-called "sick sinus syndrome" is more correctly termed *sinoatrial node (SA) dysfunction*. The clinical manifestations of SA node dysfunction have been well-described (Table 9-1.) One common clinical scenario involves runs of paroxysmal atrial fibrillation which terminates to a long sinus pause (Figure 9-2 & Figure 9-3), the so called "Tachy-Brady syndrome". The "sinus node pauses" seen with this condition may have various etiologies, ranging from arrest of the SA node impulse (rare) to various types (degrees) of exit block (Figure 9-4) (Table 9-2.) In general, these "sinus pauses" do not represent a failure of impulse generation within the SA nodal cells, but rather from conduction block of the impulse as it travels from the SA node proper through the border zone of transitional cells to the atrial muscle proper (exit block) (Figure 9-5). The replacement of transitional border zone cells with non-excitable fibrocytes may explain the *exit block* of the cardiac impulse. The fact that this represents exit block, as opposed to failure of impulse generation within the SA node proper, is often manifested by the find-

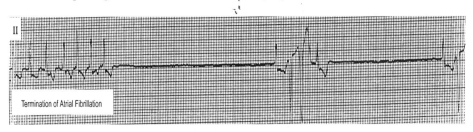

FIGURE 9-2. Sinus pause following termination of paroxysmal atrial fibrillation. Paper speed 25 mm/sec.

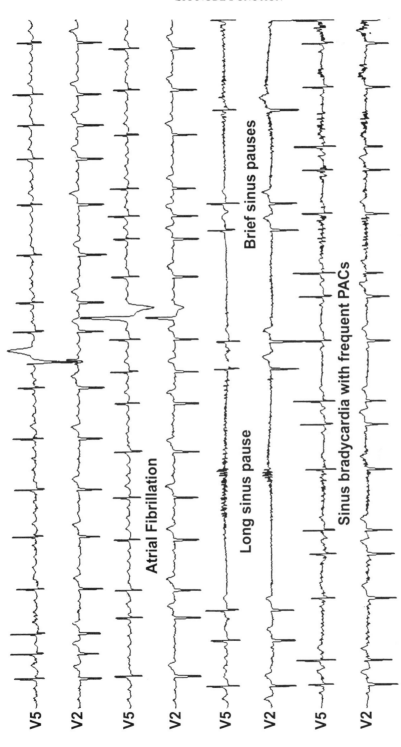

FIGURE 9-3. Long segment of continuous Holter recording (ECG leads V2 and V5 recorded) in patient with SA node dysfunction showing many of the characteristic clinical findings of this disorder, including paroxysmal atrial fibrillation, long and short sinus pauses, atrial ectopy and frequent premature atrial contractions (PACs) and sinus bradycardia. Paper speed 12.5 mm/sec.

ing that the "resumption" of P waves after the pause occur within a time interval which is a whole number multiple of the preceding P-P interval duration immediately before the pause (Figure 9-4). Even when there is not such a a whole number relationship, exit block is still almost always the cause with more complex types of block occurring at multiple sites within the pathway from the SA node proper to the atrial muscle proper. Because this disorder may result from a failure of impulse conduction through the fibrotic border zone tissue at the sinoatrial junction and not failure of action potential generation, drugs such as atropine or β-adrenergic agents which exert their effects by enhancing the ionic currents responsible SA node action potential, have little or no effect on the sinus pauses. In fact, such agents may at least theoretically worsen this disorder by increasing the rate of action potential generation which may exacerbate any exit block which has a rate-dependent component.

TABLE 9-2. Classification of sinus pauses

Type of sinus pause	ECG description
Sinus arrest	Complete quiescence of SA pacemaker cells; difficult or impossible to establish with certainty; the duration of the pause is not an exact multiple of the preceding P-P interval and is not preceded by a gradual shortening of the P-P interval
Sinoatrial exit block	
First degree sinoatrial exit block	Simple delay in conduction of impulse from SA node proper to perinodal atrial tissue (cannot diagnose from surface ECG recording because ECG does not record intranodal activity proximal to site of block).
Second degree sinoatrial exit block	
Type I (Wenckebach)	Progressive P-P interval shortening preceding exit block with "dropped P wave".
Type II (high-grade)	The duration of the pause is (approximately) an exact multiple of the preceding P-P interval (although may not be apparent due to variations on P-P imposed by sinus arrhythmia or beat-to-beat autonomic variations), the pause is not preceded by gradual shortening of the preceding P-P interval.
Third degree sinoatrial exit block	Indistinguishable from prolonged sinus arrest

There are *intrinsic* or *extrinsic* causes of SA node dysfunction. Intrinsic causes include ischemia/infarction, cardiomyopathy, trauma, inflammation (myocarditis), or postcardiac surgery, especially repair of congenital heart defects. There is an increased incidence of this disorder in the elderly, but it can be congenital as well as familial [1-7]. A common histological finding in elderly patients with this condition is replacement of normal SA nodal and perinodal tissues with fibrous tissue [8-11]. Simultaneous involvement of the AV node and its perinodal transitional zones has also been described [1].

Unlike intrinsic SA node dysfunction which implies a largely fixed, permanent dysfunction of the SA node presumed to reside within the SA node or perinodal tissue, *per*

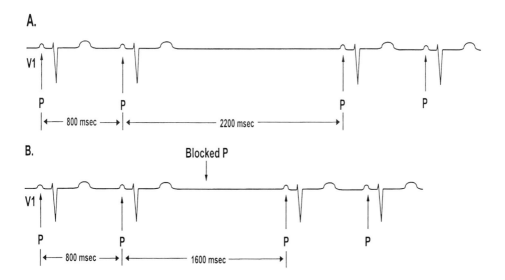

FIGURE 9-4. Schematic comparison between pauses due to SA node arrest (panel A) and SA node exit block (Panel B). With a pause due to SA node exit block (in which the SA node continues to discharge at its regular rate but conduction is blocked from the SA node proper to the surrounding atrium) resumption of normal conduction results with a P wave appearing "on time" at some multiple of the normal immediately preceding P-P interval (in this case, the P wave reappears s x the basic P-P interval of 800 ms. With SA node arrest, the P wave reappearance would be at an unpredictable time and unlikely to be a multiple of the preceding P-P interval. This distinction is hypothetical and the clinical reality is that because of probable complex types of exit block and exit delay, exit block associated with a simple multiple of the preceding P-P interval is unusual.

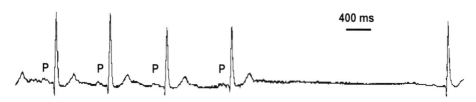

FIGURE 9-5. 69 year old man who suffered a syncopal episode and a motor vehicle accident. As part of his work-up he received a 24-hour ambulatory ECG monitor which recorded symptomatic episodes of asystole (3.5 sec shown here), probably due to sinus exit block. His symptoms resolved after implantation of a dual chamber pacemaker. Paper speed 25 mm/sec.

se, extrinsic SA node dysfunction may combine a totally functionally normal SA node with abnormal external influences. Extrinsic SA node dysfunction usually results from autonomic influences (neurally-mediated syncope, vasovagal syncope, carotid sinus hypersensitivity) (Figure 9-6) or cardioactive drugs (Table 9-3.)

TABLE 9-3. Cardioactive drugs adversely affecting SA node function

Class of drug	Examples
Cardiac glycosides	Digoxin, digitoxin, digitalis
Sympatholytic agents	α-methyldopa, reserpine, clonidine, guanethidine, bretylium
β–adrenergic blocking agents	Propranolol, atenolol, nadolol, etc.
Ca^{2+} channel blocking agents	Verapamil, diltiazem, nifedipine
Antiarrhythmic drugs	Quinidine, procainamide, flecainide, propafenone, sotalol, amiodarone,
Miscellaneous agents	Lithium carbonate, cimetidine, amitriptyline, phenothiazines

9.2 Assessment of Sinoatrial Node Function

A complete assessment of SA node function may involve simple non-invasive testing or more involved pharmacological or invasive testing in selected patients (Table 9-4.) As in all testing of any component of the cardiac conduction system, the specific evaluation of SA node function in any particular patient should be planned based upon the specific clinical presentation of the individual patient.

TABLE 9-4. Assessment of intrinsic and extrinsic sinoatrial node function

Non-invasive assessment
>   Exercise testing
>   Carotid sinus massage
>   Valsalva maneuver
>   Ambulatory electrocardiography
>   Tilt table testing

Pharmacologic assessment
>   Atropine
>   Isoproterenol
>   Propranolol
>   Intrinsic heart rate (IHR)

Invasive assessment
>   Sinoatrial conduction time (SACT)
>   Sinoatrial node recovery time (SNRT)
>   Sinoatrial node refractory period
>   Direct recording of sinoatrial node electrogram

Carotid Sinus Massage

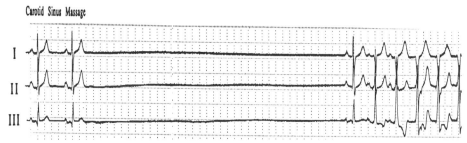

FIGURE 9-6. Effect of mild left carotid sinus massage on a patient with carotid sinus hypersensitivity. Paper speed 25 mm/sec. See text for details.

· 9.2.1 NON-INVASIVE ASSESSMENT OF SINOATRIAL NODE FUNCTION

The non-invasive tests of SA node function include exercise testing, carotid sinus massage, Valsalva maneuver, and ambulatory ECG recording. Exercise testing is useful when the clinician is attempting to evaluate *chronotropic incompetence*. Carotid sinus massage is useful when screening for *carotid sinus hypersensitivity* (Figure 9-6). A pause greater than 3 sec in response to mild to moderate left or right-sided carotid massage of up to 5 sec duration is considered a minimum positive result. Performance of the Valsalva maneuver is occasionally useful to assess autonomic function and sinus node response to it. A Valsalva maneuver is performed by forced exhalation for 10 sec against a closed glottis valve producing at least a 40-mm Hg pressure gradient. An abnormal response is the failure to produce a blood pressure overshoot and reflex bradycardia (Table 9-5.) [12,13]. Head-up tilt table testing is rapidly becoming a standard to evaluate suspected neurally-mediated syncope (vasovagal or vasodepressor), although there is still wide variability in how it is performed. Ambulatory ECG monitoring, either continuous 24-48 hr monitoring or "event-triggered" recording may be useful to uncover the ECG abnormalities associated with SA node dysfunction (Figure 9-3 & Figure 9-7).

TABLE 9-5. Four phases of the Valsalva maneuver

Phase	Physiologic Description
1	Increased arterial pressure due to transmission of the increased intrathoracic pressure
2	Fall in blood pressure due to a decrease in venous return triggering a baroreflex-mediated vasoconstriction & increase in heart rate to limit the blood pressure decline
3	Sudden decrease in blood pressure after release of forced exhalation due to transmission of decreased intrathoracic pressure to aorta
4	Reflex increase in mean & systolic blood pressure (overshoot) & slowing of heart rate

9.2.2 Pharmacologic Assessment of Sinoatrial Node Function

It is clear that the autonomic nervous system can significantly affect the activity of the SA node. In the normal SA node, β_1-adrenergic activation results in an increase in the rate of action potential development, while an increase in parasympathetic activity causes a decrease in the rate of action potential generation. Assuming no sinoatrial exit block is present, these changes result in an increase and decrease, respectively, in the atrial and ventricular rate (assuming 1:1 A-V conduction).

Pharmacological agents have been used to assess the effect of the autonomic nervous system on normal SA node function (Table 9-6.) Atropine (1-3 mg) which blocks muscarinic receptors, and therefore removes parasympathetic (vagal) influences on the SA node, results in a 20-50% increase in sinus rate over the control level [14-22]. Isoproterenol (1-3 μg/min), which binds to and activates β-adrenergic receptors, causes acceleration of the sinus rate by at least 25% [14-18,22]. β_1-Adrenergic blockade with propranolol (0.1 mg/kg)·results in a 12-22% decrease in sinus rate. Maximum pharmacologic blockade of both the parasympathetic and sympathetic systems with atropine (0.04 mg/kg) and propranolol (0.2 mg/kg) results in an estimate of the *intrinsic heart rate (IHR)* [23-29]. These studies indicate that the normal IHR is inversely proportional to age and can be calculated from the regression equation [27,28]:

$$IHR = 118.1 - (0.57 \times age) \pm 16/min$$

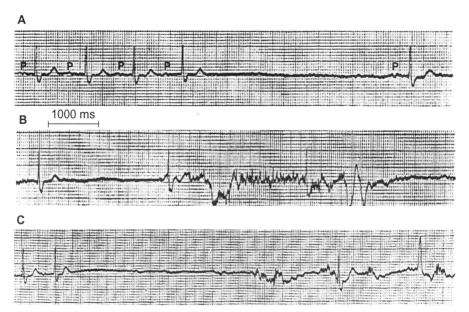

FIGURE 9-7. Seventy-four year old man with severe sinoatrial node dysfunction and recurrent episodes of syncope. Panels A, B, and C are a continuous ambulatory ECG recording during an episode of syncope. Note the artifact in panels B and C, probably due to involuntary patient movements. Patient's symptoms resolved with implantation of a dual chamber pacemaker. Paper speed 25 mm/sec.

For example, the IHR of a 50 year-old individual would be predicted to be 91 beats/min. The IHR is usually higher than the resting heart rate in the unblocked state and correlates well with the resting heart rate in patients receiving denervated cardiac transplants [30].

TABLE 9-6. Effect of pharmacologic interventions on sinus rate in normal individuals

Drug	Dose	Effect on sinus rate or cycle length	Reference
Atropine	1 mg	>17% decrease in sinus cycle length	[31]
Atropine	0.04 mg/kg	>15% increase in sinus rate	[32]
Atropine	1 mg	Sinus rate > 90/min	[33]
Atropine	0.03 mg/kg	Sinus rate > 90/min	[34-36]
Isoproterenol	3 μg/min	>25% increase in sinus rate	[17]
Isoproterenol	1-2 μg/min	Sinus rate > 90-100/min	[37]
Propranolol	0.20 mg/kg	≥ 12% decrease in sinus rate	[32]
Propranolol	0.10 mg/kg	≥ 12% decrease in sinus rate	[38]

9.2.3 INVASIVE ASSESSMENT OF SINOATRIAL NODE FUNCTION

Sinoatrial conduction time
The sinoatrial conduction time (SACT) provides one electrophysiological assessment of SA node function [21,39-43], although it is, in actuality, a composite measure of SA node function and atrial conduction. Determination of the SACT requires the introduction of conducted premature atrial stimuli (A_2) after eight or ten beats of a stable sinus rhythm (A_1-A_1). Accurate determination of the SACT requires retrograde penetration of the SA node and assumes that the retrograde conduction time into the SA node is equal to the anterograde conduction time out of the node, although this may not be true. Four possible responses can be seen in the duration of the return cycle A_2-A_3 and are compared to the sinus cycle length (A_1-A_1) (Figure 9-8). If the A_1-A_2 coupling interval is close to the spontaneous sinus rate, the late-delivered A_2 will not effect the sinus node and the next sinus beat (A_3) occurs on time. As the A_1-A_2 coupling interval is shortened, however, the SA node is reset and A_3 occurs earlier than the control sinus A_3 would have otherwise occurred, although A_2-A_3 is greater than the sinus cycle length because of the conduction time necessary between atrium and SA node. With even shorter A_1-A_2 intervals, A_3 suddenly becomes very early and is less than the A_1-A_1 interval due to interpolation of A_2. With an even earlier A_2 extrastimuli, an even earlier return cycle results such that (A_1-A_2) + (A_2-A_3) is less than A_1-A_1, indicating sinoatrial node reentry.

Assuming that retrograde conduction into the SA node is equal to anterograde conduction out of the node, the SACT is one-half of the difference between the recovery cycle (A_2-A_3) and the sinus cycle length (A_1-A_1) within the range of SA node resetting (Figure 9-8):

$$SACT = \frac{[(A_2 - A_3) - (A_1 - A_1)]}{2}$$

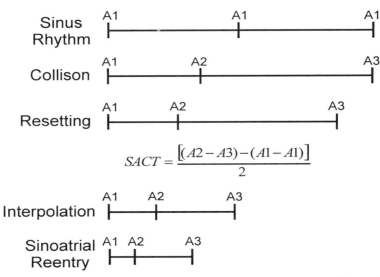

FIGURE 9-8. Schematic diagram depicting the possible atrial responses to premature atrial extrastimuli (A_2) delivered during sinus rhythm (A_1-A_1). The relative position of the first recovery sinus-derived atrial depolarization (A_3) is recorded and compared to its expected time of occurrence had sinus rhythm not been disrupted by A_2. The sinoatrial conduction time is one-half of the difference between the sinus cycle length (A_1-A_1) and the A_2-A_3 interval recorded within the zone of resetting. Adapted from [48]. See text for details.

For patients with normal SA node function, values range from approximately 40 to 150 msec (Table 9-7.) [17,21,39-47].

Sinus node recovery time
The sinus node recovery time (SNRT) [14,33,40,49-53] assesses the recovery of sinus node automaticity after overdrive suppression of the SA node pacemaker using rapid

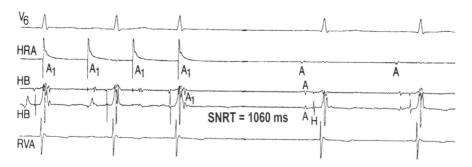

FIGURE 9-9. Surface ECG and intracardiac recording during determination of sinus node recovery time (SNRT). Shown are the surface ECG lead V_6 and intracardiac electrograms from the high right atrium (HRA), His bundle region (HB), and right ventricular apex (RVA). Fixed cycle length pacing of the HRA is performed for one minute (A_1-A_1 = 400 msec) (last four atrial stimuli shown here). The interval between the last atrial-paced event (A_1) and the appearance of the first sinus-derived atrial depolarization (A) is the uncorrected SNRT (1060 msec). H, His bundle electrogram. See text for details.

atrial pacing. The spontaneous sinus cycle length after the cessation of overdrive atrial pacing is normally prolonged for one or more cardiac cycles due to suppression of sinus node automaticity (Figure 9-9). The prolongation of the post-pacing sinus cycle length is a valid assessment of sinus node function only if the SA node is penetrated by the atrial action potentials elicited by the rapid atrial pacing. Furthermore, prolongation of the SACT can also prolong the post-drive sinus cycle length because it indicates delay in conduction of the sinus impulse to the atria. The mechanism responsible or overdrive suppression includes enhanced efflux of K^+ from SA node cells and intracellular Na^+ loading which together enhance electrogenic Na^+/K^+ pumping and decrease the rate of diastolic depolarization responsible for the pacemaker activity [54-57].

Determination of the SNRT involves rapid atrial pacing for at least one minute using a series of A_1-A_1 cycle lengths between the spontaneous sinus rate and the atrial refractory period. After cessation of the pacing, the recovery spontaneous cycle lengths are recorded and the longest cycle length noted. It is essential to establish that the subsequent spontaneous atrial activity originates from the SA node. Recovery sinus cycle lengths equal to or less than the pre-pacing spontaneous rate suggests that either the SA node is not penetrated by the atrial pacing (entrance block) or the recovery atrial impulses originate from a location other than the sinus node. Normally the SNRT is directly

TABLE 9-7. Normal values for sinoatrial conduction time (SACT)

SACT (msec)	SACT total (msec)	Reference
<82		[23,45-47]
<120		[40,49]
<172		[58]
<152		[39,59]
	<214	[60]
	<206	[29]
	<260	[61]

SACT = [(A_2-A_3) - (A_1-A_1)]/2; SACT total = (A_2-A_3) - (A_1-A_1)

proportional to the spontaneous cycle length [14,15]. The uncorrected SNRT may be very long in patients with severe SA node dysfunction (Figure 9-10). The *corrected sinus node recovery time (SNRT$_c$)* is the difference between the longest measured post-pacing recovery sinus interval (SNRT) and the baseline spontaneous cycle length (SCL):

$$SNRT_C = SNRT - SCL$$

The SNRT$_c$ is less than 500 to 600 ms in individuals with normal sinus node function (Table 9-8.) [14,33,40,49-51]. The SNRT$_c$ may be falsely normal for patients with SA

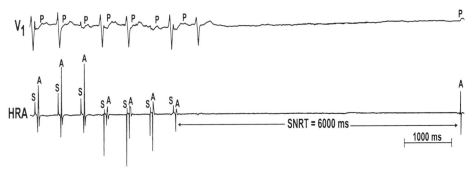

FIGURE 9-10. Markedly abnormal SNRT in a patient with SA node dysfunction and a history of syncope associated with sinus pauses. Uncorrected SNRT measures 6000 msec.

node disease and marked bradycardia (very long SCL). Atropine (1-3 mg) decreases both the SNRT and usually the SNRT$_c$ [14,40,49,50,52].

TABLE 9-8. Normal values for sinoatrial node recovery time and corrected sinoatrial node recovery time

SNRT (msec)	SNRT$_C$ (msec)	Reference
<1475	<495	[40]
<1207		[14,15,17]
<1680		[59,62]
	<354	[60]
	<525	[50]
<1250	<390	[61]
<1500	<533	[51]
	<472	[63]
	<550	[48]

SNRT, sinus node recovery time; SNRT$_C$, corrected sinus node recovery time

9.3   Treatment Strategies for Patients with SA Node Dysfunction

For patients with symptomatic SA node dysfunction of intrinsic origin, treatment invariably requires implantation with a permanent pacemaker. In general, pacemakers capable of AAIR or DDDR pacing provides optimum therapeutic benefit not only because they prevent pause-induced symptoms, but also because they provide rate-adaptive atrial and/or ventricular pacing in patients with chronotropic incompetence. In addition, patients with paroxysmal atrial tachycardia/flutter/fibrillation, may also benefit from pacemakers with programmable mode-switching. Single chamber VVI pacemakers are generally not indicated in these patients except possibly in very elderly individuals with severe disability due to chronic diseases who need protection from rare sinus pauses due to intrinsic SA node dysfunction.

Patients with SA node dysfunction due to extrinsic causes may often not require pacemaker implantation. Instead, therapy may be targeted at the specific extrinsic cause. Drug-induced SA node pauses may be treatable by withdrawing the offending agent(s). Symptomatic bradycardia due to hypothyroidism or electrolyte disturbances are readily addressed by reversing those conditions. Neurally-mediated syncope often can be treated with β_1-adrenergic blocking agents, volume expanders (mineralocorticoids), support-hose, vagolytic agents (scopolamine, disopyramide), and/or α-agonists (midodrine). However, caution and clinical judgement should be exercised especially in patients with malignant vasovagal syncope and very long sinus pauses, or those with carotid sinus hypersensitivity, who may require implantation with a dual chamber pacemaker.

References

1. Barak M, Herschkowitz S, Shapiro I, Roguin N: Familial combined sinus node and atrioventricular conduction dysfunctions. *Int J Cardiol* **15**:231-9, 1987.
2. Lorber A, Maisuls E, Palant A: Autosomal dominant inheritance of sinus node disease. *Int J Cardiol* **15**:252-6, 1987.
3. Scott O, Macartney FJ, Deverall PB: Sick sinus syndrome in children. *Arch Dis Child* **51**:100-5, 1976.
4. Surawicz B, Hariman RJ: Follow-up of the family with congenital absence of sinus rhythm. *Am J Cardiol* **61**:467-9, 1988.
5. Yabek SM, Dillon T, Berman W, Jr., Niland CJ: Symptomatic sinus node dysfunction in children without structural heart disease. *Pediatrics* **69**:590-3, 1982.
6. Yabek SM, Swensson RE, Jarmakani JM: Electrocardiographic recognition of sinus node dysfunction in children and young adults. *Circulation* **56**:235-9, 1977.
7. Yabek SM, Jarmakani JM: Sinus node dysfunction in children, adolescents, and young adults. *Pediatrics* **61**:593-8, 1978.
8. Kaplan BM, Langendorf R, Lev M, Pick A: Tachycardia-bradycardia syndrome (so-called "sick sinus syndrome"). Pathology, mechanisms and treatment. *Am J Cardiol* **31**:497-508, 1973.
9. Lev M, Watne AL: Method for routine histopathologic study of the sinoatrial node. *Arch Pathol* **57**:168-177, 1954.
10. Lev M. The conduction system. In: Gould SC, ed. *Pathology of the Heart and Blood Vessels.* 3rd ed. Springfield, Illinois: Charles C. Thomas, 180-220: 1968.
11. Lev M, Bharati S. Lesions of the conduction system and their functional significance. In: Sommers SC, ed. *Pathology Annual 1974.* New York: Appleton-Century-Crofts, 157-208: 1974.
12. Gorlin R, Knowles JH, Storey CF: The valsalva maneuver as a test of cardiac function. *Am J Med* **22**:197, 1957.
13. McIntosh JD, Burnum JF, Hickam JB, Warren JV: Circulatory changes produced by the valsalva maneuver in normal subjects, patients with mitral stenosis and autonomic nervous system alterations. *Circulation* **9**:511, 1954.
14. Mandel W, Hayakawa H, Danzig R, Marcus HS: Evaluation of sino-atrial node function in man by overdrive suppression. *Circulation* **44**:59-66, 1971.
15. Mandel WJ, Hayakawa H, Allen HN, et al.: Assessment of sinus node function in patients with the sick sinus syndrome. *Circulation* **46**:761-9, 1972.
16. Mandel WJ, Obayashi K, Laks MM: Editorial: Overview of the sick sinus syndrome. *Chest* **66**:223-4, 1974.

17. Mandel WJ, Laks MM, Obayashi K: Sinus node function; evaluation in patients with and without sinus node disease. *Arch Intern Med* **135**:388-94, 1975.

18. Mandel WJ, Jordan JL, Yamaguchi I: The sick sinus syndrome. *Adv Cardiol* **22**:71-9, 1978.

19. Craig FN: Effects of atropine, work and heat on heart rate and sweat production in man. *J Applied Physiol* **4**:826, 1952.

20. Morton HJV, Thomas ET: Effect of atropine on the heart rate. *Lancet* **2**:1313, 1958.

21. Strauss HC, Bigger JT, Saroff AL, Giardina EGV: Electrophysiologic evaluation of sinus node function in patients with sinus node dysfunction. *Circulation* **53**:763, 1976.

22. Cleaveland CR, Rangno RE, Shand DG: A standardized isoproterenol sensitivity test: The effects of sinus arrhythmia, atropine, and propranolol. *Arch Intern Med* **130**:47, 1972.

23. Jordan JL, Yamaguchi I, Mandel WJ. Function and dysfunction of the sinus node: clinical studies in the evaluation of sinus node function. In: Bonke FI, ed. *The sinus node.* he Hague, Netherlands: Nijhoff Medical Division, 3-22: 1978.

24. Jose AD: Effect of combined sympathetic and parasympathetic blockade on heart rate and cardiac function in man. *Am J Cardiol* **18**:476, 1966.

25. Jose AD, Taylor RR: Autonomic blockade by propranolol and atropine to study intrinsic myocardial function in man. *J Clin Invest* **48**:2019-31, 1969.

26. Jose AD, Stitt F: Effects of hypoxia and metabolic inhibitors on the intrinsic heart rate and myocardial contractility in dogs. *Circ Res* **25**:53-66, 1969.

27. Jose AD, Collison D: The normal range and determinants of the intrinsic heart rate in man. *Cardiovasc Res* **4**:160-7, 1970.

28. Jose AD, Stitt F, Collison D: The effects of exercise and changes in body temperature on the intrinsic heart rate in man. *Am Heart J* **79**:488-98, 1970.

29. Desai JM, Scheinman MM, Strauss HC, et al.: Electrophysiologic effects on combined autonomic blockade in patients with sinus node disease. *Circulation* **63**:953-60, 1981.

30. Mason JW: Overdrive suppression of the transplanted heart: Effect of the autonomic nervous system on human sinus rate recovery. *Circulation* **62**:688, 1980.

31. Dauchot P, Gravenstein JS: Effects of atropine on the electrocardiogram in different age groups. *Clin Pharmacol Ther* **12**:274-80, 1971.

32. Eckberg DL, Drabinsky M, Braunwald E: Defective cardiac parasympathetic control in patients with heart disease. *N Engl J Med* **285**:877-83; 1971.

33. Rosen KM, Loeb HS, Sinno MZ, et al.: Cardiac conduction in patients with symptomatic sinus node disease. *Circulation* **43**:836-44, 1971.

34. Lekieffre J, Medvedowsky JL, Thery C: Recent advances in the knowledge about the sinus node and malfunctions of the sinus. *Ann Cardiol Angeiol (Paris)* **30**:109-12, 1981.

35. Lekieffre J, Thery C, Asseman P: The sinus node. Anatomical and electrophysiological review (author's transl). *Ann Cardiol Angeiol (Paris)* **29**:1-5, 1980.

36. Lekieffre J: Sinoatrial node. *Acta Cardiol* **35**:1-9, 1980.

37. Ferrer MI: The sick sinus syndrome. *Circulation* **47**:635-41, 1973.

38. Vasquez M, Chuquimia R, Shantha N, et al.: Clinical electrophysiological effects of propranolol on normal sinus node function. *Br Heart J* **41**:709-15, 1979.

39. Dhingra RC, Wyndham C, Amat YL, et al.: Sinus nodal responses to atrial extrastimuli in patients without apparent sinus node disease. *Am J Cardiol* **36**:445-52, 1975.

40. Breithardt G, Seipel L, Loogen F: Sinus node recovery time and calculated sinoatrial conduction time in normal subjects and patients with sinus node dysfunction. *Circulation* **56**:43, 1977.

41. Breithardt G, Seipel L: The effect of premature atrial depolarization on sinus node automaticity in man. *Circulation* **53**:920, 1976.

42. Masini G, Dianda R, Grasiina A: Analysis of sinoatrial conduction in man using premature atrial stimulation. *Cardiovasc Res* **9**:498, 1975.

43. Strauss HC, Saroff AL, Bigger JT, Giardina EGV: Premature atrial stimulation as a key to the understanding of sinoatrial conduction in man. *Circulation* **47**:86, 1973.

44. Jordan J, Yamaguchi I, Mandel WJ, McCullen AE: Comparative effects of overdrive on sinus and subsidiary pacemaker function. *Am Heart J* **93**:367-74, 1977.

45. Jordan JL, Yamaguchi I, Mandel WJ: The sick sinus syndrome. *JAMA* **237**:682-4, 1977.

46. Jordan J, Yamaguchi I, Mandel WJ: Characteristics of sinoatrial conduction in patients with coronary artery disease. *Circulation* **55**:569-74, 1977.

47. Gomes JA, Kang PS, El-Sherif N: The sinus node electrogram in patients with and without sick sinus syndrome: techniques and correlation between directly measured and indirectly estimated sinoatrial conduction time. *Circulation* **66**:864-73, 1982.

48. Josephson ME. Sinus node function. *Clinical Cardiac Electrophysiology: Techniques and Interpretations*. Philadelphia: Lea & Febiger: 1993.

49. Breithardt G, Seipel L: Influence of drugs on the relationship between sinus node recovery time and calculated sinoatrial conduction time in man. *Basic Res Cardiol* **73**:68, 1978.

50. Narula OS, Samet P, Javier RP: Significance of the sinus node recovery time. *Circulation* **45**:140, 1972.

51. Kulbertus HE, Leval-Rutten F, Mary L, Casters P: Sinus node recovery time in the elderly. *Br Heart J* **37**:420, 1975.

52. Steinbeck G, Luderitz B: Comparative study of sinoatrial conduction time and sinus node recovery time. *Br Heart J* **37**:956, 1975.

53. Tonkin AM, Heddle WF: Electrophysiological testing of sinus node function. *PACE* **7**:735, 1984.

54. Kodama I, Goto J, Sando S, et al.: Effects of rapid stimulation on the transmembrane action potentials of rabbit sinus node pacemaker cells. *Circ Res* **46**:90, 1980.

55. Lu HH, Lange G, Brooks CM: Factors controlling pacemaker action in cells of the sinoatrial node. *Circ Res* **17**:460, 1965.

56. Vassalle M: The relationship among cardiac pacemakers: Overdrive suppression. *Circ Res* **41**:268-277, 1977.

57. Lange G: Action of driving stimuli from intrinsic and extrinsic sources on in situ cardiac pacemaker tissues. *Circ Res* **17**:449, 1965.

58. Crook B, Kitson D, McComish M, Jewitt D: Indirect measurement of sinoatrial conduction time in patients with sinoatrial disease and in controls. *Br Heart J* **39**:771, 1977.

59. Dhingra RC, Amat YLF, Wyndham C, et al.: The electrophysiological effects of ouabain on sinus node and atrium in man. *J Clin Invest* **56**:555-62, 1975.

60. Alboni P, Malcarne C, Pedroni P, et al.: Electrophysiology of normal sinus node with and without autonomic blockade. *Circulation* **65**:1236-42, 1982.

61. Engel TR, Bond RC, Schaal SF: First-degree sinoatrial heart block: sinoatrial block in the sick-sinus syndrome. *Am Heart J* **91**:303-10, 1976.

62. Dhingra RC, Rosen KM, Rahimtoola SH: Normal conduction intervals and responses in sixty-one patients using His bundle recording and atrial pacing. *Chest* **64**:55-9, 1973.

63. Gupta PK, Lichstein E, Chadda KD, Badui E: Appraisal of sinus nodal recovery time in patients with sick sinus syndrome. *Am J Cardiol* **34**:265-70, 1974.

CHAPTER 10

DISTURBANCES OF ATRIOVENTRICULAR CONDUCTION

Rather than a series of discrete elements, the AV conduction system is best viewed as a continuum of variably conductive tissues extending from the sinoatrial nodal/atrial junction to the Purkinje network/ventricular muscle cell junction. However, from a practical standpoint, electrophysiologists generally compartmentalize different segments of this continuum to facilitate ease of study and analysis. Consequently, study of normal and abnormal AV conduction involves an analyses of impulse conduction through the 1) sinoatrial node/atria; 2) AV node; 3) His bundle; and) infra-Hisian (His-Purkinje) system/ventricular myocardium. From a clinical standpoint, conduction disturbances residing below the central fibrous body within the His bundle and His-Purkinje system have the most pathological significance as they are often associated with clinically significant structural heart disease. In selected patients, intracardiac electrophysiology study may assist in the precise localization of the conduction disturbance thereby allowing the identification and differentiation of symptomatic high-risk patients from low-risk patients, especially when non-invasive testing has not proved useful.

10.1 Normal AV Conduction

Normal intra-atrial conduction involves spread of the high right atrial impulse to the low right atrial AV junction as well as to the left atrium. As previously noted (see "Functional Anatomy of the Conduction System" on page 1), it is debatable whether specific anatomically-identifiable "tracts" are present in the human atria to facilitate this conduction [1,2]. Normal conduction times within and between the atria has been the subject of limited investigations. The P-A interval — measured from the earliest onset of the P wave recorded by the surface ECG to the onset of atrial activation recorded by the His bundle catheter — has been used by many investigators to assess intra-atrial conduction [3-9]. However, this interval has been deemed an unreliable measure of intra-atrial conduction [10]. Instead endocardial recordings are the more reliable means to evaluate intra-atrial conduction [10]. Simultaneous multipolar intracardiac recordings within the right atrium and at the anterior and posterior AV junctions can be used to evaluate intra-atrial conduction in patients with and without atrial disease. In general, in patients lacking atrial disease, the conduction time from the high right atrium to the His bundle region is 25-35 msec [11].

The AV nodal conduction time, measured as the A-H interval (Figure 10-1), accounts for the major component of total AV conduction time during sinus rhythm. By definition, this conduction time represents the time for the cardiac impulse to conduct

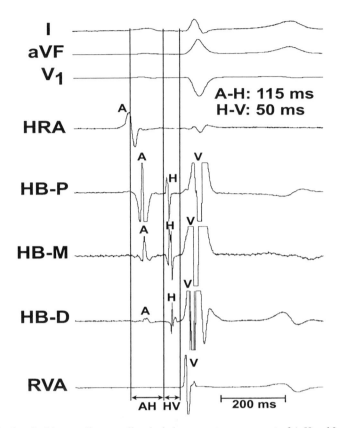

FIGURE 10-1. Standard intracardiac recording depicting correct measurement of A-H and H-V intervals. The A-H interval should be measured from the earliest reproducible rapid deflection of the atrial electrogram in the His bundle recording to the earliest activation of the His bundle. The H-V interval should be measured from the earliest deflection from baseline of a proximal His bundle electrogram to the earliest onset of ventricular activation recorded in any surface ECG or His bundle lead. See text for further discussion.

from the low right atrium at the interatrial septum through the AV node to the His bundle. Therefore it does not exclusively represent conduction time through the AV node. The A-H interval should be measured from the earliest reproducible rapid deflection of the atrial electrogram in the His bundle recording to the earliest activation of the His bundle (Figure 10-1). Consequently, the bipole on the His bundle catheter which is used to record the earliest His bundle activation should be positioned so as to record the most proximal His bundle electrogram that can be detected (usually this is the bipole that can record the largest atrial electrogram and still record a His bundle electrogram). Although very sensitive to autonomic modulation, the normal value for the A-H interval during sinus rhythm ranges from 45 to 150 msec [3-9,12-17].

During an intracardiac electrophysiologic study, typical Wenckebach periodicity can be produced in the normal AV node with increasingly rapid atrial pacing rates (Figure 10-2). With shortening of the A_1-A_1 cycle length, the A_1-H_1 interval gradually prolongs until, eventually, at a critical cycle length (the *Wenckebach block cycle length*),

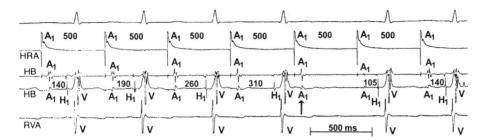

FIGURE 10-2. AV nodal Wenckebach block cycle length. Fixed cycle length pacing of the HRA (A_1-A_1 = 500 msec) results in progressive prolongation of the A_1-H_1 interval recorded by the His bundle electrographic (HB) lead. With continued pacing, conduction eventually blocks (upward arrow) in the AV node. Note that in the first paced complex following the block the A_1-H_1 interval is much shorter than in the complex occurring just before the development of block. Recording paper speed 100 mm/sec. A, atrial electrogram. H, His bundle electrogram. RVA, right ventricular apex. V, ventricular electrogram.

AV nodal conduction is blocked for one pacing cycle (A_1 not followed by H_1). AV nodal conduction resumes with the next pacing cycle but with a short A-H interval. This Wenckebach cycling can continue in a stable pattern; however, with continued shortening of the A_1-A_1 cycle length, AV nodal conduction may settle into a stable 2:1 pattern (Figure 10-3).

The conduction time from the proximal His bundle to the earliest activation of the ventricle is used to assess the functioning of the His-Purkinje conduction system. This conduction time is best approximated by the H-V interval which is measured from the earliest deflection from baseline of a proximal His bundle electrogram to the earliest onset of ventricular activation regardless of where it is recorded (surface ECG or intracardiac His bundle lead) (Figure 10-1). Care should be taken to record from the proximal His bundle region, in which case normal values for H-V are 35-55 ms in adults. If the "H-V"

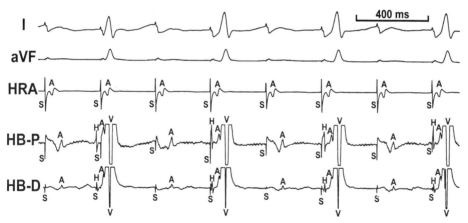

FIGURE 10-3. Mobitz type I AV conduction block with 2:1 AV conduction during rapid fixed rate atrial pacing at a cycle length of 270 msec. Note that the non-conducted atrial depolarizations are not followed by a His bundle activation.

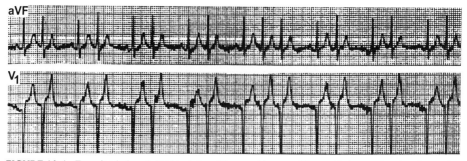

FIGURE 10-4. Exercise-induced AV block in a 52 year old man with easy fatigue and reduced exercise capacity. His clinical symptoms are reproduced at stage II of a treadmill exercise test, at which time he developed 3:2 and 4:3 AV Wenckebach periodicity. During a subsequent electrophysiology study, a markedly prolonged AV nodal refractory period, unaffected by an intravenous isoproterenol infusion, was documented. Paper speed 25 mm/sec.

interval measures at less than 35 ms, either preexcitation is present or the electrophysiologist is mistakenly recording a distal His bundle electrogram, or right bundle branch potential.

10.2   Abnormalities of AV Conduction

Disturbances of conduction of the normal pacemaker impulse may occur at any number of levels between the sinoatrial node (see "Disturbances of Sinoatrial Node Function" on page 453) and the ventricular muscles cells. Novices to ECG analyses commonly assume that virtually all AV conduction disturbances reside within the AV node proper, when in fact relatively few *clinically significant* disruptions of AV conduction involve the AV node. This is because disruptions of AV conduction of sufficient severity to require therapy with, for example, a permanent pacemaker, usually involve the regions below the AV node (except for sinoatrial node dysfunction). Rarely, severe AV node disease may clinically manifest itself with symptoms of dizziness/light-headedness, syncope, easy fatigue, reduced exercise capacity, dyspnea on exertion, and chronotropic incompetence, e.g., exercise-induced sinus tachycardia with Mobitz I (Wenckebach) second degree AV block (Figure 10-4). Under these circumstances, pacemaker therapy using the VDD mode (see Chapter 5, "Principles of Pacemaker Therapy" on page 173) is indicated, particularly in the very symptomatic and elderly patients.

10.2.1 CLASSIFICATION OF DISTURBANCES OF AV CONDUCTION

Atrioventricular conduction disturbances can be classified based upon: 1) the level within the specialized cardiac conduction system where the AV block develops, e.g., AV node, His bundle, etc., or 2) the classic system used in surface ECG analysis, e.g., first, second, and third degree AV block. Since the clinical approach to the patient often begins with a 12-lead ECG or rhythm strip, it may be most helpful to discuss AV conduction disturbances starting within that framework (Table 10-1.) Using the terminology of classical ECG analysis, abnormalities of AV conduction have been divided into *first degree* (delay in AV conduction), *second degree* (intermittent failure of AV conduction, with or without preceding delay in conduction), and *third degree* (total absence of AV conduction noted during the period of observation). Some investigators consider high grade AV block an intermediate category between second degree and third degree AV block during which two or more atrial depolarizations (P-waves) fail to conduct to the ventricles (Figure 10-5)

TABLE 10-1. Classification and diagnosis of AV conduction block

Type of AV block	ECG Diagnosis	Usual site(s) of AV block
1st degree AV block	1:1 AV conduction with P-R interval prolongation (>210 msec).	AV node, His-Purkinje system
2nd degree AV block Mobitz Type I (Wenckebach)	Intermittent conduction failure of AV conduction with either progressive P-R prolongation preceding the non-conducted P wave or the P-R interval immediately following the last non-conducted P wave is shorter than the P-R interval immediately preceding the first non-conducted P wave.	AV node
2nd degree AV block Mobitz Type II	Intermittent conduction failure of AV conduction without any detectable change in the P-R interval during cardiac cycles either immediately preceding or following the non-conducted P waves.	His-Purkinje system
3rd degree AV block	Absence of AV conduction with atrial activity dissociated from ventricular activity (if any).	AV node, His-Purkinje system

First degree AV block

Typically first degree AV block occurs most commonly at the level of the AV node and only occasionally within the atrium or the His-Purkinje system. It may be totally benign, as in the case of prolonged AV nodal conduction time secondary to an increase in parasympathetic (vagal) tone, although it may occasionally signify His-Purkinje disease, especially if it presents in the setting of intraventricular conduction system delay or bundle branch block. While conduction time from the high right atrium to the anterior or poste-

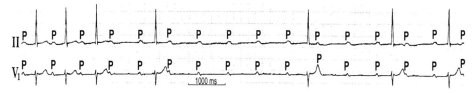

FIGURE 10-5. High degree AV block in a 51 year old man with a one year history of pre-syncopal spells. The symptoms date from surgery for mitral valve repair, and after an increase in their frequency, the patient sought medical advice. An event recorder showed frequent episodes similar to the one displayed above. Note that intermittently two or more atrial depolarizations (P-waves) are non-conducted, resulting in irregular R-R intervals.

rior AV junction may be significantly prolonged as a result of atrial disease, first degree AV block resulting solely from abnormalities of intra-atrial conduction secondary to intra-atrial disease [18] is unusual. In some cases, the appearance of first degree AV block may indicate a pathological process, such as acute myocardial ischemia. In other cases it may result from therapeutic or toxic doses of drugs especially digitalis, Ca^{++} channel blockers, or β-adrenergic antagonists.

First degree AV block is often due to prolongation of the A-H interval. Many of these cases represent functional or physiological first degree AV block due to vagal influences and they commonly resolve with vagolysis or enhancement of sympathetic tone. Corroborative evidence supporting this diagnosis includes the concomitant finding of slowing of the sinus rate (increase P-P interval). True fixed chronic first degree AV block present during sinus rhythm due to intrinsic disease of the AV node or His-Purkinje system may also occur. Furthermore, first degree AV block may represent conduction within a slow AV nodal pathway in patients with dual AV nodal pathway physiology after failure of conduction in the fast AV nodal pathway (prolonged refractoriness) upon attainment of a critical sinus cycle length.

Second degree AV block
Classically, second degree AV block has been divided into two types, Mobitz type I (or Wenckebach), and Mobitz type II. In Mobitz type I block, there is either progressive P-R prolongation preceding the non-conducted P wave or the P-R interval immediately following the last non-conducted P wave is shorter than the P-R interval immediately preceding the first non-conducted P wave (Figure 10-6). Atrioventricular conduction block which occurs without any detectable change in the P-R interval during cardiac cycles either immediately preceding or following the non-conducted P waves is termed Mobitz type II second degree AV block (Figure 10-7). The problems with this definition, of

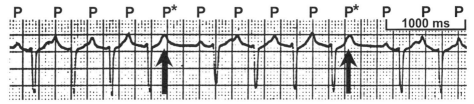

FIGURE 10-6. Mobitz type I (Wenckebach) second degree AV block during sinus tachycardia at 140 beats/min. Note the progressive lengthening of the PR interval before the non-conducted P-waves (P*, upward arrow).

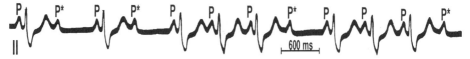

FIGURE 10-7. Mobitz type II second degree AV block. ECG lead II recording. Baseline right bundle branch block is present. The PR interval is approximately 160 ms immediately before the non-conducted P waves (P*) as well as the first conducted P wave after the conduction block. This patient had a history of recurrent of syncope which resolved with implantation of a permanent pacemaker system.

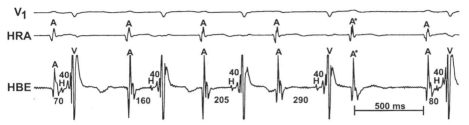

FIGURE 10-8. His bundle recording during Mobitz type I (Wenckebach) second degree AV block. ECG lead V₁ along (HRA) and His bundle region (HBE) are displayed. Note that the A-H interval progressively prolongs (e.g., from 70 ms to 290 ms) before there is a total failure of AV conduction of an atrial depolarization (A*). The H-V interval remains constant throughout at 40 ms. A, atrial electrogram H, His bundle electrogram; V, ventricular electrogram.

course, is that very small differences in the duration of the P-R interval may either simply go undetected, or in practical terms, are unmeasurable given limitations in visually determining the precise onset of the P wave and the QRS complex when viewed using the common recording speed of 25 mm/sec. Consequently, it is entirely possible that some cases of Mobitz type I second degree AV block are mis-diagnosed as Mobitz type II AV block.

Second degree AV block resulting from conduction block within the atrium proper appears to be extremely rare and has only been observed during atrial pacing [8,9,19,20].

Mobitz type I second degree AV block is usually due to conduction block within the AV node proper. In these patients, intracardiac His bundle recordings show that there is progressive lengthening of the A-H interval before the non-conducted atrial depolarization and the atrial electrogram is not followed by a normal His bundle electrogram (Figure 10-8). Conduction block at the level of the AV node is usually due to functional or physiological modulation of AV nodal conduction by the autonomic nervous system and does not usually imply the presence of any fixed intrinsic conduction system disease (See "The Autonomic Nervous System and Functional Conduction Block" on page 419.) Since this type of block is generally due to enhancement of the activity of the parasympathetic nervous system relative to that of the sympathetic nervous system, careful ECG evaluation usually reveals corroborating evidence such as P-P interval prolongation (sinus slowing) occurring around the same time as the appearance of the non-conducted P waves (Figure 10-9) or occurrence during sleep when vagal tone is naturally high. In addition, in these cases, the AV block generally immediately resolves with exercise or pharmacological treatments with atropine or isoproterenol. Patients with Mobitz type I AV block generally exhibit a benign course with an excellent prognosis. However, as previously mentioned (Figure 10-4), severe AV nodal disease may cause clinically significant symptoms and, may therefore, require treatment with a permanent pacemaker. Mobitz type I (Wenckebach) AV block may rarely occur in the diseased His-Purkinje system due to degeneration, myocardial ischemia, and/or antiarrhythmic drugs, such as class I and class III agents, that prolong His-Purkinje refractoriness (Figure 10-10).

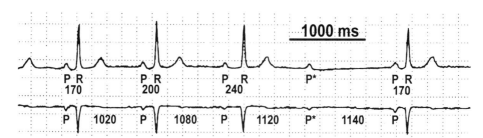

FIGURE 10-9. Mobitz Type 1 (Wenckebach) second degree AV block due to hypervagotonia. During the Wenckebach cycle shown here, the P-R interval increases from 170 ms to 240 ms before AV conduction block occurs. A solitary atrial depolarization (P*) fails to conduct to the ventricle. Following this block, conduction resumes with the PR interval much shorter (170 ms) than it is during the last conducted beat before the block (240 ms). Also note that the P-P interval increases from 1020 ms to 1140 ms. This prolongation of the P-P interval (decrease in sinus rate) with P-R prolongation with eventual AV conduction block is consistent with vagally-induced Wenckebach type AV conduction block.

Mobitz II second degree AV block (Figure 10-7) is usually (but not always) due to conduction block below the AV node, generally within the His bundle proper or just distal to it. In these patients, intracardiac His bundle recordings may show that at the time of the non-conducted P-wave the atrial and His bundle electrograms are inscribed but

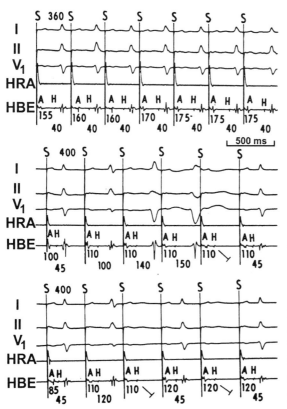

FIGURE 10-10. Conduction disturbance in His-purkinje system caused by N-acetylprocainamide (NAPA). From top to bottom in each panel are shown ECG leads I, II, and V1, along with intracardiac electrograms from the high right atrium (HRA) and the His bundle region (HBE). Panel A: During atrial pacing at a cycle length (S-S) of 360 msec, AV conduction is 1:1. The corresponding AV nodal conduction time (A-H interval) ranges from 155 to 175 msec, while the conduction time in the His-Purkinje system (H-V interval) is 40 msec. Panel B: Following NAPA infusion, the atrium is paced at a cycle length of 400 msec. Note the development of 5:4 AV block below the level of the His bundle. This is preceded by prolongation of the H-V interval from 45 to 150 msec. Associated with this is the progression of the bundle branch block with the development of incomplete right bundle branch block (second QRS complex), incomplete left bundle branch block (third QRS complex), and complete left bundle branch block (fourth QRS complex). Panel C: Further progression to 3:2 and 2:1 AV block in the His-Purkinje system. S, stimulus artifact, A, atrial electrogram, H, His bundle electrogram. From [33] with permission.

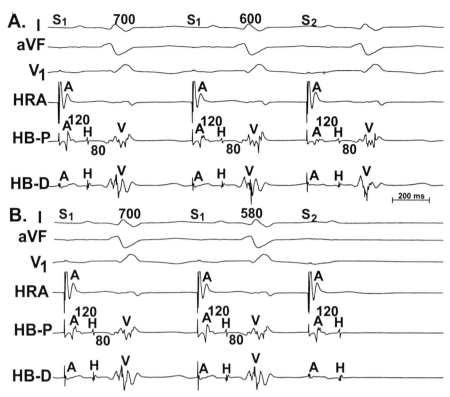

FIGURE 10-11. Infra-Hisian conduction block in a 68-year old man with a history of syncope. From top to bottom in each panel is shown surface ECG leads I, aVF, and V₁ along with intracardiac recordings from the high right atrium (HRA) and proximal (HB-P) and distal (HB-D) His bundle region. At baseline, the patient's 12-lead ECG shows first degree AV block along with a right bundle branch block and left anterior fascicular block. His baseline H-V interval is prolonged at 80 ms. An eight beat drive train (S₁-S₁) is delivered to the HRA at a cycle length of 700 ms is followed by a single premature extrastimulus at a coupling interval (S₁-S₂) of 600 ms (panel A) or 580 ms (panel B). Note that despite the absence of any change in the A-H or the H-V interval (120 ms and 80 ms, respectively) during the drive and extrastimulus, the premature extrastimulus delivered at a coupling interval of 580 ms blocked below the His bundle (note H without following V in panel B). A, atrial electrogram; H, His bundle electrogram; V, ventricular electrogram.

without subsequent activation of the ventricles (Figures 10-11 & 10-12). Almost invariably, therefore, these patients have significant His-Purkinje system disease. These patients may exhibit baseline prolongation of the P-R interval on their electrocardiograms (Figure 10-12) associated with intraventricular conduction disease or bundle branch/fascicular blocks (Figures 10-7 & 10-11). The QRS duration during the escape rhythm is generally prolonged (>120 msec). Finally, these patients may present with episodes of near-syncope, syncope, or even sudden death. Consequently, identification and differentiation of these high risk patients with Mobitz type II AV block from those low risk patients with Mobitz type I block is essential. Atrioventricular block with 2:1 AV conduction may occur either at the level of the AV node or at the His-Purkinje system. Intracardiac His bundle recordings with pharmacological testing may be required for definitive differential diagnosis in these cases (Figures 10-3 & 10-13). A number of clini-

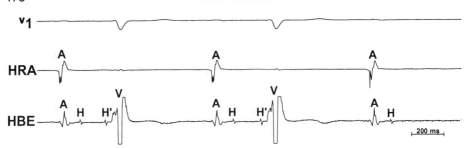

FIGURE 10-12. Intra-Hisian conduction block with widely split His bundle potentials recorded in a 75-year old woman with a history of syncope and Mobitz Type II second degree AV block. From top to bottom are displayed ECG lead V_1 and intracardiac recordings from the high right atrium (HRA) and His bundle region (HBE). The patient's surface ECG displays first degree AV block with a PR interval approaching 400 ms. The QRS duration is normal. The first and second (from the left) sinus beats are conducted to the ventricle with first degree AV block. The third sinus beat blocks between within the His bundle (note proximal H with out distal H' or V).

TABLE 10-2. Findings which favor an AV nodal site of block in patients with second degree AV block

Block is associated with increase in P-P interval, reflecting hypervagotonia

Block is associated with normal QRS complexes (without intraventricular/bundle branch conduction defect)

Pre-block P-R interval is longer than first post-block P-R interval

Resolution of block with exercise or administration of isoproterenol or atropine

Exacerbation of block during/following carotid sinus massage

Presence of AV nodal blocking drugs (digoxin, β-adrenergic blockers, Ca^{2+} channel blockers) or sympatholytic agents (α-methyldopa, clonidine)

History of athletic training

Presence of 1:1 AV conduction during sinus rhythm even in presence of PR interval prolongation ≥ 210 ms

cal and pharmacological features favor the AV node as the site of block over the His-Purkinje system in patients with second degree AV block (Table 10-2.)

Third degree AV block
Short of surgically-produced intra-atrial conduction disturbances, naturally-occurring third degree AV block resulting from atrial disease is unknown in humans. In most patients with naturally occurring third degree AV block, the level of block is within the His-Purkinje system and less commonly the AV node These patients often have evidence of significant conduction system disease with intraventricular conduction delay, bundle branch block, and bifascicular block, as well as significant first degree AV block due to prolongation of the H-V interval. When these patients develop complete AV block, the escape rhythm (if present) is usually ventricular in origin and exhibits a wide QRS complex (Figure 10-14). Patients with complete AV block at the level of the AV node generally exhibit a narrow QRS complex escape rhythm originating either very proximal within the His-Purkinje system or within the AV node region. Complete AV

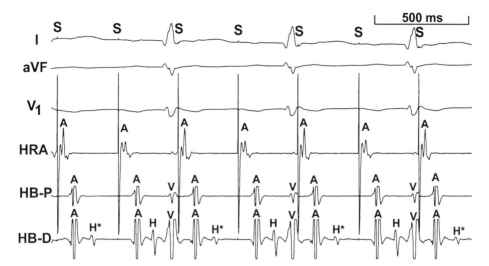

FIGURE 10-13. Surface ECG and intracardiac recordings showing 2:1 AV conduction block in the infra-Hisian region. Displayed from top to bottom are surface ECG leads I, aVF, V₁ and intracardiac recordings from the high right atrium (HRA), proximal (HBE-P) and distal (HBE-D) region. Fixed rate atrial pacing is performed at a cycle length (S-S) of 310 msec. Note that every other atrial depolarization fails to conduct to the ventricle. Although during each of these cardiac cycles, the His bundle is activated (H*), conduction fails to proceed to the ventricle. A, atrial electrogram, H, His bundle electrogram during AV conduction, H*, His bundle electrogram during AV block, V, ventricular electrogram.

block occurring during atrial fibrillation is characterized by regularization of the R-R intervals (Figure 10-15). The escape rhythm can exhibit either a narrow or wide QRS complex, depending upon its origin. A narrow QRS complex would be expected if the escape rhythm originates in the AV node or proximal His bundle region, while a wide QRS complex would be expected if the rhythm arises from the His-Purkinje system.

10.2.2 RATE-DEPENDENT CONDUCTION BLOCK

During normal AV conduction, ventricular activation begins nearly simultaneously at three left ventricular endocardial sites – high anteroseptal, mid-septal, and lower posteroseptal [21-24]. Normal right ventricular activation begins 5-10 ms later at the base of the anterior papillary muscle. In adults, biventricular activation is normally complete

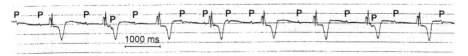

FIGURE 10-14. Third degree (complete) AV block. Note that there is dissociation of the atrial and ventricular activity with the P-P interval = 680 ms and the R-R interval = 1600 ms. Some of the P waves cannot be visualized as they are "buried" in the T waves or QRS complexes. The regular and wide QRS complexes (QRS duration 160 ms) with bizarre repolarization (deep T wave inversion) originate from an escape pacemaker located in the ventricle.

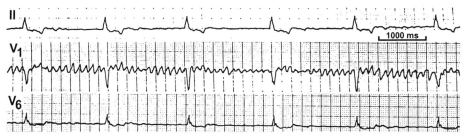

FIGURE 10-15. Regularization of the R-R interval in a patient with atrial fibrillation and complete AV block with a wide QRS complex escape rhythm. See text for additional discussion.

within <100 ms. "Complete" bundle branch block is arbitrarily defined as biventricular activation requiring more than 120 msec (QRS duration ≥ 120 msec). Biventricular activation is said to be "delayed" when biventricular activation time is between 100 and 120 msec. However, slow conduction in one or more of the fascicles of the His-Purkinje system (resulting from, for example, disease, drugs, or markedly premature impulses) can readily prolong biventricular activation to this degree without fixed complete conduction block in any single fascicle actually being present. Therefore, a QRS duration ≥ 120 ms does not necessarily imply fixed block, but instead may merely indicate markedly slowed conduction in one or more fascicles.

In a patient with a normal His-Purkinje system, anterograde AV conduction block normally occurs in the AV node before refractoriness of the His bundle or bundle branches is reached. In the presence of antiarrhythmic drugs or exogenous catecholamines (isoproterenol) the functional refractory period of the AV node may be less than the effective refractory period of the His-Purkinje system. Rapid atrial pacing under these conditions may result in intra- or infra-Hisian anterograde conduction block before block appears in the AV node. This may not by itself indicate a diseased or abnormal His-Purkinje conduction system.

If conduction through the AV node is not limiting, the premature atrial extrastimuli may conduct to the His bundle and bundle branches and *functional bundle branch block* may develop. Conduction delay or block in the His bundle, or one or more of the fascicles, can occur if the input coupling interval into the tissue is greater than the effective refractory period of that tissue. For example, in the absence of limiting conduction delay through the AV node, atrial extrastimuli can conduct in a 1:1 fashion without delay to the His bundle. Assuming no delay or block in the His bundle, the impulses emerging from the His bundle will encounter the branching fascicles of the ventricular conduction system. If the H_1-H_2 interval resulting from any A_1-A_2 interval is shorter than the effective refractory period of one of the fascicles (Figure 10-16), slower than normal conduction may occur in that fascicle resulting in a bundle branch block pattern recorded by the surface 12-lead ECG. The exact bundle branch block pattern that is recorded will depend upon which fascicles are involved and which areas of ventricular myocardium have their activation most delayed. In patients able to exhibit aberrant His-Purkinje conduction of premature atrial extrastimuli, a large majority (up to 93%) exhibit a right bundle branch block pattern, up to 44% may have a left bundle branch block pattern, and up to 19% exhibit both patterns [25-28].

Rate-dependent bundle branch blocks
Two types of rate-dependent bundle branch block are recognized: *tachycardia-dependent bundle branch block (phase 3 block)* and *bradycardia-dependent bundle branch block (phase 4 block)*. In phase 3 block [29-31], conduction block develops in one of the bundle branches because the cycle length of the supraventricular impulse encroaches on the refractory period of the bundle branch, which occurs during phase 3 (late repolarization) of the action potential. This can readily occur in the Purkinje fibers of the bundle branches because the duration of their action potentials and their refractory periods are relatively long. When the subsequent action potential of the tachycardia arrives while fibers in the bundle branch are still refractory in phase 2 or 3, anterograde conduction is blocked in that bundle and activation of the ventricle must occur via the other bundle branch resulting in a wide QRS complex. Phase 3 block involving the right bundle branch is more common than in the left bundle. Right bundle branch block aberration is more frequently noted at long drive cycle lengths while shorter drive cycle lengths more often results in left bundle branch block aberration (Figure 10-17) [30,31].

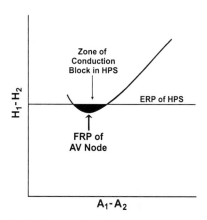

FIGURE 10-16. AV nodal input-output relationship and functional His-Purkinje conduction block. Functional conduction block in the His-Purkinje system (HPS) results when the extra-stimuli output coupling interval from the AV node is less than the effective refractory period (ERP) of the HPS (black shaded region). The A_1-A_2 coupling interval at which the shortest H_1-H_2 occurs is the functional refractory period (FRP) of the AV node (upward arrow).

Phase 4 block can develop during bradycardia because the long periods of diastole between QRS complexes permits phase 4 depolarization to develop in the Purkinje fibers

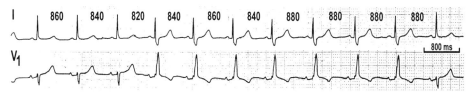

FIGURE 10-17. Tachycardia-dependent (phase 3) block. Shown are surface ECG recordings using leads I and V_1. With a decrease in sinus cycle length from 860 to 820 ms (increase in sinus rate from 70 to 73 beats/min), the QRS contour changes from normal to one with a right bundle branch block (RBBB) morphology. As the sinus rate declines, the RBBB QRS morphology resolves, but only after the sinus cycle length increases to 880 msec (68 beats/min). The persistence of RBBB aberrancy at longer cycle lengths is probably due to trans-septal concealed conduction from left to right with retrograde activation of the right bundle branch (*linking*). This perpetuates refractoriness of the right bundle branch until sinus cycle length slows sufficiently to allow dissipation of refractoriness of the retrograde-activated right bundle branch.

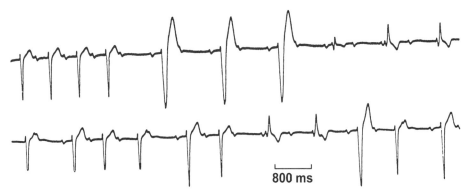

FIGURE 10-18. Bradycardia-dependent (phase 4) block. Continuous ECG recording of lead V$_1$. The rhythm is sinus with Wenckebach AV block of varying periodicity. QRS complexes with the shortest R-R intervals (680 -840 msec) are conducted without aberration. QRS complexes following slightly longer R-R intervals (1080 msec) exhibit incomplete left bundle branch block (LBBB) aberration. Conducted QRS complexes closing the longest R-R cycles (1260 msec) demonstrate complete LBBB aberration.

of the bundle branches (most often the left bundle branch which apparently has a faster rate of diastolic depolarization) [32]. This reduction of membrane potential may result in the development of refractoriness in the bundle branch, thereby blocking conduction within the bundle branch during a subsequent supraventricular impulse. This produces a wide QRS complex with a bundle branch block morphology at slow supraventricular rates (Figure 10-18).

The *Ashman's phenomenon* is a special case of right bundle branch block (very rarely left bundle branch block) associated with a short cardiac cycle following a long R-R interval. In this case, the long R-R interval is associated with an action potential of long duration. A subsequent early atrial depolarization (short cycle length) will either completely fail to conduct within the right bundle branch, or conduct very slowly, because the Purkinje fibers in the bundle branch are still refractory due to the preceding long duration action potential (most Na$^+$ channels still inactive). The right bundle branch block pattern is perpetuated even if the R-R interval again somewhat lengthens because trans-septal conduction from the left to right ventricle maintains refractoriness in the right bundle branch, a phenomenon known as linking. Only after the R-R interval prolongs sufficiently to allow time for recovery of excitability in the right bundle branch does the aberrancy resolve.

Rate-dependent complete AV block
Complete AV block may also occur as a result of acceleration (phase 3) or deceleration (phase 4) of the sinus rate with mechanisms similar to those responsible for rate-dependent bundle branch block as discussed above. The site of block is usually located within the His-Purkinje system but at times in the AV node. Clinically, rate-dependent complete AV block is often called "paroxysmal AV block" and most commonly occurs in situations when sinus rate accelerates, such as during exercise or an anxiety reaction (Figure 10-19).

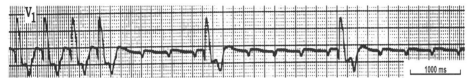

FIGURE 10-19. Paroxysmal AV block in a patient with complete right bundle branch block and left anterior fascicular block associated with previous myocardial infarction. The rhythm strip (lead V_1) shows acceleration of sinus rate with shortening of sinus cycle length to 520 msec (111 beats/min) is followed by development of high degree and complete AV block. From [34] with permission.

10.2.3 PSEUDO AV BLOCK

Pseudo AV block (Figure 10-20) is characterized by the development of an AV conduction disturbance due to extra-depolarizations originating at the AV junction but that are not recorded by the surface ECG (concealed junctional extrasystoles). In this situation, both anterograde and retrograde conduction of these junctional depolarizations is blocked and the phenomenon can only be recognized as isolated His bundle depolarizations during intracardiac recordings at the AV junction (Figure 10-21). Because the surface ECG recording fails to detect the intracardiac manifestation of the concealed conduction, the physician may mistakenly interpret the recording as showing a genuine disruption of AV conduction. Consequently, this phenomenon is referred to as "pseudo AV block" since it may be erroneously interpreted as a true pathological AV block.

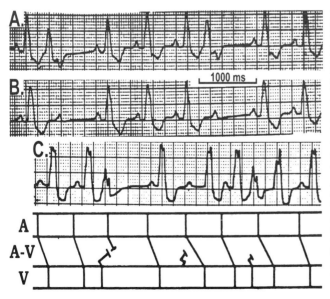

FIGURE 10-20. Example of pseudo AV block in a patient with manifest and concealed extra-depolarizations. Panel A: ECG rhythm strip (lead II) showing "complete" left bundle branch block with manifest ventricular premature depolarizations. Panel B: Mobitz type II 2nd degree AV block resulting from concealed extra-depolarizations. Based upon the frequent premature ventricular depolarizations recorded (panel A), pseudo AV block may be inferred as the mechanism in panel B. Panel C: Unexpected prolongation of the P-R interval in the same patient. A ladder diagram is constructed to explain the sudden appearance of first degree AV block caused by concealed AV junctional extra-depolarizations. From [34] with permission.

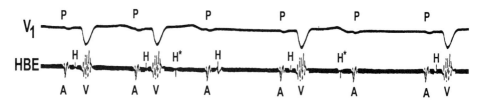

FIGURE 10-21. His bundle recording (HBE) showing pseudo Mobitz type II AV block due to concealed extra-depolarizations emanating from the region of the His bundle. A, atrial electrogram; H, His bundle electrogram resulting from normal AV conduction; H*, electrogram resulting from extra-His bundle depolarization; V, ventricular depolarization; P, atrial depolarization recorded by lead V_1 of the surface ECG. From [34] with permission.

10.3   Management of AV Conduction Disturbances

First degree AV block alone generally does not require treatment. In most patients, Mobitz type I (Wenckebach) second degree AV block usually indicates a conduction disturbance within the AV node. Usually in these cases the conduction problem is either caused by enhanced vagal tone or drugs that suppress AV nodal function. Consequently, most patients with Wenckebach block do not require pacemaker therapy. However, some patients with chronic AV node disease may exhibit Mobitz type I second degree AV block and be highly symptomatic with fatigue, chronotropic incompetence (Figure 10-4), or syncope, and may, therefore, require treatment with a permanent pacemaker. Mobitz type II second degree AV block is usually due to disease within the His-Purkinje system; consequently, implantation of a pacemaker system is often necessary. Pacemaker therapy is generally recommended even in asymptomatic patients because they are at high risk of progression to complete AV block. Patients with high degree AV block may require insertion of a temporary pacemaker followed by implantation of a permanent pacemaker if the disease process involves the His-Purkinje system rather than the AV node (Figure 10-5). Patients presenting with complete (third degree) AV block generally require emergent insertion of a temporary pacemaker or placement of a transcutaneous (transthoracic) external pacemaker. Urgent treatment is generally necessary because complete AV block causes near-syncope, syncope, dyspnea, angina pectoris, congestive heart failure, or torsade de pointes. Unless the cause of third degree block can be identified and reversed, implantation of a permanent pacemaker is generally required.

In all patients with second or third degree AV block, diagnostic evaluation should include a search for reversible causes such as: 1) acute myocardial ischemia or infarction, 2) metabolic acidosis with or without hyperkalemia, 3) infection (including sepsis, lyme disease, infective endocarditis), 4) drug reaction or toxicity (e.g., digoxin, β-adrenergic blocking agents, Ca^{++} channel blocking drugs, or class I, II, or III antiarrhythmic drugs), and mechanical factors such as catheter-induced trauma (e.g., pulmonary artery flotation catheter) to the right bundle branch in a patient with complete left bundle branch block or surgery for mitral or aortic valve replacement.

In patients with complete AV block associated with digitalis intoxication, placement of a transcutaneous external pacemaker and establishment of central venous access for temporary transvenous pacing is recommended (See "Temporary Pacing" on page 423.). Intracardiac pacing may provoke fatal ventricular tachyarrhythmias in patients with digitalis toxicity. Under these circumstances, urgent treatment with digoxin antibodies along with correction of metabolic derangements may be necessary. Theoretically, antiarrhythmic agents can be used to suppress AV junctional extra-depolarizations in symptomatic patients with pseudo AV block. Unfortunately, these patients often have associated intraventricular conduction system disease (Figures 10-20 & 10-21); consequently, the use of antiarrhythmic agents in this setting may exacerbate the AV conduction disturbance, potentially producing complete AV block. Therefore, pacemaker therapy may be necessary in this subset of patients.

References

1. Sherf L: The atrial conduction system: clinical implications. *Am J Cardiol* **37**:814, 1976.
2. Rossi L: Interatrial, internodal and dual reentrant atrioventricular nodal pathways: an anatomical update of arrhythmogenic substrates. *Cardiologia* **41**:129-134, 1996.
3. Damato AN, Lau SH, Patton RD, et al.: A study of atrioventricular conduction in man using premature atrial stimulation and His bundle recordings. *Circulation* **40**:61-9, 1969.
4. Damato AN, Lau SH, Helfant RH, et al.: Study of atrioventricular conduction in man using electrode catheter recordings of His bundle activity. *Circulation* **39**:287-96, 1969.
5. Damato AN, Lau SH, et al.: Recording of specialized conducting fibers (A-V nodal, His bundle, and right bundle branch) in man using an electrode catheter technic. *Circulation* **39**:435-47, 1969.
6. Damato AN, Lau SH: Clinical value of the electrogram of the conduction system. *Prog Cardiovasc Dis* **13**:119-40, 1970.
7. Castellanos A, Castillo C, Agha A: Contribution of the His bundle recording to the understanding of clinical arrhythmias. *Am J Cardiol* **28**:499, 1971.
8. Narula OS, Scherlag BJ, Samet P, Javier RP: Atrioventricular block: Localization and classification by His bundle recordings. *Am J Med* **50**:146, 1971.
9. Narula OS, Cohen LS, Samet P, et al.: Localization of A-V conduction defects in man by recording of the His bundle electrogram. *Am J Cardiol* **25**:288, 1970.
10. Josephson ME. Electrophysiologic investigation: General concepts. *Clinical Cardiac Electrophysiology: Techniques and Interpretations*. Philadelphia: Lea & Febiger, 28-70: 1993.
11. Josephson ME. Atrioventricular conduction. *Clinical Cardiac Electrophysiology: Techniques and Interpretations*. 2nd ed. Philadelphia: Lea & Febiger, 96-116: 1993.
12. Damato AN, Lau SH, Helfant R, et al.: A study of heart block in man using His bundle recordings. *Circulation* **39**:297-305, 1969.
13. Schuilenburg RM, Durrer D: Conduction disturbances located within the His bundle. *Circulation* **45**:612, 1972.
14. Bekheit S, Murtagh JG, Morton P, Fletcher E: Measurements of sinus impulse conduction from electrogram of bundle of His. *Br Heart J* **33**:719, 1971.
15. Bekheit S, Murtagh JG, Morton P, Fletcher E: Studies of heart block with His bundle recordings. *Br Heart J* **34**:717, 1972.
16. Rosen KM: Evaluation of cardiac conduction in the cardiac catheterization laboratory. *Am J Cardiol* **30**:701-3, 1972.
17. Rosen KM, Scherlag BJ, Samet P, Helfant RH: His bundle electrogram. *Circulation* **46**:831-2, 1972.
18. Fisher JD, Lehmann MH: Marked intra-atrial conduction delay with split atrial electrograms: substrate for reentrant supraventricular tachycardia. *Am Heart J* **111**:781-4, 1986.
19. Castellanos A, Sung RJ, Aldrich JL, et al.: Alternating Wenckebach periods occurring in the atria, His-Purkinje system, ventricles and Kent bundle. *Am J Cardiol* **40**:853-9, 1977.

20. Castellanos A, Iyengar R, Agha AS, Castillo CA: Wenckebach phenomenon within the atria. *Br Heart J* **34**:1121-6, 1972.

21. Durrer D, Dam RTV, Freud GE, et al.: Total excitation of the isolated human heart. *Circulation* **41**:899-912, 1970.

22. Cassidy DM, Vassallo JA, et al.: Endocardial mapping in humans in sinus rhythm with normal left ventricles: activation patterns and characteristics of electrograms. *Circulation* **70**:37-42, 1984.

23. Wyndham CR: Epicardial activation in bundle branch block. *PACE Pacing and Clinical Electrophysiology* **6**:1201-9, 1983.

24. Roos JP, van Dam RT, Durrer D: Epicardial and intramural excitation of normal heart in six patients 50 years of age and older. *Br Heart J* **30**:630-7, 1968.

25. Denker S, Shenasa M, Gilbert CJ, Akhtar M: Effects of abrupt changes in cycle length on refractoriness of the His-Purkinje system in man. *Circulation* **67**:60-8, 1983.

26. Elizari MV, Lazzari JO, Rosenbaum MB: Phase-3 and phase-4 intermittent left anterior hemiblock. Report of first case in the literature. *Chest* **62**:673-7, 1972.

27. Elizari MV, Lazzari JO, Rosenbaum MB: Phase-3 and phase-4 intermittent left bundle branch block occurring spontaneously in a dog. *Eur J Cardiol* **1**:95-103, 1973.

28. Elizari MV, Nau GJ, Levi RJ, et al.: Experimental production of rate-dependent bundle branch block in the canine heart. *Circ Res* **34**:730-42, 1974.

29. Akhtar M, Gilbert C, Al-Nouri M, Denker S: Site of conduction delay during functional block in the His-Purkinje system in man. *Circulation* **61**:1239-48, 1980.

30. Chilson DA, Zipes DP, Heger JJ, et al.: Functional bundle branch block: discordant response of right and left bundle branches to changes in heart rate. *Am J Cardiol* **54**:313-6, 1984.

31. Wellens HJ, Ross DL, Farre J, Brugada P. Functional bundle branch block during supraventricular tachycardia in man: Observations on mechanisms and their incidence. In: Zipes DP, Jalife J, eds. *Cardiac Electrophysiology and Arrhythmias*. Orlando: Grune and Stratton, Inc.: 1985.

32. Rosenbaum MB, Lazzara JO, Elizari MV. The role of phase 3 and phase 4 block in clinical electrocardiography. In: Wellens HJJ, Lie KI, Janse MJ, eds. *The Conduction System of the Heart: Structure, Function, and Clinical Implications*. Philadelphia: Lea & Febiger: 1976.

33. Sung RJ, Juma Z, Saksena S: Electrophysiologic properties and antiarrhythmic mechanisms of intravenous N-acetylprocainamide in patients with ventricular dysrhythmias. *Am Heart J* **105**:811-9, 1983.

34. Castellanos A, Sung RJ, Mallon SM, et al.: His bundle electrocardiography in manifest and concealed right bundle branch extrasystoles. *Am Heart J* **94**:307-15, 1977.

CHAPTER 11

ATRIOVENTRICULAR NODAL REENTRANT TACHYCARDIA

Atrioventricular (AV) nodal reentrant tachycardia is a common cause of paroxysmal supraventricular tachycardia. Based on observations made in animal experiments, the mechanism of AV nodal reentrant tachycardia was postulated to be due to "longitudinal dissociation" of the AV node [1-5] in which two AV nodal pathways with different functional properties – fast and slow converge proximally and distally to form proximal and distal common pathways. An atrial or ventricular premature impulse may thus induce a reentrant phenomenon, utilizing one pathway for anterograde conduction and the other pathway for retrograde conduction (Figures 11-1 through 11-3) [6-11].

Using the technique of intracardiac mapping, it was subsequently demonstrated that the fast and slow pathways had anatomically distinct atrial insertions during retrograde conduction in patients with dual AV node pathway physiology [12]. The retrograde atrial exit of the fast pathway was located at the low septal right atrium near the His bundle recording site, while that of the slow pathway at or near the coronary sinus ostium, inferior and posterior to the fast pathway (Figure 11-4). Thus, dual AV node pathway physiology is not only functional, but also anatomical. Intraoperative mapping of the AV junction has confirmed these findings in patients with AV nodal reentrant tachycardia [13-15].

Building upon the above framework, open-heart surgical and percutaneous catheter techniques were developed to provide a curative treatment for patients with AV nodal re-

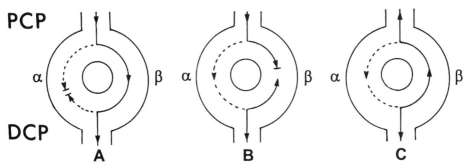

FIGURE 11-1. Schematic representation of the occurrence of a reentrant phenomenon. A reentrant circuit is composed of a proximal common pathway (PCP), two conduction pathways (α and b), and a distal common pathway (DCP). The β pathway has a faster conduction time (solid line) with a longer refractory period, and the α pathway has a slower conduction time (dash line) with a shorter refractory period. (A) An impulse is conducted over both α and β pathways without initiation of a reentrant phenomenon. (B) A premature impulse is blocked in the β pathway but is conducted slowly (slow conduction) by way of the α pathway. (C) The slow conduction in the α pathway is sufficient to allow recovery of excitability of the previously blocked β pathway (unidirectional block). The premature impulse can thus be conducted over the β pathway in a retrograde direction initiating a reentrant phenomenon.

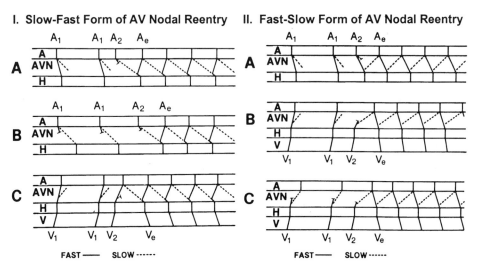

FIGURE 11-2. Ladder diagrams summarizing the modes of induction of AV nodal reentrant tachycardia of the slow-fast form (I, left panels) and fast-slow form (II, right panels) during programmed electrical stimulation. In the left figure (I), the slow-fast form of AV nodal reentrant tachycardia is induced with atrial (Panels IA and IB) and ventricular (Panel IC) extrastimulation. Panel IA: Induction of tachycardia associated with discontinuous A_1-A_2/A_2-H_2 and A_1-A_2/H_1-H_2 curves. Panel IB: Induction of tachycardia associated with smooth A_1-A_2/A_2-H_2 and A_1-A_2/H_1-H_2 curves. Panel IC: Induction of tachycardia associated with smooth V_1-V_2/V_2-A_2 and V_1-V_2/A_1-A_2 curves. In the right figure (II) the fast-slow form of AV nodal reentry is induced with atrial (Panel IIA) and ventricular (Panels IIB and IIC) extrastimulation. Panel IIA: Induction of tachycardia associated with smooth A_1-A_2/A_2-H_2 and A_1-A_2/H_1-H_2 curves. Panel IIB: Induction of tachycardia associated with discontinuous V_1-V_2/V_2-A_2 and V_1-V_2/A_1-A_2 curves. Panel IIC: Induction of tachycardia associated with smooth V_1-V_2/V_2-A_2 and V_1-V_2/A_1-A_2 curves. A, atrium; AVN, AV node; H, His bundle; V, ventricle. A_1 and V_1 basic atrial and ventricular drives, respectively. A_2 and V_2, atrial and ventricular premature complexes, respectively. Ae and Ve, atrial and ventricular echoes, respectively. Solid and dashed lines denote fast and slow AV node pathways, respectively.

entrant tachycardia. Both peri-"nodal" cryosurgery and dissection, respectively, were effective in preventing sustained AV node reentry [16,17], and delivery of DC countershock proximal to the His bundle recording site through a transvenous electrode catheter could result in selective ablation of fast pathway conduction [18]. With the development of the radiofrequency (RF) energy source [19-23], coupled with the transvenous catheter technique, selective fast or slow pathway ablation (Figure 11-5) has become less morbid and simpler to perform [25-37]. In particular, the techniques of selective ablation of slow pathway conduction not only has provided a relatively safe and noninvasive means to cure AV nodal reentrant tachycardia, but also because the size of the endocardial lesion produced by RF energy is small and discrete, this technology has proven that the fast and slow AV node pathways are anatomically distinct.

11.1   Cellular Electrophysiology of the AV Node

For details of the gross and microscopic anatomy of the AV node the reader is referred to "Functional Anatomy of the Conduction System" on page 1.

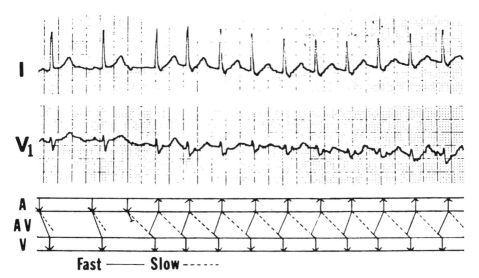

FIGURE 11-3. Initiation of reentrant supraventricular tachycardia with an atrial premature beat. During sinus rhythm at a cycle length of 760 ms, an atrial premature beat (third P wave) with a premature coupling interval of 400 ms conducts to the ventricles with a markedly prolonged P-R interval (0.38 sec) and initiates an onset of supraventricular tachycardia with a cycle length of 460 ms. The ladder diagram illustrates the development of unidirectional block in a fast-conducting pathway with resultant slow pathway conduction (dash line) before the initiation of the reentrant supraventricular tachyarrhythmia. ECG leads I and V₁ are simultaneously recorded. A = atrium; AV = atrioventricular junction; V = ventricle.

Using microelectrode and voltage clamp techniques, the cellular electrophysiological properties of the AV junction and AV nodal cells have been characterized in mammalian hearts [38-47]. Based upon cellular electrophysiological properties, the AV node has been divided into the AN, N, and NH cell zones; and even smaller subdivisions [38,39] (Figure 1-4 on page 5). The AN region consists of large Purkinje-like cells comprising the internodal pathways with a large portion of the slender transitional cells. The N region corresponds primarily to the mass of interweaving and interconnected transitional cells of all types, while the NH region appears to be where P cells and some transitional cells connect with large Purkinje-type cells of the His bundle [48]. The disparity in cell types and arrangements accounts for anisotropic conduction demonstrated at the AV junction [49].

Cells in the N-zone (roughly corresponding to the mid-nodal area of the compact AV node) exhibit the lowest resting potentials and have action potentials with slow upstrokes similar to those seen in the sinoatrial node. AN cells, found in the transitional zone between the atrium and the compact node, have variable resting potentials and action potentials with upstroke velocities ranging from fast, as with atrial fibers, to slow, as with cells from the N-zone or sinoatrial node. NH cells, which reside between the compact node and the His bundle proper, have high negative resting potentials and action potentials with fast upstrokes, similar to those seen in the His-Purkinje system (Figure 1-4 on page 5). In all cases, the transition from one cell zone to the next is gradual, with some cells showing intermediate levels of resting potential and action potential upstroke velocities.

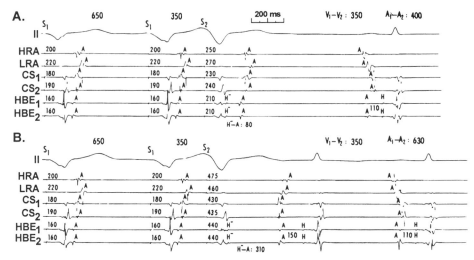

FIGURE 11-4. Retrograde atrial activation sequence resulting from retrograde dual AV node pathway conduction. In each panel, top to bottom, are shown surface ECG lead II along with intracardiac recordings from the high right atrium (HRA), lateral right atrium (LRA), coronary sinus ostium (CS₁), distal coronary sinus (CS₂), and proximal and distal His-bundle regions (HBE1 and HBE2, respectively). In each panel, the right ventricle is driven at a cycle length (S₁S₁) of 650 ms. Panel A: A ventricular premature depolarization with a premature coupling interval (S₁-S₂) of 350 ms results in ventriculoatrial conduction using a fast AV node pathway with retrograde atrial activation recorded earliest at the His bundle region. Panel B: In this case, a ventricular premature depolarization with a premature coupling interval (S₁-S₂) of 350 ms results in ventriculoatrial conduction using a slow AV node pathway with retrograde atrial activation recorded earliest at the ostium of the coronary sinus [12].

During anterograde and retrograde AV node conduction, the majority of the conduction time is spent traversing the AN region (approximately 20%-80%), with about 10% of the time due to conduction through the NH zone and approximately 20% of the total AV nodal conduction time resulting from conduction through the N-zone [38,50,51] (Figure 1-4 on page 5). However, the greatest increase in conduction delay during anterograde AV conduction occurs in the N cell zone. Finally, while AV node conduction block can occur at any level during anterograde and retrograde conduction, the N cell zone appears to be the usual site of block.

As with cells in the sinoatrial node, AV node cells in the N-zone, and many cells in the AN-zone, exhibit low levels of resting potential in the range of −40 to −50 mV [43,44]. This compares to the resting potential found in working myocardial cells from the atrium, ventricles, or specialized conducting cells in the His-Purkinje system of −80 to −90 mV. The ionic basis for this difference appears primarily to result from low density of the inwardly rectifying K⁺ channels, I_{K1}, in these AV node cells [46]. Because these channels are open at high negative levels membrane potential and close at more positive potentials, the high density of I_{K1} channels in atrial or ventricular cells is responsible for the normal resting potential of these fibers approaching the K⁺ equilibrium potential (-80 to −90 mV). Virtually lacking this channel, AV node cells in the N-zone (and to a lesser degree, the AN region) have resting potentials regulated by the balance between a variety of background and pump currents, the voltage dependent delayed rectifi-

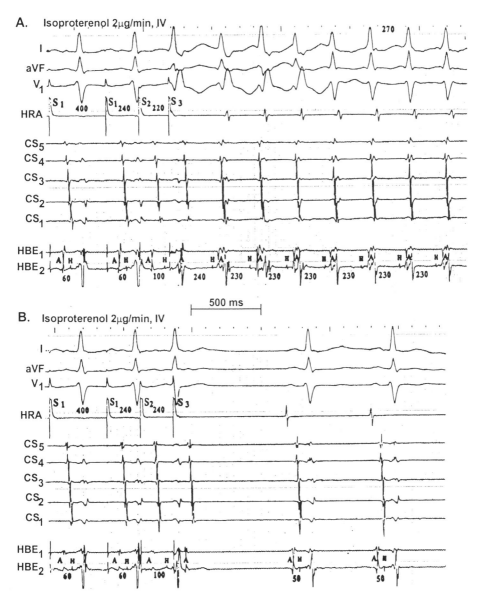

FIGURE 11-5. Selective ablation of slow AV node pathway conduction. From top to bottom in each panel are surface ECG leads I, aVF, and V_1, along with intracardiac recordings from the high right atrium (HRA), proximal to distal coronary sinus (CS_1 is distal, CS_5 is proximal), and proximal and distal His bundle regions (HBE_1 and HBE_2, respectively). Panel A: At baseline in the presence of an isoproterenol infusion at 2 µg/min, two extrastimuli (S_2 and S_3) during high right atrial pacing (S_1–S_1 = 400 ms) are required to expose anterograde slow AV nodal pathway conduction (A-H interval of 240 ms) and induce AV nodal reentrant tachycardia of the slow-fast form (cycle length = 270 ms). Panel B: After selective RF catheter ablation of an atrial site near the ostium of the coronary sinus, anterograde slow pathway conduction disappears and AV nodal reentrant tachycardia is no longer inducible despite double atrial extrastimulation during isoproterenol infusion.

er K$^+$ current (I$_{Kr}$) and probably significantly by the acetylcholine-dependent K$^+$ current (I$_{K(Ach)}$) [52,53].

It is not clear if AV node cells with low resting potentials possess fast Na$^+$ channels in any significant numbers. Regardless, however, at their normally reduced resting potential, any fast Na$^+$ channels present will be inactivated, and action potential conduction will occur not by I$_{Na}$, but rather will be dependent upon the L-type Ca^{++} current (I$_{Ca-L}$) (slow response action potentials) [43,45]. Repolarization proceeds with activation of the delayed rectifier K$^+$ current (I$_{Kr}$) after depolarization of the membrane resulting from activation of I$_{Ca-L}$.

11.2 Neuropharmacologic Responses of the AV Node

Autonomic tone significantly affects the action potentials of slowly conducting AV node cells. Specifically, the parasympathetic neurotransmitter, acetylcholine, can activate the acetylcholine-dependent K$^+$ current, I$_{K(Ach)}$ [54-56]. Activation of these channels is mediated through agonist binding to membrane bound muscarinic receptors, which triggers an increase in the active form of the intracellular G-protein, G$_i$. This G-protein enhances I$_{K(Ach)}$. This same channel appears to be activated by the purinergic agonist, adenosine, by coupling G$_i$ to membrane bound adenosine A$_1$ receptors [57]. Activation of the outward current I$_{K(Ach)}$ may be responsible for the vagal and adenosine- induced negative dromotropic effect and termination of supraventricular tachycardias that use the AV node as part of the reentrant circuit [58,59]. Adenosine appears to block slow response type action potential conduction within myocytes residing in the N-zone [60,61]. It is known that adenosine (or acetylcholine) can reverse the catecholamine-induced increase in I$_{Ca-L}$ and I$_f$ and enhance I$_{K(Ach)}$ [62-65], and that adenosine does not appear to affect the basal, non-catecholamine-stimulated, levels of I$_{Ca-L}$ and I$_f$. Adenosine, therefore may block AV node action potential conduction by either increasing the outward current I$_{K(Ach)}$, or decreasing the magnitude of inward currents. It is believed that the activation of outward I$_{K(Ach)}$ is the most important factor in reducing the net inward depolarizing current and blocking action potential propagation since adenosine appears to have little effect upon the basal (non-catecholamine-stimulated) levels of inward currents (such as I$_{Ca-L}$, I$_f$, or the background inward Na$^+$ leak current). Clinically adenosine is equally effective in terminating catecholamine-dependent and -independent forms of supraventricular tachycardia [59].

Sympathetic tone can also alter the electrophysiological behavior of AV node cells. While β-adrenergic agonists have little effect on the resting potential, they do enhance the pacemaker current, I$_f$, the L-type Ca^{++} current, I$_{Ca-L}$, and the voltage dependent delayed rectifier K$^+$ current (I$_{Kr}$), through a G-protein dependent mechanisms possibly involving both the protein kinase A and C systems [66-72]. These ionic changes enhance Ca^{++}-dependent action potential conduction in the AV node, shorten the action potential duration, shorten the AV node effective refractory period, and increase the rate of diastolic depolarization. These β-adrenergic stimulation-induced cellular electrophysiological changes are responsible for the isoproterenol-induced facilitation of induction of AV nodal reentrant tachycardia [73]. Verapamil and diltiazem are also effective in terminating catecholamine-dependent supraventricular tachycardias by virtue of their inhibitory action on I_{Ca-L} [73,74].

11.3   Clinical Electrophysiology

The definition of the "AV node" needs to be clarified and a consensus achieved among anatomists, clinicians, and electrophysiologists. If the compact node is regarded as the sole component of the AV node, then descriptions about functional properties of the AV node and tissue components of the AV nodal reentrant circuit must include not only the compact node but also "extra-nodal" structures such as the transitional cell zones (atrionodal bundles). Basic electrophysiologists often use the term "AV node" "in a loose sense to mean the entire complex of fibers functionally interposed between atrial fiber proper and His bundle fibers" [42]. Hence, from a functional standpoint, the "AV node" may be considered as a network structure comprised of the compact node and those transitional cell zones. However, some clinical electrophysiologists suggest that the term "atrionodal" or "AV junctional" reentry may be more appropriate than "AV nodal reentry" in describing the underlying mechanism of this arrhythmia [75,76]. For practical purposes, most investigators continue to use the term "AV nodal reentry."

11.3.1 ANTEROGRADE DUAL AV NODAL PATHWAY CONDUCTION

With the method of atrial extrastimulation, AV node conduction curves are depicted by plotting conduction times (A_2-H_2) and output intervals (H_1-H_2) as a function of increasingly premature input intervals (A_1-A_2). Normally, AV node conduction is characterized by gradual conduction time (A-H) prolongation with atrial extrastimulation or with incremental atrial pacing. Normal AV node conduction curves (A_1-A_2/A_2-H_2 and A_1-A_2/H_1-H_2) so generated are smooth, and with progressive prolongation of AV node conduction time, the A_1-A_2/H_1-H_2 curve may demonstrate an exponential increase in H_1-H_2 intervals at short A_1-A_2 intervals until AV node conduction is limited by atrial refractoriness [77-79]. Discontinuous AV node conduction curves (A_1-A_2/A_2-H_2 and A_1-A_2/H_1-H_2) are suggestive of anterograde dual AV node pathway conduction (Figure 11-2, Figure 11-6, Figure 11-7) [6-9,80-83]. The discontinuity of these curves is caused by sudden increment of AV node conduction time (A_2-H_2) and, consequently, of the H_1-H_2 interval in response to critically timed premature atrial extrastimulation. An increment of 50 ms or more in the A_2-H_2 interval resulting from a decrement of 10 msec in the A_1-A_2 interval is considered diagnostic of anterograde dual AV node pathway conduction [7]. This discontinuity in the AV node conduction curves reflects a shift of conduct from a fast pathway with a long refractor period to a slow pathway with a short refractory period. Hence, the curves (A_1-A_2/A_2-H_2 and A_1-A_2/H_1-H_2) to the right of the discontinuity represent fast pathway conduction, and those to the left represent slow pathway conduction.

The demonstration of discontinuous AV node conduction curves depends on selection of atrial pacing cycle lengths at which AV node conduction is not limited by atrial

refractoriness and at which the anterograde effective refractory period of the fast pathway is longer than that of the slow pathway. Anterograde conduction properties of the
fast and slow pathways are analyzed from these conduction curves. The effective refractory period of the fast pathway is defined as the longest A_1-A_2 interval in which conduction fails in the fast pathway, and its functional refractory period is the shortest attainable
H_1-H_2 interval on the fast pathway conduction curves. Similarly, the effective refractory
period of the slow pathway is the longest A_1-A_2 interval in which conduction fails in the
slow pathway, and its functional refractory period is the shortest attainable H_1-H_2 interval
on the slow pathway conduction curves. When complete exposure of slow pathway conduction is limited by atrial refractoriness, the effective refractory period of the slow pathway is less than the functional refractory period of the atrium (shortest attainable A_1-A_2
interval), and its functional refractory period may not be measurable if the slope of the
slow pathway conduction curve (H_1-H_2) points downward. When the functional properties of the AV node are assessed as a whole, the effective refractory period of the slow

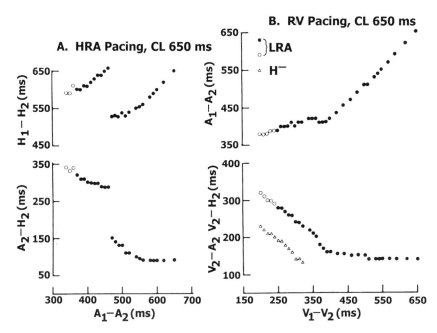

FIGURE 11-6. Panel A: A_1-A_2/H_1-H_2 and A_1-A_2/A_2-H_2 curves during high right atrial (HRA) pacing at a
cycle length (CL) of 650 ms. Note discontinuity due to a sudden increase in AV node conduction time (A_2-
H_2) at a premature coupling interval (A_1-A_2) of 460 ms. Black dots represent responses without atrial echoes,
while open circles represent responses with atrial echoes. The curves to the right of discontinuity represent
anterograde fast pathway conduction, and those to the left represent anterograde slow pathway conduction.
Panel B: V_1-V_2/A_1-A_2 and V_1-V_2/V_2-A_2 curves during right ventricular (RV) pacing at a cycle length (CL) of
650 ms. Black dots represent responses without ventricular echoes, while open circles represent responses
with ventricular echoes. Retrograde His-bundle potentials (H^-) are depicted as open triangles. Both V_1-V_2/
A_1-A_2 and V_1-V_2/V_2-A_2 curves are smooth. Retrograde AV node conduction time (H_2-A_2) ranges from 90 to
100 ms. Induction of AV nodal reentrant tachycardia of the slow-fast form coincides with the ventricular
echo zone between premature coupling intervals (V_1-V_2) of 240 and 220 ms. The corresponding intracardiac
recordings for panel A are illustrated in Figure 11-7 and those for panel B in Figure 11-9. From [10] with permission.

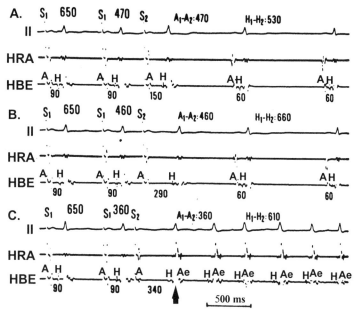

FIGURE 11-7. Atrial premature stimulation with induction of AV nodal reentrant tachycardia of the slow-fast form. ECG lead II and high right atrial (HRA) and His-bundle (HBE) electrographic leads are shown. S_1 and S_2 are pacing and premature stimuli. A and H are atrial and His-bundle electrograms, respectively. The high right atrium is driven at a cycle length (S_1-S_1) of 650 ms. Panel A: An atrial premature stimulus at a coupling interval (S_1-S_2) of 470 ms lengthens the A-H interval from 90 to 150 ms. Panel B: An atrial premature stimulus at a coupling interval (S_1-S_2) of 460 ms suddenly prolongs the A-H interval to 290 ms, producing a discontinuous AV nodal conduction curve (Figure 11-6, panel A). Panel C: An atrial premature stimulus at a coupling interval (S_1-S_2) of 360 ms further prolongs the A-H interval to 340 ms and induces AV nodal reentrant tachycardia of the slow-fast form (arrow). Note that the ratio of the atrial-His conduction time to the His-atrial conduction time (Ae-H/H-Ae) is greater than one during the tachycardia. From [10] with permission.

pathway is the AV node effective refractory period, and the functional refractory period of the fast pathway is the AV node functional refractory period.

The method of incremental atrial pacing without atrial extrastimulation may also reveal dual AV node pathway conduction. At critical atrial pacing cycle lengths, a sudden rather than progressive increment of AV node conduction time can result in a discontinuous A-A/A-H curve or an atypical Wenckebach periodicity, or both [80-83]. These phenomena are commonly seen in patients with dual AV node pathway physiology and are also suggestive of anterograde conduction failure of the fast pathway with a resultant anterograde conduction shift to the slow pathway. Likewise, electrocardiographic manifestation of two sets of P-R intervals during sinus or atrial-paced rhythm are consistent with dual AV node pathway conduction in which the anterograde effective refractory period of the fast pathway is long relative to the sinus or atrial cycle length. A shift of conduction from anterograde fast to anterograde slow pathway conduction may be followed by repetitive retrograde concealed conduction to the fast pathway, thereby

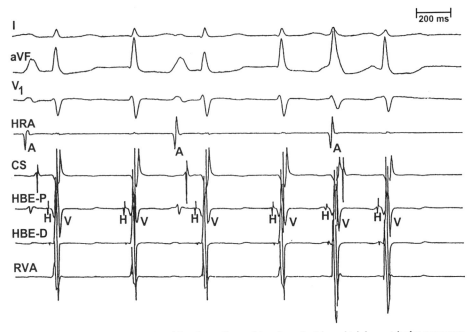

FIGURE 11-8. Non-reentrant AV nodal tachycardia resulting from double and triple ventricular responses. Note that the first atrial (A) depolarization (from the left) is conducted through anterograde fast and a slow AV nodal pathways and the second atrial depolarization is conducted though an anterograde fast and two anterograde slow AV nodal pathways. ECG leads I, aVF, and V$_1$ are simultaneously recorded with a high right atrial (HRA), coronary sinus (CS), and the proximal (HBE-P) and distal (HBE-D) His bundle intracardiac electrograms. [121].

maintaining anterograde slow pathway conduction. Rarely, a sinus or atrial impulse may produce simultaneous fast and slow pathway conduction, resulting in double ventricular responses [80-83]. Repetition of such a phenomenon produces a form of non-reentrant tachycardia [84] (Figure 11-8). Electrophysiological conditions favoring the occurrence of this non-reentrant form of tachycardia include: 1) retrograde unidirectional block in both fast and slow pathways and, 2) sufficient anterograde slow pathway conduction delay to allow sequential conduction of the impulse over both pathways.

11.3.2 AV NODAL REENTRANT TACHYCARDIA OF THE SLOW-FAST FORM

The initiation of AV nodal reentrant tachycardia depends on differences in functional properties of the fast and slow pathways in both anterograde and retrograde directions. The usual form of AV nodal reentrant tachycardia is the slow-fast form using a slow pathway for anterograde conduction and a fast pathway for retrograde conduction [7]. Sustained reentry of this form requires the ability for repetitive anterograde slow pathway and repetitive retrograde fast pathway conduction [85]. Characteristically during tachycardia, the ratio of the atrial-His (AeH) conduction time to the His-atrial (HAe) conduction time is greater than one (Figure 11-7, Figure 11-9). During atrial extrastimulation or incremental atrial pacing, the induction of AV nodal reentrant tachycardia of the

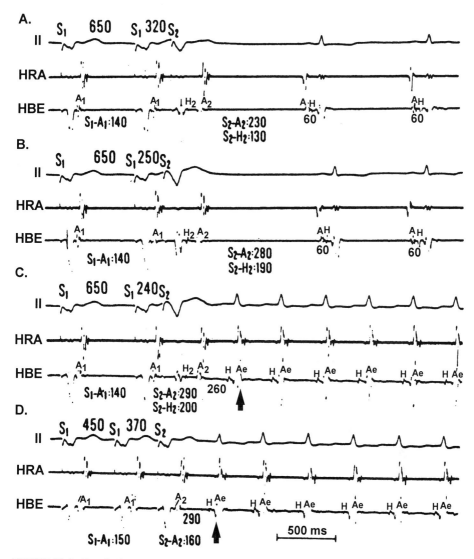

FIGURE 11-9. Ventricular premature stimulation with induction of AV nodal reentrant tachycardia of the slow-fast form. The right ventricle is driven at a cycle length of 650 ms. Panels A-C: Ventricular premature beats (S_2) at coupling intervals of 320, 250, and 240 ms induce retrograde atrial activation with a gradual prolongation of ventriculoatrial conduction time (S_2-A_2 = 230, 280, and 290 ms, respectively). The corresponding V_1-V_2/A_1-A_2 and V_1-V_2/V_2-A_2 curves are smooth (Figure 11-6, panel B). Retrograde AV node conduction time (H_2-A_2) is 90 ms. Panel C: The ventricular premature stimulus (S_2) elicits not only a ventricular echo beat but also AV nodal reentrant tachycardia of the slow-fast form (arrow). Note that during the tachycardia the ratio of the atrial-His conduction time to the His-atrial conduction time (Ae-H/H-Ae) is greater than one. Panel D: When the ventricular pacing cycle length (S_1-S_2) is decreased to 450 ms, a ventricular premature depolarization (S_2) induces AV nodal reentrant tachycardia of the slow-fast form (arrow), beginning at a coupling interval (S_1-S_2) of 370 ms. From [10] with permission.

slow-fast form requires: 1) achievement of anterograde slow pathway conduction; 2) attainment of a critical AH interval; and 3) adequate retrograde fast pathway conduction. Both of these first two conditions may be fulfilled if the slow pathway has an anterograde effective refractory period shorter than that of the fast pathway and if AV node conduction is not limited by atrial refractoriness. A critical AH interval is needed to allow the fast pathway that is blocked in the anterograde direction to recover for retrograde excitation – an atrial echo phenomenon. The atrial echo phenomenon, when perpetuated, leads to the slow-fast form of AV nodal reentrant tachycardia. The critical AH interval varies among patients and depends on fast pathway conduction properties in the retrograde direction. The atrial echo zones may thus not coincide with the entire slow pathway conduction curves.

The induction of AV nodal reentrant tachycardia of the slow-fast form is rarely observed during either ventricular extrastimulation or incremental ventricular pacing [10]. Such a mode of tachycardia induction requires that the slow pathway has a retrograde effective refractory period longer than that of the fast pathway. Ventriculoatrial conduction thus proceeds exclusively over the fast pathway during ventricular extrastimulation producing smooth ventriculoatrial conduction curves (V_1-V_2/V_2-A_2 and V_1-V_2/A_1-A_2) (Figures 11-2, 11-6, & 11-9). At a critical premature coupling interval, a ventricular premature beat, being blocked in the retrograde slow pathway, is conducted over the fast pathway in the retrograde direction and may, in turn, activate slow pathway in the anterograde direction resulting in a ventricular echo beat. This ventricular echo phenomenon, when perpetuated, leads to the slow-fast form of AV nodal reentrant tachycardia. The rarity of induction of sustained reentry of the slow-fast form during programmed ventricular stimulation can be explained by 1) difficulty in attaining critical (sufficient) retrograde conduction delay in the fast pathway; 2) the slow pathway having a retrograde effective refractory period nearly equal to that of the fast pathway (narrow window); and 3) limitation of retrograde conduction by retrograde effective and functional refractory periods of the fast pathway, the His-Purkinje system and the ventricular myocardium.

11.3.3 RETROGRADE DUAL AV NODAL PATHWAY CONDUCTION

Retrograde dual AV node pathway conduction is suggested by demonstration of discontinuous ventriculoatrial conduction curves (V_1-V_2/V_2-A_2 and V_1-V_2/A_1-A_2) during programmed ventricular extrastimulation (Figures 11-2 & 11-10) [10,79-83,86]. The demonstration of discontinuous ventriculoatrial conduction curves requires that the slow pathway have a retrograde effective refractory period shorter than that of the fast pathway. At critically-timed ventricular premature coupling intervals (V_1-V_2), failure of retrograde propagation via the fast pathway is followed by a shift in conduction over the slow pathway in the retrograde direction, resulting in a sudden increase in ventriculoatrial conduction times (V_2-A_2) and, consequently, discontinuous ventriculoatrial conduction curves (V_1-V_2/V_2-A_2 and V_1-V_2/A_1-A_2). Similar to anterograde dual AV node pathway conduction, the curves to the right of discontinuity represent fast pathway conduction, and those to the left represent slow pathway conduction.

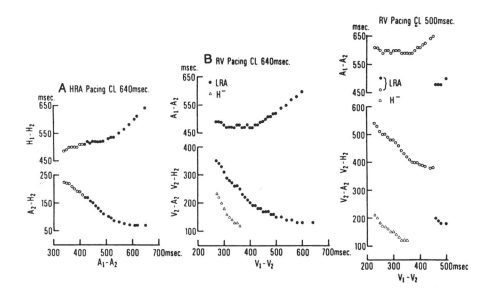

FIGURE 11-10. Panel A: A_1-A_2/H_1-H_2 and A_1-A_2/A_2-H_2 and curves during high right atrial (HRA) pacing at a cycle length (CL) of 640 msec. Black dots represent responses without atrial echoes, while open circles represent responses with atrial echoes. Both A_1-A_2/H_1-H_2 and A_1-A_2/A_2-H_2 curves are smooth. Note progressive lengthening of AV node conduction time (A_2-H_2) as the atrial premature coupling interval (A_1-A_2) gradually shortened. Panel B: V_1-V_2/A_1-A_2 and V_1-V_2/V_2-A_2 curves during right ventricular (RV) pacing at a cycle length (CL) of 640 msec. Black dots represent responses without ventricular echoes. Retrograde His-bundle potentials (H^-) are depicted as open triangles. Both V_1-V_2/A_1-A_2 and V_1-V_2/V_2-A2 curves are smooth. Retrograde AV node conduction time (V_2-H_2) ranges from 120 to 130 ms. No ventricular echo phenomenon or AV nodal reentrant tachycardia can be induced. Panel C: V_1-V_2/A_1-A_2 and V_1-V_2/V_2-A_2 curves during right ventricular (RV) pacing at a cycle length (CL) of 500 msec. Note curve discontinuity due to a sudden increase in ventriculoatrial conduction time (V_2-A_2) at a ventricular premature coupling interval (V_1-V_2) of 450 msec. Black dots represent responses without ventricular echoes, while open circles represent responses with ventricular echoes. Retrograde His-bundle potentials are depicted as open triangles. The curves to the right of the discontinuity represent retrograde fast pathway conduction, and those to the left represent retrograde slow pathway conduction. Retrograde slow pathway conduction time (H_2-A_2) ranges from 300 to 330 ms. Induction of AV nodal reentrant tachycardia of the fast-slow form coincides with the entire retrograde slow AV node pathway conduction curves. Corresponding intracardiac recording for panel A is in Figure 11-12 and for panel C is in Figure 11-11. From [10] with permission.

During programmed ventricular stimulation, the difficulty and uncertainty in recording retrograde His bundle potentials frequently handicap delineation of the exact route of ventriculoatrial conduction. Therefore, retrograde conduction properties of the fast and slow pathways can only be assumed from analysis of these conduction curves (V_1-V_2/V_2-A_2 and V_1-V_2/A_1-A_2). The longest V_1-V_2 interval in which conduction fails in the fast pathway is the retrograde effective refractory period of the fast pathway, and the shortest attainable A_1-A_2 interval on the fast pathway conduction curves is its functional refractory period. Likewise, the longest V_1-V_2 interval in which conduction fails in the slow pathway is the retrograde effective refractory period of the slow pathway, and the shortest attainable A_1-A_2 interval on the slow pathway conduction curves is its functional refractory period.

The demonstration of discontinuous ventriculoatrial conduction curves (V_1-V_2/V_2-A_2 and V_1-V_2/A_1-A_2) depends on selection of ventricular pacing cycle lengths at which ventriculoatrial conduction is not limited by ventricular refractoriness and at which the slow pathway exhibits a retrograde effective refractory period shorter than that of the fast pathway (Figures 11-10 & 11-11). Retrograde dual AV node pathways are also suggested by the occurrence of double atrial responses during single ventricular extrastimulation [87] and by the development of an atypical ventriculoatrial Wenckebach periodicity with a sudden rather than progressive increment of ventriculoatrial conduction time (discontinuous V-V/V-A curve) during incremental ventricular pacing [12]. These phenomena are suggestive of a shift of ventriculoatrial conduction from retrograde fast to retrograde slow pathway conduction.

11.3.4 AV NODAL REENTRANT TACHYCARDIA OF THE FAST-SLOW FORM

The unusual form of AV nodal reentrant tachycardia is the fast-slow form in which a fast pathway is used for anterograde conduction and a slow pathway for retrograde conduction, reversing the impulse direction as compared with the slow-fast form of AV node re-entry [10,11,88]. To Sustain AV nodal reentrant tachycardia of the fast-slow form requires the capability of repetitive anterograde fast pathway and repetitive retrograde slow pathway conduction. Characteristically, the AeH/HAe ratio is less than 1 during tachycardia (Figures 11-11 & 11-12) [86,89,90].

During programmed atrial extrastimulation, the initiation of AV nodal reentrant tachycardia of the fast-slow form is only possible when the slow pathway has an anterograde effective refractory period longer than that of the fast pathway. The anterograde effective refractory period of the slow pathway cannot be measured because all the atrial impulses are exclusively conducted over the fast pathway in the anterograde direction. The AV node conduction curves (A_1-A_2/A_2-H_2 and A_1-A_2/H_1-H_2) so generated are smooth (Figures 11-2, 11-10 & 11-12). The critical AV node conduction delay (A_2-H_2) required for the induction of an atrial echo phenomenon or sustained AV nodal reentrant tachycardia of the fast-slow form (or both) is minimal, because the A_2-H_2 interval is within the range of anterograde fast pathway conduction times. In situations in which the slow pathway has markedly prolonged anterograde refractoriness relative to that of the fast pathway (wide window), late atrial premature beats or spontaneous acceleration of the sinus rate can easily instigate an onset of AV nodal reentrant tachycardia of the fast-slow form. Clinically, AV nodal reentrant tachycardia of the fast-slow form is one of the causes of incessant supraventricular tachycardias [91,92].

In contrast to AV nodal reentrant tachycardia of the slow-fast form, the induction of the fast-slow form is commonly observed during programmed ventricular extrastimulation [10]. This mode of tachycardia induction occurs when ventriculoatrial activation shifts from retrograde fast to retrograde slow pathway conduction at critically timed ventricular premature coupling intervals (V_1-V_2), as evidenced by the sudden increment of ventriculoatrial conduction times, with resultant discontinuous V_1-V_2/V_2-A_2 and V_1-V_2/A_1-A_2 curves (Figures 11-2, 11-10 & 11-11). Under these circumstances, a ventricular premature beat being retrogradely blocked in the fast pathway, is conducted over the

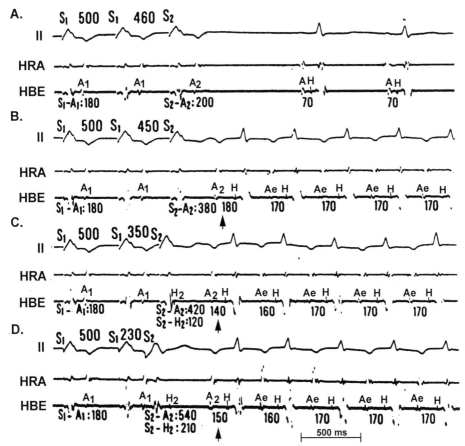

FIGURE 11-11. Ventricular premature stimulation with induction of AV nodal reentrant tachycardia of the fast-slow form. The right ventricle is driven at a cycle length (S_1-S_1) of 500 ms. Panel A: A ventricular premature beat (S_2) at a coupling interval (S_1-S_2) of 460 ms lengthens ventriculoatrial conduction time (S_2-A_2 or V_2-A_2) from 180 to 200 ms. Panel B: A ventricular premature stimulus (S_2) at a coupling interval (S_1-S_2) of 450 ms suddenly increases ventriculoatrial conduction time (S_2-A_2 or V_2-A_2) from 180 to 380 ms. This produces discontinuous ventriculoatrial conduction curves (V_1-V_2/A_1-A_2) (Figure 11-10, panel C) with induction of AV nodal reentrant tachycardia of the fast-slow form (arrow). Panels C and D: Ventricular premature stimuli (S_2) at coupling intervals (S_1-S_2) of 350 and 230 ms further lengthen ventriculoatrial conduction time (S_2-A_2 or V_2-A_2) to 420 and 540 ms, respectively, and induce AV nodal reentrant tachycardia of the fast-slow form (arrow). Retrograde AV node conduction times (H_2-A_2) are 300 and 330 ms, respectively. Note that during the tachycardia the ratio of the atrial-His conduction time to the His-atrial conduction time (AeH/ HAe) is less than one. From [10] with permission.

slow pathway in the retrograde direction. After attainment of a critical ventriculoatrial conduction delay (V_2-A_2, more precisely, H_2-A_2), the impulse activates the fast pathway in the anterograde direction and produces a ventricular echo phenomenon. This ventricular echo phenomenon, when perpetuated, leads to AV nodal reentrant tachycardia of the fast-slow form. The ventricular echo zone may or may not coincide with the entire retrograde slow pathway conduction curves, because the ventricular myocardium and His-

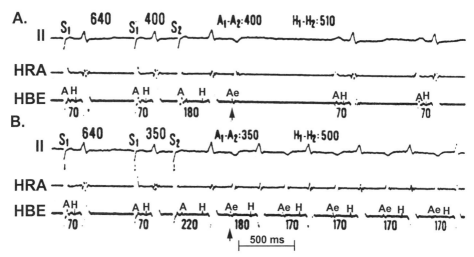

FIGURE 11-12. Atrial premature stimulation with induction of AV nodal reentrant tachycardia of the fast-slow form. The high right atrium is driven at a cycle length (S_1-S_1) of 640 ms. The AV node conduction time (A-H) progressively lengthened as the atrial premature coupling interval (S_1-S_2) gradually shortened. The corresponding A_1-A_2/H_1-H_2 and A_1-A_2/A_2-H_2 curves are smooth (see Figure 14A). Panel A: An atrial premature stimulus at a coupling interval (S_1-S_2) of 400 ms lengthens the A-H interval from 70 to 180 ms and elicits the late appearance of an atrial echo (Ae, arrow). Panel B: An atrial premature beat at a coupling interval of 350 ms elicits not only an atrial echo (Ae) phenomenon but also AV nodal reentrant tachycardia of the fast-slow form (arrow). Note that during the tachycardia the ratio of atrial-His conduction time to the His-atrial conduction time (AeH/HAe) is less than one. From [10] with permission.

Purkinje system may exhibit conduction delay in response to ventricular extrastimulation thereby precluding maintenance of critical H_2-A_2 delay required for the initiation of AV node reentry.

11.3.5 EFFECT OF PACING SITES, CYCLE LENGTHS, & MODES

In addition to the high right atrium and right ventricle, the left atrium can also serve as a site of stimulation from the coronary sinus. The refractory periods of the fast and slow pathways so measured are not significantly altered, however the A-H intervals are generally shorter than those generated by high right atrial extrastimulation [93,94]. These findings may be accounted for by having a different input into the AV node. The closer proximity of the coronary sinus to the AV junction facilitates induction of the AV node reentry, but the shorter conduction time (A-H interval) resulting from coronary sinus pacing disfavors AV node reentry. Overall, the ease with which left atrial extrastimulation initiates AV nodal reentrant tachycardia is not different from that of right atrial extrastimulation.

Proper selection of an atrial or ventricular pacing cycle length is essential for demonstration of either anterograde or retrograde dual pathway conduction as well as induction of AV nodal reentrant tachycardia of either form during programmed atrial or ventricular extrastimulation. At least two cycle lengths (600 and 400 ms) should be employed. Delivery of double and triple extrastimuli may be necessary for exposing slow pathway conduction and for inducing critical conduction delay required for the initiation of AV nodal reentrant tachycardia.

Both incremental atrial pacing and incremental ventricular pacing may facilitate induction of AV nodal reentrant tachycardia of either form. Shorter pacing cycle lengths prolong conduction time of one pathway (induction of slow conduction) and may simultaneously lengthen refractoriness of the other pathway (development of unidirectional block). Consequently, the atrial or ventricular echo zone is widened, and self-initiation (requiring no atrial or ventricular extrastimulation) of either form may become possible at shorter pacing cycle lengths.

11.3.6 SMOOTH VERSUS DISCONTINUOUS AV NODAL CONDUCTION CURVES

The induction of AV nodal reentrant tachycardia may be accompanied by smooth rather than discontinuous AV nodal conduction/ventriculoatrial conduction curves depending on functional properties of the two pathways relative to the driving cycle length.

During programmed atrial extrastimulation, the initiation of AV nodal reentrant tachycardia may be associated with smooth AV node conduction curves (A_1-A_2/A_2-H_2 and A_1-A_2/H_1-H_2): 1) exclusive fast pathway conduction may induce the fast-slow form of AV nodal reentrant tachycardia (Figures 11-2, 11-10 & 11-12); 2) exclusive slow pathway conduction may initiate the slow-fast form of AV nodal reentrant tachycardia (Figure 11-2); and 3) smooth transition from a fast pathway with a long refractory period to a slow pathway with a short refractory period occurs because the minimal conduction time (AH interval) of the slow pathway approximates the maximum conduction time (AH interval) of the fast pathway; consequently, there is no jump or discontinuity between the fast and slow pathway conduction curves, and AV nodal reentrant tachycardia of the slow-fast form is induced during anterograde slow pathway conduction. Of note, the anatomical location of respective fast and slow pathways in this latter group of patients is not different than those with discontinuous AV nodal conduction curves [95,96].

During programmed ventricular stimulation, the initiation of AV nodal reentrant tachycardia may also be associated with smooth rather than discontinuous ventriculoatrial conduction curves (V_1-V_2/V_2-A_2 and V_1-V_2/A_1-A_2): 1) exclusive fast pathway conduction may rarely provoke an onset of the slow-fast form of AV nodal reentrant tachycardia (Figures 11-2, 11-6 & 11-9); 2) exclusive slow pathway may result in the induction of the fast-slow form of AV nodal reentrant tachycardia (Figure 11-2); and 3) smooth transition from a fast pathway with a long retrograde refractory period to a slow pathway with a short retrograde refractory period may theoretically be followed by initiation of the fast-slow form of AV nodal reentrant tachycardia.

Hence, the induction of AV nodal reentrant tachycardia can be accompanied by smooth AV nodal conduction/ventriculoatrial conduction curves depending on functional properties (i.e., refractory period and conduction time) of the two pathways relative to the drive cycle length.

11.3.7 NEUROPHARMACOLOGIC EFFECTS ON DUAL AV NODAL CONDUCTION

Functional properties of the AV node are heavily influenced by the autonomic nervous system. Vagal maneuvers such as carotid sinus massage, gag reflex, and the Valsalva maneuver may abruptly increase AV node refractoriness and thereby terminate AV nodal reentrant tachycardia [97]. Both intravenous atropine and isoproterenol may facilitate the inducibility of the slow-fast form of AV nodal reentrant tachycardia by enhancing anterograde slow and retrograde fast pathway conduction [73,98]. Isoproterenol, in addition, decreases atrial refractoriness, thereby allowing delivery of atrial extrastimuli of greater prematurity which may further enhance the inducibility of AV nodal reentrant tachycardia.

AV node depressive agents such as digitalis, β-adrenergic blocking agents, adenosine, and Ca^{++}-channel blocking drugs depress fast and slow pathway conduction in both anterograde and retrograde directions [59,74,87,99-103]. In the slow-fast form of AV nodal reentrant tachycardia, these agents shift the dual AV node pathway conduction curves upward and to the right (Figure 11-13). Effects of these agents on the echo zone are variable. Intravenous ouabain, digoxin, propranolol, verapamil, and diltiazem usually terminate AV nodal reentrant tachycardia of the slow-fast form by blocking anterograde slow pathway conduction (Figure 11-14, panel A), but may at times, terminate the tachycardia by blocking retrograde fast pathway conduction [74]. These agents usually terminate AV nodal reentrant tachycardia of the fast-slow form by blocking retrograde conduction of the slow pathway (Figure 11-14, panel B) [74]. These AV node depressive agents exert no effects on conduction of anomalous AV connections except for those with decremental conduction properties similar to those of the AV node (e.g., nodoventricular, atriofascicular connections, and AV connections with decremental conduction properties) [104-106]. Adenosine, an intermediate metabolite of many biochemical pathways, possesses a depressive action on the sinus node and the upper portion of the AV node and has also been shown to be an effective agent for terminating AV nodal reentrant tachycardia (Figure 11-15) [58-65]. The negative chronotropic and dromotropic effects of adenosine are probably mediated by depression of L-type Ca^{++} channel (I_{Ca-L}) and/or by activation of the adenosine-sensitive K$^+$ channel, $I_{K(Ado)}$, which enhances K$^+$ conductance resulting in hyperpolarization of the cell membrane [58-65].

Class I antiarrhythmic agents such as quinidine, procainamide, disopyramide, ethmozine, flecainide, and propafenone prolong refractoriness of atrial, His-Purkinje, and ventricular tissues, as well as anomalous AV connections [89,107-111]. However, intravenous forms of these agents have also been shown to be effective in terminating AV nodal reentrant tachycardia of the slow-fast form by blocking retrograde fast pathway conduction. Class IC agents – encainide, flecainide, and propafenone – also depress AV node conduction and may, at times, terminate AV nodal reentrant tachycardia of the slow-fast form by blocking anterograde slow pathway conduction [110].

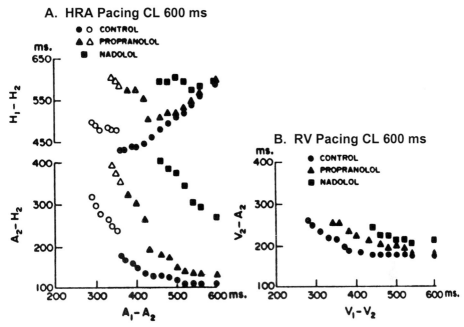

FIGURE 11-13. Effects of intravenous propranolol and oral nadolol on dual AV node pathway conduction. Panel A: A_1-A_2/A_2-H_2 and A_1-A_2/H_1-H_2 curves during high right atrial (HRA) pacing at a cycle length (CL) of 600 ms. The circles represent responses during the control study (black circles, responses without atrial echoes; open circles, responses with atrial echoes), the triangles represent responses after intravenous propranolol (black triangles, responses without atrial echoes, open triangles, responses with atrial echoes), and the squares represent responses after oral nadolol (black squares, responses without atrial echoes). During the control study, the AV node conduction time (A-H) is 110 ms; the effective and functional refractory periods of the fast pathway are 350 and 430 ms, respectively; and those of the slow pathway are 280 and 480 ms, respectively. Induction of atrial echoes (290 to 350 ms) is followed by initiation of AV nodal reentrant tachycardia of the slow-fast form. After intravenous infusion of propranolol, the AV node conduction time (A-H) is 120 ms and the effective and functional refractory periods of the fast pathway are 420 and 455 ms, respectively. Induction of single atrial echoes (340 to 360 ms) is not followed by AV nodal reentrant tachycardia. After oral nadolol therapy, the AV nodal conduction time (A-H) is lengthened to 270 ms, and the A_1-A_2/A_2-H_2 and A_1-A_2/H_1-H_2 curves become smooth, suggesting only slow pathway conduction. The effective and functional refractory periods of the slow pathway are 450 and 575 ms, respectively. No atrial echoes are induced. Panel B: V_1-V_2/V_2-A_2 curves during right ventricular (RV) pacing at a cycle length of 600 ms. The black circles represent responses during the control study, the black triangles represent responses after intravenous propranolol, and the black squares represent responses after oral nadolol. Note prolongation of ventriculoatrial conduction time (V-A) and retrograde effective refractory period of the ventriculoatrial conduction system after administration of intravenous propranolol and oral nadolol. No ventricular echoes are induced during the control study, after intravenous propranolol or after nadolol. From [87] with permission.

11.3.8 DIFFERENTIAL DIAGNOSIS

Reentrant supraventricular tachycardias induced during an electrophysiology study include AV nodal reentrant tachycardia, sinoatrial reentrant tachycardia (high cristal focal atrial tachycardia), and AV reciprocating tachycardia involving an anomalous AV connection for retrograde conduction:

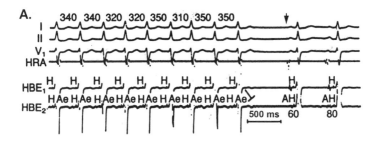

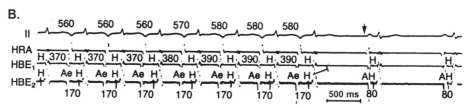

FIGURE 11-14. Termination of AV nodal reentrant tachycardia with intravenous verapamil. Panel A: During AV nodal reentrant tachycardia of the slow-fast form, verapamil induces prolongation of the tachycardia cycle length with erratic tachycardia cycle length variation ranging from 310 to 350 ms with eventual conduction block in the anterograde slow pathway. The tachycardia cycle length is 300 ms before administration of verapamil (not shown). Panel B: During AV nodal reentrant tachycardia of the fast-slow form, verapamil induces gradual prolongation of the tachycardia cycle length from 490 to 580 ms with eventual conduction block in the retrograde slow pathway. The tachycardia cycle length is 490 ms before administration of verapamil (not shown). In both panels A and B, the arrow points to the resumption of normal sinus rhythm. Ae, retrograde atrial activity during AV nodal reentrant tachycardia. From [74] with permission.

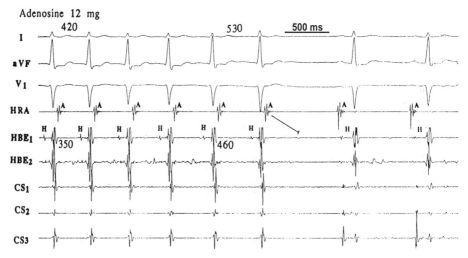

FIGURE 11-15. Effects of adenosine on AV nodal reentrant tachycardia. Intravenous bolus of adenosine (12 mg) is given during sustained AV nodal reentrant tachycardia of the slow-fast form. Within 10 sec of administration, the tachycardia is terminated. Note that adenosine exerts its depressive effects primarily on the anterograde slow pathway by prolonging its conduction time (A-H interval increased from 350 ms to 460 ms) before finally inducing conduction block thereby reverting the rhythm to sinus. Also note that ventriculoatrial conduction remains unchanged before conversion. A, atrial electrogram; CS, coronary sinus; H, His bundle potential; HBE$_1$ and HBE$_2$, distal and proximal His bundle electrographic leads, respectively; HRA, high right atrium.

1.   In patients with AV nodal reentrant tachycardia, both fast and slow pathway conduction in either anterograde or retrograde direction should exhibit progressive decremental conduction in response to programmed extrastimulation [77-79,112]. In contrast, an atrio-His connection is characterized by the lack of progressive decremental conduction during incremental atrial pacing and atrial extrastimulation. The A_1-A_2/A_2-H_2 curve representing anterograde conduction of the atrio-His connection is flat, and its corresponding A_1-A_2/H_1-H_2 curve should coincide with the line of identity. Similarly, retrograde conduction over an anomalous AV connection is characterized by a lack of progressive decremental conduction during incremental ventricular pacing and ventricular extrastimulation. The V_1-V_2/V_2-A_2 curve representing retrograde conduction of the anomalous connection is relatively flat, and its corresponding V_1-V_2/A_1-A_2 curve should coincide with the line of identity except for its terminal portion, which may be deviated because of conduction delay in the ventricular myocardium [113] occurring below the level of the His bundle [114-116]. Recording of the retrograde His bundle potential at short ventricular premature coupling intervals (V_1-V_2) is of value in delineating the site of ventriculoatrial conduction delay. Prolongation of the retrograde His bundle to low atrium conduction time (H-A) indicates that retrograde conduction delay occurs within the AV node (Figures 11-10 & 11-11).

2.   Retrograde conduction over an anomalous AV connection generally produces an eccentric retrograde atrial activation sequence distinctly different than that of retrograde normal AV (fast) pathway conduction in which the earliest site of activation is located near the right anterior septum at the His bundle potential recording site [113,117]. However, an anomalous septal AV connection may exhibit retrograde atrial activation sequence similar to that of retrograde fast pathway of AV nodal reentrant tachycardia (the slow-fast form). In general, ventriculoatrial conduction time is shorter during the slow-fast form of AV nodal reentrant tachycardia compared to that of AV reciprocating tachycardia. In fact, ventriculoatrial activation often precedes or coincides with ventricular depolarization (QRS complex) resulting in a non-discernible retrograde P wave during AV nodal reentrant tachycardia of the slow-fast form. In contrast, the retrograde P wave is often clearly inscribed immediately after the QRS complex during AV reciprocating tachycardia as the ventricle is a part of the reentrant circuit [113,117]. Nevertheless, AV nodal reentrant tachycardia of the slow-fast form may exhibit clearly identifiable retrograde P waves behind the QRS complex when conduction velocity in the retrograde fast pathway is reduced because of intrinsic or extrinsic factors (e.g., aging process, ischemia, drugs, etc.) [118]. Additionally, ventricular extrastimulation can be delivered at the time of anterograde His bundle depolarization during the tachycardia. Premature activation of the atrium, referred to as "atrial preexcitation," may occur via retrograde conduction through an anomalous AV connection. Finally, intravenous infusion of adenosine (6-12 mg) may be of

some value in differential diagnosis as it is more likely to suppress conduction of the retrograde fast AV nodal pathway than an anomalous AV connection [119,120].

3. Complicated situations may be encountered: 1) dual AV nodal pathway conduction with or without inducible AV nodal reentrant tachycardia may coexist with an overt or concealed anomalous AV or nodoventricular connection with or without inducible AV reciprocating tachycardia [104] and 2) AV nodal reentrant tachycardia of the slow-fast form may display the earliest retrograde atrial exit site to be near the coronary sinus ostium (Figure 11-16). In this subgroup of patients, the AV nodal reentrant tachycardia has also been referred to as the slow-intermediate (or slow-slow) form of AV nodal reentrant tachycardia [76]. In fact, multiple AV nodal pathways are not uncommon and may functionally affect patterns of both anterograde and retrograde AV conduction as well as electrophysiological behaviors of AV nodal reentrant tachycardia (Figure 11-8 & Figures 11-17 through 11-20) [121].

4. AV nodal reentrant tachycardia of the fast-slow type needs to be differentiated from atrial tachycardia. Atrial tachycardia is usually induced from programmed atrial stimulation and its onset requires no critical AV conduction delay. Atrial tachycardia is rarely suppressible with adenosine or verapamil and it cannot be terminated by ventricular premature stimulation without ventriculoatrial conduction. Ventricular pacing (in the absence of ventriculoatrial conduction) usually produces AV dissociation while the atrial tachycardia continues.

5. Differentiation between AV nodal reentrant tachycardia of the fast-slow form and orthodromic AV reciprocating tachycardia using an anomalous AV connection with decremental conduction properties (often referred to as the permanent form of AV junctional tachycardia) [92] is difficult when the anomalous AV connection is located near the septum at the AV junction. Atrial preexcitation with ventricular premature stimulation during anterograde His bundle depolarization favors the diagnosis of the permanent form of AV junctional tachycardia. However, transient AV block occurring during tachycardia should prove that the ventricle is not part of the tachycardia circuit and thus exclude the involvement of a slowly conducting septal AV connection [12]. During an application of RF energy, successful ablation of the slow AV nodal pathway — but not an anomalous AV connection — is signaled by the emergence of an AV junctional rhythm [122-125].

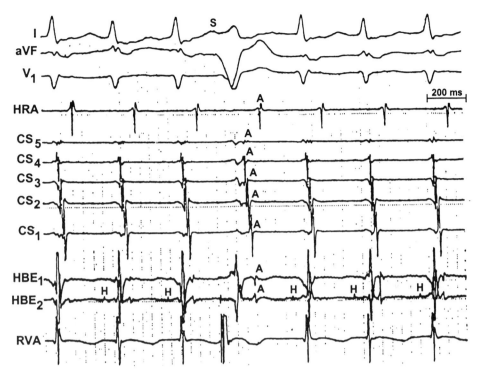

FIGURE 11-16. Unusual atrial activation sequence during retrograde conduction through the fast AV nodal conduction pathway. A premature stimulus (S) is delivered at the right ventricular apex (RVA) during the slow-fast form of AV nodal reentrant tachycardia (ventriculoatrial interval < 90 ms). The resultant ventricular premature depolarization separates the local atrial electrogram from the local ventricular electrogram thereby allowing analysis of the retrograde atrial activation sequence. Note that the atrial electrogram recorded from the coronary sinus ostium (CS$_5$) precedes low septal right atrial (HBE) and high right atrial (HRA) activation. This may be a form of the so-called "slow-intermediate" (or "slow-slow") AV nodal reentrant tachycardia. A, atrial electrogram; H, His bundle potential. CS$_1$-CS$_5$: distal-to-proximal coronary sinus.

11.4   Catheter Ablation of AV Nodal Reentrant Tachycardia

11.4.1   ELECTROPHYSIOLOGIC MAPPING

A 7 Fr. Quadripolar (2 mm interelectrode distance) steerable catheter with a 4 mm deflectable tip electrode is introduced from the right femoral vein and placed in the right atrium for atrial mapping (this 4 mm electrode is later used for selective ablation of slow pathway conduction). The two pairs of electrode (proximal pair and distal pair containing the 4 mm electrode) are used for mapping and are, respectively, designated as ME1 and ME2 (ME: mapping electrodes). During mapping, the tip of the 4 mm electrode is place in four positions along the tricuspid annulus (Figures 11-21, 11-22 & 11-23): The anterior (A) region is located in the upper third, the middle (M) region in the middle third, and the posterior (P1) region in the lower third of the HBE-CSO axis (HBE, the

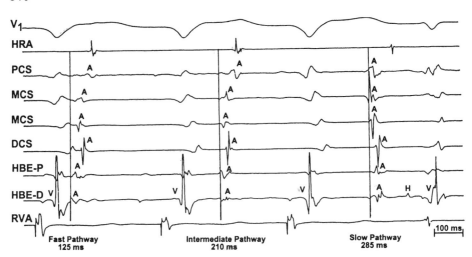

FIGURE 11-17. Three discrete retrograde AV nodal conduction pathways uncovered during ventricular pacing. From top to bottom, in each panel are shown standard ECG leads V_1 and intracardiac recordings high right atrium (HRA), proximal, middle, and distal coronary sinus (PCS, MCS, and DCS, respectively), proximal and distal His bundle regions (HBE-P and HBE-D, respectively), and right ventricular apex (RVA). During ventricular pacing at a cycle length of 450 ms, the site of earliest atrial activation during retrograde fast pathway conduction is recorded at the upper third of the triangle of Koch, close to the His bundle recording site. The earliest atrial activation during retrograde intermediate pathway conduction is recorded within the middle one-third of Koch's triangle, while the earliest retrograde atrial activation during slow pathway conduction is recorded within the lowest one-third of the triangle, close to the ostium of the coronary sinus. A ventricular echo beat (last QRS complex) conducts through the retrograde slow pathway followed by anterograde AV nodal conduction, probably through the fast pathway. The millisecond times at the bottom of the figure represent ventriculoatrial conduction measured from the ventricular-paced stimulus to the earliest onset of atrial activation in these three AV nodal pathways. From [121] with permission.

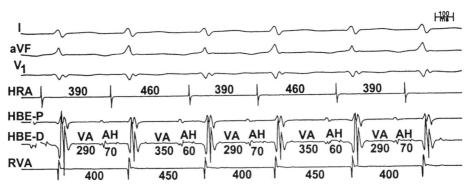

FIGURE 11-18. Fast-slow form of AV nodal reentrant tachycardia showing cycle length alternans due to alternation in ventriculoatrial intervals. The intermediate and slow pathways are used as the retrograde limb of the tachycardia circuit during alternate beats. 2:1 block in the retrograde intermediate pathway allows the retrograde slow pathway to participate in and perpetuate the tachycardia in every other beat. All intervals in milliseconds. From [121] with permission.

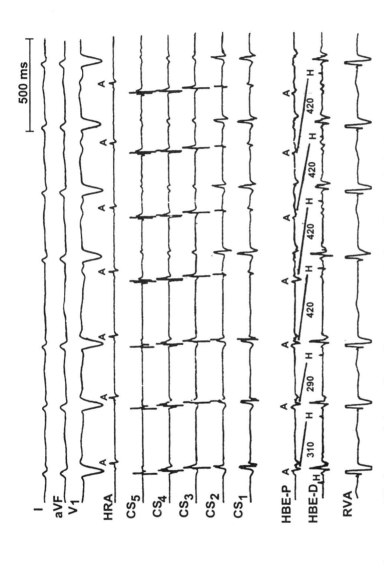

FIGURE 11-19. Spontaneous shift of anterograde intermediate pathway to anterograde slow pathway conduction during the slow-fast form of AV nodal reentrant tachycardia. Following induction of AV nodal reentrant tachycardia, the first three beats of the tachycardia uses an intermediate pathway for anterograde conduction and a fast pathway for retrograde conduction. An accommodation of intermediate pathway conduction occurs, with its conduction time (A-H) decreasing from 310 to 290 ms resulting in conduction block in the intermediate pathway followed by a shift of anterograde conduction to a slower pathway. During the latter slow-fast form of AV nodal reentrant tachycardia, the anterograde conduction time (A-H) is increased to 420 ms. Consequently, the retrograde P wave is inscribed before the QRS complex. Note that the retrograde atrial activation sequence remains unchanged throughout with the septal atrial activation in the His bundle electrogram (HBE) preceding those recorded at the ostium of the coronary sinus (CS₅) and the high right atrium (HRA). ECG leads I, aVF, and V₁ simultaneously recorded. RVA, right ventricular apex; P, proximal; D, distal.

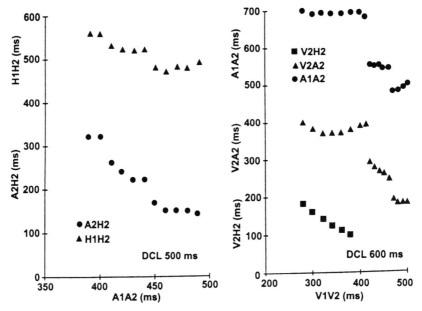

FIGURE 11-20. Conduction curves suggestive of triple AV nodal pathway conduction. Panel A: Anterograde AV nodal conduction curves (A_1-A_2/A_2-H_2 and A_1-A_2/H_1-H_2). Panel B: Retrograde ventriculoatrial (AV nodal) conduction curves (V_1-V_2/V_2-H_2, V_1-V_2/V_2-A_2 and V_1-V_2/A_1-A_2). Note two discrete discontinuities in both anterograde and retrograde directions indicating the presence of three distinct anterograde and retrograde AV nodal conduction pathways. From [121] with permission.

His bundle recording site, and CSO, the coronary sinus ostium, correspond to the upper and lower parts of the triangle of Koch). In addition, the region approximately 1 cm inferior and posterior to the CSO (designated as P2) is also mapped. Atrial mapping in

FIGURE 11-21. Schematic diagram of a right anterior oblique projection illustrating the anterior (A), middle (M), and posterior (P) regions along the tricuspid annulus within the triangle of Koch. The P region is often divided into an anterior half (P1) and a posterior half (P2).

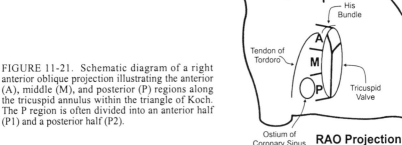

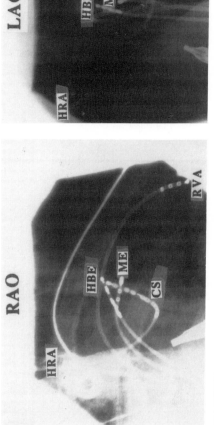

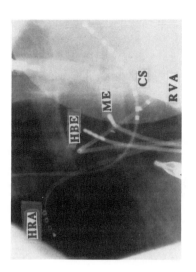

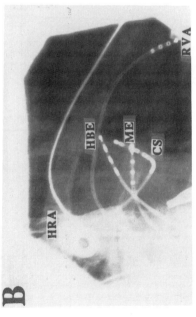

FIGURE 11-22. Fluoroscopic radiograph of the position of the mapping electrode (ME) as seen from the right anterior oblique (RAO) and left anterior oblique (LAO) views. Panel A: The 4-mm distal electrode of ME is positioned in the upper third of Koch's triangle (A region), the long axis of which extends along an imaginary line drawn from the point of recording the His bundle electrogram posteriorly to the ostium of the coronary sinus. Panel B: ME is positioned in the middle third of Koch's triangle (M region). CS, coronary sinus; HBE, His bundle electrographic lead; HRA, high right atrium; RVA, right ventricular apex.

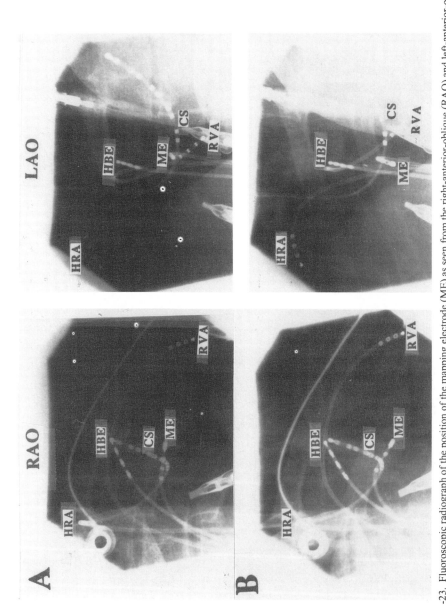

FIGURE 11-23. Fluoroscopic radiograph of the position of the mapping electrode (ME) as seen from the right-anterior-oblique (RAO) and left-anterior-oblique (LAO) views. Panel A: The 4-mm distal electrode ME is in the posterior region corresponding to the lower third of the His bundle electrographic lead (HBE)–coronary sinus (CS) ostium axis. Panel B: The ME is in the region approximately 1-cm inferior and posterior to the CS ostium. Abbreviations as Figure 11-22.

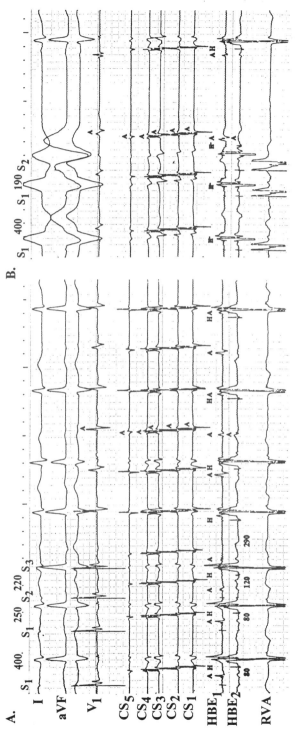

FIGURE 11-24. Comparison between the retrograde atrial activation sequence of a slow-fast form of AV nodal reentrant tachycardia and that induced by programmed ventricular pacing with extrastimulation. Panel A: An AV nodal reentrant tachycardia is induced by two atrial extrastimuli (S_2 and S_3) during high right atrial pacing (S_1S_1) at a cycle length of 400 ms. The S_1S_2 and S_2S_3 intervals are 250 and 220 ms, respectively. Failure of S_3 (A_3) conduction in the anterograde fast pathway with resultant conduction by way of the anterograde slow pathway (A-H interval lengthened from 80 to 290 ms) is followed by initiation of a sustained episode of AV nodal tachycardia of the slow-fast form. The tachycardia manifests transient 2:1 AV block, thereby allowing clear visualization of the retrograde atrial activation sequence by way of the fast pathway. Panel B: Programmed ventricular extrastimulation (S_2) during right ventricular apical (RVA) pacing (S_1S_1) at a cycle length of 400 ms. Note decremental conduction properties of ventriculoatrial conduction induced by S_2 with a premature coupling interval (S_1S_2) of 190 ms. The sequence of retrograde atrial activation induced by programmed RVA stimulation (S_1 and S_2) is identical to that observed during AV nodal reentrant tachycardia with 2:1 AV block in which the low septal right atrial activity in the His bundle electrographic lead (HBE) precedes atrial activation at the ostium of the coronary sinus (CS_5) and the high right atrium (HRA). A; atrial electrogram; CS_1-CS_5; distal to proximal coronary sinus leads; H, anterograde His bundle potential; H$^-$, retrograde His bundle potential. Paper speed: 100 mm/sec.

each region is performed while the right ventricular apex is paced at cycle lengths during which the ventriculoatrial Wenckebach periodicity can be reproducibly induced.

Retrograde fast pathway

In the slow-fast form of AV nodal reentrant tachycardia, the retrograde atrial activation sequence resulting from retrograde fast pathway conduction can only be clearly discernible during tachycardia with 2:1 AV block (Figure 11-24) or when the retrograde P wave is inscribed in front of the QRS complex (Figure 11-19). Thus, in the majority of patients, programmed ventricular extrastimulation is required to separate the atrial electrogram from the ventricular electrogram during tachycardia for analysis of the retrograde atrial activation sequence (Figure 11-16). The retrograde atrial activation sequence of the slow-fast form of AV nodal reentrant tachycardia is identical to that of retrograde fast pathway conduction induced by programmed ventricular stimulation (Figure 11-24). During both incremental ventricular pacing and ventricular extrastimulation, ventriculoatrial conduction resulting from retrograde fast pathway conduction should display decremental conduction properties, even though the site of conduction delay often occurs between the His bundle and the ventricular pacing site (Figure 11-25).

Retrograde slow pathway

Right ventricular pacing at cycle lengths between 300 and 450 ms may induce an abrupt alteration of the retrograde atrial activation sequence associated with a ventriculoatrial Wenckebach periodicity is suggestive of retrograde dual AV nodal pathway conduction [12,126]. As shown in Figure 11-25 (panel B), right ventricular apical (RVA) pacing at a cycle length of 360 ms induces a ventriculoatrial Wenckebach periodicity (3:2 for the 1st to 3rd and 2:1 for the 4th and 5th ventricular-paced beats). The long ventriculoatrial conduction time produced by the 2nd and 4th ventricular-paced beats is accompanied by an abrupt change in the sequence of retrograde atrial activation compared to that of the 1st and 6th ventricular-paced beats with relatively short ventriculoatrial conduction time (the 3rd and 5th ventricular paced-beats induce no ventriculoatrial conduction). The sequence of retrograde atrial activation in these two (2nd and 4th ventricular-paced) beats reveals that the earliest atrial activation is in the coronary sinus ostium (CS_5) rather than in the low septal right atrium of the His bundle recording site (HBE), and that the temporal relationship among all atrial activities (high right atrium — HRA, distal to proximal coronary sinus — CS_1-CS_5) and lower septal right atrium (HBE) is also altered. The increased conduction time from the retrograde His bundle (H^-) potential to the atrium (A) suggests that the sudden prolongation of ventriculoatrial conduction time is caused by a shift from retrograde fast to retrograde slow pathway conduction [12].

Localization of the earliest retrograde atrial exit site of fast & slow pathways

Mapping of the retrograde atrial exit site can be systematically performed beginning in the A region near the His bundle recording site, followed sequentially by the M, P1, and P2 regions during ventricular-paced rhythm at cycle lengths between 300 and 450 ms [126]. The earliest retrograde atrial exit site of the fast pathway can usually be identified

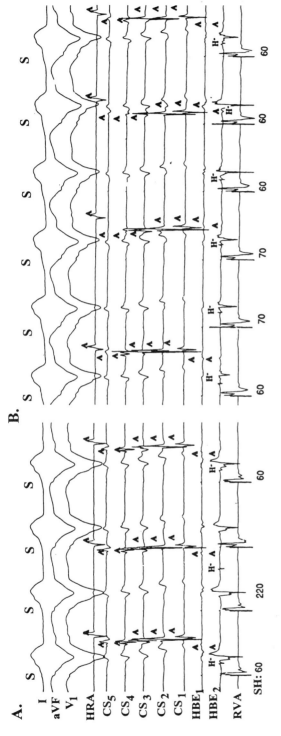

FIGURE 11-25. Retrograde atrial activation sequence with induction of ventriculoatrial Wenckebach periodicity. Panel A: Right ventricular apical (RVA) pacing at a cycle length of 340 ms induces a 3:2 ventriculoatrial conduction pattern. Note that the retrograde atrial activation sequence remains unchanged as the low septal right atrial activity recorded from the His bundle electrographic lead (HBE) precedes atrial activation recorded near the ostium of the coronary sinus (CS₅) and the high right atrium (HRA). Registration of the retrograde His bundle electrogram (H⁻) suggests that retrograde atrial activation is by way of the retrograde fast pathway and that the Wenckebach periodicity occurs in the structure below the level of the His bundle. Panel B: RVA pacing at a cycle length of 360 ms in the same patient induces 3:2 and 2:1 ventriculoatrial conduction patterns (3:2 for the 1st - 3rd and 2:1 for the 4th and 5th ventricular-paced beats). Note that the sequence of retrograde atrial activation abruptly changes in the 2nd and 4th ventricular-paced beats with markedly prolonged ventriculoatrial conduction time compared to that induced by the 1st and 6th ventricular-paced beats; ostium of the coronary sinus (CS₅) atrial activity precedes the low septal right atrial (HBE) and HRA activation. Also note that the temporary relationship among atrial activities is altered compared to that induced by the 1st and 6th ventricular-paced beats. Registration of H⁻ suggests that ventriculoatrial conduction with markedly prolonged ventriculoatrial conduction is caused by conduction through the retrograde slow pathway. The 3rd and 5th ventricular-paced beats are believed to have no ventriculoatrial conduction and the 6th ventricular-paced beat resumes ventriculoatrial conduction by way of the retrograde fast pathway. Paper speed: 150 mm/sec. A, atrial electrogram; CS₁-CS₅, distal-to-proximal coronary sinus; H⁻, retrograde His bundle electrogram.

in all (100%) patients with inducible slow-fast AV nodal reentrant tachycardia and its distribution is 72%, 18%, 10%, and 0% in the A, M, P1, and P2 regions, respectively. In contrast, the earliest retrograde atrial exit site of the slow pathway can only be identified in approximately 30% of patients who exhibit ventriculoatrial Wenckebach periodicity with retrograde dual AV nodal pathway physiology, and its distribution is 0%, 32%, 48%, and 20% in the A, M, P1, and P2 regions, respectively. Hence, the earliest retrograde atrial exit site of each pathway varies in its anatomical location. However, the earliest retrograde atrial exit site of the slow pathway is always inferior and posterior relative to that of the fast pathway [126]. For example, Figures 11-26 & 11-27 show the fast pathway has its earliest retrograde atrial exit site located in the M region 13 ms before the atrial reference point in the His bundle recording site (HBE), whereas the slow pathway has its earliest retrograde atrial exit site in the P1 region 17 ms before the atrial reference point in the proximal coronary sinus (CS_5). Figures 11-28 & 11-29 reveal that the earliest retrograde exit site of the fast pathway is in the A region while that of the slow pathway is in the M region. Rarely, the earliest retrograde atrial exit site of the fast pathway (may be an intermediate or additional slow pathway) can be located in the P1 region and that of the slow pathway in the P2 region as shown in Figure 11-16 and Figure 11-30

Slow pathway potentials
It has been suggested that intracardiac recording of the so-called "slow pathway potentials" may be used as a guide for selective ablation of slow pathway conduction [28,29]. However, experimental studies have provided conflicting data regarding the nature of "slow pathway potentials." "Slow potentials" can be recorded directly from the posterior extensions of the AV node, but can also be generated by asynchronous arrival of wave fronts in different coupled layers of transitional cells [127,128]. Clinical studies have indicated that these "slow pathway potentials" (of either low or high frequency) are inconsistent markers for selective ablation of slow pathway conduction [126]. Of note, using high resolution intraoperative mapping of the endocardial surface in the region of the triangle of Koch, both low and high frequency potentials can be recorded from overlapping regions (M, P1 and P2) at the site of, as well as distant from, the earliest retrograde atrial exit site of the slow pathway. It is suggested that low frequency potentials are probably far-field signals from nearby regions while the high frequency potentials may represent local atrial activity [129-130].

Radiofrequency catheter ablation of slow pathway conduction
The application of RF energy to the cardiac tissues results in resistive heating of tissue and the development of coagulation necrosis [19-23]. The spread of the heating appears equal in all directions, producing a concentric, spherical or hemispherical type lesion radiating from the RF source. The effect on directly adjacent cardiac cells exposed to this type of heating is immediate depolarization and death. The technique of catheter RF ablation in the treatment of AV nodal reentrant tachycardia has been well described [25-37]. Currently selective ablation of slow pathway conduction is the preferred method. Between the 4-mm electrode and an adhesive skin electrode in the right thigh, RF current

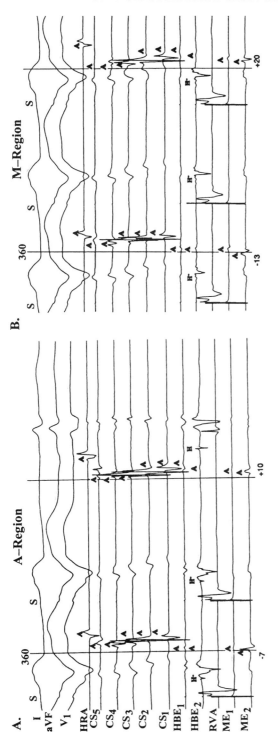

FIGURE 11-26. Mapping of the retrograde atrial exit site of both the fast and slow pathways (same patient as in Figure 11-25). The right ventricular apex (RVA) is paced (S-S) at a cycle length of 360 ms. Panel A: The atrial electrogram recorded from the distal mapping electrode (ME$_2$) in the A–region is inscribed 7 ms before the low septal right atrial electrogram recorded from the His bundle electrographic lead (HBE) during retrograde fast pathway conduction (the first ventricular-paced beat with ventriculoatrial conduction). The atrial electrogram recorded from (ME$_2$) in the A–region occurs 10 ms after the atrial electrogram recorded near the ostium of the coronary sinus (CS$_5$) during retrograde slow pathway conduction (the 2nd ventricular-paced beat). A ventricular echo beat conducted within the anterograde fast AV nodal pathway was induced following retrograde conduction through the slow pathway. Panel B: The atrial electrogram recorded from ME$_2$ in the M–region is inscribed 13 ms before the atrial electrogram recorded from CS$_5$ during retrograde fast pathway conduction (the first ventricular-paced beat with ventriculoatrial conduction) and at the same time as the atrial electrogram is inscribed in the anterior His bundle recording (HBE) during retrograde fast pathway conduction. The atrial electrogram recorded from ME$_2$ in the M–region occurs 20 ms after the proximal coronary sinus (CS$_5$) during retrograde slow conduction. H′: retrograde His bundle potential. Paper speed: 150 mm/sec.

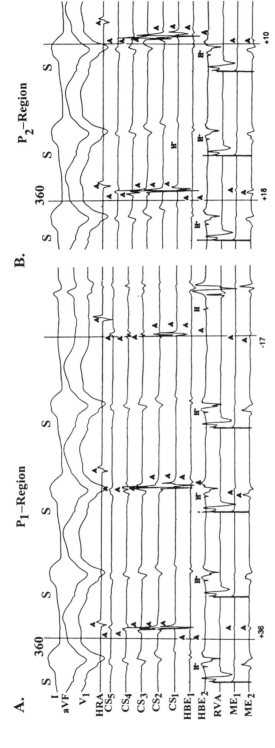

FIGURE 11-27. Mapping of the retrograde atrial exit site of both the fast and slow pathways (same patient as in Figure 11-25 & Figure 11-26). The right ventricular apex (RVA) is paced (S-S) at a cycle length of 360 ms. Panel A: The atrial electrogram recorded from the distal mapping electrode (ME₂) in the P₁ region (the first ventricular-paced beat with ventriculoatrial conduction) is +36 ms relative to the low septal right atrial electrogram (vertical line) recorded from the His bundle electrographic lead (HBE) during retrograde fast pathway conduction, and it is −17 ms (the 2nd and 4th ventricular-paced beats with ventriculoatrial conduction) relative to the atrial electrogram (vertical line) recorded near the ostium of the coronary sinus (CS₅) during retrograde slow pathway conduction. Note that the 3rd ventricular-paced beat induces no ventriculoatrial conduction because of 3:2 ventriculoatrial Wenckebach periodicity, and that the 4th ventricular-paced beat induces a ventricular (AV node) echo beat. Panel B: The atrial electrogram recorded from ME₂ in the P₂ region is +18 ms (the first ventricular-paced beat with ventriculoatrial conduction) relative to the low septal right atrial electrogram (vertical line) recorded from HBE during retrograde fast pathway conduction, and is +10 ms (the second ventricular-paced beat with ventriculoatrial conduction) relative to the atrial electrogram (vertical line) recorded from CS₅ during retrograde slow pathway conduction. P₁, the posterior (lower) third region of the HBE-CS₅ axis; P₂, the region approximately 1 cm inferior/posterior to the CS₅ along the tricuspid annuls; H⁻, retrograde His bundle potential. Figure 11-26 and Figure 11-27 illustrate that the earliest retrograde atrial exit site of the fast pathway is in the M region and that of the slow pathway is in the P₁ region in this patient. Paper speed: 150 mm/sec.

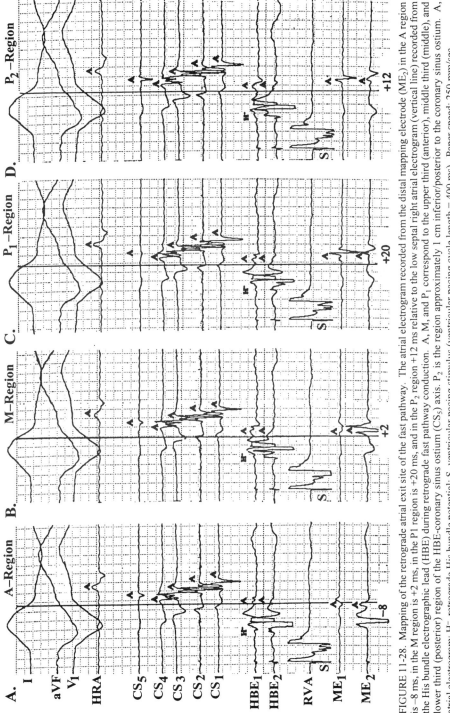

FIGURE 11-28. Mapping of the retrograde atrial exit site of the fast pathway. The atrial electrogram recorded from the distal mapping electrode (ME$_2$) in the A region is −8 ms, in the M region is +2 ms, in the P1 region is +20 ms, and in the P$_2$ region +12 ms relative to the low septal right atrial electrogram (vertical line) recorded from the His bundle electrographic lead (HBE) during retrograde fast pathway conduction. A, M, and P$_1$ correspond to the upper third (anterior), middle third (middle), and lower third (posterior) region of the HBE-coronary sinus ostium (CS$_5$) axis. P$_2$ is the region approximately 1 cm inferior/posterior to the coronary sinus ostium. A, atrial electrogram; H−, retrograde His bundle potential; S, ventricular pacing stimulus (ventricular pacing cycle length = 400 ms). Paper speed: 250 mm/sec.

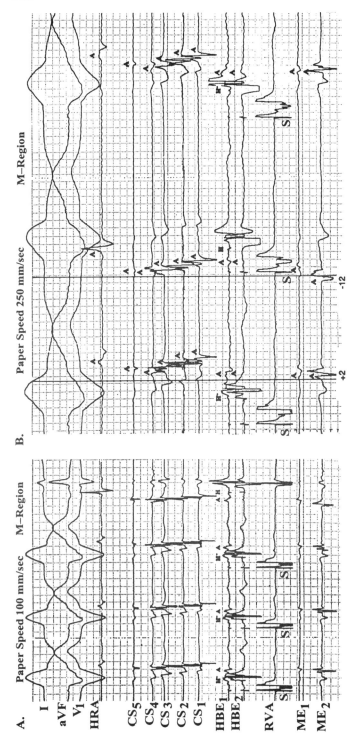

FIGURE 11-29. Mapping of the retrograde atrial exit site of the slow pathway. Same patient as in Figure 11-28. Panel A and B: the right ventricular apex (RVA) is paced (S-S) at a cycle length of 400 ms. Panel A: Paper speed 100 mm/sec. The third (last) ventricular-paced beat induces double atrial responses with simultaneous retrograde fast pathway and retrograde slow pathway conduction which is in the A region. However, during retrograde slow pathway conduction, the earliest retrograde atrial activation site is in the M region. Panel B: Paper speed 250 mm/sec. The first ventricular-paced beat also produces double ventriculoatrial responses with two different retrograde atrial activation sequences identical to those seen in Panel A. Note that the atrial electrogram recorded from ME_2 in the M region is +2 ms relative to the low septal right atrial electrogram (vertical line) recorded from the HBE during retrograde fast pathway conduction, and it is –12 ms relative to the atrial electrogram recorded near the ostium of the coronary sinus ostium (CS_5) during retrograde slow pathway conduction. Based upon data in Figure 11-28 and Figure 11-29, the earliest retrograde atrial exit site of the fast pathway is in the A–region and that of the slow pathway is in the M–region in this patient. A, atrial electrogram; H, His bundle potential; H⁻, retrograde His bundle potential.

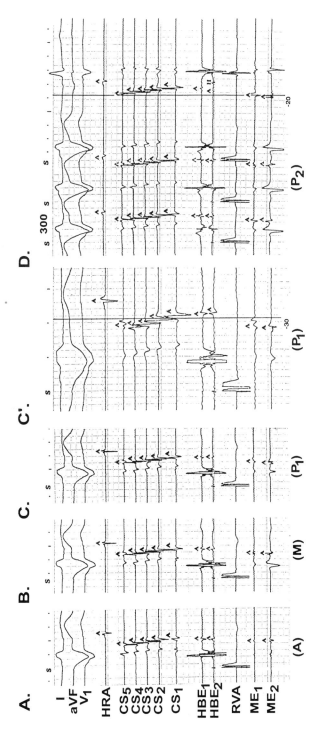

FIGURE 11-30. Mapping of the retrograde atrial exit site of both the fast and slow pathways in the same patient as in Figure 11-16. The atrial electrograms are recorded from the distal mapping electrode (ME$_2$) in the A, M, P$_1$, and P$_2$ regions during ventricular pacing (S). Paper speed in panels A, B,C, and D is 100 mm/sec and 250 mm/sec in Panel C'. Of note, the atrial electrogram (vertical line) recorded from HBE during retrograde fast pathway conduction. As seen in Panel C' the earliest retrograde atrial exit site of the fast pathway is in the P$_1$ region. In panel D, the right ventricular apex (RVA) is paced (S–S) at a cycle length of 300 ms. The third ventricular-paced beat induces ventriculoatrial conduction with markedly prolonged ventriculoatrial conduction time followed by a ventricular (AV node) echo beat. Note the change in the retrograde atrial activation sequence following the shift from retrograde fast (the first and second ventricular-paced beats) to retrograde slow pathway conduction (the third ventricular-paced beat). The atrial electrogram record from ME$_2$ in the P$_2$ region is −30 ms relative to the low septal right atrial electrogram recorded from the His bundle electrographic lead (HBE) during retrograde fast pathway conduction, and it is −20 ms in reference to the atrial electrogram recorded from the coronary sinus ostium (CS$_5$) (vertical line) during retrograde slow pathway conduction. Thus, in this patient, the P$_1$ and P$_2$ positions are the earliest sites of retrograde atrial exit activation during fast and slow pathway conduction, respectively. The retrograde fast pathway may be interpreted as a retrograde "intermediate pathway". A, atrial electrogram, H, His bundle potential.

is delivered via a power supply as a continuous, unmodulated sine wave output at 500-kHz for selective ablation of slow pathway conduction. For patients in whom the earliest retrograde atrial exit site of the slow pathway can be identified, RF energy is applied directly to that site. On the other hand, in patients who exclusively exhibit retrograde fast pathway conduction, RF energy is always applied to an area inferior and posterior to the earliest retrograde exit of the fast pathway (usually the P1, P2, or low M region). No attempt is made to search for the so-called "slow potentials" [76,126]. A stable recording of the His bundle potential is essential while attempting selective ablation of slow pathway conduction. In all patients, the electrogram obtained from the distal pair of mapping electrodes (ME2) before ablation should exhibit an atrial to ventricular electrogram ratio of ≤ 0.25. A brief period of bipolar pacing (4-6 beats) through the distal pair of mapping electrodes (ME2) may be performed to assure capture of the atrial tissue. Radiofrequency energy to achieve an electrode-tissue interface temperature of 50-60 °C for 30 sec is applied in each attempt. Failure to note an AV junctional rhythm within 10-15 sec after initiating RF energy delivery should prompt termination of the RF application and catheter repositioning [125]. If the electrode-tissue interface temperature is less than 50 °C, multiple applications of RF energy are often required for successful ablation of slow pathway conduction. The end point of catheter RF ablation is the non-inducibility of AV nodal reentrant tachycardia with programmed electrical stimulation with or without isoproterenol infusion (Figure 11-5). Inducible single echo beats are allowed [29-33], although the disappearance of anterograde and retrograde slow pathway conduction is considered to be a better endpoint.

11.4.2 LESSONS LEARNED FROM AV NODAL MAPPING & CATHETER ABLATION

Anatomic substrates
That AV nodal reentrant tachycardia involves tissues outside of the AV node proper (compact node) is evidenced by successful abolition of the tachycardia inducibility following selective ablation of slow pathway conduction. Furthermore, the excitable gap of AV nodal reentrant tachycardia has been demonstrated to be significantly wider in both the fast and slow pathway areas ($34 \pm 9\%$ and $33 \pm 11\%$, respectively) than the high right atrium, proximal coronary sinus, and right ventricular apex ($3 \pm 5\%$, $24 \pm 11\%$, and $4 \pm 6\%$, respectively) [131]. Hence, the transitional cell zones corresponding to the antero-superior atrionodal (fast pathway area) and postero-inferior atrionodal bundles (slow pathway area) are very likely to be parts of the reentrant circuit. Indeed, early atrial extrastimulation from these two areas can affect not only the subsequent but also the preceding tachycardia cycle length. As shown in Figure 11-31, an atrial premature depolarization conducts in the orthodromic direction through the anterograde slow pathway, thereby affecting the subsequent H-H interval. However, shortening of the preceding H-H interval can be accounted for by two possible different routes for the transmission of the antidromic impulse of the atrial premature beat. First, the antidromic impulse can conduct through the anterograde fast pathway to collide with the previous tachycardia impulse from the anterograde slow pathway at the lower turn-around tissue (distal common pathway). The impulse collision at the lower turn-around tissue produces

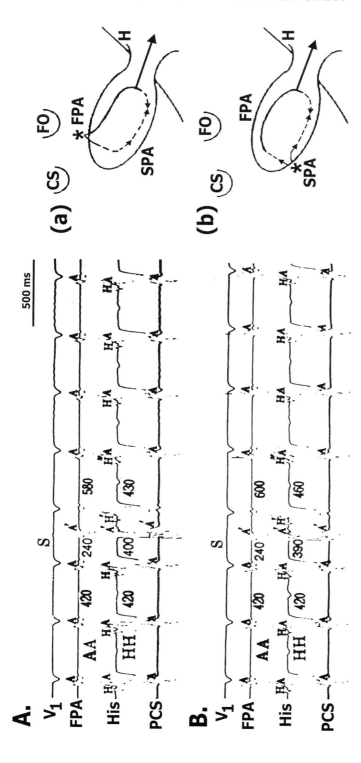

FIGURE 11-31. Tracings showing tachycardia resetting with interference during the following and preceding tachycardia beats. The slow-fast AV nodal reentrant tachycardia has a basic cycle length of 420 ms. A single extrastimulus (S) delivered from either the fast pathway area (FPA) or the slow pathway area (SPA) can reset the tachycardia. When the premature beat is delivered from the FPA (panel A) and SPA (panel B), the H-H" interval preceding the premature beat shortens from 420 to 400 ms and from 420 to 390 ms, respectively, while the H'-H" interval following the premature beat prolongs from 420 to 430 ms and from 420 to 460 ms, respectively. (a) and (b) are accessory figures illustrating schematically that the premature beat (asterisk) captures the fast pathway and antidromically collides with the slow pathway in the slow pathway path, but it also captures the slow pathway and orthodromically conducts within the slow pathway to reach the His bundle (H). The former process shortens the preceding H-H interval and the latter process lengthens the subsequent H-H interval. His, His bundle electrographic lead; PCS, proximal coronary sinus. From [131] with permission.

impulse summation that consequently shortens the preceding H-H interval. Second, the antidromic impulse not only prematurely depolarizes the whole anterograde fast pathway but also passes the lower turnaround tissue to activate the His bundle and simultaneously to collide with the previous tachycardia wave-front from the anterograde slow pathway within the slow pathway. Activation of the His bundle by the antidromic impulse from the anterograde fast pathway results in shortening of the preceding H-H interval. Also, the finding that the excitable gap is significantly wider in both the fast and slow pathway areas compared to the proximal coronary sinus suggests that the left atrial input to the AV node may not participate in the reentrant circuit of the tachycardia [131].

Despite clear delineation of fast and slow pathway conduction areas and subsequent successful techniques of selection ablation of either fast or slow pathway conduction [12,18,28], an actual path of reentry has not been demonstrated either electrophysiologically or morphologically [75,76,132]. Impulse propagation through the atrionodal bundles and the compact AV node may take the form of anisotropic conduction [49]. As a consequence, a broad wavefront of activation enters the three-dimensional non-homogeneous AV junctional structure and the preferred route of impulse transmission is determined by its orientation relative to the functional properties of the tissues involved. The retrograde atrial activation sequence may thus not necessarily represent a linear or sequential activation by a discrete pathway. In fact, results of pharmacologic testing and detailed electrophysiological mapping suggest that the fast and slow anterograde and retrograde conduction pathways may be anatomically and/or functionally distinct [37,76,119-121,133-135].

The renewed interests in the AV nodal structure depicting its posterior extensions may have an impact on the concept of AV node reentry [136]. Specifically, the presence of posterior AV node extensions is a consistent finding in humans, and experimental studies in rabbit hearts have confirmed that these posterior extensions are an independent substructure of the normal AV node with specific anatomic and functional characteristics similar to those of compact AV node. These experimental studies have further shown that activation of transitional cells is fast rather than slow and provides only a trigger of activation of these posterior AV nodal extensions. Thus, the posterior extensions of the AV node may participate in the genesis of AV node reentry, and the issue of AV nodal reentry being intranodal or extra-nodal remains to be settled.

Significance of AV junctional rhythm during ablation of slow pathway conduction
An accelerated AV junctional rhythm is frequently seen while attempting selective ablation of either fast or slow pathway conduction using RF energy [26,28,29]. The appearance of this rhythm often heralds a successful modification of AV node reentry. Since the ablation site of slow pathway conduction is usually significantly distant from the compact node ($\cong 1.0 - 1.5$ cm), it is generally regarded as a safer site for AV junctional ablation. During ablation of slow pathway conduction, the emergence of AV junctional activity occurs during 98% of successful ablations, but in only 43% of the unsuccessful attempts (sensitivity, 98%; specificity, 57%; negative predictive value, 99%) [125]. The mean time to the appearance of AV junctional beats is 8.8 ± 4.1 sec (mean $\pm$ SD) after the onset of RF energy application. Furthermore, atrial mapping has revealed that the

retrograde atrial activation sequence of the RF-induced AV junctional beats is earliest in the anterior atrial septum identical to that seen during pacing from the right ventricular apex [125]. Thus, RF energy application at the site of slow pathway conduction (posterior triangle of Koch) results in the development of an AV junctional rhythm which exists distantly from the retrograde atrial exit site of the fast conduction pathway (anterior triangle of Koch). This finding favors the notion that the slow pathway area (the posterior transitional cell zone) is connected to AV node-His bundle which has been demonstrated to possess automatic activities (diastolic depolarizations) [42]. The slow pathway area must possess specialized conduction properties (lower intracellular and/or extracellular resistivity) different than those of atrial tissues as RF energy applied to the atrial tissues does not induce a similar AV junctional rhythm. It can be hypothesized that the injury amount resulting from RF energy conducts decrementally from its site of origin in the slow pathway near the ostium of the coronary sinus to the anteriorly located AV node-His bundle and in turn, instigates the emergence of an automatic AV junctional rhythm. Of note, experimental studies have shown that the rate of automatic AV junctional rhythm is a temperature-dependent phenomenon [137]. A proximity to the compact AV node and a better tissue contact with resultant achievement of a higher temperature will instigate a faster automatic AV junctional rhythm.

While the development of an AV junctional rhythm during attempted RF ablation of slow pathway conduction is not necessarily indicative of a successful ablation, the absence of such activity is a sensitive marker of an unsuccessful ablation attempt. During attempted ablation of slow pathway conduction, failure to note an AV junctional within 10-15 sec of initiating RF energy delivery should prompt termination of the RF application and catheter repositioning. Early termination of inevitably unsuccessful RF applications may result in reduced procedure time, less radiation exposure to patients, physicians, and laboratory staff and may limit unnecessary and unintended RF-induced damage to the AV junction.

Electrophysiologic mapping rather than simple anatomic approach
Anatomical variation of the earliest retrograde atrial exit site of both AV nodal pathways does exist [76,126]. The existence of anatomical variation explains why selective ablation of each pathway may be achieved in various positions and different results may occur if applying the electrical energy to one particular region without detailed mapping in certain patients. Thus, the so-called "anterior" and "posterior" approaches appear to be oversimplified. Moreover, the dimensions of Koch triangle vary considerably among individuals [138] and the apex of the Koch triangle is really cephalad and anterior, and the base of the triangle between the ostium of the coronary sinus and the tricuspid annulus is really caudal and posterior. A potentially high risk of producing complete AV block can be expected in those patients with unusual location of the earliest retrograde atrial exit site of each pathway, and those with an especially narrow triangle of Koch with the earliest retrograde atrial exit sites of both pathways in proximity. This also explains why there is still a 2% incidence of producing complete AV block during attempts of selective ablation of slow pathway conduction.

The anatomical variation can also be caused by the posterior/inferior placement of the His bundle such as in ostium primum atrial septal or endocardial cushion defect, anterior rotation of heart rendering the apparent length of the region between the His bundle and the ostium of the coronary sinus short, and complex AV junctional structure with multiple pathways exhibiting either intermediate conduction times or unusually rapid slow pathway [76]. Therefore, the so-called "anterior" and "posterior approaches cannot be equated with selective fast and selective slow pathway ablations, respectively. To avoid producing complete AV block, a stable recording of the His bundle potential is essential. This is followed by selection of the targeted area with appropriate A/V electrogram ration (≤ 0.25) and the retrograde A electrogram (ventricular pace rhythm) being later than that recorded in HBE lead. The targeted area is usually located in the P1 region toward the low M region. Additionally, using emergence of automatic AV junctional rhythm within 10-15 sec as a guide will narrow the region within the triangle of Koch where the slow pathway will be found.

TABLE 11-1. Potential proarrhythmic effects of catheter ablation at the atrioventricular junction

Conduction Pathway	Anterograde	Retrograde	Potential Proarrhythmia Mechanism (Reentry)
Fast	+	−	Slow-Fast
Fast	−	+	Fast-Slow
Fast	+	+	Slow-Accessory Pathway (concealed)
Slow	+	−	Unlikely*
Slow	−	+	Unlikely
Slow	+	+	Unlikely

* Retrograde conduction by way of slow pathway. +, ablation successful; −, ablation unsuccessful

Proarrhythmia

Selective ablation of slow pathway conduction is less likely to be proarrhythmic compared to selective ablation of fast pathway conduction [76], consistent with the theoretical basis underlying the mechanism of AV nodal reentrant tachycardia. While attempting selective ablation of fast pathway conduction, several potential adverse consequences may occur. These include (Table 11-1.):

1. Elimination of anterograde fast pathway conduction alone can result in development of incessant slow-fast AV nodal reentrant tachycardia.

2. Elimination of retrograde fast pathway conduction alone can result in the development of the fast-slow form of AV nodal reentrant tachycardia (Figure 11-32). In either case, repeated attempts at ablation of the remaining retrograde or anterograde fast pathway conduction could further increase the incidence of complete AV block.

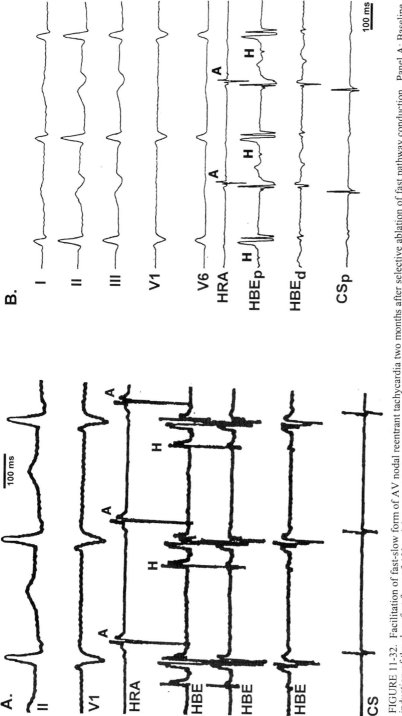

FIGURE 11-32. Facilitation of fast-slow form of AV nodal reentrant tachycardia two months after selective ablation of fast pathway conduction. Panel A: Baseline induction of the slow-fast form of AV nodal reentrant tachycardia before ablation of fast pathway conduction. Panel B: Recurrence of supraventricular tachycardia two months after ablation of fast pathway conduction is documented to be a fast-slow form of AV nodal reentrant tachycardia. Anterograde, but not retrograde, fast pathway. fast pathway conduction has recovered after attempted selected ablation of fast pathway conduction. HRA, high right atrium; HBE, His bundle electrographic lead; CS, coronary sinus; p, proximal; d, distal.

3. Elimination of anterograde and retrograde fast pathway conduction may uncover a previously clinically silent AV reciprocating tachycardia using the anterograde slow pathway for anterograde conduction and a concealed accessory AV connection for retrograde conduction (Figure 11-33). This would necessitate further ablation attempts to eliminate the anomalous AV connection.

Rarely while attempting selective ablation of slow pathway conduction, biophysical derangements caused by the RF applications may uncover other retrograde slow conduction pathways triggering the appearance of clinically significant atypical (fast-slow) form of AV nodal reentrant tachycardia [139].

11.4.3 FUTURE REFINEMENT OF THE CATHETER ABLATION TECHNIQUE

The structure of the human AV junction is complex. Up to date, the exact reentrant circuit of AV nodal reentrant tachycardia remains to be defined. Correlation between electrophysiologic characteristics and the morphological structure of the AV junction can only be speculative. The distinctly separated earliest retrograde atrial exit sites of the fast and slow pathways can be accounted for by the presence of the antero-superiorly located and postero-inferiorly located fast pathway and slow pathway areas, respectively. These two areas somehow transmit electrical impulses to the "compact node." The fact that AV nodal reentrant tachycardia may not recur despite inducible single atrial (AV node) echo beats following attempted ablation of slow pathway conduction in certain patients suggests that sustained AV nodal reentry can be achieved by ablation-induced damage to the slow pathway area or the upper turnaround tissue between the fast and slow pathways. Future investigations should be directed toward studying the anatomical location and morphological structure of this upper turnaround tissue – perinodal atrial tissues, transitional cell zones and posterior AV node extensions. The technique of catheter RF ablation of AV nodal reentrant tachycardia can then be refined, and the risk of AV block be further reduced.

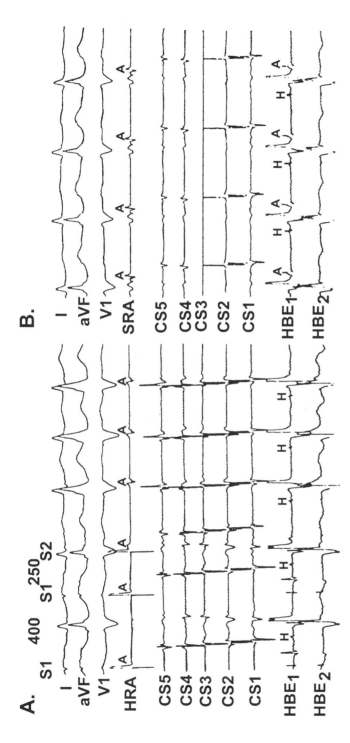

FIGURE 11-33. Facilitation of induction of AV reciprocating tachycardia one month after selective ablation of fast pathway conduction. Panel A: Baseline induction of a slow-fast form of AV nodal reentrant tachycardia before selective ablation of fast pathway conduction. Panel B: Recurrence of supraventricular tachycardia one month later is documented to be AV reciprocating tachycardia with anterograde conduction by way of the anterograde slow AV nodal pathway and retrograde conduction by way of a (concealed) right anteroseptal accessory AV connection. Note that activation of the anterior septal right atrium (SRA) precedes atrial activation recorded in the His bundle electrogram (HBE) as well as the proximal (CS1) and distal (CS5) coronary sinus. This sequence of retrograde atrial activation is distinctly different from that of the slow-fast form of AV nodal reentrant tachycardia. HRA: high right atrium; SRA: anterior septal right atrium; A: atrial electrogram; H: His bundle electrogram. Paper speed 100 mm/sec.

References

1.   Janse MJ, Capelle FJV, Freud GE, Durrer D: Circus movement within the AV node as a basis for su-praventricular tachycardia as shown by multiple microelectrode recording in the isolated rabbit heart. *Circ Res* **28**:403-14, 1971.

2.   Mendez C, Moe GK: Demonstration of a dual A-V nodal conduction system in the isolated rabbit heart. *Circ Res* **19**:378-393, 1966.

3.   Moe GK, Preston JB, Burlington H: Physiologic evidence for a dual A-V transmission system. *Circulation* **4**:357-375, 1956.

4.   Moe GK, Mendez C: The physiologic basis of reciprocal rhythm. *Progress in Cardiovascular Disease* **8**:461-482, 1966.

5.   Scherf D: An experimental study of reciprocating rhythm. *Arch Intern Med* **67**:372-382, 1941.

6.   Casta A, Wolff GS, Mehta AV, et al.: Dual atrioventricular nodal pathways: a benign finding in arrhyth-mia-free children with heart disease. *Am J Cardiol* **46**:1013-8, 1980.

7.   Denes P, Wu D, Dhingra RC, Chuquimia R, Rosen KM: Demonstration of dual A-V nodal pathways in patients with paroxysmal supraventricular tachycardia. *Circulation* **48**:549-55, 1973.

8.   Denes P, Wu D, Dhingra R, et al.: Dual atrioventricular nodal pathways. A common electrophysiologi-cal response. *Br Heart J* **37**:1069-76, 1975.

9.   Rosen KM, Mehta A, Miller RA: Demonstration of dual atrioventricular nodal pathways in man. *Am J Cardiol* **33**:291-4, 1974.

10.   Sung RJ, Styperek JL, Myerburg RJ, Castellanos A: Initiation of two distinct forms of atrioventricular nodal reentrant tachycardia during programmed ventricular stimulation in man. *Am J Cardiol* **42**:404-15, 1978.

11.   Wu D, Denes P, Amat YLF, et al.: An unusual variety of atrioventricular nodal re-entry due to retro-grade dual atrioventricular nodal pathways. *Circulation* **56**:50-9, 1977.

12.   Sung RJ, Waxman HL, Saksena S, Juma Z: Sequence of retrograde atrial activation in patients with dual atrioventricular nodal pathways. *Circulation* **64**:1059-67, 1981.

13.   Ross DL, Johnson DC, Denniss AR, et al.:: Curative surgery for atrioventricular junctional ("AV nod-al") reentrant tachycardia. *J Am Coll Cardiol* **6**:1383-92, 1985.

14.   Keim S, Werner P, Jazayeri M, et al.: Localization of the fast and slow pathways in atrioventricular nod-al reentrant tachycardia by intraoperative ice mapping. *Circulation* **86**:919-25, 1992.

15.   Chang JP, Chang CH, Yeh SJ, et al.: Surgical cure of automatic atrial tachycardia by partial left atrial isolation. *Ann Thorac Surg* **49**:466-8, 1990.

16.   Cox JL, Holman WL, Coin ME: Cryosurgical treatment of atrioventricular node reentrant tachycardia. *Circulation* **76**:1329-1336, 1987.

17.   Johnson DC, Nunn GR, Meldrum-Hanna W: Surgery for atrioventricular node reentrant tachycardia: The surgical dissection technique. *Semin Thorac Cardiovasc Surg* **1**:53-57, 1989.

18.   Haissaguerre M, Warin JF, Lemetayer P, et al.: Closed-chest ablation of retrograde conduction in pa-tients with atrioventricular nodal reentrant tachycardia. *N Engl J Med* **320**:426-33, 1989.

19.   Huang SK, Graham AR, Hoyt RH, Odell RC: Transcatheter desiccation of the canine left ventricle us-ing radiofrequency energy: a pilot study. *Am Heart J* **114**:42-8, 1987.

20.   Huang SK, Bharati S, et al.: Closed chest catheter desiccation of the atrioventricular junction using ra-diofrequency energy--a new method of catheter ablation. *J Am Coll Cardiol* **9**:349-58, 1987.

21.   Huang SK, Bazgan ID, Marcus FI, Ewy GA: Endocardial catheter ablation for refractory ventricular ta-chycardia associated with coronary artery disease. *Pacing Clin Electrophysiol* **10**:1071-80, 1987.

22.   Huang SK, Bharati S, Lev M, Marcus FI: Electrophysiologic and histologic observations of chronic atrioventricular block induced by closed-chest catheter desiccation with radiofrequency energy. *Pacing Clin Electrophysiol* **10**:805-16, 1987.

23.   Borggrefe M, Budde T, Podczeck A, Breithardt G: High frequency alternating current ablation of an ac-cessory pathway in humans. *J Am Coll Cardiol* **10**:576-582, 1987.

25.   Calkins H, Sousa J, El-Atassi R, et al.: Diagnosis and cure of the Wolff-Parkinson-White syndrome or paroxysmal supraventricular tachycardia during a single electrophysiologic test. *New Engl J Med* **324**:1612-1618, 1991.

26. Goy JJ, Fromer M, Schlaepfer J, Kappenberger L: Clinical efficacy of radiofrequency current in the treatment of patients with atrioventricular node reentrant tachycardia. *J Am Coll Cardiol* **16**:418-23, 1990.

27. Lee MA, Morady F, Kadish A, et al.: Catheter modification of the atrioventricular junction with radiofrequency energy for control of atrioventricular nodal reentry tachycardia. *Circulation* **83**:827-35, 1991.

28. Jackman WM, Beckman KJ, McClelland JH, et al.: Treatment of supraventricular tachycardia due to atrioventricular nodal reentry, by radiofrequency catheter ablation of slow-pathway conduction. *N Engl J Med* **327**:313-8, 1992.

29. Haissaguerre M, Gaita F, Fischer B, et al.: Elimination of atrioventricular nodal reentrant tachycardia using discrete slow potentials to guide application of radiofrequency energy. *Circulation* **85**:2162-75, 1992.

30. Jazayeri MR, Hempe SL, Sra JS, et al.: Selective transcatheter ablation of the fast and slow pathways using radiofrequency energy in patients with atrioventricular nodal reentrant tachycardia. *Circulation* **85**:1318-28, 1992.

31. Jazayeri MR, Sra JS, Akhtar M: Transcatheter modification of the atrioventricular node using radiofrequency energy. *Herz* **17**:143-50, 1992.

32. Kay GN, Epstein AE, Dailey SM, Plumb VJ: Selective radiofrequency ablation of the slow pathway for the treatment of atrioventricular nodal reentrant tachycardia. Evidence for involvement of perinodal myocardium within the reentrant circuit. *Circulation* **85**:1675-88, 1992.

33. Mitrani RD, Klein LS, Hackett FK, et al.: Radiofrequency ablation for atrioventricular node reentrant tachycardia: comparison between fast (anterior) and slow (posterior) pathway ablation. *J Am Coll Cardiol* **21**:432-41, 1993.

34. Langberg JJ: Radiofrequency catheter ablation of AV nodal reentry: the anterior approach. *Pacing Clin Electrophysiol* **16**:615-22, 1993.

35. Langberg JJ, Leon A, Borganelli M, et al.: A randomized, prospective comparison of anterior and posterior approaches to radiofrequency catheter ablation of atrioventricular nodal reentry tachycardia. *Circulation* **87**:1551-6, 1993.

36. Wathen M, Natale A, Wolfe K, et al.: An anatomically guided approach to atrioventricular node slow pathway ablation. *Am J Cardiol* **70**:886-9, 1992.

37. Wu D, Yeh SJ, Wang CC, et al.: A simple technique for selective radiofrequency ablation of the slow pathway in atrioventricular node reentrant tachycardia. *J Am Coll Cardiol* **21**:1612-21, 1993.

38. Janse MJ, van Capelle FJL, Anderson RH, et al.: Electrophysiology and structure of the atrioventricular node of the isolated rabbit heart. In: Wellens HJJ, Lie KI, Janse MJ, eds. *The Conduction System of the Heart: Structure, Function and Clinical Implication*. Leiden, The Netherlands: Sterfest Kroese BV, 296-315: 1976.

39. Meijler FL, Janse MJ: Morphology and electrophysiology of the mammalian atrioventricular node. *Physiol Rev* **68**:608-47, 1988.

40. Hoffman BF, Paes de Carvalho A, De Mello WC: Transmembrane potentials of single fibres of the atrio-ventricular node. *Nature* **181**:66-67, 1958.

41. Hoffman BF, Paes de Carvalho A, De Mello WC, al. e: Electrical activity of single fibers of the atrioventricular node. *Circ Res* **7**:11-18, 1959.

42. Hoffman BF, Cranefield PF: *Electrophysiology of the Heart*. 1st ed. New York, NY: McGraw-Hill Book Company, 1960.

43. Kokubun S, Nishimura M, Noma A, Irisawa H: Membrane currents in the rabbit atrioventricular node cell. *Pflugers Arch* **393**:15-22, 1982.

44. Kokubun S, Nishimura M, Noma A, Irisawa H: The spontaneous action potential of rabbit atrioventricular node cells. *Jpn J Physiol* **30**:529-40, 1980.

45. Nakayama T, Kurachi Y, Noma A, Irisawa H: Action potential and membrane currents of single pacemaker cells of the rabbit heart. *Pflugers Arch* **402**:248-57, 1984.

46. Noma A, Nakayama T, Kurachi Y, Irisawa H: Resting K conductances in pacemaker and non-pacemaker heart cells of the rabbit. *Jpn J Physiol* **34**:245-54, 1984.

47. Paes de Carvalho A, de Almeida DF: Spread of activity through the atrioventricular node. *Circ Res* **8**:801-809, 1960.

48. Sherf L, James TN, Woods WT: Function of the atrioventricular node considered on the basis of observed histology and fine structure. *J Am Coll Cardiol* **5**:770-780, 1985.

49. Spach MS, Josephson ME: Initiating reentry: the role of nonuniform anisotropy in small circuits. *J Cardiovasc Electrophysiol* **5**:182-209, 1994.

50. Janse MJ, Capelle FJV, Anderson RH, et al.: Correlation between electrophysiologic recordings and morphologic findings in the rabbit atrioventricular node. *Arch Int Physiol Biochim* **82**:331-2, 1974.

51. Janse MJ: Influence of the direction of the atrial wave front on A-V nodal transmission in isolated hearts of rabbits. *Circ Res* **25**:439-49, 1969.

52. Irisawa H, Noma A: Pacemaker currents in mammalian nodal cells. *J Mol Cell Cardiol* **16**:777-81, 1984.

53. Irisawa H, Giles WR. Sinus and atrioventricular node cells. In: Zipes DP, Jalife J, eds. *Cardiac Electrophysiology: From Cell to Bedside*. 1st ed. Philadelphia, PA: W.B. Saunders, Co., 95-102: 1990.

54. Breitwieser GE, Szabo G. Nature 317:538-540: Coupling of cardiac muscarinic and beta-adrenergic receptors from ions channels by a guanine nucleotide analogue. *Nature* **317**:538-540, 1985.

55. Pfaffinger PJ, Martin JM, Hunter DD, et al.: GTP-binding proteins couple cardiac muscarinic receptors to a K channel. *Nature* **317**:536-8, 1985.

56. Soejima M, Noma A: Mode of regulation of the ACh-sensitive K-channel by the muscarinic receptor in rabbit atrial cells. *Pflugers Arch* **400**:424-31, 1984.

57. Kurachi Y, Nakajima T, Sugimoto T: On the mechanism of activation of muscarinic K+ channel by adenosine in isolated atrial cells: Involvement of GTP-binding proteins. *Pflügers Archiv* **407**:264-274, 1986.

58. Lai W-T, Lee C-S, Wu S-N: Rate-dependent properties of adenosine-induced negative dromotropism in humans. *Circulation* **90**:1832-1839, 1994.

59. Lauer MR, Young C, Liem LB, Sung RJ: Efficacy of adenosine in terminating catecholamine-dependent supraventricular tachycardia. *Am J Cardiol* **73**:38-42, 1994.

60. Clemo HF, Belardinelli L: Effect of adenosine on atrioventricular conduction. II: Modulation of atrioventricular node transmission by adenosine in hypoxic isolated guinea pig hearts. *Circ Res* **59**:437-46, 1986.

61. Clemo HF, Belardinelli L: Effect of adenosine on atrioventricular conduction. I: Site and characterization of adenosine action in the guinea pig atrioventricular node. *Circ Res* **59**:427-36, 1986.

62. Belardinelli L, Linden J, Berne RM: The cardiac effects of adenosine. *Prog Cardiovasc Dis* **32**:73-97, 1989.

63. Belardinelli L, Wu S-N, Visentin S. Adenosine regulation of cardiac electrical activity. In: Zipes DP, Jalife J, eds. *Cardiac Electrophysiology: From Cell to Bedside*. Philadelphia, PA: W.B. Saunders, 513-525: 1990.

64. Belardinelli L, Lerman BB: Electrophysiological basis for the use of adenosine in the diagnosis and treatment of cardiac arrhythmias. *Br Heart J* **63**:3-4, 1990.

65. Belardinelli L, Lerman BB: Adenosine: cardiac electrophysiology. *Pacing Clin Electrophysiol* **14**:1672-80, 1991.

66. DiFrancesco D, Ferroni A, Mazzanti M, Tromba C: Properties of the hyperpolarizing-activated current (if) in cells isolated from the rabbit sino-atrial node. *J Physiol (Lond)* **377**:61-88, 1986.

67. DiFrancesco D, Tromba C: Inhibition of the hyperpolarization-activated current (if) induced by acetylcholine in rabbit sino-atrial node myocytes. *J Physiol (Lond)* **405**:477-91, 1988.

68. DiFrancesco D, Tromba C: Muscarinic control of the hyperpolarization-activated current (if) in rabbit sino-atrial node myocytes. *J Physiol (Lond)* **405**:493-510, 1988.

69. Kameyama M, Hofmann F, Trautwein W: On the mechanism of beta-adrenergic regulation of the Ca channel in the guinea-pig heart. *Pflugers Arch* **405**:285-93, 1985.

70. Tohse N, Kameyama M, Irasawa I: Intracellular Ca2+ and protein kinase C modulate K+ current in guinea pig heart cells. *Am J Physiol* **253**(5 Pt 2):H1321-H1324, 1987.

71. Trautwein W, Kameyama M: Intracellular control of calcium and potassium currents in cardiac cells. *Jpn Heart J* **27 Suppl 1**:31-50, 1986.

72. Walsh KB, Kass RS: Regulation of a heart potassium channel by protein kinase A and C. *Science* **242**:67-69, 1988.

73. Huycke EC, Lai WT, Nguyen NX, et al.: Role of intravenous isoproterenol in the electrophysiologic in-
     duction of atrioventricular node reentrant tachycardia in patients with dual atrioventricular node path-
     ways. *Am J Cardiol* **64**:1131-7, 1989.
74. Sung RJ, Elser B, McAllister RG, Jr.: Intravenous verapamil for termination of re-entrant supraventric-
     ular tachycardias: intracardiac studies correlated with plasma verapamil concentrations. *Ann Intern Med*
     93:682-9, 1980.
75. McGuire MA, Janse MJ, Ross DL: "AV nodal" reentry. Part II: AV nodal, AV junctional, or atrionodal
     reentry? *J Cardiovasc Electrophysiol* **4**:573-86, 1993.
76. Sung RJ, Lauer MR, Chun H: Atrioventricular node reentry: current concepts and new perspectives.
     Pacing Clin Electrophysiol **17**:1413-30, 1994.
77. Hoffman BF, Moore EN, Stuckey JH, et al.: Functional properties of the atrioventricular conduction
     system. *Circ Res* **13**:308-328, 1963.
78. Ferrier GR, Dresel PE: Role of the atrium in determining the functional and effective refractory periods
     and the conductivity of the atrioventricular transmission system. *Circ Res* **33**:375-385, 1973.
79. Wit AL, Weiss MB, Berkowitz WD, et al.: Patterns of atrioventricular conduction in the human heart.
     Circ Res **27**:345-59, 1970.
80. Wu D, Denes P, Wyndham C, Amat-y-Leon F, et al.: Demonstration of dual atrioventricular nodal path-
     ways utilizing a ventricular extrastimulus in patients with atrioventricular nodal re-entrant paroxysmal
     supraventricular tachycardia. *Circulation* **52**:789-98, 1975.
81. Wu D, Denes P, Dhingra R, et al.: New manifestations of dual A-V nodal pathways. *Eur J Cardiol*
     2:459-66, 1975.
82. Wu D, Denes P, Wyndham C, et al.: Demonstration of dual atrioventricular nodal pathways utilizing a
     ventricular extrastimulus in patients with atrioventricular nodal re- entrant paroxysmal supraventricular
     tachycardia. *Circulation* **52**:789-98, 1975.
83. Wu D, Denes P, Dhingra R, et al.: Determinants of fast- and slow-pathway conduction in patients with
     dual atrioventricular nodal pathways. *Circ Res* **36**:782-90, 1975.
84. Csapo G: Paroxysmal nonreentrant tachycardia due to simultaneous conduction in dual atrioventricular
     nodal pathways. *Am J Cardiol* **43**:1033-1045, 1979.
85. Denes P, Wu D, Amat-y-Leon F, et al.: The determinants of atrioventricular nodal re-entrance with pre-
     mature atrial stimulation in patients with dual A-V nodal pathways. *Circulation* **56**:253-9, 1977.
86. Wu D, Denes P, Bauernfeind R, et al.: Effects of procainamide on atrioventricular nodal re-entrant par-
     oxysmal tachycardia. *Circulation* **57**:1171-9, 1978.
87. Chang MS, Sung RJ, Tai TY, et al.: Nadolol and supraventricular tachycardia: an electrophysiologic
     study. *J Am Coll Cardiol* **2**:894-903, 1983.
88. Wu D, Amat-y-Leon F, Simpson RJ, Jr., et al.: Electrophysiological studies with multiple drugs in pa-
     tients with atrioventricular re-entrant tachycardias utilizing an extranodal pathway. *Circulation* **56**:727-
     36, 1977.
89. Wu D, Denes P, Amat-y-Leon F, et al.: Clinical, electrocardiographic and electrophysiologic observa-
     tions in patients with paroxysmal supraventricular tachycardia. *Am J Cardiol* **41**:1045-51, 1978.
90. Sung RJ, Gelband H, Castellanos A, et al.: Clinical and electrophysiologic observations in patients with
     concealed accessory atrioventricular bypass tracts. *Am J Cardiol* **40**:839-47, 1977.
91. Sung RJ: Incessant supraventricular tachycardia. *Pacing Clin Electrophysiol* **6**:1306-26, 1983.
92. Coumel P, Cabrol C, Fabiato A, et al.: Tachycardie permanente par rhythme reciproque. *Arch Mal Co-
     eur* **60**:1830-1849, 1967.
93. Batsford WP, Akhtar M, Caracta AR, et al.: Effect of atrial stimulation site on the electrophysiological
     properties of the atrioventricular node in man. *Circulation* **50**:283-92, 1974.
94. Ross DL, Brugada P, Bar FW, et al.: Comparison of right and left atrial stimulation in demonstration of
     dual atrioventricular nodal pathways and induction of intranodal reentry. *Circulation* **64**:1051-8, 1981.
95. Brugada P, Vanagt EJ, Dassen WR, et al.: Atrioventricular nodal tachycardia with and without discon-
     tinuous anterograde and retrograde atrioventricular nodal conduction curves: a reappraisal of the dual
     pathway concept. *Eur Heart J* **1**:399-407, 1980.
96. Sheahan RG, Klein GJ, Yee R, et al.: Atrioventricular node reentry with 'smooth' AV node function
     curves: a different arrhythmia substrate? *Circulation* **93**:969-72, 1996.

97. Waxman MB, Wald RW, Sharma AD, et al.: Vagal techniques for termination of paroxysmal supraventricular tachycardia. *Am J Cardiol* **46**:655-64, 1980.
98. Wu D, Denes P, Bauernfeind R, et al.: Effects of atropine on induction and maintenance of atrioventricular nodal reentrant tachycardia. *Circulation* **59**:779-88, 1979.
99. Bauernfeind RA, Wyndham CR, Dhingra RC, et al.: Serial electrophysiologic testing of multiple drugs in patients with atrioventricular nodal reentrant paroxysmal tachycardia. *Circulation* **62**:1341-9, 1980.
100. Reddy CP, McAllister RG: Effect of verapamil on retrograde conduction in atrioventricular nodal reentrant tachycardia. *Am J Cardiol* **54**:535-543, 1984.
101. Wellens HJ, Duren DR, Liem DL, Lie KI: Effect of digitalis in patients with paroxysmal atrioventricular nodal tachycardia. *Circulation* **52**:779-88, 1975.
102. Wu D, Denes P, Dhingra R, et al.: The effects of propranolol on induction of A-V nodal reentrant paroxysmal tachycardia. *Circulation* **50**:665-77, 1974.
103. Wu D, Wyndham C, Amat-y-Leon F, et al.: The effects of ouabain on induction of atrioventricular nodal re-entrant paroxysmal supraventricular tachycardia. *Circulation* **52**:201-7, 1975.
104. Sung RJ, Styperek JL: Electrophysiologic identification of dual atrioventricular nodal pathway conduction in patients with reciprocating tachycardia using anomalous bypass tracts. *Circulation* **60**:1464-76, 1979.
105. Tai DY, Chang MS, Svinarich JT, et al.: Mechanisms of verapamil-induced conduction block in anomalous atrioventricular bypass tracts. *J Am Coll Cardiol* **5**:311-7, 1985.
106. Anderson RH, Becker AE, Brechenmacher C, et al.: Ventricular preexcitation: A proposed nomenclature for its substrates. *European Journal of Cardiology* **3**:27, 1975.
107. Bexton RS, Hellestrand KJ, Nathan AW, et al.: A comparison of the antiarrhythmic effects on AV junctional re-entrant tachycardia of oral and intravenous flecainide acetate. *Eur Heart J* **4**:92-102, 1983.
108. Chazov EI, Rosenshtraukh LV, Shugusher KK: Ethmozine. II. Effects of intravenous drug administration on atrioventricular nodal reentrant tachycardia. *Am Heart J* **108**:483-489, 1984.
109. Sethi KK, Jaishankar S, Khalilullah M, Gupta MP: Selective blockade of retrograde fast pathway by intravenous disopyramide in paroxysmal supraventricular tachycardia mediated by dual atrioventricular nodal pathways. *Br Heart J* **49**:532-43, 1983.
110. Shen EN, Keung E, Huycke E, et al.: Intravenous propafenone for termination of reentrant supraventricular tachycardia. A placebo-controlled, randomized, double-blind, crossover study. *Ann Intern Med* **105**:655-61, 1986.
111. Wu D, Hung JS, Kuo CT, et al.: Effects of quinidine on atrioventricular nodal reentrant paroxysmal tachycardia. *Circulation* **64**:823-31, 1981.
112. Svenson RH, Miller HC, Gallagher JJ, Wallace AG: Electrophysiological evaluation of the Wolff-Parkinson-White syndrome: problems in assessing antegrade and retrograde conduction over the accessory pathway. *Circulation* **52**:552-62, 1975.
113. Sung RJ, Castellanos A, Mallon SM, et al.: Mode of initiation of reciprocating tachycardia during programmed ventricular stimulation in the Wolff-Parkinson-White syndrome. With reference to various patterns of ventriculoatrial conduction. *Am J Cardiol* **40**:24-31, 1977.
114. Akhtar M, Damato AN, Caracta AR, et al.: The gap phenomena during retrograde conduction in man. *Circulation* **49**:811-7, 1974.
115. Akhtar M, Damato AN, Batsford WP, et al.: Unmasking and conversion of gap phenomenon in the human heart. *Circulation* **49**:624-30, 1974.
116. Akhtar M, Damato AN, Caracta AR, et al.: The gap phenomenon during retrograde conduction in man. *Circulation* **49**:811, 1974.
117. Sung RJ, Castellanos A, Mallon SM, et al.: Mechanisms of spontaneous alternation between reciprocating tachycardia and atrial flutter-fibrillation in the Wolff-Parkinson-White syndrome. *Circulation* **56**:409-16, 1977.
118. Sung RJ: Can alteration of dual atrioventricular nodal pathway physiology be related to sinus node dysfunction?. *J Cardiovasc Electrophysiol* **9**:479-80, 1998.
119. Keim S, Curtis AB, Belardinelli L, et al.: Adenosine-induced atrioventricular block: a rapid and reliable method to assess surgical and radiofrequency catheter ablation of accessory atrioventricular pathways. *J Am Coll Cardiol* **19**:1005-12, 1992.

120. Souza JJ, Zivin A, Flemming M, et al.: Differential effect of adenosine on anterograde and retrograde fast pathway conduction in patients with atrioventricular nodal reentrant tachycardia. *J Cardiovasc Electrophysiol* **9**:820-4, 1998.
121. Lee KL, Chun HM, et al.: Multiple atrioventricular nodal pathways in humans: Electrophysiologic demonstration and characterization. *Journal of Cardiovascular Electrophysiology* **9**:129-140, 1998.
122. Alison JF, Yeung-Lai-Wah JA, et al.: Characterization of junctional rhythm after atrioventricular node ablation. *Circulation* **31**:84-90, 1995.
123. Jentzer JH, Goyal R, Williamson BD, et al.: Analysis of junctional ectopy during radiofrequency ablation of the slow pathway in patients with atrioventricular nodal reentrant tachycardia. *Circulation* **90**:2820-6, 1994.
124. Kelly PA, Mann DE, Adler SW, et al.: Predictors of successful radiofrequency ablation of extranodal slow pathways. *PACE Pacing and Clinical Electrophysiology* **17**:1143-1148, 1994.
125. Yu JC, Lauer MR, Young C, et al.: Localization of the origin of the atrioventricular junctional rhythm induced during selective ablation of slow-pathway conduction in patients with atrioventricular node reentrant tachycardia. *Am Heart J* **131**:937-46, 1996.
126. Kuo CT, Lauer MR, Young C, et al.: Electrophysiologic significance of discrete slow potentials in dual atrioventricular node physiology: implications for selective radiofrequency ablation of slow pathway conduction. *Am Heart J* **131**:490-8, 1996.
127. de Bakker JMT, Loh P, et al.: Double component action potentials in the posterior approach to the AV node: do they reflect activation delay in the slow pathway? *J Am Coll Cardiol* **34**:570-7, 1999.
128. Medkour D, Becker AE, Khalife K, Billette J: Anatomic and functional characteristics of a slow posterior AV nodal pathway. Role in dual-pathway physiology and reentry. *Circulation* **98**:164-174, 1998.
129. McGuire MA, Lau KC, Johnson DC, et al.: Patients with two types of atrioventricular junctional (AV nodal) reentrant tachycardia. Evidence that a common pathway of nodal tissue is not present above the reentrant circuit. *Circulation* **83**:1232-46, 1991.
130. de Bakker JM, Coronel R, McGuire MA, et al.: Slow potentials in the atrioventricular junctional area of patients operated on for atrioventricular node tachycardias and in isolated porcine hearts. *J Am Coll Cardiol* **23**:709-15, 1994.
131. Lai WT, Lee CS, Sheu SH, et al.: Electrophysiological manifestations of the excitable gap of slow-fast AV nodal reentrant tachycardia demonstrated by single extrastimulation. *Circulation* **92**:66-76, 1995.
132. Janse MJ, Anderson RH, McGuire MA, Ho SY: "AV nodal" reentry: Part I: "AV nodal" reentry revisited. *J Cardiovasc Electrophysiol* **4**:561-72, 1993.
133. Anselme F, Frederiks J, Papageorgiou P, et al.: Nonuniform anisotropy is responsible for age-related slowing of atrioventricular nodal reentrant tachycardia. *J Cardiovasc Electrophysiol* **7**:1145-53, 1996.
134. Wu D: Dual atrioventricular nodal pathways: a reappraisal. *Pacing Clin Electrophysiol* **5**:72-89, 1982.
135. Wu D, Yeh SJ, Wang CC, et al.: Nature of dual atrioventricular node pathways and the tachycardia circuit as defined by radiofrequency ablation technique. *J Am Coll Cardiol* **20**:884-95, 1992.
136. Inoue S, Becker AE: Posterior extensions of the human compact atrioventricular node: a neglected anatomic feature of potential clinical significance. *Circulation* **97**:188-93, 1998.
137. Thibault B, de Bakker JM, Hocini M, et al.: Origin of heat-induced accelerated junctional rhythm. *J Cardiovasc Electrophysiol* **9**:631-41, 1998.
138. Ueng KC, Chen SA, Chiang CE, et al.: Dimension and related anatomical distance of Koch's triangle in patients with atrioventricular nodal reentrant tachycardia. *J Cardiovasc Electrophysiol* **7**:1017-23, 1996.
139. Kalbfleisch SJ, Strickberger SA, Hummel JD, et al.: Double retrograde atrial response after radiofrequency ablation of typical AV nodal reentrant tachycardia. *J Cardiovasc Electrophysiol* **4**:695-701, 1993.

CHAPTER 12

VENTRICULAR PREEXCITATION SYNDROMES: THE WOLFF-PARKINSON-WHITE SYNDROME AND VARIANTS

The Wolff-Parkinson-White syndrome is a clinical constellation of recurrent supraventricular tachycardia and/or atrial flutter-fibrillation associated with the electrocardiographic features of a short PR interval and a broad QRS complex [1-4]. The presence of an accessory AV connection has been demonstrated to be primarily responsible for the syndrome. Since its description, the Wolff-Parkinson-White syndrome has provided a clinical model for advancing our understanding of electrophysiological mechanisms of reentrant arrhythmias [5], for refining the techniques of electrophysiology study and intraoperative mapping, and for developing curative surgical and electrode catheter ablation procedures [6]. Moreover, it has inspired investigation to unravel and characterize different types of accessory connections causing ventricular preexcitation [7-10], and to study reentrant arrhythmias caused by various anatomical substrates [6].

12.1   The Physiology of Ventricular Preexcitation

Most accessory AV connections consist of working atrial or ventricular myocardial bridging the atria and the ventricles [8-10]. These accessory connections totally bypass the normal AV conduction pathway and often are called "bundles of Kent" [11]. Unlike AV nodal tissue, conduction over these accessory connections is rapid and does not, in general, show decremental properties [12,13], although such is not always the case [8]. If a rapidly conducting accessory connection is present, then some areas of ventricular myocardium will be activated via the accessory connection, while other regions will continue to be activated through the normal AV conduction system. When viewed with the surface ECG, two pathway activation of the ventricles results in a shortened P-R interval, slurring of the QRS complex upstroke (*delta wave*), increased duration of the QRS complex, and, often, an atypical QRS complex axis. Fast conduction over the AV connection bypassing the AV node–His–Purkinje system accounts for the short P-R interval, while the resulting ventricular preexcitation is responsible for generation of the delta wave and prolongation of the QRS complex duration [14-16]. Thus, this abnormal two-pathway activation of the ventricles, a form of *ventricular fusion*, results in a hybrid QRS complex which is different from that generated by exclusive conduction over either the normal or accessory pathway alone.

Varying degrees of ventricular preexcitation with dynamic variations in the QRS complex configuration can be observed in the same patient at different times. The degree of ventricular preexcitation is determined by the time relation of the two different wavefronts from the normal and accessory AV conduction pathways arriving at the ventricles [12,17,18].

Ventricular preexcitation during sinus rhythm is often more pronounced with right-sided than left-sided accessory AV connections, because right-sided accessory connections are relatively closer to the sinus node, thereby diminishing the time available for fusion to occur via the AV node–His–Purkinje system pathway. A shift in the location of an ectopic atrial impulse or pacing site can also change the degree of ventricular preexcitation. The closer the site of the ectopic impulse to the accessory AV connection, the greater the degree of ventricular preexcitation. A change in the cardiac cycle length may also cause variation in the degree of ventricular preexcitation. Before reaching the anterograde effective refractory period of an accessory AV connection, atrial pacing at faster rates and atrial premature stimulation with progressively shorter coupling intervals increase the degree of ventricular preexcitation (concertina effect) (Figure 12-1).

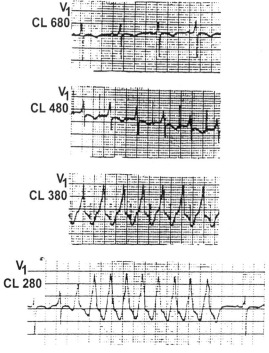

FIGURE 12-1. Increasing degree of ventricular preexcitation during incremental atrial pacing in a patient with a left-sided accessory AV connection. A burst of rapid atrial pacing from the coronary sinus at a cycle length (CL) of 280 ms produces 1:1 AV conduction over the accessory AV connection mimicking ventricular tachycardia (bottom tracing). Electrocardiographic lead V_1 is recorded.

This is because the progressive lengthening of AV nodal conduction time associated with shortening of the cardiac cycle length permits more ventricular excitation to occur through the accessory connection. Despite the increasing degree of ventricular preexcitation, the atrial stimulus artifact-to-delta wave (P-R interval) remains constant, characteristic of conduction over an accessory AV connection. Vagal stimulation may also be expected to increase the degree of preexcitation by prolonging AV nodal conduction time, thereby promoting the contribution of accessory pathway conduction to ventricular excitation.

Normalization of the QRS complex morphology with disappearance of ventricular preexcitation may occur under a variety of situations. A reduction in vagal tone during exercise or blocking vagal effects with atropine facilitates normal pathway conduction, thereby lessening (or possibly eliminating) preexcitation with normalization of the QRS

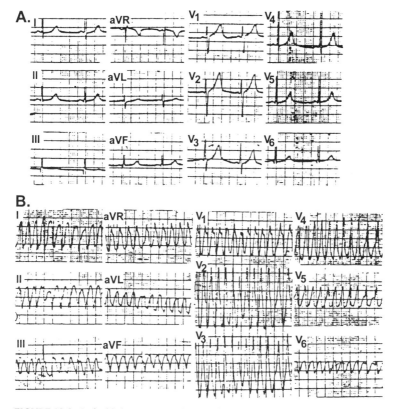

FIGURE 12-2. Left-sided accessory AV connection in a 23-year-old man. 12-lead ECG recorded during sinus rhythm (panel A) and during atrial flutter (panel B). During sinus rhythm ventricular preexcitation is not evident despite a short PR interval of 0.12 sec. During atrial flutter, ventricular preexcitation becomes evident with 1:1 AV conduction within the accessory AV connection at a rate of 300/min (confirmed by electrophysiology study).

complex and lengthening of the P-R interval. These paradoxical effects of vagal influence on the P-R interval in patients with an accessory AV connection have been noted since the original description of the Wolff-Parkinson-White syndrome [1]. Other situations associated with the disappearance of preexcitation and normalization of ventricular activation include [12,17-19]: late activation of the accessory AV connection relative to the normal AV pathway conduction (latent ventricular preexcitation) (Figure 12-2) and ineffective atrial conduction at the entrance (anterograde block) of the accessory AV connection, which may be rate dependent [19].

12.2 Electrophysiology Study

The electrophysiologic properties of accessory connections are usually different from those of the normal AV conduction system and they vary greatly among patients, as well as being influenced by age, heart rate, autonomic tone, pharmacologic agents, and their anatomic locations. Using the technique of programmed electrical stimulation, intracardiac recordings, and pharmacologic agents, some of the electrophysiologic properties of these accessory connections can be characterized.

12.2.1 REFRACTORY PERIODS

Both the atria and the right ventricular apical endocardium are stimulated at one or two cycle lengths (A_1-A_1 or V_1-V_1). Following every eighth spontaneous or paced beats (A_1 or V_1), single premature atrial or ventricular beats (A_2 or V_2) are delivered at progressively shorter coupling intervals until the effective refractory period (ERP) of the atrium or the ventricle is encountered. Using programmed stimulation from the high right atrium or coronary sinus, anterograde conduction is studied in order to analyze the following electrophysiological parameters:

1. *Effective refractory period of the atrium*: The longest S_1-S_2 interval that fails to generate an atrial response.

2. *Functional refractory period of the atrium*: The shortest attainable A_1-A_2 interval achieved during programmed atrial stimulation.

3. *Anterograde effective refractory period of the accessory AV connection*: The longest A_1-A_2 interval near the accessory AV connection which fails to conduct with a ventricular preexcitation pattern [12,20,21].

4. *Atrial vulnerability*: A premature stimulus (S_2) delivered close to the effective refractory period of the atrium (within its relative refractory period) may elicit short-lived repetitive atrial responses (mean atrial cycle length of 300 ms or less) or a paroxysm of atrial flutter-fibrillation (mean atrial cycle length of less than 250 ms) [22,23].

Using programmed stimulation from the right ventricular apex, retrograde conduction is studied in order to analyze the following electrophysiological parameters:

1. *Effective refractory period of the ventricle*: The longest S_1-S_2 interval that fails to generate a ventricular response.

2. *Functional refractory period of the ventricle*: The shortest attainable V_1-V_2 interval achieved during programmed ventricular stimulation.

3. *Retrograde effective refractory period of the accessory AV connection*: The longest V_1-V_2 interval near the accessory AV connection which fails to conduct with an eccentric retrograde atrial activation sequence [12,20,21].

12.2.2 INDUCTION OF AV RECIPROCATING TACHYCARDIA

The atrium (right or left), the two AV conduction pathways (normal and accessory), and the ventricle (right or left) constitute a reentry circuit. A premature atrial or ventricular stimulus can initiate *AV reciprocating (circus movement) tachycardia* as a result of differences in the electrophysiologic properties of the two AV conduction pathways [12,24,-26]. In most instances, an *orthodromic* form of AV reciprocating tachycardia is induced, utilizing the normal AV conduction pathway for anterograde conduction and an accessory AV connection for retrograde conduction. The initiation of this form of AV reciprocating tachycardia is usually related to conduction block of an atrial premature depolarization in the accessory AV connection (Figure 12-3), when the anterograde effective refractory period of the accessory AV connection is longer than that of the normal AV conduction pathway. Conversely, the initiation of an orthodromic AV reciprocating tachycardia during ventricular pacing is associated with conduction block of a ventricular premature depolarization in the normal AV conduction pathway [27]. This occurs when the retrograde effective refractory period of the accessory pathway is shorter than that of the normal AV conduction pathway. The site of block induced by the ventricular premature depolarization is frequently located in the infra-His structure or the AV node. The QRS complex is narrow during orthodromic AV reciprocating tachycardia (unless there is functional or preexisting bundle branch block) because activation of

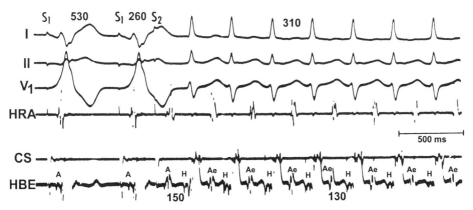

FIGURE 12-3. Initiation of AV reciprocating tachycardia with programmed atrial extrastimulation in the Wolff-Parkinson-White syndrome. ECG leads I, II, and V_1 are simultaneously recorded along with high right atrial (HRA), coronary sinus (CS), and His bundle electrograms (HBE). The CS is driven at a cycle length (S_1-S_1) of 530 ms. Note the ventricular preexcitation with a positive QRS deflection in V_1 during the atrial-paced rhythm (first and second QRS complexes), suggesting the presence of a left-sided accessory AV connection. An atrial premature stimulus (S_2) with a premature coupling interval (S_1-S_2) of 260 ms fails to conduct over the accessory AV connection, but it does conduct slowly to the ventricle through the normal AV conduction pathway. The sudden disappearance of the ventricular preexcitation pattern is followed by prolongation of the P-R interval, normalization of the QRS complex, and an onset of AV reciprocating tachycardia with a cycle length of 310 ms. During tachycardia, the AV node-His-Purkinje system is used for anterograde conduction, and the left-sided accessory AV connection is used for retrograde conduction. Note that left atrial activation precedes low septal right atrial and high right atrial activation during retrograde atrial activation. A = atrial electrogram. H = His bundle electrogram. Ae = atrial echo.

the ventricles results from anterograde conduction through the normal AV node-His-Purkinje system.

An *antidromic* form of an AV reciprocating tachycardia, on the other hand, is associated with a wide QRS complex because the ventricles are activated by anterograde conduction through the accessory AV connection with the circuit completed using the normal AV conduction pathway for retrograde conduction [28]. In order to initiate this form of AV reciprocating tachycardia with programmed atrial stimulation, an atrial premature depolarization must fail to conduct over the normal AV conduction pathway but be capable of anterograde conduction by way of the accessory AV connection. This can occur when the anterograde effective refractory period of the normal AV conduction pathway is greater than that of the accessory AV connection. Conversely, to initiate an antidromic reciprocating tachycardia using programmed ventricular stimulation, a premature ventricular depolarization must fail to conduct in the accessory AV connection, but be capable of retrograde conduction by way of the normal AV conduction pathway. This occurs when the retrograde effective refractory period of the accessory AV connection is longer than that of the normal AV conduction pathway. During an antidromic AV reciprocating tachycardia there is no ventricular activation through the normal AV node-His-Purkinje system and there is maximal ventricular preexcitation (broad bizarre QRS complex) resulting from exclusive ventricular activation from the accessory AV connection reminiscent of ventricular tachycardia (Figures 12-4 & 12-5).

Electrocardiographically, antidromic AV reciprocating tachycardia is difficult to differentiate from (1) atrial flutter or atrial tachycardia with 1:1 or 2:1 AV conduction over an accessory AV connection (Figure 12-2); (2) AV nodal reentrant tachycardia with a 1:1 AV conduction over a bystander accessory AV connection; (3) AV reciprocating tachycardia involving two accessory AV connections; (4) supraventricular tachycardia associated with functional or preexisting bundle branch block; and (5) ventricular tachycardia [29-33]. AV reciprocating tachycardia involving two or more accessory AV connections is exceedingly rare [31-33]. In this case, the tachycardia uses one accessory AV connection for anterograde conduction and another accessory AV connection for retrograde conduction (Figure 12-6). If different accessory connections function as the anterograde limb of the reentrant circuit at different times it will result in multiple tachycardia morphologies [32].

12.2.3 PATTERNS OF VENTRICULOATRIAL CONDUCTION

Increasingly premature cardiac impulses entering the normal AV conduction pathway in either the anterograde or retrograde direction normally experience decremental conduction, resulting in a progressive increase in atrioventricular or ventriculoatrial conduction time. On the other hand, anterograde or retrograde conduction within most accessory connections is rapid and non-decremental [12,13]. The decremental conduction properties of the normal AV conduction pathway in the retrograde direction result from both the intrinsic characteristics of the AV node as well as the retrograde conduction properties at the junction of the Purkinje and working myocardial fibers. The purkinje fibers exhibit action potentials with durations longer than those found in adjacent myocardial

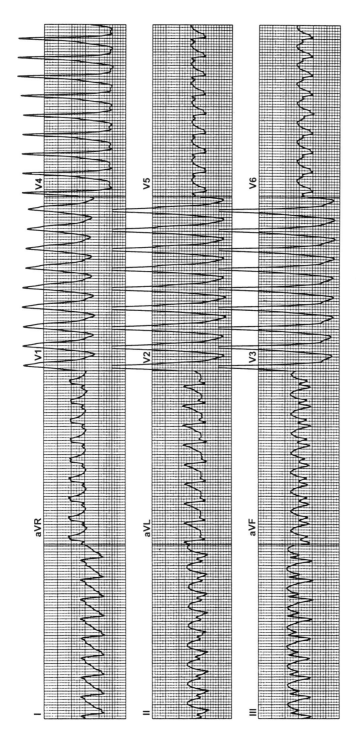

FIGURE 12-4. Surface 12-lead ECG recording of antidromic AV reciprocating tachycardia involving a left posterior accessory AV connection. During the tachycardia, anterograde conduction within the left-sided posterior accessory pathway results in a positive QRS complex in lead V_1 (right bundle branch block pattern) with left/superior frontal plane axis. The mechanism of the tachycardia is confirmed by electrophysiology study (Figure 12-5). Paper speed 25 mm/sec.

fibers. This creates a gating mechanism that accounts for the infra-Hisian decremental conduction frequently seen during programmed ventricular extrastimulation.

Four patterns of ventriculoatrial conduction may be induced during programmed ventricular stimulation and these patterns determine the inducibility of AV reciprocating tachycardia from the ventricle [27,34]. First, there may be a total absence of ventriculoatrial conduction due to retrograde block in both the normal AV conduction system and the accessory AV connection. In this case, AV reciprocating tachycardia cannot be elicited. Second, there may be persistent retrograde atrial fusion due to wavefronts of depolarization conducting through both the normal and accessory AV pathways. In this case, both pathways have identical effective refractory periods and an AV reciprocating tachycardia cannot be induced. Third, predominant or exclusive retrograde activation of the atria via the normal AV conduction pathway may occur (Figures 12-7 & 12-8). In this case, the normal AV conduction system has a retrograde effective refracting period

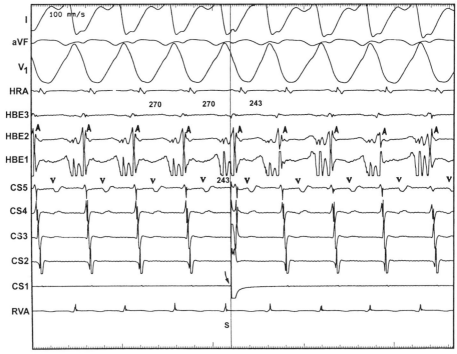

FIGURE 12-5. Atrial extrastimulus testing during antidromic AV reciprocating tachycardia (same patient as in Figure 12-4). During antidromic AV reciprocating tachycardia, a left posterior accessory AV connection is utilized for anterograde conduction producing a positive QRS complex in lead V₁ with a left/superior frontal plane axis. Note that retrograde atrial activation is by way of the normal AV conduction system with the earliest atrial electrogram in the His bundle electrographic lead (HBE) preceding retrograde atrial activation in the proximal coronary sinus (CS) and high right atrium (HRA). Atrial premature stimulation (S) delivered at the distal coronary sinus (CS1) (see arrow) causes atrial fusion and prematurely activates the posterior left ventricle (V-V cycle length shortened from 270 to 243 ms), resetting the antidromic AV reciprocating tachycardia. Advancement of ventricular depolarization favors antidromic AV reciprocating tachycardia rather than AV nodal reentrant tachycardia with a bystander accessory AV connection. CS1-5, distal to proximal coronary sinus, respectively; RVA, right ventricular apex. Surface ECG leads I, aVF and V₁ displayed at the top.

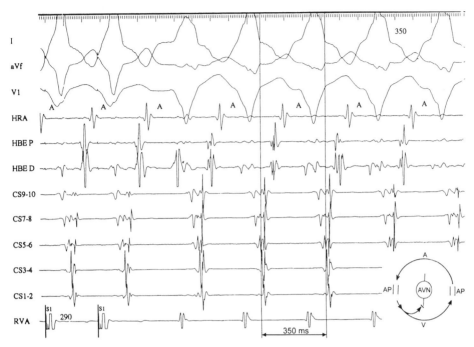

FIGURE 12-6. Antidromic AV reciprocating tachycardia involving two accessory AV connections. Ventricular pacing (S1-S1) at a cycle length of 290 ms (first two QRS complexes) elicits an antidromic AV reciprocating tachycardia (CL 350 ms) utilizing a right-sided posterolateral accessory AV connection for anterograde conduction and a left-sided posterolateral accessory AV connection for retrograde conduction (see inset schematic diagram in right lower coroner). Note that during the tachycardia anterograde conduction within the right-sided posterolateral accessory connection results in a negative QRS complex in lead V1 with a superior frontal plane axis and retrograde conduction within the left-sided posterolateral accessory AV connection results in earliest retrograde atrial activation in the distal coronary sinus (CS3-4) (vertical lines). A, atrial electrogram; HBEP and HBED, proximal and distal His bundle electrographic leads, respectively; CS1-2 to CS9-10, distal to proximal coronary sinus, respectively; RVA, right ventricular apex. (Courtesy of Dr. George Van Hare).

shorter than that of the accessory AV connection and an antidromic AV reciprocating tachycardia may be induced. Finally, predominant or exclusive retrograde activation of the atria via the accessory AV connection may occur. In this case, the accessory AV connection has a retrograde effective refractory period shorter than that of the normal AV conduction system and an orthodromic AV reciprocating AV tachycardia may be induced (Figures 12-9 through 12-11).

During programmed ventricular stimulation, the induction of a sustained episode of orthodromic AV reciprocating tachycardia requires: (1) an accessory AV connection capable of conduction in the retrograde direction with a shorter retrograde effective refractory period compared to that of the normal AV conduction system; (2) minimal retrograde concealed conduction in the normal AV conduction system induced by ventricular premature depolarization; and (3) sufficient anterograde conduction delay with a short anterograde effective refractory period of the AV node-His Purkinje system. On the other hand, the induction of a sustained episode of an antidromic AV reciprocating tachycardia with programmed ventricular stimulation requires: (1) the normal AV con-

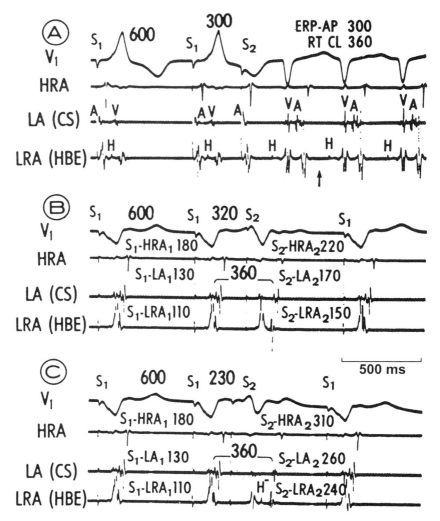

FIGURE 12-7. Initiation of AV reciprocating tachycardia following anterograde conduction block in accessory AV connection. Panel A: During left atrial (LA) pacing from the coronary sinus at a cycle length (S_1-S_1) of 600 ms, atrial extrastimulation with a coupling interval (S_1-S_2) of 300 ms results in the disappearance of ventricular preexcitation and initiates AV reciprocating tachycardia (RT) (arrow). Thus, the anterograde effective refractory period of the accessory pathway (ERP-AP) is 300 ms (LA_1-LA_2 = S_1-S_2). The tall R wave in lead V_1 during left atrial pacing and the sequence of atrial activation during reciprocating tachycardia suggest that the accessory pathway is left-sided. Panels B & C: During right ventricular pacing (S_1-S_1) at a cycle length of 600 ms, there is progressive lengthening of V-A conduction time at all three recording sites (LRA = low septal right atrium, LA = left atrium (via coronary sinus), HRA = high right atrium) in response to increasing prematurity of ventricular coupling intervals (S_1-S_2). The low septal right atrium (in His bundle electrographic lead, HBE) is constantly activated 20 to 70 ms before the LA and HRA, respectively, suggesting retrograde conduction within the normal AV conduction pathway. Note LA_1-LA_2 intervals at S_1-S_2 of both 320 and 230 ms are 360 ms, which is beyond the anterograde ERP-AP at a comparable cycle length of 600 ms; however, no reciprocating tachycardia is elicited. The latter findings suggest that retrograde concealed conduction of the accessory pathway in response to the ventricular premature beats prevents the transmission of the impulse across the accessory pathway in an anterograde direction. H^- = retrograde His bundle potential [27].

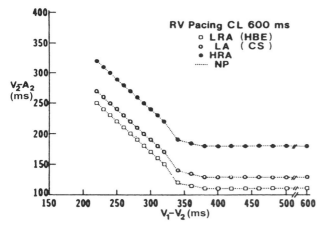

FIGURE 12-8. Retrograde conduction time of premature ventricular beats (V_2-A_2) as a function of premature coupling intervals (V_1-V_2) demonstrating exclusive ventriculoatrial conduction through the normal pathway (NP). Same patient as in Figure 12-7. Note the progressive lengthening of retrograde atrial activation time in three atrial recording sites (high right atrium, HRA; left atrium, LA; low septal right atrium, LRA). CL = cycle length. CS = coronary sinus. HBE = His bundle electrogram. RV = right ventricle. From [27] with permission.

duction system has a shorter retrograde effective refractory period compared to that of an accessory AV connection; (2) minimal retrograde concealed conduction in the accessory AV connection induced by ventricular premature depolarization; and (3) sufficient retrograde conduction delay of the AV node-His Purkinje system along with an accessory AV connection having a short anterograde effective refractory period. Of note, retrograde concealed conduction in the accessory AV connection during premature ventricular stimulation often prevents a retrograde impulse conducted to the atria through the normal AV conduction system to be conducted in an anterograde fashion through the accessory

FIGURE 12-9. During right ventricular pacing (S_1-S_1) at a cycle length of 600 ms, high right atrial (HRA) activation precedes left atrial (LA) activation by 20 ms (S_1-HRA_1 = 140 ms, S_1-LA_1 = 160 ms). However, when the premature coupling interval (S_1-S_2) is shortened to 400 ms (Panel A) or less (Panel B), the low septal right atrial (LRA) electrogram (in the His bundle electrocardiographic lead, HBE) becomes discernible. The sequence of atrial activation then reveals that the left atrium is constantly activated 20 and 40 ms, respectively, before the LRA and HRA, suggesting a shift in the pattern of ventriculoatrial conduction from retrograde atrial fusion to exclusive retrograde atrial activation through the left-sided accessory pathway. Abbreviations as in Figure 12-7. From [27] with permission.

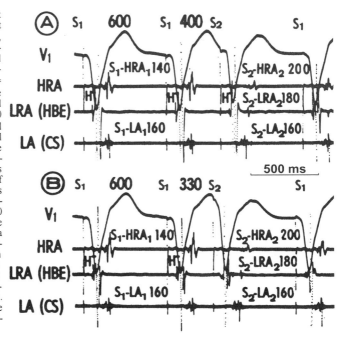

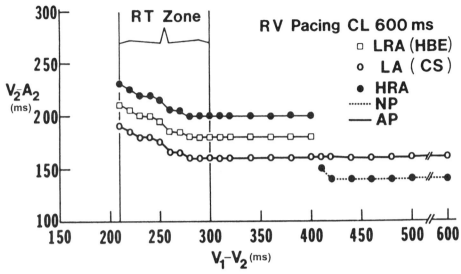

FIGURE 12-10. Retrograde conduction time of premature ventricular depolarizations (V_2-A_2) as a function of premature coupling intervals (V_1-V_2), demonstrating a shift of the ventriculoatrial conduction pattern from retrograde atrial fusion to exclusive retrograde atrial activation through the left-sided accessory pathway (AP). A reciprocating tachycardia (RT) zone is defined between premature coupling intervals (V_1-V_2) of 300 and 210 ms and, in each instance, the onset of RT is related to repetitive ventricular responses (see Figure 12-9). Same patient as in Figure 12-9. From [27] with permission.

AV connection. This explains why antidromic AV reciprocating tachycardia is rarely seen clinically (Figure 12-7 & 12-8) [27].

12.2.4 INDUCTION OF ATRIAL FLUTTER-FIBRILLATION

The genesis of atrial flutter-fibrillation is related to the presence of atrial vulnerability which, in turn, is related to tissue inhomogeneity [22,23,35]. Atrial vulnerability is defined as the induction of repetitive atrial activity or a paroxysm of atrial flutter-fibrillation in response to an atrial premature stimulus delivered close to the functional refractory period of the atrium (Figure 12-12). During atrial flutter-fibrillation, three types of AV conduction patterns may be observed: (1) exclusive conduction through the normal AV conduction system with normal QRS complex morphology; (2) exclusive conduction through the accessory pathway with a maximally preexcited QRS complex; and (3) a fusion QRS complex resulting from conduction through both the normal and accessory pathways.

The rate of ventricular response during atrial flutter-fibrillation is determined by the electrophysiologic properties of both AV conduction pathways (normal and accessory), the interplay between AV conduction over these two pathways, the electrophysiologic properties of the ventricles, and the state of autonomic tone [36-39]. Generally, the shorter the effective refractory period of the accessory AV connection, the faster the resultant ventricular response during atrial flutter-fibrillation. As a very fast ventricular

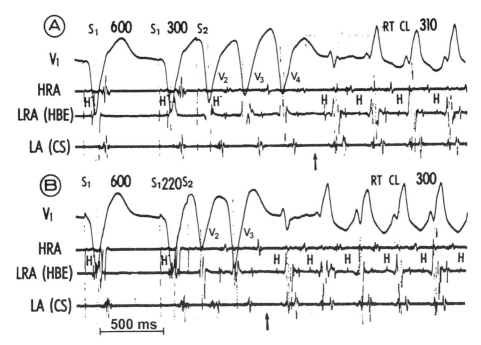

FIGURE 12-11. During right ventricular pacing (S₁-S₂) at a cycle length (CL) of 600 ms, repetitive ventricular responses (V₂-V₃-V₄ in Panel A or V₂-V₃ in Panel B) at short premature coupling intervals (S₁-S₂) initiate the onset of reciprocating tachycardia (RT) (arrows). Note persistent retrograde atrial activation from the accessory pathway (AP) during repetitive ventricular responses and the development of a functional complete right bundle branch block pattern during reciprocating tachycardia. It is assumed that decremental depolarization of the normal pathway in the retrograde direction induced by repetitive ventricular responses facilitates initiation of reciprocating tachycardia. Same patient as in Figure 12-9 & 12-10. Abbreviation as in Figure 12-7. From [27] with permission.

rate (e.g., 250/min) is approached, atrial flutter-fibrillation may degrade into ventricular fibrillation [36-39]. Clinical studies have demonstrated that determining the duration of the anterograde effective refractory period of the accessory connection is of value in identifying patients at high risk of developing a life-threatening rapid ventricular response during atrial flutter-fibrillation [36,38].

Although the genesis of atrial flutter-fibrillation in patients with preexcitation syndromes is not directly caused by the presence of an accessory AV connection, rapid ventriculoatrial conduction via an accessory pathway during the atrial vulnerable phase can trigger an onset of atrial flutter-fibrillation. During electrophysiologic study, this may be observed while attempting to terminate AV reciprocating tachycardia or while assessing ventriculoatrial conduction using the technique of ventricular extrastimulation or ventricular overdrive pacing (Figure 12-13). Of note, a spontaneously occurring atrial or ventricular premature beat with fast ventriculoatrial conduction through an accessory AV connection can also trigger the onset of atrial flutter-fibrillation (Figures 12-14 & 12-15) [40,41]. Clinically, the frequency with which the onset of atrial flutter-fibrillation is triggered by such a mechanism may be more common than is generally believed.

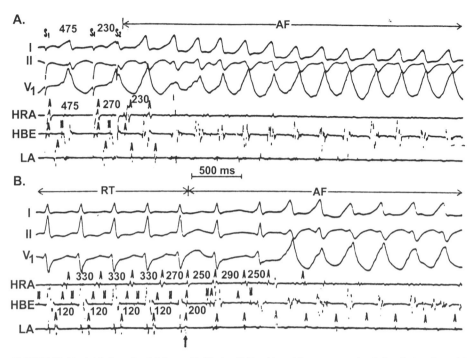

FIGURE 12-12. Initiation of atrial flutter-fibrillation (AF) with atrial premature stimulation during the atrial vulnerable phase (Panel A). ECG leads I, II, and V_1 are recorded simultaneously with high right atrial (HRA), His bundle (HBE), and left atrial (LA) electrograms through coronary sinus. The HRA is driven at a cycle length (S_1-S_1) of 475 ms: An atrial premature stimulus (S_2) with a premature coupling interval (S_1-S_2) of 230 ms initiates the onset of atrial flutter-fibrillation with a mean cycle length of 210 ms. During atrial flutter-fibrillation, the accessory AV connection maintains anterograde conduction for all propagated beats. The corresponding ventricular rate is approximately 290/min. Panel B: Spontaneous conversion of AV reciprocating tachycardia (RT) to atrial flutter-fibrillation initiated by an atrial premature depolarization to the HRA (arrow) (same patient as in Panel A). Note that LA activation precedes HBE and HRA activation during AV reciprocating tachycardia, suggesting the presence of a left-sided accessory AV connection. A = atrial electrogram, H = His bundle potential. From [35] with permission.

Atrial vulnerability is enhanced during AV reciprocating tachycardia because of its associated short cycle length and loss of AV synchrony with resultant atrial stretch [22,42,43]. This may account for the common occurrence of spontaneous conversion of AV reciprocating tachycardia to atrial flutter-fibrillation. Electrophysiology study has demonstrated that the abrupt transition from AV reciprocating tachycardia to atrial flutter-fibrillation is usually precipitated by an atrial premature depolarization (Figures 12-12 & 12-16) [41,44]. The spontaneous occurrence of atrial premature depolarization during AV reciprocating tachycardia can be explained by (1) atrial automaticity or atrial reentry induced by atrial stretch or shortened atrial cycle length of the tachycardia and (2) the potential presence of multiple accessory AV connections, allowing ventriculoatrial conduction over different conduction pathways.

Atrial flutter-fibrillation may also spontaneously convert to AV reciprocating tachycardia (Figures 12-16 through 12-18) [41]. For this electrophysiological phenomenon to occur, it requires the presence or development of anterograde unidirectional block

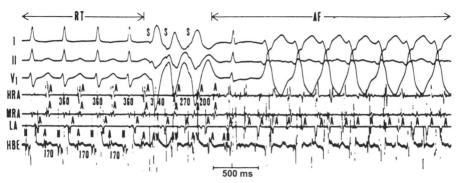

FIGURE 12-13. Conversion of AV reciprocating tachycardia (RT) to atrial flutter-fibrillation (AF) while attempting to terminate RT with ventricular premature stimulation. Note that the sequence of retrograde atrial activation produced by the three successive ventricular premature depolarizations is identical to that recorded during RT; i.e., left atrial (LA) activation (via the coronary sinus) precedes low septal right atrial activation (in HBE lead), middle right atrial (MRA) and high right atrial activation suggestive of ventriculoatrial conduction via a left-sided accessory AV connection. Abbreviations as in Figure 12-7.

in the accessory AV connection prior to spontaneous cessation of atrial flutter-fibrillation. The last atrial impulse of atrial flutter-fibrillation, which conducts anterograde through the normal AV conduction system, enters the accessory AV connection in a retrograde direction and then reactivates the atrium, initiating an AV reciprocating tachycardia. As expected, this phenomenon occurs more commonly in patients with an accessory AV connection which is capable only of retrograde conduction (concealed Wolff-Parkinson-White syndrome) [41]. Under these circumstances, the depth of anterograde penetration of the accessory AV connection, the conduction time through the AV node–His–Purkinje system, the effective refractory period of the atrium, and effective refractory period of the accessory AV connection in the retrograde direction will influence the occurrence of this phenomenon. Specifically, a decrease in the depth of anterograde penetration of the accessory AV connection associated with a preexisting or development of bundle branch block ipsilateral to the accessory connection and shortening of the

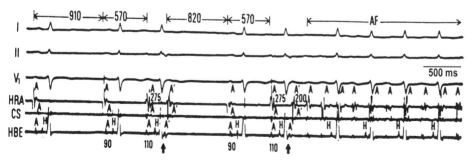

FIGURE 12-14. Atrial premature depolarization-induced AV reciprocal rhythm and atrial flutter-fibrillation (AF) in a patient with a right-sided septal accessory AV connection. CS = coronary sinus. Other abbreviations as in Figure 12-13. Arrows indicate ventriculoatrial activation following atrial premature beats. From [41] with permission.

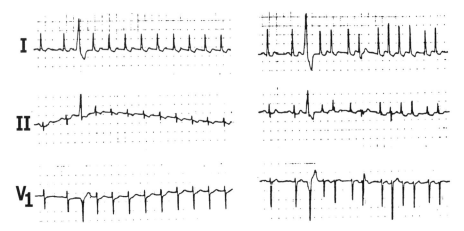

FIGURE 12-15. Initiation of paroxysmal supraventricular tachycardia and atrial fibrillation by spontaneous ventricular premature depolarizations in a patient with concealed Wolff-Parkinson-White syndrome. (Left Panel) During sinus rhythm at a cycle length of 650 ms, a ventricular premature depolarization (3rd QRS complex) with a premature coupling interval of 400 ms initiates the onset of supraventricular tachycardia (cycle length 450 ms). (Right Panel) During sinus rhythm at a cycle length of 700 ms, a ventricular premature depolarization (3rd QRS complex) with a premature coupling interval of 340 ms precipitates the onset of atrial fibrillation. From [40] with permission.

effective refractory periods of the atrium and the accessory AV connection favors the conversion of atrial flutter-fibrillation to AV reciprocating tachycardia following spontaneous termination of flutter-fibrillation.

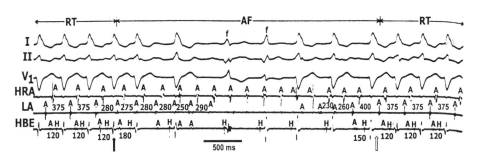

FIGURE 12-16. Spontaneous conversion between reciprocating tachycardia (RT) and atrial flutter-fibrillation (AF) in a patient with a left-sided accessory AV connection. The left atrial depolarization (A-A interval of 280 ms) following the fourth QRS complex (solid arrow) is premature with respect to the expected reciprocating rhythm (A-A interval of 375 ms) during RT. The corresponding A-H interval is lengthened from 120 ms to 180 ms following the atrial premature depolarization. A short run of AF with a mean atrial cycle length of 240 ms is then initiated. During AF, the atrial electrograms are fairly regular in the HRA lead but are fractionated in both left atrial (LA, via coronary sinus) and His bundle electrographic (HBE) leads. The seventh and eighth QRS complexes are fusion beats (f) as evidenced by the inscription of delta wave (ventricular pre-excitation) before the His bundle potential (H). The eleventh QRS complex is the last AF conducted beat which then enters the left atrium (hollow arrow) initiating an onset of RT. Note that prior to the conversion of AF to RT, anterograde conduction within the accessory AV connection of the last three AF conducted beats (ninth, tenth and eleventh QRS complexes) is blocked as evidenced by disappearance of the delta wave and normalization of the H-V interval (50 ms). A complete left bundle branch block pattern is present during RT. From [41] with permission.

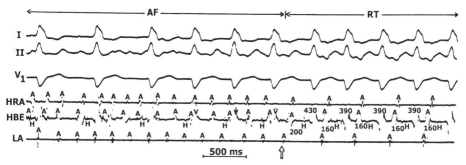

FIGURE 12-17. Spontaneous conversion of atrial flutter-fibrillation (AF) to reciprocating tachycardia (RT) in a patient with a left-sided accessory AV connection. The sixth QRS complex is the last AF conducted beat which then enters the left atrium (hollow arrow), initiating an onset of RT. A complete left bundle branch block pattern with an H-V interval of 55 ms is present during both AF and RT. Persistent anterograde unidirectional block in left-sided accessory AV connection has been demonstrated during an electrophysiological study in this patient. Abbreviations as in Figure 12-16. From [41] with permission.

12.2.5 DOUBLE VENTRICULAR RESPONSES

Rarely, an atrial impulse conducted simultaneously over the normal and accessory pathways may produce a double ventricular response (1:2 AV conduction) [45,46] similar to that occurring in patients with dual AV nodal pathways [47] or atriofascicular accessory connection [48]. This can occur because of the marked difference in conduction time between the two AV conduction pathways, with an atrial impulse first activating the ventricle through the accessory AV connection and then reactivating the ventricle through the AV node-His Purkinje system. The difference in conduction time between the two AV conduction pathways must therefore be longer than the effective refractory period of the His-Purkinje system and the ventricles. Slow conduction in the AV node, a minimal degree of retrograde concealed conduction of the His-Purkinje system induced by ventricular preexcitation, and a short effective refractory period of the ventricle favor the development of this phenomenon. Repetition of double ventricular responses during sinus rhythm or an atrial arrhythmia may theoretically generate a non-reentrant form of tachycardia similar to that of patients with dual AV node pathway physiology [49].

12.2.6 CONCEALED CONDUCTION WITHIN ACCESSORY AV CONNECTIONS

Concealed conduction occurs when a non-propagated impulse influences the conduction of a subsequent impulse [50]. In the human heart, this unique electrophysiologic phenomenon has been shown to occur in the atrium, AV node-His-Purkinje system as well as accessory AV connections [51-56]. Concealed conduction in accessory AV connections can systematically be demonstrated to occur in both anterograde and retrograde directions using the technique of programmed electrical stimulation (Figures 12-19 & 12-20) [56]. The occurrence of concealed conduction in accessory AV connections in both anterograde and retrograde directions is one of the factors modulating the initiation of AV reciprocating tachycardia by an atrial or ventricular premature depolarization and

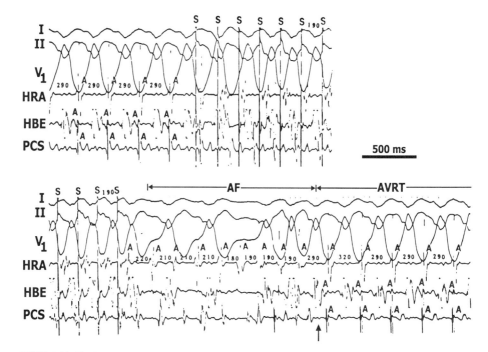

FIGURE 12-18. Spontaneous conversion of atrial flutter to antidromic atrioventricular (AV) reciprocating tachycardia. Panel A: An antidromic AV reciprocating tachycardia manifests ventricular preexcitation with a positive deflection in lead V₁ and a negative deflection in leads I and II, with a cycle length of 290 ms. Note the sequence of retrograde atrial activation is first in the low septal atrial electrogram in the His bundle electrographic lead (HBE), followed by proximal coronary sinus atrial (PCS) and high right atrial (HRA) activities. Rapid atrial stimulation (S) at a cycle length of 190 ms is attempted to terminate the antidromic AV reciprocating tachycardia. Panel B: The tracing is continuous from that in panel A. Rapid atrial stimulation inadvertently provokes the onset of atrial flutter with a cycle length of 190 to 220 ms. The atrial flutter (AF) is short-lived, as it spontaneously reverts to the antidromic form of AV reciprocating tachycardia (AVRT) (up arrow), with a cycle length of 290 to 320 ms. Note that the sequence of retrograde atrial activation is identical to that of antidromic AV reciprocating tachycardia before rapid atrial stimulation (panel A). A, atrial electrogram. From [148] with permission.

regulating the rate of ventricular response during atrial flutter-fibrillation in the Wolff-Parkinson-White syndrome [36,38].

12.3   Concealed Wolff-Parkinson-White Syndrome

The classical electrocardiographic features of ventricular preexcitation (a short P-R interval and a broad QRS complex with a delta wave) are absent in patients with accessory AV connections capable only of retrograde conduction (i.e., accessory AV connection with anterograde unidirectional block). Such patients are also prone to the development of supraventricular tachycardia and atrial flutter-fibrillation and are often said to have the *concealed Wolff-Parkinson-White syndrome* [35,57-59].

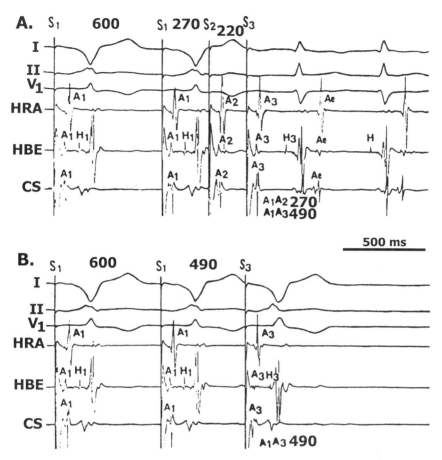

FIGURE 12-19. Anterograde concealed conduction in an accessory AV connection. Panel A: Two consecutive atrial premature beats (A_2 and A_3) are blocked in a left-sided accessory AV connection during coronary sinus (CS) pacing at a basic drive cycle length (A_1-A_1) of 600 ms. The A_1-A_2 and A_2-A_3 intervals are 270 ms and 220 ms, respectively. Note that A_2 is blocked in both the normal AV pathway and accessory AV connection and that A_3 is conducted over the normal AV pathway initiating an AV reciprocating tachycardia using the accessory AV connection for retrograde conduction (Panel B). Conduction of A_3 is restored in the accessory AV connection with removal of A_2. Also note that A_3 no longer can initiate AV reciprocation. These findings suggest that A_2 has conducted in a concealed fashion in the accessory AV connection, thereby preventing subsequent A_3 conduction in the same conduction pathway as in Panel A. HRA, high right atrium; HBE, His bundle electrographic lead; CS, coronary sinus. From [56] with permission.

In the presence of a concealed accessory AV connection, neither right nor left atrial pacing is capable of producing ventricular preexcitation. However, the sequence of retrograde atrial activation and retrograde AV conduction properties induced by programmed ventricular stimulation are those of an accessory AV connection i.e., an eccentric atrial activation sequence showing right or left atrial preexcitation and a relatively constant ventriculoatrial conduction time without refractory-dependent conduction delay (non-decremental conduction properties) [12,27,34,35,38,41]. Although "impedance mismatch" has been used to explain the development of anterograde unidirectional conduction block in these accessory AV connections [60], the pathophysiology responsible for such development remains unknown. Some of these accessory AV connections may have extremely long anterograde effective refractory periods, as ventricular preexcitation may become overt during sinus bradycardia induced by vagal maneuvers or during intravenous isoproterenol infusion [61,62]. During electrophysiology study, adenosine bolus can be administered during isoproterenol infusion to enhance anterograde conduction through the accessory AV connection, thereby maximizing the degree of ventricular preexcitation.

Electrophysiologic manifestations of concealed accessory AV connections can include any or all of the following (Figure 12-21) [41]: (1) retrograde atrial activation by

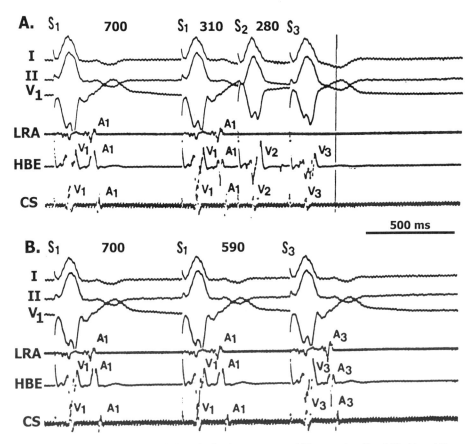

FIGURE 12-20. Retrograde concealed conduction in an accessory AV connection (Panel A). V_2 and V_3 are blocked in a right-sided accessory AV connection during right ventricular pacing at a basic cycle length (V_1-V_1) of 700 ms. The V_1-V_2 and V_2-V_3 intervals are 310 ms and 280 ms, respectively (Panel B). Conduction of V_3 is restored in the accessory AV connection with removal of V_2. These findings suggest that V_2 has concealed conduction in the accessory AV connection, thereby preventing subsequent V_3 conduction in the same conduction pathway as in Panel A. Note atrial preexcitation in which lateral right atrial (LRA) activation precedes low septal right atrial (HBE, His bundle electrographic lead) and left atrial activation (CS, coronary sinus) during the basic drive. From [56] with permission.

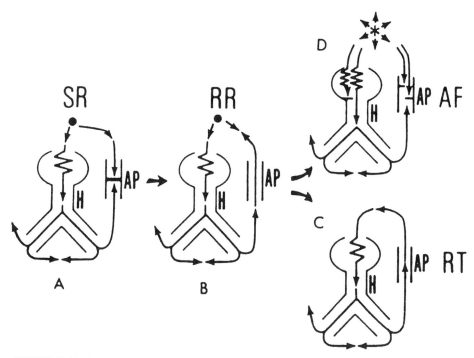

FIGURE 12-21. Schematic representation of the electrophysiologic manifestation of a concealed accessory AV connection. Panel A: During sinus rhythm (SR), the impulse conducts over the normal AV conduction pathway (AV node-His-Purkinje system) to the ventricle. There is no ventricular preexcitation, because the accessory AV connection (AP) is capable only of retrograde conduction (anterograde unidirectional block). Panel B: Retrograde atrial activation by way of the AP results in an AV reciprocal rhythm (RR). Panel C: Perpetuation of the AV reciprocal rhythm (RR) leads to AV reciprocating tachycardia (RT). Panel D: During AV RR, retrograde atrial activation during the atrial vulnerable phase may provoke onset of atrial flutter or atrial fibrillation (AF). H = His bundle. From [41] with permission.

way of the accessory AV connection, resulting in one non-conducted atrial "echo" beat referred to as an AV reciprocal rhythm; (2) perpetuation of an AV reciprocal rhythm leading to an orthodromic AV reciprocating tachycardia (Figure 12-22); or (3) retrograde atrial activation during the atrial vulnerability period resulting in an onset of atrial flutter-fibrillation (Figure 12-14). Furthermore, with preexisting anterograde unidirectional conduction block in the accessory AV connection, acceleration of sinus rhythm can in itself instigate an onset of AV reciprocating tachycardia (Figure 12-23) [41,63]. This is because shortening of the sinus cycle length decreases effective refractory periods of both the atrium and the accessory AV connection, thereby favoring the occurrence of retrograde atrial activation (atrial preexcitation) which then leads to AV reciprocating tachycardia. In addition, the development of functional bundle branch block ipsilateral to the accessory AV connection may facilitate the initiation of AV reciprocating tachycardia by delaying the impulse arrival at the ventricular end of the accessory AV connection (Figure 12-24). The ease with which AV reciprocation (circus movement) can be initiated in the presence of a concealed accessory AV connection explains why the concealed

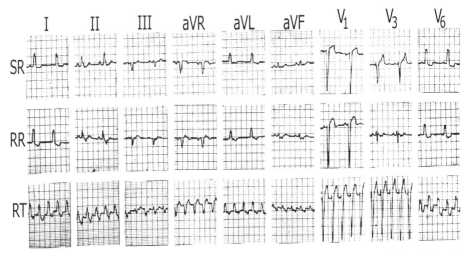

FIGURE 12-22. Sinus rhythm (SR), AV reciprocal rhythm (RR) (i.e., non-conducted atrial "echo" beats), and AV reciprocating tachycardia (RT) in a 71 year old woman with concealed Wolff-Parkinson-White syndrome. Complete left bundle branch block is present in all three rhythms. The retrograde P wave (negative in leads II, III, and aVF) has a configuration identical to those seen during AV RR and AV RT. Note the R-P interval is shorter than the P-R interval during the AV RR (R-P = 0.13 sec vs. P-R = 0.16 sec) and AV RT (R-P = 0.13 sec vs. P-R = 0.22 sec). From [41] with permission.

FIGURE 12-23. Incessant supraventricular tachycardia in a 38 year old man with complete left bundle branch block associated with a concealed left-sided accessory pathway. Panel A: Carotid sinus massage temporarily interrupts the supraventricular tachycardia. Note that the retrograde P wave is upright in the aVR lead, and the R-P interval is shorter than the P-R interval during the tachycardia. Panel B: Spontaneous initiation of the tachycardia after acceleration of the sinus rate (shortening of the sinus cycle length from 1040 to 1010 ms). Panel C: The tachycardia is finally controlled by right ventricular pacing at a cycle length of 540 ms. The first pacemaker-captured beat with a ventricular premature coupling interval of 330 ms terminates the tachycardia. Because of preexisting complete left bundle branch block, the right bundle branch and right ventricle are a part of the AV reciprocating tachycardia circuit. By depolarizing the right ventricle, right ventricular pacing is effective in terminating the AV reciprocating tachycardia. From [63] with permission.

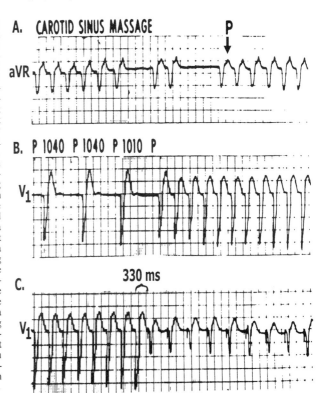

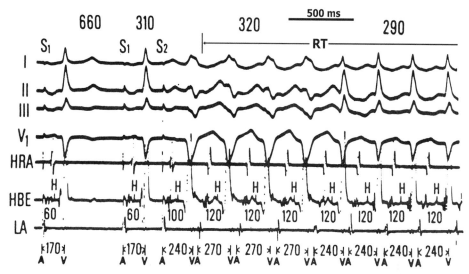

FIGURE 12-24. Initiation of AV reciprocating tachycardia (RT) during development of functional left bundle branch block in the presence of a concealed accessory AV connection on the left side. During atrial (left atrium) pacing at a cycle length (S_1-S_1) of 660 ms, an atrial premature depolarization (S_2) with a premature coupling interval (S_1-S_2) of 310 ms initiates an onset of AV reciprocating tachycardia. A concealed accessory AV connection on the left side is used for retrograde conduction during tachycardia. The presence of a concealed accessory AV connection is demonstrated by the presence of retrograde left atrial (LA, from coronary sinus) activation preceding low septal right atrial (HBE) and high right atrial (HRA) activation during tachycardia. The cycle length of tachycardia is 320 ms with, 290 ms without the complete left bundle branch block pattern. From [41] with permission.

Wolff-Parkinson-White syndrome is one of the causes of incessant supraventricular tachycardia (Figure 12-23) [64,65].

12.4   Accessory Connections with Decremental Conduction Properties

Accessory nodoventricular and fasciculoventricular connections classically are thought to arise from the AV node and the His bundle or bundle branches, respectively, and insert into the right ventricle. These accessory connections are often referred to as Mahaim fibers [7,66,-71]. Aside from producing a fixed QRS pattern of ventricular fusion (ventricular preexcitation through both the accessory connection and the normal AV conduction system), fasciculoventricular (His bundle or bundle branches to the ventricle) connections are usually not involved in the genesis of AV reciprocating tachycardia [69]. In contrast, a nodoventricular connection often participates in the initiation of an antidromic AV reciprocating tachycardia mimicking ventricular tachycardia. The antidromic AV reciprocating tachycardia uses the accessory nodoventricular connection for anterograde conduction and the normal AV conduction system for retrograde conduction. The atria are not a necessary link for the reentrant circuit and AV dissociation may occur during this form of antidromic AV reciprocating tachycardia.

The nodoventricular connection exhibits decremental conduction properties so that it can be associated with either a short or normal PR interval depending on the precise exit point of the accessory connection relative to the area of AV nodal conduction delay. At baseline, the QRS complex can be either normal or showing varying degrees of ventricular preexcitation resulting from fusion of impulse propagation through the normal and accessory conduction pathways. Incremental atrial pacing and progressive atrial premature stimulation prolong the PR and A-H (AV nodal conduction time) intervals and increase the degree of ventricular preexcitation while decreasing the H-V interval. The prolongation of the PR interval is less than that of the A-H interval. Consequently, the His bundle deflection is displaced into the ventricular electrogram and the degree of AV conduction over the nodoventricular connection (ventricular preexcitation) is increased. Total ventricular preexcitation observed during this form of antidromic reciprocating tachycardia has been typically characterized by a left bundle branch block pattern [19,26,69,72,73], suggesting insertion of the accessory nodoventricular connection into the right ventricle (right ventricular preexcitation). Characteristically, His bundle pacing at the same rate as that of atrial pacing which induces total ventricular preexcitation will normalize the QRS complex (disappearance of ventricular preexcitation). Rarely, a nodoventricular connection can be inserted in the left ventricle or its specialized conduction system [74].

12.4.1 ANTIDROMIC AV RECIPROCATING TACHYCARDIA

Anatomically there may be two varieties of accessory nodoventricular connections [75,76]: one emerging from the fast AV nodal pathway area (anterior transitional cell zone) and the other from the slow AV nodal pathway area (posterior transitional cell zone) of the AV junction. The latter variety may also be referred to as Paladino fibers [7]. An accessory nodoventricular connection bridging the fast pathway and the right ventricle exhibit right ventricular preexcitation during sinus rhythm, which becomes more marked with gradual prolongation of the PR interval with atrial extrastimulation (Figure 12-25). Furthermore, during programmed atrial stimulation, a shift from fast to slow AV nodal pathway conduction results in a sudden disappearance of right ventricular preexcitation. Discontinuous AV nodal conduction curves (A_1A_2, A_2H_2 and A_1A_2, H_1H_2) may be exposed [76].

An accessory nodoventricular connection bridging the slow pathway and the right ventricle has distinctly different electrophysiologic characteristics [76]. Firstly, right ventricular preexcitation is usually absent during sinus rhythm. Secondly, during programmed atrial stimulation, a shift from fast to slow pathway conduction results in a sudden appearance of complete left bundle branch block QRS pattern (right ventricular preexcitation) disrupting AV conduction curves (A_1A_2, V_1V_2) (Figure 12-26 & 12-27). This may be followed by induction of an antidromic AV reciprocating tachycardia using the slow pathway-accessory nodoventricular connection for anterograde conduction and the fast pathway-His-Purkinje system for retrograde conduction. These findings are in keeping with the observation that both fast and slow AV nodal pathways at the AV junc-

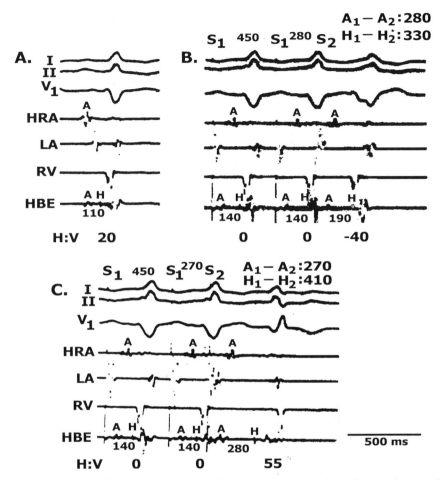

FIGURE 12-25. Effects of atrial premature stimulation in the presence of a fast pathway-nodoventricular connection. Panel A: Right ventricular preexcitation is evident during sinus rhythm with an A-H interval of 110 ms and a P-R interval of 150 ms. Panel B: During left atrial pacing at a cycle length of 450 ms, the A-H interval is increased to 140 ms and the P-R interval is increased to 160 ms, whereas the H-V interval is short-ened from 20 to 0 ms with more right ventricular preexcitation. An atrial premature stimulation with a pre-mature coupling interval of 280 ms prolongs the A-H interval to 190 ms and the P-R interval to 180 ms and produces a greater degree of right ventricular preexcitation. Note that the H-V interval is decreased to –40 ms. Panel C: Atrial premature stimulation with a premature coupling interval of 270 ms suddenly increased the A-H interval to 280 ms (a shift from a fast to slow AV nodal pathway conduction) and is followed by total disappearance of ventricular preexcitation (the third QRS complex with a right bundle branch block pattern and an H-V interval of 55 ms). A, atrial electrogram, H, His bundle electrogram; RV, right ventricle; other abbreviations as in Figure 12-24.

tion have anatomically separate locations in either anterograde or retrograde direction [77,78].

The concept of Mahaim fibers has been extended to include accessory atriofasciu-lar and accessory AV connections with decremental conduction properties [79,80]. In fact, some connections previously thought to be accessory nodoventricular connections have been shown to be either accessory atriofascicular or AV connections with decre-

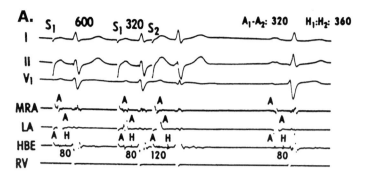

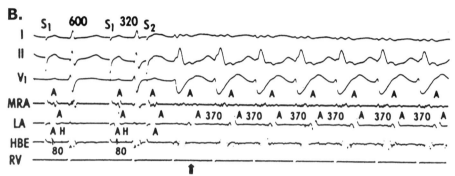

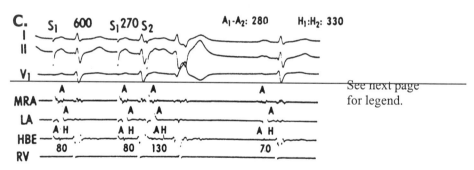

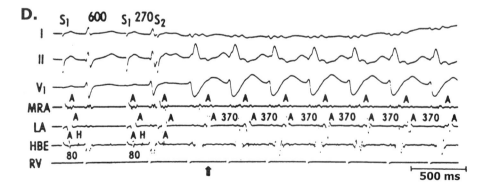

See next page for legend.

500 ms

mental conduction properties. In most cases, these accessory connections are right-sided, crossing the tricuspid annulus and inserting in the right bundle branch or right ventricle [81-83]. Electrophysiology study has demonstrated that the portion of these accessory atriofascicular or AV connections exhibiting decremental conduction properties is most likely located in the tissue above the AV annulus. The electrophysiologic basis for decremental conduction properties exhibited by these accessory connections is not well understood. It is tempting to postulate that there is a group of cells with functional characteristics similar to those found in the AV node, such as Kent nodes representing the remnants of the embryologic "specialized" myocardial ring [84-87] bridging the atrium and the fascicle or ventricular myocardium. Other possibilities include (1) tortuosity of the fiber course in connection to the ventricle and (2) nonhomogenous electrophysiologic properties of individual myocardial fibers which make up the accessory connections. These atriofascicular fibers with decremental conduction properties are often localized at the posterolateral wall of the right atrium (Figure 12-28) [80,88]. In patients with an accessory atriofascicular connection, the frequent recording of Purkinje potentials preceding the right ventricular preexcitation pattern (complete left bundle branch block), implicates a connection between the right atrium and a fascicle of the right bundle branch in the genesis of ventricular preexcitation. However, the specificity of these Purkinje potentials recorded in association with ventricular preexcitation needs to be determined as they are frequently recorded in the ventricles.

12.4.2 THE PERMANENT FORM OF THE JUNCTIONAL RECIPROCATING TACHYCARDIA

The permanent form of junctional reciprocating tachycardia (PJRT) [89-91] is caused by orthodromic AV reciprocation using an accessory AV connection exhibiting decremental conduction properties in the retrograde direction [91-95]. Because of anterograde unidirectional block in the accessory AV connection, there is no evidence of ventricular

FIGURE 12-26. *(Preceding page)* Atrial premature stimulation with intermittent induction of sustained reciprocating tachycardia in a patient with an accessory slow pathway-nodoventricular connection. The high right atrium is driven at a cycle length (S_1-S_1) of 600 ms. The AV nodal conduction time (A-H) lengthens progressively as the atrial premature coupling interval (S_1-S_2) gradually shortens. Sustained reciprocating tachycardia could be intermittently induced between premature coupling intervals (S_1-S_2) of 320 and 270 ms. Panel A: An atrial premature depolarization at a coupling interval (S_1-S_2) of 320 ms is conducted to the ventricle with an incomplete right bundle branch block pattern. The corresponding A-H and H-V intervals are 120 and 50 ms, respectively. Panel B: An atrial premature depolarization at the same coupling interval (S_1-S_2) of 320 ms is conducted to the ventricle with complete left bundle branch block pattern followed by initiation of a sustained reciprocating tachycardia (arrow). Note the sudden disappearance of the His bundle potential and prolongation of AV conduction time (A_2-V_2) before ventricular activation with a complete left bundle branch block pattern. Panel C: An atrial premature depolarization at a coupling interval (S_1-S_2) of 270 ms is conducted to the ventricle with a complete right bundle branch block pattern and a superior axis. The corresponding A-H and H-V intervals are 130 and 65 ms, respectively. Panel D: An atrial premature depolarization at the same coupling interval (S_1-S_2) of 270 ms is conducted to the ventricle with a complete left bundle branch block pattern, followed by initiation of sustained reciprocating tachycardia (arrow). Also note the sudden disappearance of the His bundle potential and prolongation of the AV conduction time A_2-V_2 before ventricular activation with a complete left bundle branch block pattern similar to that seen in Panel B. The sudden disappearance of the His bundle potential is caused by an abrupt shift from fast to slow pathway with resultant slow pathway-accessory nodoventricular preexcitation (complete left bundle block pattern). During reciprocating tachycardia (both Panels B and D), the low septal right atrial electrogram cannot clearly be separated from the ventricular electrogram. However, the mid-right atrial electrogram (MRA) activation precedes the left atrial (LA) activation, and the ventriculoatrial conduction time is constant after initiation of tachycardia. Abbreviations as in Figure 12-13 and Figure 12-25. From [75] with permission.

preexcitation during either sinus or an atrial paced rhythm. During AV reciprocating tachycardia, the RP interval is longer than the PR interval (a form of long RP tachycardia) [64,92] because of decremental conduction of the accessory AV connection in the retrograde direction. This is in contrast to the typical orthodromic AV reciprocating tachycardia in which the RP interval is shorter than the PR interval due to the lack of refractory-dependent conduction delay of the accessory AV connection. This form of long RP tachycardia [92] needs to be distinguished from ectopic atrial tachycardia and the atypical form of AV nodal reentrant tachycardia [96,97].

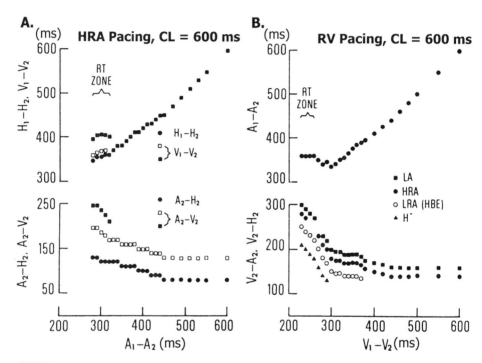

FIGURE 12-27. A_1-A_2, H_1-H_2 (A_1-A_2, V_1-V_2) and A_1-A_2, A_2-H_2 (A_1-A_2, A_2-V_2) curves during high right atrial (HRA) pacing at a cycle length (CL) of 600 ms (panel A) (same patient as in Figure 12-26). There is gradual prolongation of AV nodal conduction time (A_2-H_2) as the atrial premature coupling interval (A_1-A_2) progressively shortens, compatible with AV nodal properties. However, between premature coupling intervals (A_1-A_2) of 320 and 270 ms, an atrial premature depolarization (A_2) is conducted to the ventricle with either an incomplete-to-complete right bundle branch block pattern (open squares) or a complete left bundle branch block pattern (closed squares). Of note, when the incomplete-to-complete right bundle branch pattern appears, it is always preceded by a His bundle potential with an H-V interval of 50-65 ms. When the complete left bundle branch block pattern appears, the His bundle potential suddenly disappears and it is followed by initiation of a sustained reciprocating tachycardia (RT) (Figure 12-26). The sudden disappearance of the His bundle potential is caused by an abrupt shift from fast to slow pathway with resultant slow pathway-accessory nodoventricular preexcitation (complete left bundle branch block pattern). Panel B: V_1-V_2, V_2-A_2, and V_1-V_2, A_1-A_2 curves during right ventricular (RV) pacing at a cycle length of 600 ms. Note that the sequence of ventriculoatrial conduction is the low septal right atrium (LRA) initially, followed by the HRA, and then the left atrium (LA) compatible with retrograde conduction by way of the AV node (fast pathway)-His-Purkinje system. Additionally, the progressive ventriculoatrial conduction delay as the ventricular premature coupling interval (V_1-V_2) gradually shortens is in keeping with the retrograde conduction properties of the AV node-His-Purkinje system. RT could be elicited between ventricular premature coupling intervals of 260 and 230 ms. From [75] with permission.

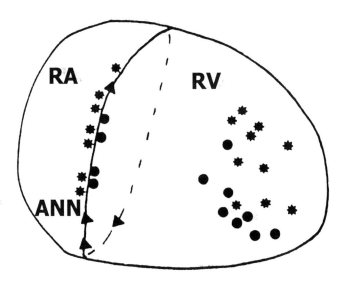

FIGURE 12-28. Schematic illustration of the different types of anterograde decrementally conducting accessory AV connections as viewed in the right anterior oblique projection. Black stars indicate the long atriofascicular accessory connections; black-filled circles represent the long accessory AV connections; black-filled triangles denote the location of the short accessory AV pathways. ANN, septal border of the tricuspid annulus; RA, right atrium; RV, right ventricle. From [88] with permission.

Participation of such a concealed accessory AV connection with decremental conduction properties capable only of retrograde conduction is analogous to the situation in which a concealed accessory AV connection without decremental conduction properties is used for retrograde conduction during orthodromic reciprocating tachycardia [41,57-59]. These accessory AV connections are commonly located at the mid-septum of the atrium and close to the coronary sinus ostium (Figure 12-29) [15,69,91-95], and have

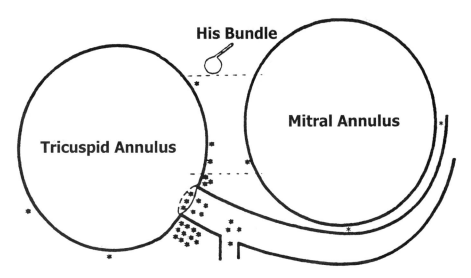

FIGURE 12-29. Schematic diagram drawn in 60° left anterior oblique view displaying the successful site (asterisks) of radiofrequency catheter ablation of 33 accessory connections exhibiting retrograde decremental conduction and participating in long RP tachycardias. Dashed lines denote the mid-septal region. From [144] with permission.

been, therefore, called accessory AV nodes because of their proximity to the AV node near the slow AV nodal pathway area. Nevertheless, they have also been localized to be in the right and left atrial free walls (Figures 12-30 & 12-31) [88,98] and responds to verapamil similar to AV nodal tissue [98]. Hence, the term "PJRT" should be referred to as "orthodromic AV reciprocating tachycardia with a long RP interval." Of note, intermittent ventricular preexcitation with anterograde decremental conduction properties has also been demonstrated in few patients with the so-called PJRT tachycardia. These findings suggest a unified mechanism for both antidromic and orthodromic AV reciprocating tachycardia in patients with accessory connections with decremental conduction properties. It is tempting to postulate that there may be an involvement of Kent nodes, the remnants of embryologic "specialized" myocardial ring, in both anterograde and retrograde directions responsible for PJRT, and for antidromic AV reciprocating tachycardia involving an atriofascicular or AV connection with decremental conduction properties [84-87].

12.4.3 ATRIAL FLUTTER-FIBRILLATION & NODOVENTRICULAR CONNECTIONS

During atrial flutter or fibrillation, anterograde conduction via an accessory nodoventricular connection usually exhibits a complete left bundle branch block pattern (right ventricular preexcitation). However, if there is preexisting or functional right bundle branch block, the QRS complexes may show intermittent complete right and left bundle branch block patterns mimicking bilateral bundle branch block (Figure 12-32) [75]. Intracardiac recordings should reveal that the QRS complex of the complete right bundle branch block pattern is always preceded by a His bundle potential with an H-V interval equal to, or longer than, the baseline H-V interval of the sinus rhythm. In contrast, the QRS complex of a complete left bundle branch block pattern is either not preceded by a His bundle potential or is preceded by a His bundle potential but with an H-V interval shorter than the baseline H-V interval during sinus rhythm.

12.4.4 ACCESSORY ATRIO-HISIAN AND ATRIO-NODAL CONNECTIONS

The presence of an accessory atrio-Hisian or atrio-nodal connection is characterized by a short PR interval ($\leq$ 120 msec in adult subjects) and a normal QRS complex [99-101]. In response to programmed atrial stimulation (incremental atrial pacing and atrial premature extrastimulation), three types of AV conduction curves may be observed: (1) a subnormal prolongation of the A-H interval suggestive of an intranodal (atrionodal) bypass tract or a small AV node; (2) no lengthening of the A-H interval suggestive of an atrio-Hisian connection; and (3) no lengthening of the A-H interval at slow pacing rates, but normal prolongation of the A-H interval at fast pacing rates, suggestive of an accessory atrio-Hisian connection in conjunction with dual AV nodal pathway conduction.

The association of paroxysmal supraventricular and atrial flutter-fibrillation with a short PR interval ($\leq$ 0.12 seconds) and a normal QRS complex during sinus rhythm is referred to as the Lown-Ganong-Levine syndrome [102-108]. Of note, the electrophysiologic mechanism of supraventricular tachycardia associated with the so-called Lown-

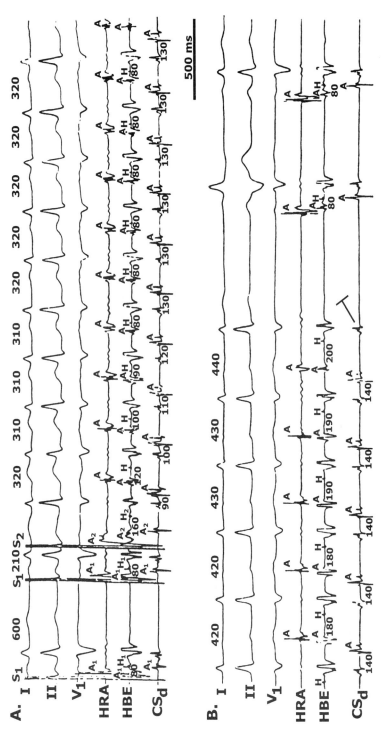

FIGURE 12-30. Termination of AV reciprocating tachycardia by the direct depressive effect of verapamil on the accessory AV connection. Panel A: AV reciprocating tachycardia is initiated by an atrial premature beat (S2) with a premature coupling interval (S₁-S₂) of 210 ms after a basic drive cycle length of (S₁-S₁) of 600 ms. During the tachycardia, the earliest retrograde atrial activation is recorded at the distal coronary sinus (CSd). Note that the ventriculoatrial (V-A) conduction time measured from the CSd progressively lengthens from 90 to 130 ms as the AV nodal conduction time (A-H interval) gradually shortens from 160 to 80 ms. Panel B: Verapamil prolongs AV nodal conduction time (A-H interval increases from 180 to 200 ms) and V-A conduction time (140 ms) and terminates AV reciprocating tachycardia by inducing retrograde conduction block in the accessory connection. HRA, high right atrium; HBE, His bundle electrographic lead. From [98] with permission.

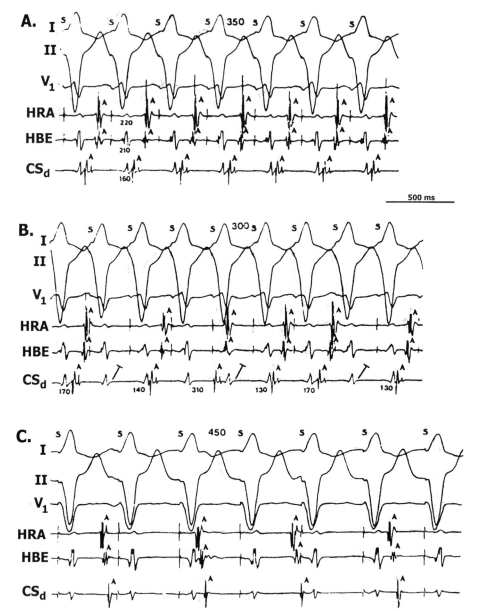

FIGURE 12-31. Effects of intravenous verapamil on ventriculoatrial (V-A) conduction during incremental ventricular pacing (same patient as in Figure 12-30). Panel A: During right ventricular (RV) pacing at a cycle length (S$_1$-S$_1$) of 350 ms, there is a 1:1 VA conduction. The sequence of retrograde atrial activation is identical to that observed during AV reciprocating tachycardia (Figure 12-30). The sequence of retrograde atrial activation is recorded earliest at the distal coronary sinus (CS$_d$), followed by the His bundle (HBE), and finally at the high right atrium (HRA). V-A conduction time measured at the CS$_d$ is 160 ms. Panel B: RV pacing at a cycle length (S$_1$-S$_1$) of 300 ms induces a second degree (Wenkebach) V-A block in the accessory AV connection. Panel C: After intravenous infusion of verapamil, complete V-A block develops during RV pacing at a cycle length (S$_1$-S$_1$) of 450 ms. From [98] with permission.

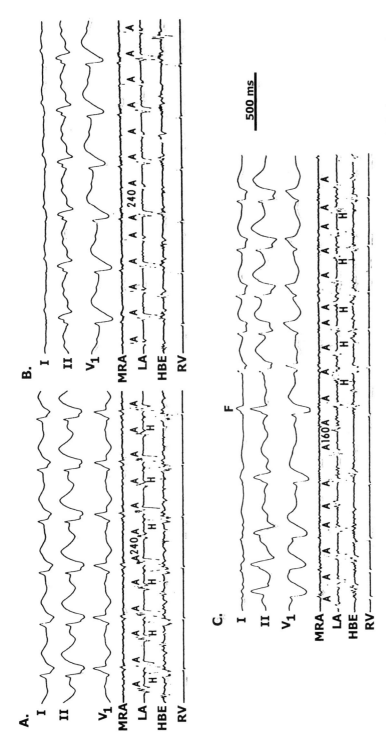

FIGURE 12-32. Intermittent AV conduction by way of the fast AV node-His-Purkinje system pathway and the slow AV node-nodoventricular bypass tract pathway during atrial flutter-fibrillation. Panels A and B: Atrial flutter (atrial cycle length of 240 ms) manifests 2:1 AV block. Note that the QRS complex of a complete right bundle branch block pattern is always preceded by the His bundle potential with an H-V interval of 65 ms (Panel A). In contrast, when the QRS complex shows a complete left bundle branch block pattern, no His bundle activity can be identified (Panel B). Similar phenomena occur during atrial fibrillation with a mean cycle length of 160 ms (Panel C). F = fusion beat. Abbreviations as in Figure 12-26. From [75] with permission.

Ganong-Levine syndrome has been shown to be either AV nodal reentry due to dual AV nodal pathway physiology or AV reciprocation using a concealed accessory AV connection for retrograde conduction (Figure 12-33). There has been no involvement of an accessory atrio-Hisian or atrionodal connection in the tachycardia circuit demonstrated. The rates of tachycardia are significantly higher than those of the same arrhythmias in patients without a baseline short PR interval [88]. Furthermore, the combination of short AV nodal conduction time and abbreviated AV nodal refractory period may result in a very rapid ventricular rate during atrial flutter-fibrillation. Theoretically, atrial flutter-fibrillation with a fast ventricular response may degenerate into ventricular fibrillation leading to sudden cardiac death similar to the Wolff-Parkinson-White syndrome [99-101,108-109].

12.5   Pharmacological Effects on Accessory Connections

Various antiarrhythmic agents have been shown to depress conduction and increase refractoriness of accessory AV connections. These include class I and class III agents, e.g., quinidine, procainamide, disopyramide, lidocaine, mexiletine, encainide, flecainide, propafenone [110,111], sotalol [112], and amiodarone [113]. Intravenous digitalis and verapamil may decrease the effective refractory periods of accessory AV connections. The effect of digitalis on AV connections is probably mediated by its direct pharmacologic action [114], whereas that of verapamil is secondary to a reflex increase in adrenergic tone resulting from its peripheral vasodilation [115,116]. Besides, both digitalis and verapamil depress AV nodal conduction. Hence, intravenous preparations of both agents may enhance and accelerate the rate of conduction over accessory AV connections during atrial flutter-fibrillation (Figure 12-34), leading to degeneration into ventricular fibrillation [114].

Rarely verapamil may exert a depressive action on accessory AV connections and terminate AV reciprocating tachycardia by inducing conduction block in these accessory AV connections [98]. This is in contrast to the usual mechanism by which it terminates AV reciprocating tachycardia, namely by blocking AV nodal conduction [117]. Depending on functional properties of accessory AV connections, intravenous verapamil may: (1) directly prolong conduction and refractoriness of accessory AV connections with decremental conduction properties (Figures 12-30 & 12-31), or (2) indirectly induce alternating long and short cycle lengths (slow and fast AV nodal pathway conduction) which, in turn, leads to conduction block in accessory AV connections associated with an Ashman phenomenon (Figure 12-35).

Changes in autonomic tone can influence functional properties of accessory AV connections [61,62] and affect the rate of ventricular response during atrial flutter-fibrillation. Isoproterenol infusion can shorten anterograde effective refractory periods of the atrium, accessory AV connection, and the ventricle and thereby increase the rate of conduction over the accessory AV connection during atrial flutter-fibrillation [37,38]. β-adrenergic blockade reverses the effects induced by isoproterenol (Figures 12-36 & 12-37) [118]. Furthermore, β-adrenergic blockade depresses AV nodal conduction, thereby

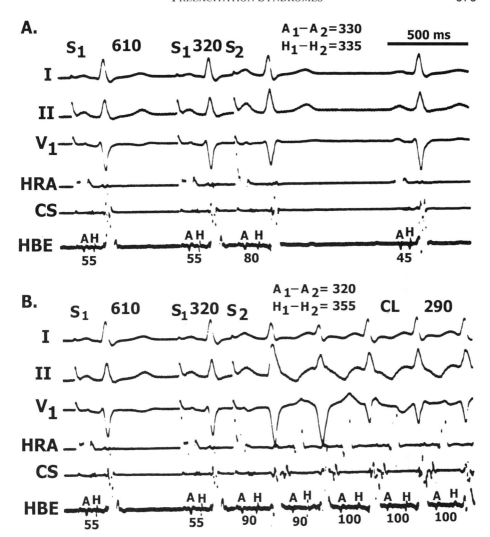

FIGURE 12-33. Induction of AV reciprocating tachycardia involving a concealed left-sided accessory AV connection in a patient with the Lown-Ganong-Levine syndrome. Panel A: Atrial premature stimulation at a driving cycle length of 610 ms produces subnormal prolongation of AV nodal conduction time (A-H interval). Note that the baseline A-H interval of 55 ms and atrial premature stimulation with a coupling interval of 330 ms lengthen the A-H interval to only 80 ms. Panel B: Atrial premature stimulation with a coupling interval of 320 ms increases the A-H interval to 90 ms, provokes development of a functional left bundle branch block, and initiates the onset of AV reciprocating tachycardia using a concealed left-sided accessory AV connection for retrograde conduction. HRA, high right atrium; CS, coronary sinus; HBE, His bundle electrographic lead.

slowing the rate of AV reciprocating tachycardia and may thus reduce the atrial vulnerability [22]. Although β-adrenoceptor blocking agents are not useful for acute treatment of atrial flutter-fibrillation with ventricular preexcitation, chronic treatment with these agents may be beneficial in patients with the Wolff-Parkinson-White syndrome prone to

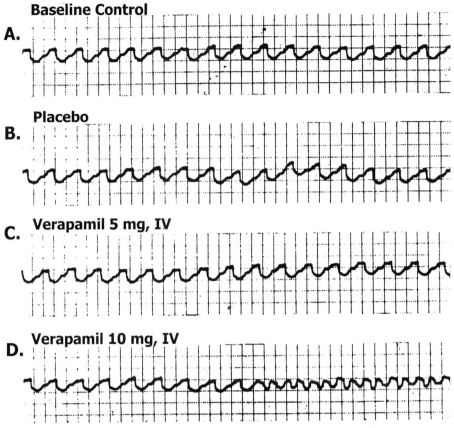

FIGURE 12-34. Acceleration of ventricular responses during atrial flutter in a patient with left-sided accessory AV conduction. Panel A shows atrial flutter with 2:1 conduction over the accessory AV connection. Intravenous infusion with either a placebo (Panel B) or 5 mg verapamil (Panel C) exhibits no effect. However, intravenous infusion of 10 mg verapamil (Panel D) accelerates AV conduction from 2:1 to 1:1 conduction over the accessory AV connection.

atrial flutter-fibrillation by virtue of: 1) reducing atrial vulnerability; 2) preventing catecholamine-induced acceleration of ventricular rate; and 3) depressing catecholamine-induced triggering factors (e.g., atrial or ventricular premature depolarizations [118].

Intravenous bolus infusion of adenosine, an A_1-receptor agonist, can terminate both AV nodal reentrant tachycardia and AV reciprocating tachycardia by depressing conduction in the AV node [119-121]. However, adenosine may also induce conduction block in accessory AV connections, especially those exhibiting decremental conduction properties (Figures 12-38 & 12-39) [122,123].

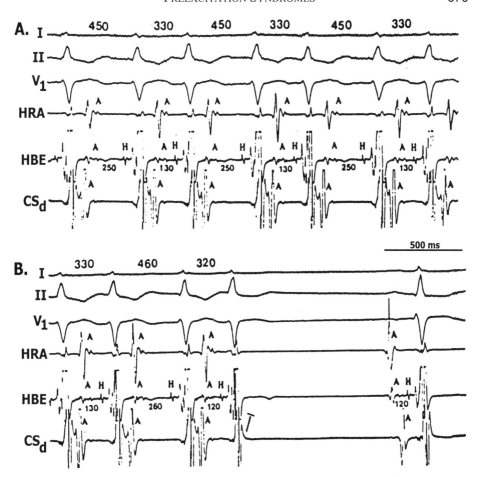

FIGURE 12-35. Termination of AV reciprocating tachycardia by an indirect depressive effect of verapamil on the accessory AV connection. Tracings in panels A and B are continuous. Panel A: After intravenous infusion of verapamil, there is development of alternating long and short AV nodal conduction times (A-H intervals) of 250 and 130 ms resulting in alternating long and short cycle lengths of 450 and 350 ms during the tachycardia. Panel B: The tachycardia is terminated by subsequent development of retrograde conduction block in the anomalous AV bypass tract. Note that the development of this conduction block follows a short cycle length of 460 ms (A-H interval of 260 ms), consistent with the Ashman phenomenon. Abbreviations as in Figure 12-30 and Figure 12-31. From [98] with permission.

12.6 Differential Diagnosis

AV reciprocating tachycardia is the best clinical model in which reentry (circus movement) can be demonstrated to be the underlying mechanism responsible for a sustained tachyarrhythmia. During the tachycardia, the anatomic path is longer than the wavelength of the reentrant depolarization-repolarization wavefront. Between the advancing "head" and the receding "tail" of the reentrant wave there exists an excitable gap that allows a premature depolarization to enter the reentrant circuit, resetting or entraining the

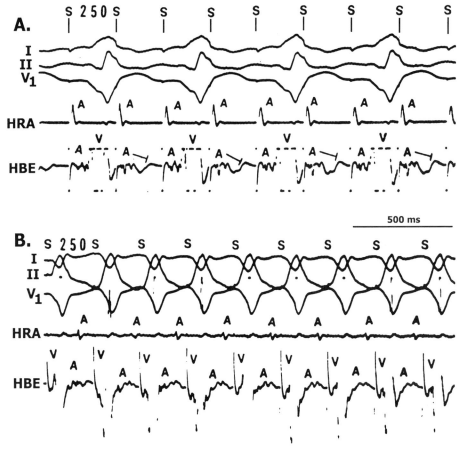

FIGURE 12-36. During high right atrial pacing at a cycle length of 250 ms, there is a 2:1 AV conduction over a right-sided accessory AV connection (Panel A). During right ventricular pacing at the same cycle length of 250 ms, there is 1:1 ventricular capture (Panel B). These findings suggest that 2:1 AV conduction is due to 2:1 conduction block in the accessory AV connection at the cycle length of 250 ms. HRA, high right atrium; CS, coronary sinus; HBE, His bundle electrographic lead; S, electrical stimulus.

tachycardia, or terminating it due to the production of bidirectional block (orthodromic and antidromic) (Figures 12-40, 12-41 & 12-42).

Typically orthodromic AV reciprocating tachycardia has a short RP interval with a retrograde P wave (negative in leads II, III, and aVF) which is inscribed immediately behind the QRS complex. The RP interval is shorter than the PR interval. In contrast, typical AV nodal reentrant tachycardia of the slow-fast form has no discernible retrograde P wave because it is often buried within the QRS complex (it can be inscribed slightly before or behind the QRS complex). Exceptions do exist as accessory septal AV connections may have a retrograde P wave partially buried within the QRS complex and a retrograde fast pathway of AV nodal reentrant tachycardia may manifest relatively slow conduction [124], thereby allowing the retrograde P wave to become clearly discernible. During electrophysiology study, an accessory septal AV connection has a retrograde atri-

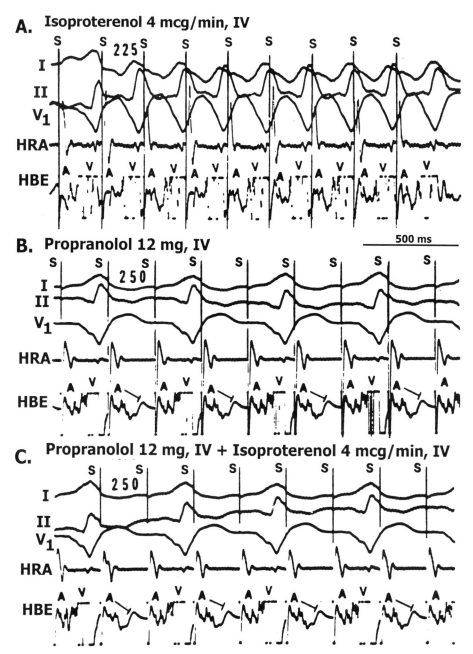

A. Isoproterenol 4 mcg/min, IV

B. Propranolol 12 mg, IV

500 ms

C. Propranolol 12 mg, IV + Isoproterenol 4 mcg/min, IV

FIGURE 12-37. Isoproterenol infusion at 4 μg/min enhances AV conduction over the accessory AV connection with 1:1 conduction up to a cycle length of 225 ms (panel A) (same patient as in Figure 12-36). Panel B: After intravenous infusion of 12 mg propranolol, AV conduction over the accessory pathway is decreased to 2:1. Panel C: Rechallenge with isoproterenol infusion after propranolol fails to enhance AV conduction over the accessory AV connection. HRA, high right atria; HBE, His bundle electrographic lead.

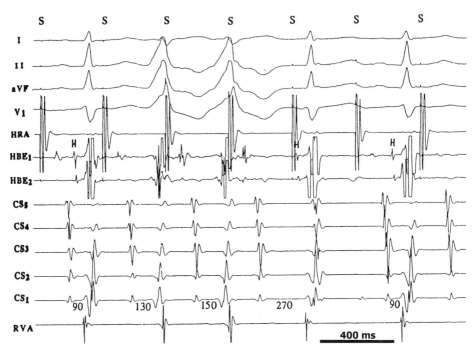

FIGURE 12-38. A left-sided accessory AV connection with decremental conduction properties located in the anterior paraseptal region. Note the Wenkebach periodicity in both the accessory AV connection and the AV node during high right atrial pacing (HRA) pacing at a cycle length of 340 ms (S-S interval). The 2nd and 3rd stimuli (S) induce progressive prolongation of the AV interval (AV interval in the distal coronary sinus lead, CS_1, increased from 130 to 150 ms) and increasing degrees of preexcitation before development of conduction block in the accessory AV connection (the 4th stimulus). The 5th stimulus captures the atria but the impulse is blocked in both the accessory AV connection and the AV node. The 6th stimulus is also blocked in the accessory AV connection but does conduct within the normal AV nodal pathway. HBE, His bundle electrographic lead; H, His bundle potential; CS_1 to CS_5, distal to proximal coronary sinus.

al activation sequence similar to that of retrograde fast AV nodal pathway conduction — septal atrial activation at the His bundle recording site precedes proximal coronary sinus and high right atrial activation. The diagnosis of an accessory septal AV connection conducting in a retrograde direction is supported by (1) atrial preexcitation induced by a ventricular premature beat during the tachycardia (Figure 12-43) and (2) the lack of refractory-dependent conduction delay demonstrated by programmed ventricular stimulation. Moreover, adenosine is more likely to suppress a retrograde fast AV nodal pathway than a retrograde conducting accessory septal AV connection without decremental conduction properties [125,126].

Lengthening of the tachycardia cycle length associated with development of bundle branch block suggests AV reciprocating tachycardia is more likely to be the underlying mechanism (Figure 12-24). Furthermore, it suggests that the location of the accessory AV connection is ipsilateral to the side of the bundle branch block which delays impulse arrival at the ventricular end of the accessory AV connection during orthodromic AV reciprocating tachycardia. Nevertheless, this phenomenon is less likely to be observed in the presence of a septal accessory AV connection or during oscillation of AV nodal con-

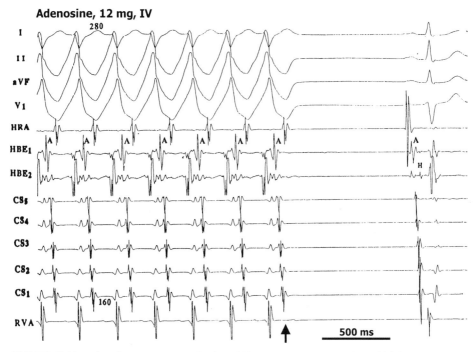

FIGURE 12-39. Adenosine suppresses conduction within accessory AV connection exhibiting decremental conduction properties. Same patient as in Figure 12-38. An antidromic AV reciprocating tachycardia (CL 280 ms) uses a left–sided anterior paraseptal accessory AV connection for anterograde conduction and the AV node-His-Purkinje system for retrograde conduction. The AV interval from the distal coronary sinus, CS_1, is 160 ms. An intravenous bolus of adenosine, 12 mg, terminates the tachycardia by blocking antero-grade conduction of the accessory AV connection (arrow). A, atrial electrogram; H, His bundle electrogram, CS_1 to CS_5, distal to proximal coronary sinus; HBE, His bundle electrographic lead; HRA, high right atrium; RVA, right ventricular apex

duction (A-H interval). In fact, the existence of dual AV nodal pathway conduction may negate or even produce a paradoxical effect on the cycle length of an orthodromic AV re-ciprocating tachycardia. (Figure 12-44).

In orthodromic AV reciprocating tachycardia with a long PR interval, the so-called PJRT, should be differentiated from the atypical (fast-slow) form of AV nodal reentrant tachycardia and atrial tachycardia. The ability of a ventricular premature beat to induce atrial preexcitation while anterograde His bundle potential is depolarized during the ta-chycardia favors the presence of a retrograde conducting AV connection with decremen-tal conduction properties. Unfortunately, the absence of this phenomenon does not exclude its diagnosis. AV nodal depressive agents such as adenosine and verapamil are of no use in differential diagnosis as these agents depress slow AV nodal pathway as well as accessory AV connections with decremental conduction properties. However, spontaneous development of 2:1 AV block during tachycardia supports the diagnosis of either atrial tachycardia or AV nodal reentrant tachycardia of the fast-slow form, and the induction of AV dissociation or lack of ventriculoatrial conduction with programmed ventricular stimulation favors the diagnosis of an atrial tachycardia.

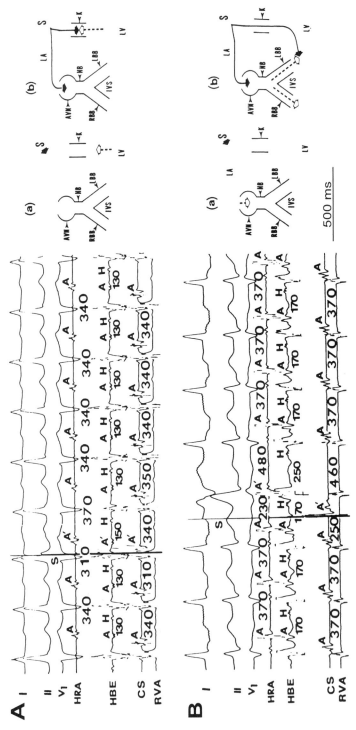

FIGURE 12-40. Variable sites of antidromic impulse collision during single extrastimulus-induced resetting of atrioventricular (AV) reciprocating tachycardia. Panel A: An extrastimulus (S) captures the left atrium (A′) from the coronary sinus with a premature coupling interval (A-A′) of 310 ms and resets the AV reciprocating tachycardia which uses a left-sided anomalous AV bypass tract for retrograde conduction and has a basic tachycardia cycle length of 340 ms. The antidromic impulse collision occurs at the anomalous AV bypass tract. Panel B: An extrastimulus (S) captures the left atrium (A′) from the coronary sinus (CS) with a premature coupling interval of 250 ins, and resets the AV reciprocating tachycardia which uses a left-sided anomalous AV by-pass tract for retrograde conduction and has a basic tachycardia cycle length of 370 ms. Antidromic impulse collision occurs at the ventricular myocardium as the QRS morphology corresponding to the extrastimulus (S) is a form of ventricular fusion. Accessory figures (a) and (b) are schematic representations of the electrophysiologic events demonstrated in each tracing. AVN, atrioventricular node; HB, His bundle; IVS, interventricular septum; K, Kent bundle (anomalous AV bypass tract); LA, left atrium; LV, left ventricle; LBB, left bundle branch; RBB, right bundle branch; S, stimulus artifact. Solid arrowhead shows the direction of stimulus-induced impulse; open arrowhead shows the direction of tachycardia-induced impulse. From [149] with permission.

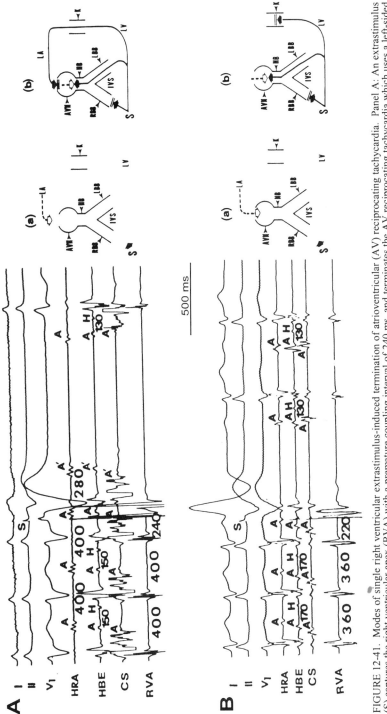

FIGURE 12-41. Modes of single right ventricular extrastimulus-induced termination of atrioventricular (AV) reciprocating tachycardia. Panel A: An extrastimulus (S) captures the right ventricular apex (RVA) with a premature coupling interval of 240 ms, and terminates the AV reciprocating tachycardia which uses a left-sided anomalous AV bypass tract for retrograde conduction and has a basic tachycardia cycle length of 400 ms. While the site of antidromic impulse collision cannot be determined exactly, the site of orthodromic conduction block appears to be in the AV node. Panel B: An extrastimulus (S) captures the right ventricular apex (RVA) with a premature coupling Interval of 220 ms, and terminates the AV reciprocating tachycardia which uses a left-sided anomalous AV bypass tract for retrograde conduction and has a basic tachycardia cycle length of 360 ms. While the site of antidromic impulse collision cannot be determined exactly, the site of orthodromic conduction block appears to be in the anomalous AV bypass tract. Accessory figures (a) and (b) are schematic representations of the electrophysiologic events demonstrated in each tracing. Abbreviations as in Figure 12-40. From [149] with permission.

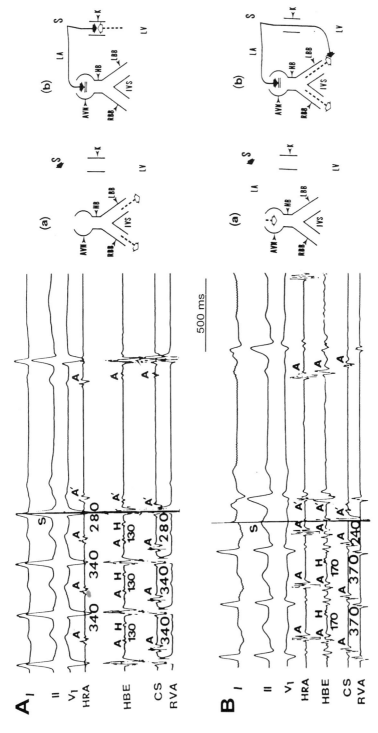

FIGURE 12-42. Modes of single left atrial extrastimulus-induced termination of atrioventricular (AV) reciprocating tachycardia. Panel A: An extrastimulus (S) captures the left atrium through coronary sinus (CS) with a premature coupling interval (A-A) of 280 ms, and terminates an AV reciprocating tachycardia which uses a left-sided anomalous AV bypass tract for retrograde conduction and has a basic tachycardia cycle length of 340 ms. While antidromic impulse collision occurs at the anomalous AV bypass tract, the site of orthodromic conduction block appears to be in the AV node. Panel B: An extrastimulus (S) captures the left atrium through the coronary sinus (CS) with a premature coupling interval of 240 ms, and terminates an AV reciprocating tachycardia which uses a left-sided anomalous AV bypass tract for retrograde conduction and has a basic tachycardia cycle length of 370 ms. While antidromic impulse collision occurs at the ventricular myocardium, the site of orthodromic conduction block appears to be in the AV node. Accessory figures (a) and (b) are schematic representations of the electrophysiologic events demonstrated in each tracing. Abbreviations as in Figure 12-40. From [149] with permission.

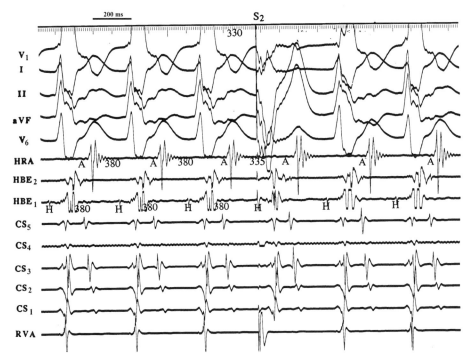

FIGURE 12-43. Atrial preexcitation induced by ventricular extrastimulation during AV reciprocating tachycardia. An orthodromic AV reciprocating tachycardia uses an accessory anteroseptal AV connection for retrograde conduction. The sequence of retrograde atrial activation is identical to that observed during retrograde fast AV nodal pathway conduction (i.e., retrograde atrial activation recorded from His bundle electrographic lead (HBE) precedes the proximal coronary sinus (CS_5) and high right atrial (HRA) activation. The cycle length (A-A) of the tachycardia is 380 ms. A premature ventricular stimulus (S_2) delivered from the right ventricular apex (RVA) with a coupling interval of 330 ms at the time of anterograde His bundle depolarization (H) preexcites the atria with resultant resetting and shortening of the A-A interval from 380 ms to 335 ms. This finding is indicative of the presence of a septal bypass tract rather than fast AV node pathway as the retrograde limb of the tachycardia circuit. CS_1 to CS_5, distal to proximal coronary sinus.

Antidromic AV reciprocating tachycardia should be separated from ventricular tachycardia, supraventricular tachycardia with aberrant conduction, and AV nodal reentrant tachycardia with a bystander accessory AV connection. Under these circumstances, the finding of AV dissociation favors the diagnosis of ventricular tachycardia. In supraventricular tachycardia with aberrant conduction, the QRS complex is preceded by a His bundle potential (anterograde) with an HV interval equal to or longer than that of the sinus QRS complex. In antidromic AV reciprocating tachycardia, the His bundle potential (retrograde) is usually buried within the QRS complex. AV nodal reentrant tachycardia with a bystander accessory AV connection is difficult to be distinguished from antidromic AV reciprocating tachycardia. However, atrial premature stimulation during the tachycardia may be useful for differential diagnosis. An atrial premature beat which is blocked in the accessory AV connection should terminate antidromic AV reciprocating tachycardia, but may not terminate AV nodal reentrant tachycardia with a bystander accessory AV connection (Figures 12-4, 12-5, 12-45 & 12-46).

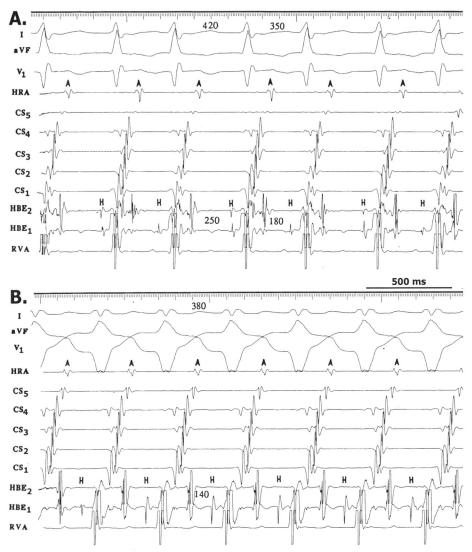

FIGURE 12-44. Dual AV nodal pathway physiology and bundle branch block during orthodromic AV reciprocating tachycardia. Panel A: An orthodromic AV reciprocating tachycardia uses the AV node–His–
Purkinje system for anterograde conduction and a left-lateral accessory AV connection for retrograde conduction. Note the cycle length alternans between 420 and 350 ms due to alternation of AV nodal conduction (A-
H interval) between 250 and 180 ms (oscillation between anterograde slow and fast AV nodal pathway conduction). Panel B: Development of complete left bundle branch block during the orthodromic AV reciprocating tachycardia (same patient as in panel A). Note that the tachycardia cycle length is 380 ms associated with
a stable AV nodal conduction time (A-H interval) of 140 ms. CS_1 to CS_5, distal to proximal coronary sinus.

Also in support of a diagnosis of AV reciprocating tachycardia is the observation that an
atrial premature stimulus delivered near the reentry circuit advances the tachycardia
while the right atrial septum (recorded by the His bundle catheter) is already committed
to activation by the preceding tachycardia cycle (Figure 12-47). Finally, responses to

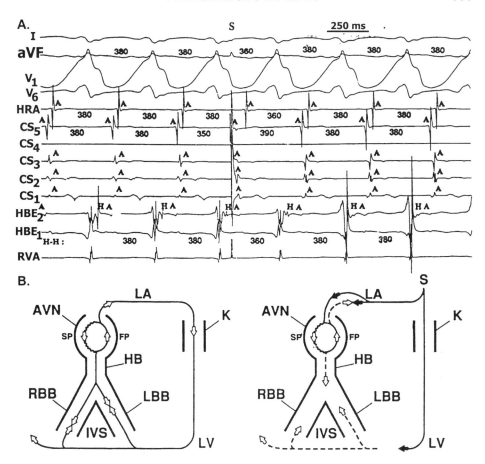

FIGURE 12-45. Effect of left atrial (LA) extrastimulation on preexcited tachycardia resulting from the slow-fast form of AV nodal (AVN) reentrant tachycardia with anterograde AV conduction using a bystander left free-wall accessory AV connection. Panel A: (top to bottom) surface electrocardiographic leads I, aVF, V_1, and V_6 and intracardiac electrograms from high right atrium (HRA), proximal (CS_5) to distal (CS_1) coronary sinus, proximal (HBE_2) and distal (HBE_1) His bundle region, and right ventricular apex (RVA). Panel B: Schematic diagrams illustrate events occurring before delivery of atrial extrastimulus (panel B, left) and resulting from atrial extrastimulus (panel B, right). Black arrows show direction of stimulus-induced impulse; white arrows show direction of tachycardia-induced impulse. A, atrial electrogram; FP, fast AV nodal conduction pathway; H, His bundle electrogram; HB, His bundle; IVS, interventricular septum; K, Kent bundle (accessory AV connection); LBB, left bundle branch; LV, left ventricle; RBB, right bundle branch; S, stimulus artifact; SP, slow AV nodal conduction pathway. From [145] with permission.

catheter ablation may separate accessory nodoventricular connection from accessory AV connection with decremental conduction properties. Successful ablation of the former, but not the latter, is signaled by an emergence of an AV junctional rhythm with a retrograde atrial activation sequence identical to that of the retrograde fast AV node pathway conduction — a phenomenon similar to that observed during selective ablation of slow AV nodal pathway conduction (Figures 12-48 through 12-50).

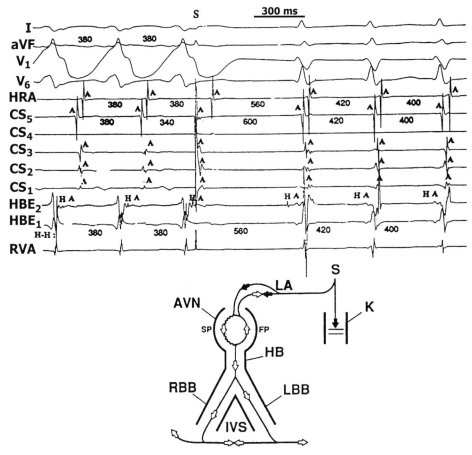

FIGURE 12-46. Effect of atrial extrastimulation on preexcited tachycardia resulting from the slow-fast form of AV nodal reentrant tachycardia with anterograde AV conduction using a bystander left free-wall accessory AV connection. Abbreviations as in Figure 12-45. From [145] with permission.

12.7   Radiofrequency Catheter Ablation

Radiofrequency catheter ablation of accessory pathway conduction is a safe and highly effective curative procedure that can be offered to patients suffering from recurrent AV reciprocating tachycardia or atrial flutter/fibrillation with rapid ventricular rate due to ventricular preexcitation [127,128]. Because the lesion size produced by radiofrequency energy is relatively small, the critical component of any ablative attempt is mapping the precise location of the accessory connection. Although the manifest ventricular preexcitation pattern as displayed on the surface 12-lead ECG is useful for predicting the location of the accessory AV connection (Figure 12-51 and Table 12-1.), an electrophysiology study is required for its precise localization. A decapolar electrode catheter positioned in the coronary sinus and great cardiac vein can greatly assist in de-

FIGURE 12-47. Advancement of antidromic AV reciprocating tachycardia by atrial premature stimulation. Surface ECG leads I, aVF, and V₁ are displayed along with intracardiac recordings from the proximal (HBE-P), middle (HBE-M), and distal (HBE-D) His bundle regions as well as the proximal (MAP-P) and distal (MAP-D) mapping/ablating electrode catheter positioned at the right lateral tricuspid annulus, and the right ventricular apex (RVA). An antidromic AV reciprocating tachycardia using a right-lateral accessory AV connection for antidromic conduction and the AV node-His-Purkinje system for retrograde conduction has a cycle length of 260 ms. An atrial premature extrastimulus (S₂) with a coupling interval of 240 ms is delivered to the lateral right atrium using the mapping/ablating catheter. Delivery of this extrastimulus is timed to occur after the septal right atrium, recorded by the His bundle catheter, is already committed to activation (A-A interval = 260 ms, same as the tachycardia cycle length) by the preceding tachycardia cycle. Consequently, the tachycardia is reset and advanced as evidenced by the shortening of the A-A and V-V intervals to 230 ms followed by continuation of the tachycardia and return to the previous cycle length of 260 ms. The principle illustrated here is that delivery of an extrastimulus close to the reentry circuit of a tachycardia with a wide excitable gap allows advancement and resetting of the tachycardia. However, advancement and resetting would not occur if the excitable gap is narrow and the tachycardia circuit is far away from the site of extrastimulus delivery. If this tachycardia were AV node reentrant tachycardia using the right-sided accessory connection for bystander AV conduction, it would not have been possible to advance and reset the tachycardia with this extrastimulus given the timing and location of its delivery. The reason, of course, is because the AV node reentry circuit is very small, has a narrow excitable gap, and is located far from the right lateral atrial site at which the premature extrastimulus is delivered.

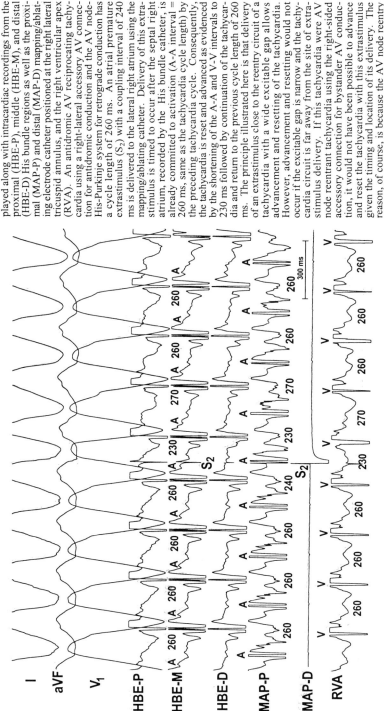

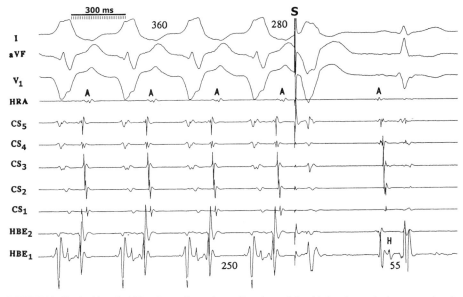

FIGURE 12-48. Antidromic AV reciprocating tachycardia using a right-sided nodoventricular connection for anterograde conduction and a fast AV nodal pathway for retrograde conduction. The cycle length of the tachycardia is 360 ms. The AV interval, measured from the low septal right atrium (HBE), is 250 ms. A ventricular premature depolarization delivered with a coupling interval of 280 ms (without ventriculoatrial conduction) terminates the tachycardia. The retrograde atrial activation sequence is consistent with a fast AV nodal pathway (retrograde atrial activation in the HBE lead precedes the activation near the ostium of the coronary sinus (CS_5) and high right atrium (HRA)). Also note that there is no evidence of ventricular preexcitation during the sinus conducted beat (the last QRS complex, HV = 55 ms). CS_1 to CS_5: distal to proximal coronary sinus.

termining the general location of left-sided accessory connections. Localization of right-sided accessory connections can be achieved by using a steerable catheter positioned around the tricuspid annulus or a small electrode catheter positioned in the right coronary artery. Once identified to the right or left side of the heart, the accessory connection must be further localized precisely around the respective AV groove in order to eliminate conduction using the minimum number of radiofrequency energy applications (Figures 12-52 through 12-62).

TABLE 12-1. Localization of accessory AV connections based upon the delta wave/QRS complex polarity

ECG Lead	Left-Sided Accessory AV Connection			Right-Sided Accessory AV Connection		
	Anterior/Lateral	Posterolateral	Posterior	Posterior	Posterolateral	Anterior/Lateral
I	−	+	+	+	+	+
II/III	+	±	−	−	±	+
V_1	+	+	+	−	−	−

+, positive deflection; −, negative deflection; ±, biphasic

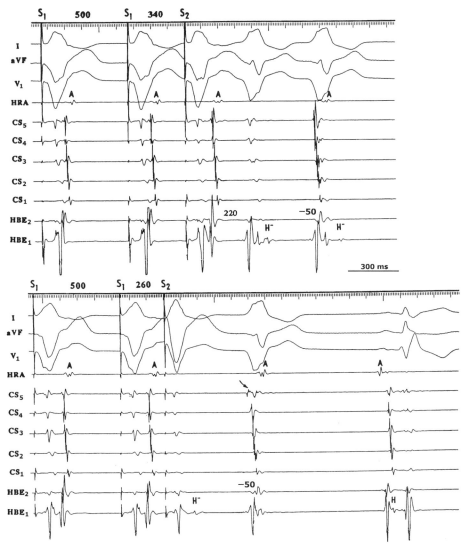

FIGURE 12-49. Slow AV node–nodoventricular connection (same patient as in Figure 12-48. Panel A: During ventricular pacing at a cycle length (S_1-S_1) of 500 ms a ventricular premature stimulus (S_2) is delivered with a coupling interval (S_1-S_2) of 340 ms provokes two AV reciprocal beats (the 4th and 5th QRS complexes). The ventricular premature stimulus (S_2) induces ventriculoatrial conduction within a fast AV node pathway which then activates the ventricle by way of a nodoventricular connection with an AV interval (measured in HBE) of 220 ms. Retrograde conduction proceeds through the His–Purkinje system (H⁻) and activates the slow AV nodal pathway which then preexcites the ventricle with an AV interval of -50 ms. The negative A-H interval is caused by earliest activation of the proximal coronary sinus (CS_5), close to where the slow AV nodal pathway is located. Panel B: At the ventricular pacing cycle length (S_1-S_1) of 500 ms, a ventricular premature stimulus (S_2) delivered at a coupling interval (S_1-S_2) of 260 ms provokes long ventriculoatrial conduction through slow AV nodal pathway followed by ventricular preexcitation. Note that atrial activity in the proximal coronary sinus (CS_5) precedes activation in the HBE and HRA. Also note that the atrial and ventricular activations recorded at the proximal coronary sinus (CS_5) are continuous with a high frequency potential suggestive of an accessory pathway potential (arrow) and that the AV interval measured from in the HBE lead is -50 ms. CS_1-CS_5: distal to proximal coronary sinus electrode pairs.

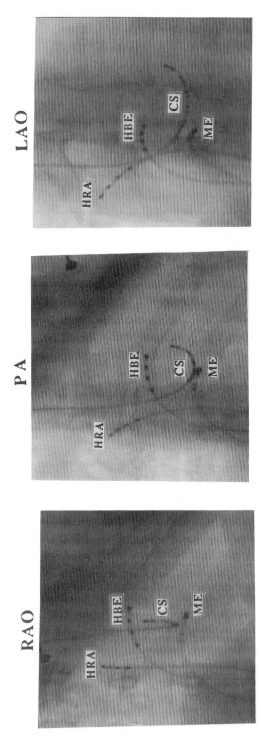

FIGURE 12-50. Fluoroscopic views showing the site of successful catheter ablation of the slow AV node–nodoventricular connection as described in Figure 12-48 and Figure 12-49. Radiofrequency energy delivered to the atrium anterior and inferior to the coronary sinus ostium generates AV junctional rhythm and abolishes slow AV nodal pathway conduction as well as ventricular preexcitation (not shown). CS: coronary sinus; HBE: His bundle electrographic lead; HRA: high right atrium; ME: mapping and ablation electrode.

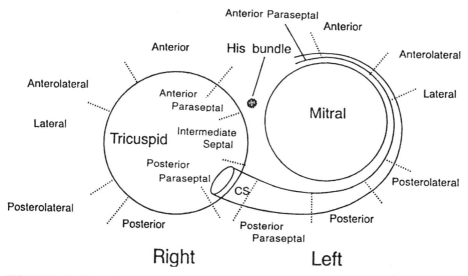

FIGURE 12-51. Schematic representation of various locations of accessory AV connections. CS, coronary sinus.

12.7.1 CATHETER ABLATION OF MANIFEST ACCESSORY AV CONNECTIONS

For manifest accessory AV connections capable of anterograde conduction, the technique of ventricular-paced mapping (Figures 12-52 through 12-55) can be utilized to map the sites of their ventricular insertion precisely, allowing radiofrequency energy ablation with a minimum of failed attempts. Using this technique, a 12-lead ECG template is recorded during maximal preexcitation. In general, this can be achieved by using a short cycle length pacing (e.g., 400 msec) of the atrium using a catheter positioned near the site of the accessory AV connection. For example, for a left-sided accessory connection, pacing from a pair of electrodes in the coronary sinus catheter often is adequate (Figure 12-55). If atrial pacing at a short cycle length alone is not sufficient to eliminate ventricular fusion, adenosine bolus injection during an atrial pacing cycle length of 600 msec or during isoproterenol infusion may assist in revealing the maximal preexcitation pattern.

Once obtained in this fashion, the template is the body surface 12-lead ECG representation of the ventricular activation resulting *solely* from anterograde accessory pathway conduction, and thus it will be different for accessory connections located at different positions. An electrode catheter is then positioned in the appropriate ventricular cavity along the AV groove near the presumptive ventricular insertion of the accessory AV connection. Access to the right ventricle is through the inferior or superior vena cava and the left ventricle from the aorta (retrograde). Pacing from this site (ventricular pacing) will result in a surface 12-lead ECG QRS complexes identical to those of the template (Figure 12-55). Radiofrequency energy application achieving an electrode-tissue interface temperature of 60°-70°C for 30 to 40 seconds at the site will eliminate accessory AV pathway conduction. If the ablating/pacing catheter is positioned at a site at

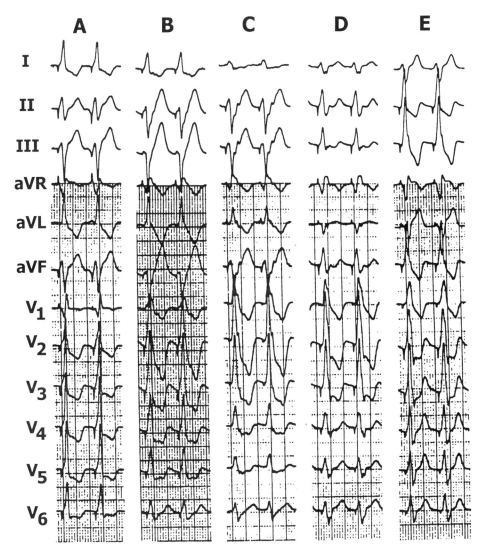

FIGURE 12-52. ECG recordings of ventricular pace-mapping in patient with left free wall accessory connection. ECG recordings are obtained during left ventricular pacing along mitral annulus, beginning at left lateral free wall and proceeding posteriorly to left posterior septal/paraseptal region. ECG in panel A is recorded at most proximal location in posterior septal/paraseptal region whereas 12-lead ECG in panel E is obtained during ventricular pacing of the left free wall near site of distal pair of electrodes in coronary sinus. Panels B to D are ECG recordings obtained during pacing at intervening sites (second, third and fourth pairs of electrodes, respectively). Note that as ventricular pacing proceeds from left free wall to left septum, frontal-plane QRS axis gradually shifts from right to left axis, and there is loss of initial positive deflection of QRS complex in lead V_1 with development of distinct rSR or QR pattern in lead V_1 at the posterior septal/paraseptal area. Paper speed 25 mm/sec. From [146] with permission.

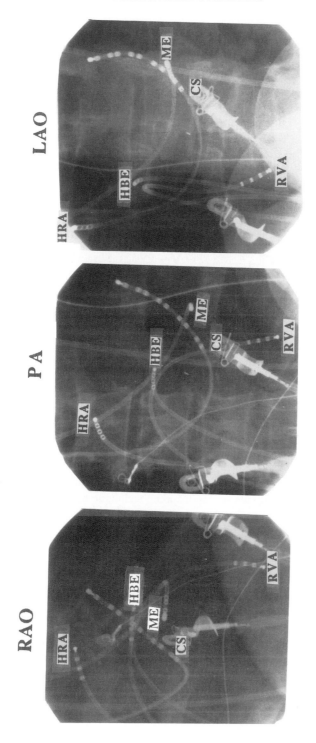

FIGURE 12-53. Fluoroscopic radiograph displaying relation of intracardiac catheters during mapping and ablation procedure in a patient with a left-sided posterior accessory AV connection. Note positioning of tip of mapping electrode (ME) in leftward and posterior position. CS, coronary sinus ostium; HBE, His bundle electrodes; HRA, high right atrium; LAO, 30° left anterior oblique projection; PA, posteroanterior projection; RAO, 30° right anterior oblique projection; RVA = right ventricular apex.

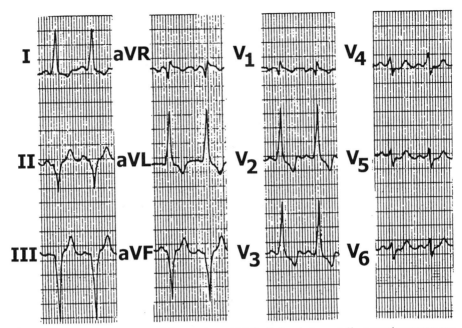

FIGURE 12-54. Surface 12-lead ECG from patient with left-sided posterior septal/paraseptal accessory connection during sinus rhythm. Patient has marked ventricular preexcitation and QR morphology in lead V_1. Frontal plane QRS is approximately -50°. Ventricular insertion of this pathway is successfully ablated in the left posterior septal/ paraseptal region using the ventricular pace-mapping technique (see Figure 12-52). Paper speed 25 mm/sec. From [146] with permission.

which ventricular pacing results in an ECG pattern which is even slightly different than the template, the application of radiofrequency energy will usually fail to eliminate conduction in the accessory AV connection. The precise location is usually signaled by the disappearance of the ventricular preexcitation pattern within 5–6 QRS complexes after beginning the application of radiofrequency energy (Figure 12-60). Strict adherence to these criteria makes the ventricular-paced mapping technique highly effective at reducing the number of ineffective radiofrequency energy applications when ablating anterograde conducting accessory AV connections.

12.7.2 CATHETER ABLATION OF CONCEALED ACCESSORY AV CONNECTIONS

For accessory connections that conduct only in the retrograde direction, ventricular-paced mapping cannot be utilized. Instead, the technique of earliest retrograde atrial activation must be used to determine the optimum catheter position for radiofrequency catheter ablation. Using this technique, the site along the appropriate AV groove at which earliest retrograde atrial activation occurs, is determined preferably during orthodromic AV reciprocating tachycardia rather than right ventricular pacing. Positioning of the ablating catheter in the AV groove at the site of the accessory AV connection will result in the earliest appearing retrograde atrial activation. Radiofrequency energy is deliv-

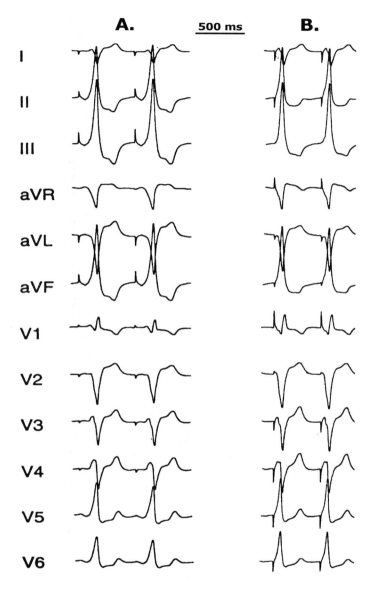

FIGURE 12-55. Surface 12-lead ECG recorded during coronary sinus atrial pacing and maximal preexcitation in patient with accessory AV connection inserting into left anterior paraseptal region of left ventricle (panel A). Surface 12-lead ECG recorded during ventricular pacing at left anterior paraseptal region of AV junction in same patient (panel B). Note that 12-lead QRS pattern during ventricular pacing at this left paraseptal location is identical to that obtained during atrial pacing with maximal preexcitation, indicating that the accessory AV connection inserts into left anterior paraseptal region at a ventricular site marked by tip of pacing catheter. From [147] with permission.

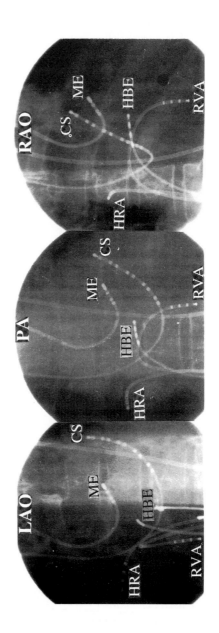

FIGURE 12-56. Fluoroscopic view of location of anterior paraseptal accessory AV connections showing position of mapping electrode (ME) catheter with its tip at left anterior paraseptal AV annulus. RAO, right anterior oblique view; PA, posteroanterior view; LAO, left anterior oblique view; HRA, high right atrial catheter, CS, coronary sinus catheter; HBE, His bundle catheter; RVA, right ventricular apical catheter. From [147] with permission.

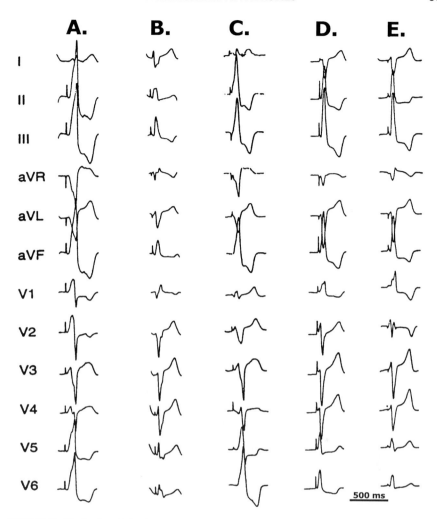

FIGURE 12-57. Surface 12-lead EGG recordings in five patients (panels A–E) during ventricular pacing from left anterior paraseptal region of mitral valve annulus as shown in Figure 12-56. In each case note similarity to 12-lead ECG pattern obtained during maximal ventricular preexcitation in patient with manifest left anterior paraseptal accessory connection depicted in Figure 12-55.

ered in the ventricle at or near the site during a relatively slow ventricular-paced rhythm (usually 600 ms). A successful ablation is signaled by disappearance of retrograde conduction through the accessory AV connection within 5–6 QRS complexes. Several attempts are often necessary for successful ablation. Alternatively, an atrial approach may be used to ablate accessory AV connections. For left-sided accessory AV connections, the left atrium above the mitral annulus may be reached retrogradely from the left ventricle, or by the transeptal technique from the right atrium. Some investigators prefer the atrial approach for all forms of AV reciprocating tachycardia to the ventricular approach regardless of the conduction properties of accessory connections. The notion is to avoid

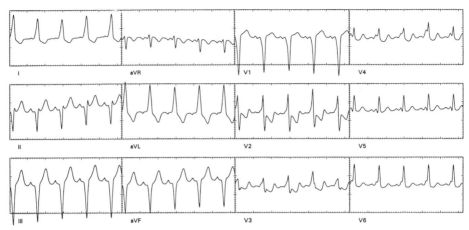

FIGURE 12-58. Surface 12-lead ECG recording from a patient with a right-sided posterior septal/paraseptal accessory AV connection. Note the typical QS pattern in lead V_1 and a left superior frontal plane axis. Paper speed 25 mm/sec.

creating any lesions in the ventricular cavity in fear of its potential arrhythmogenicity. As a rule, in patients with aortic regurgitation or prosthetic valve, the atrial approach is the only method recommended for ablating left-sided accessory connections. The transeptal technique should be performed by an experienced person to avoid accidental puncture of the neighboring aorta which often causes acute and excessive bleeding requiring emergency surgical intervention.

Other potentially significant complications while attempting catheter ablation of accessory connections include disruption of the aortic valve causing acute aortic regurgi-

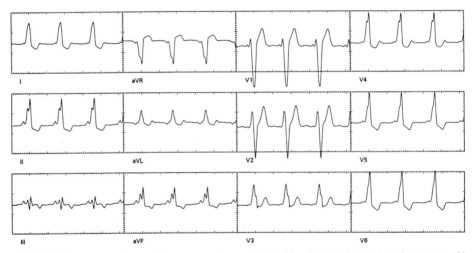

FIGURE 12-59. Surface 12-lead ECG recording from a patient with a right-sided anterolateral accessory AV connection. Note the rS pattern in lead V_1 and a left inferior frontal plane axis. Paper speed 25 mm/sec.

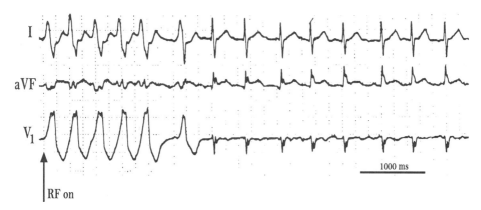

I

aVF

V_1

RF on

1000 ms

FIGURE 12-60. Radiofrequency catheter ablation of a left posterolateral accessory AV connection using a ventricular approach (retrograde transaortic) during atrial fibrillation. Note the disappearance of ventricular preexcitation after the 6th QRS complex. RF: radiofrequency energy.

tation, atrial or ventricular perforation resulting in excessive bleeding and cardiac tamponade, injury to the neighboring coronary artery leading to bleeding and/or myocardial infarction, damage to the mitral valve producing mitral regurgitation and the development of thromboembolism (pulmonary and systemic) and complete AV block. Many of the above potential complications can be avoided by precise placement of the electrode catheter and the use of a temperature-controlled and impedance-controlled delivery system of radiofrequency energy.

12.7.3 PARASEPTAL ACCESSORY AV CONNECTIONS

Posterior paraseptal accessory AV connections may actually have their atrial insertion sites located in the coronary sinus or the proximal mid-cardiac vein. Electrocardiographically, the ventricular preexcitation pattern often manifests a superior frontal plane axis with a negative deflection in V_1. However, there is a rapid transition to a positive deflection in lead V_2 (Figure 12-54). Detailed mapping within these latter structures is required before application of radiofrequency energy. Caution should be given to the possibility of perforating the venous structure and injuring the neighboring coronary arterial system. Right-sided anterior paraseptal accessory AV connections may be located near the AV node and the His bundle referred to as "intermediate accessory AV connections." The method of ablation can be either an atrial or ventricular approach (Figures 12-60 & 12-61). However, because of the proximity to the AV node and His bundle, the incidence of producing complete AV block is high in attempting to ablate these "intermediate accessory AV connections". Patients with this variety of accessory connections should be warned of the possibility of requiring implantation of a permanent pacemaker following the catheter ablation procedure.

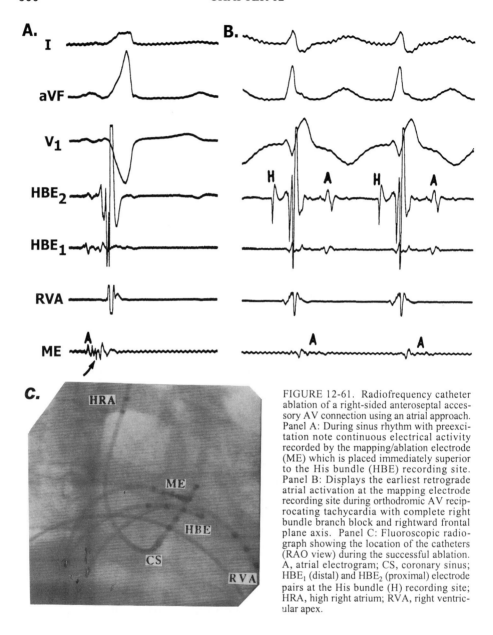

FIGURE 12-61. Radiofrequency catheter ablation of a right-sided anteroseptal accessory AV connection using an atrial approach. Panel A: During sinus rhythm with preexcitation note continuous electrical activity recorded by the mapping/ablation electrode (ME) which is placed immediately superior to the His bundle (HBE) recording site. Panel B: Displays the earliest retrograde atrial activation at the mapping electrode recording site during orthodromic AV reciprocating tachycardia with complete right bundle branch block and rightward frontal plane axis. Panel C: Fluoroscopic radiograph showing the location of the catheters (RAO view) during the successful ablation. A, atrial electrogram; CS, coronary sinus; HBE$_1$ (distal) and HBE$_2$ (proximal) electrode pairs at the His bundle (H) recording site; HRA, high right atrium; RVA, right ventricular apex.

12.7.4 ACCESSORY NODOVENTRICULAR AND ATRIOFASCICULAR CONNECTIONS

Accessory nodoventricular and atriofascicular connections usually have their ventricular insertion located in the right ventricle. However, the sites of ventricular insertion can be arborized 0.5 to 2.0 cm in diameter making them difficult to be precisely localized from

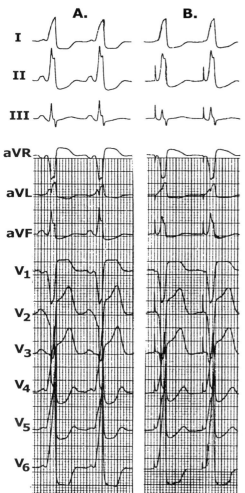

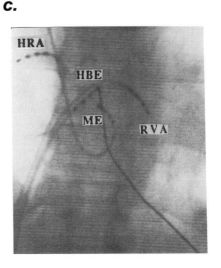

FIGURE 12-62. Radiofrequency catheter ablation of a right-sided anteroseptal accessory AV connection by a ventricular approach. Panel A: 12-lead ECG recorded during sinus rhythm. Panel B: 12-lead ECG recording during ventricular pacing from the tip of the mapping/ablation electrode (ME) placed beneath the His bundle recording site in the right ventricle. Panel C: Fluoroscopic radiograph (shallow LAO projection) illustrating the position of the ME catheter on the ventricular side of the tricuspid annulus (using a right internal jugular approach) at the successful site of ablation near the His bundle. HRA, high right atrial catheter; HBE, His bundle catheter, RVA right ventricular apex catheter. Paper speed 25 mm/sec.

the ventricle (Figure 12-28) [88]. Therefore, the atrial approach is the recommended method for radiofrequency catheter ablation. With decremental conduction properties, the shortest AV interval (atrial- or stimulus-to-delta) during a sinus or atrial-paced rhythm is regarded as the atrial insertion site of the accessory connection (Figure 12-49). Other electrophysiologic parameters include premature stimulation during tachycardia searching for the maximal resetting of ventricular activation and a direct recording of the Mahaim fiber potential (Figures 12-49 & 4-11) [88,129-135]. Multiple attempts may be required to abolish the ventricular preexcitation pattern and to render antidromic AV reciprocating tachycardia becoming non-inducible.

12.8 Surgery

Accessory connections can be interrupted by surgical incision via either an epicardial or endocardial approach [136-143]. Detailed intraoperative mapping during induced AV reciprocating tachycardia is required before the surgical incision. Because radiofrequency catheter ablation is a safe and highly effective procedure, nowadays it is seldom necessary to refer patients with the ventricular preexcitation syndrome (Wolff-Parkinson-White syndrome and its variants) for surgical intervention. Surgery is reserved for those with accessory connections not amenable to radiofrequency catheter ablation such as certain posterior sepal and paraseptal, or subepicardially located pathways.

References

1. Wolff L, Parkinson J, White PD: Bundle branch block with short P-R interval in healthy young people prone to paroxysmal tachyarrhythmia. *Am Heart J* **5**:685, 1930.
2. Newman BJ, Donoso E, Friedberg CK: Arrhythmias in the Wolff-Parkinson-White syndrome. *Progress in Cardiovascular Disease* **9**:147, 1966.
3. Gallagher JJ, Gilbert M, Svenson RH, et al.: Wolff-Parkinson-White syndrome. The problem, evaluation, and surgical correction. *Circulation* **51**:767-85, 1975.
4. Durrer D, Wellens HJ: The Wolff-Parkinson-White syndrome anno 1973. *Eur J Cardiol* **1**:347-67, 1974.
5. Mines GR: On circulating excitations in heart muscles and their possible relation to tachycardia and fibrillation. *Proc Roy Soc Can* **IV**:43, 1914.
6. Gallagher JJ: Wolff-Parkinson-White syndrome: surgery to radiofrequency catheter ablation. *Pacing Clin Electrophysiol* **20**:512-33, 1997.
7. Anderson RH, Becker AE, Brechenmacher C, et al.: Ventricular preexcitation: A proposed nomenclature for its substrates. *Eur J Cardiol* **3**:27, 1975.
8. Becker AE, Anderson RH, Durrer D, Wellens HJ: The anatomical substrates of Wolff-Parkinson-White syndrome. A clinicopathologic correlation in seven patients. *Circulation* **57**:870-9, 1978.
9. Lev M, Kennamer R, Prinzmetal M, de Mesquita RH: A histopathologic study of the atrioventricular communication in 2 hearts with the Wolff-Parkinson-White syndrome. *Circulation* **24**:41, 1961.
10. Lunel AAV: Significance of annulus fibrosis of heart in relation to AV conduction and ventricular activation in case of Wolff-Parkinson-White syndrome. *Br Heart J* **34**:1263, 1972.
11. Kent AFS: Researches on structure as a function of the mammalian heart. *J Physiol* **14**:233, 1893.
12. Svenson RH, Miller HC, Gallagher JJ, Wallace AG: Electrophysiological evaluation of the Wolff-Parkinson-White syndrome: problems in assessing antegrade and retrograde conduction over the accessory pathway. *Circulation* **52**:552-62, 1975.
13. Wellens HJJ. The electrophysiologic properties of the accessory pathway in the Wolff-Parkinson-White syndrome. In: Wellens HJJ, Lie KI, Janse MJ, eds. *The Conduction System of the Heart: Structure, Function and Clinical Implication.* Philadelphia,PA: Lea & Febiger, 567-587: 1976.
14. Castellanos A, Jr., Chapunoff E, Castillo C, et al.: His bundle electrograms in two cases of Wolff-Parkinson-White (pre-excitation) syndrome. *Circulation* **41**:399-411, 1970.
15. Gallagher JJ, Pritchett EL, Sealy WC, et al.: The preexcitation syndromes. *Prog Cardiovasc Dis* **20**:285-327, 1978.
16. Moore EN, Spear JE, Boineau JP: Electrophysiological studies on preexcitation in the dog using an electrically stimulated atrioventricular bypass pathway. *Circ Res* **31**:74, 1972.
17. Boineau JP, Moore EN, Spear JF, Sealy WC: Basis of static and dynamic electrocardiographic variations in Wolff-Parkinson-White syndrome. Anatomic and electrophysiologic observations in right and left ventricular preexcitation. *Am J Cardiol* **32**:32, 1973.

18. Rosenbaum FF, Hecht HH, Wilson FN, Johnston FD: The potential variations of the thorax and esophagus in anomalous atrioventricular excitation (Wolff-Parkinson-White syndrome). *Am Heart J* **29**:281, 1945.

19. Gallagher JJ, Sealy WC, Kasell J, Wallace AG: Multiple accessory pathways in patients with the preexcitation syndrome. *Circulation* **54**:571-91, 1976.

20. Tonkin AM, Gallagher JJ, Svenson RH, et al.: Anterograde block in accessory pathways with retrograde conduction in reciprocating tachycardia. *Eur J Cardiol* **3**:143-52, 1975.

21. Tonkin AM, Miller HC, Svenson RH, et al.: Refractory periods of the accessory pathway in the Wolff-Parkinson-White syndrome. *Circulation* **52**:563-9, 1975.

22. Wyndham CRC, Amat-y-Leon F, Wu D, et al.: Effects of cycle length on atrial vulnerability. *Circulation* **55**:260-7, 1977.

23. Andrus EC, Carter EP: The refractory period of the normally beating dog's auricle; with a note on the occurrence of auricular fibrillation following a single stimulus. *J Exp Med* **51**:357, 1930.

24. Durrer D, Schoo L, Schuilenburg RM, Wellens HJ: The role of premature beats in the initiation and the termination of supraventricular tachycardia in the Wolff-Parkinson-White syndrome. *Circulation* **36**:644-62, 1967.

25. Wellens HJ, Schuilenberg RM, Durrer D: Electrical stimulation of the heart in patients with Wolff-Parkinson-White syndrome, type A. *Circulation* **43**:99-114, 1971.

26. Wellens HJ, Schuilenburg RM, Durrer D: Electrical stimulation of heart in study of patients with the Wolff-Parkinson-White syndrome type A. *Br Heart J* **33**:147, 1971.

27. Sung RJ, Castellanos A, Mallon SM, et al.: Mode of initiation of reciprocating tachycardia during programmed ventricular stimulation in the Wolff-Parkinson-White syndrome. With reference to various patterns of ventriculoatrial conduction. *Am J Cardiol* **40**:24-31, 1977.

28. Fontaine G, Frank R, Coutte R, et al.: Rhythme reciproque antidromique dans un syndrome de Wolff-Parkinson-White de type A. *Ann Cardiol Angeiol* **24**:59, 1975.

29. Benditt DG, Pritchett EL, Gallagher JJ: Spectrum of regular tachycardias with wide QRS complexes in patients with accessory atrioventricular pathways. *Am J Cardiol* **42**:828-38, 1978.

30. Benson DW, Jr., Smith WM, Dunnigan A, et al.: Mechanisms of regular, wide QRS tachycardia in infants and children. *Am J Cardiol* **49**:1778-88, 1982.

31. Cinca J, Valle V, Gutierrez L, et al.: Reciprocating tachycardia using bilateral accessory pathways: Electrophysiological and clinical implications. *Circulation* **62**:657, 1980.

32. Bardy GH, Packer DL, German LD, Gallagher JJ: Preexcited reciprocating tachycardia in patients with Wolff-Parkinson-White syndrome: incidence and mechanisms. *Circulation* **70**:377-91, 1984.

33. Denes P, Amat YLF, Wyndham C, et al.: Electrophysiologic demonstration of bilateral anomalous pathways in a patient with Wolff-Parkinson-White syndrome. *Am J Cardiol* **37**:93-101, 1976.

34. Wellens HJ, Durrer D: Patterns of ventriculo-atrial conduction in the Wolff-Parkinson-White syndrome. *Circulation* **49**:22-31, 1974.

35. Sung RJ, Castellanos A, Mallon SM, et al.: Mechanisms of spontaneous alternation between reciprocating tachycardia and atrial flutter-fibrillation in the Wolff-Parkinson-White syndrome. *Circulation* **56**:409-16, 1977.

36. Castellanos A, Jr., Myerburg RJ, Craparo K, et al.: Factors regulating ventricular rates during atrial flutter and fibrillation in pre-excitation (Wolff-Parkinson-White) syndrome. *Br Heart J* **35**:811-6, 1973.

37. German LD, Gallagher JJ, Broughton A, et al.: Effects of exercise and isoproterenol during atrial fibrillation in patients with Wolff-Parkinson-White syndrome. *Am J Cardiol* **51**:1203-6, 1983.

38. Wellens HJ, Durrer D: Wolff-Parkinson-White syndrome and atrial fibrillation. Relation between refractory period of accessory pathway and ventricular rate during atrial fibrillation. *Am J Cardiol* **34**:777-82, 1974.

39. Wellens HJ, Brugada P, Roy D, et al.: Effect of isoproterenol on the anterograde refractory period of the accessory pathway in patients with the Wolff-Parkinson-White syndrome. *Am J Cardiol* **50**:180-4, 1982.

40. Shen EN, Sung RJ: Initiation of atrial fibrillation by spontaneous ventricular premature beats in concealed Wolff-Parkinson-White syndrome. *Am Heart J* **103**:911-2, 1982.

41. Sung RJ, Gelband H, Castellanos A, et al.: Clinical and electrophysiologic observations in patients with concealed accessory atrioventricular bypass tracts. *Am J Cardiol* **40**:839-47, 1977.

42. Klein LS, Miles WM, Zipes DP: Effect of atrioventricular interval during pacing or reciprocating tachycardia on atrial size, pressure, and refractory period. Contraction-excitation feedback in human atrium. *Circulation* **82**:60-8, 1990.

43. Satoh T, Zipes DP: Unequal atrial stretch in dogs increases dispersion of refractoriness conducive to developing atrial fibrillation. *J Cardiovasc Electrophysiol* **7**:833-42, 1996.

44. Campbell RW, Smith RA, Gallagher JJ, et al.: Atrial fibrillation in the preexcitation syndrome. *Am J Cardiol* **40**:514-20, 1977.

45. Grolleau R, Puech P, Cabasson J, et al.: Particularities de la conduction auriculo-ventriculare dans un syndrome de Wolff-Parkinson-White. *Arch Mal Coeur* **67**:13, 1974.

46. Neuss H, Schelpper M, Spies HF: Double ventricular response to an atrial extrasystole in a patient with Wolff-Parkinson-White syndrome type C. *Eur J Cardiol* **2**:175, 1974.

47. Wu D, Denes P, Dhingra R, et al.: New manifestations of dual A-V nodal pathways. *Eur J Cardiol* **2**:459-66, 1975.

48. Motte G, Oster G, Coumel P, Slama R: Tachycardia caused by reciprocal rhythm between normal pathways and a rapid atrial-His pathway. *Arch Mal Coeur Vaiss* **68**:673-82, 1975.

49. Csapo G: Paroxysmal nonreentrant tachycardia due to simultaneous conduction in dual atrioventricular nodal pathways. *Am J Cardiol* **43**:1033-1045, 1979.

50. Langendorf R: Concealed A-V conduction: The effect of blocked impulses on the formation and conduction of subsequent impulses. *Am Heart J* **35**:542, 1948.

51. Cohen HC, D'Cruz I, Pick A: Concealed intraventricular conduction in the His bundle electrogram. *Circulation* **53**:776, 1976.

52. Damato AN, Lau SH, Berkowitz WD, et al.: Recording of specialized conducting fibers (A-V nodal, His bundle, and right bundle branch) in man using an electrode catheter technic. *Circulation* **39**:435-47, 1969.

53. Damato AN, Lau SH, Patton RD, et al.: A study of atrioventricular conduction in man using premature atrial stimulation and His bundle recordings. *Circulation* **40**:61-9, 1969.

54. Damato AN, Lau SH, Helfant RH, et al.: Study of atrioventricular conduction in man using electrode catheter recordings of His bundle activity. *Circulation* **39**:287-96, 1969.

55. Sung RJ, Myerburg RJ, Castellanos A: Electrophysiological demonstration of concealed conduction in the human atrium. *Circulation* **58**:940-6, 1978.

56. Svinarich JT, Tai DY, Mickelson J, et al.: Electrophysiologic demonstration of concealed conduction in anomalous atrioventricular bypass tracts. *J Am Coll Cardiol* **5**:898-903, 1985.

57. Coumel P, Attuel P: Reciprocating tachycardia in overt and latent preexcitation. Influence of functional bundle branch block on the rate of the tachycardia. *Eur J Cardiol* **1**:423-36, 1974.

58. Slama R, Coumel P, Bouvrain Y: Type A Wolff-Parkinson-White syndromes, inapparent or latent in sinus rhythm. *Arch Mal Coeur Vaiss* **66**:639-53, 1973.

59. Zipes DP, DeJoseph RL, Rothbaum DA: Unusual properties of accessory pathways. *Circulation* **49**:1200-11, 1974.

60. De la Fuente D, Sasyniuk B, Moe GK: Conduction through a narrow isthmus in isolated canine atrial tissue. A model of the W-P-W syndrome. *Circulation* **44**:803-9, 1971.

61. Przybylski J, Chiale PA, Halpern MS, et al.: Unmasking of ventricular preexcitation by vagal stimulation or isoproterenol administration. *Circulation* **61**:1030-7, 1980.

62. Przybylski J, Chiale PA, Elizari MV, Rosenbaum MB. Physiological properties of accessory pathways. In: Rosenbaum MB, Elizari MV, eds. *Frontiers of Cardiac Electrophysiology*. Boston, MA: Martinus Nijhoff Publishers, 702-823: 1983.

63. Sung RJ, Castellanos A, Gelband H, Myerburg RJ: Mechanism of reciprocating tachycardia initiated during sinus rhythm in concealed Wolff-Parkinson-White syndrome: report of a case. *Circulation* **54**:338-44, 1976.

64. Sung RJ: Incessant supraventricular tachycardia. *Pacing Clin Electrophysiol* **6**:1306-26, 1983.

65. Parkinson J, Papp C: Repetitive paroxysmal tachycardia. *Br Heart J* **9**:241, 1947.

66. Mahaim I, Benatt A: Nouvelles recherches sur les connexions superieures de la branche gauche du faisceau de His-Tawara avec cloison interventriculaire. *Cardiologia* **1**:61, 1968.

67. Lev M, Fox SMd, Bharati S, et al.: Mahaim and James fibers as a basis for a unique variety of ventricular preexcitation. *Am J Cardiol* **36**:880-8, 1975.

68. Neuss H, Thormann J: Functional properties of Mahaim fibers. *Klin Wochenschr* **55**:1031, 1977.
69. Gallagher JJ, Smith WM, Kasell JH, et al.: Role of Mahaim fibers in cardiac arrhythmias in man. *Circulation* **64**:176-89, 1981.
70. Tonkin AM, Dugan FA, Svenson RH, et al.: Coexistence of functional Kent and Mahaim-type tracts in the pre-excitation syndrome. Demonstration by catheter techniques and epicardial mapping. *Circulation* **52**:193-200, 1975.
71. Ward DE, Carson AJ, Spurrell RAJ: Ventricular preexcitation due to anomalous nodoventricular pathways: Report of 3 patients. *Eur J Cardiol* **9**:111, 1979.
72. Wellens HJJ. Tachycardias related to the preexcitation syndrome. In: Wellens HJJ, ed. *Electrical Stimulation of the Heart in the Study and Treatment of Tachycardias.* Baltimore, MD: University Park Press, 70-121: 1971.
73. Sung RJ, Castellanos A: Preexcitation syndrome. *Cardiovasc Clin* **11**:103-12, 1980.
74. Yamabe H, Okumura K, Minoda K, Yasue H: Nodoventricular Mahaim fiber connecting to the left ventricle. *Am Heart J* **122**:232, 1991.
75. Sung RJ, Styperek JL: Electrophysiologic identification of dual atrioventricular nodal pathway conduction in patients with reciprocating tachycardia using anomalous bypass tracts. *Circulation* **60**:1464-76, 1979.
76. Juma Z, Saksena S, Levy S, et al.: Electrophysiologic characteristics of nodoventricular bypass tract conduction in patients with dual atrioventricular nodal pathways. *Circulation* **60**:III-47, 1980.
77. Young C, Lauer MR, Liem LB, et al.: Demonstration of a posterior atrial input to the atrioventricular node during sustained anterograde slow pathway conduction. *J Am Coll Cardiol* **31**:1651-21, 1998.
78. Sung RJ, Waxman HL, Saksena S, Juma Z: Sequence of retrograde atrial activation in patients with dual atrioventricular nodal pathways. *Circulation* **64**:1059-67, 1981.
79. Klein GJ, Guiraudon GM, Kerr CR, et al.: "Nodoventricular" accessory pathway: evidence for a distinct accessory atrioventricular pathway with atrioventricular node-like properties. *J Am Coll Cardiol* **11**:1035-40, 1988.
80. Tchou P, Lehmann MH, Jazayeri M, Akhtar M: Atriofascicular connection or a nodoventricular Mahaim fiber? Electrophysiologic elucidation of the pathway and associated reentrant circuit. *Circulation* **77**:837-48, 1988.
81. Gillette PC, Garson A, Cooley DA, McNamara DG: Prolonged and decremental antegrade conduction properties in right anterior accessory connections: Wide QRS antidromic tachycardia of left bundle branch block pattern without Wolff-Parkinson-White configuration in sinus rhythm. *Am Heart J* **103**:66, 1982.
82. Murdock CJ, Leitch JW, Klein GJ, et al.: Epicardial mapping in patients with "nodoventricular" accessory pathways. *Am J Cardiol* **68**:208-14, 1991.
83. Murdock CJ, Leitch JW, Teo WS, et al.: Characteristics of accessory pathways exhibiting decremental conduction. *Am J Cardiol* **67**:506-10, 1991.
84. Anderson RH, Janse MJ, van Capelle FJ, et al.: A combined morphological and electrophysiological study of the atrioventricular node of the rabbit heart. *Circ Res* **35**:909-22, 1974.
85. Anderson RH, Wilkinson JL, Arnold R, et al.: Morphogenesis of bulboventricular malformations. II. Observations on malformed hearts. *Br Heart J* **36**:948-70, 1974.
86. Anderson RH, Wilkinson JL, Arnold R, Lubkiewicz K: Morphogenesis of bulboventricular malformations. I. Consideration of embryogenesis in the normal heart. *Br Heart J* **36**:242-55, 1974.
87. Inoue S, Becker AE: Posterior extensions of the human compact atrioventricular node: a neglected anatomic feature of potential clinical significance. *Circulation* **97**:188-93, 1998.
88. Haissaguerre M, Cauchemez B, Marcus F, et al.: Characteristics of the ventricular insertion sites of accessory pathways with anterograde decremental conduction properties. *Circulation* **91**:1077-85, 1995.
89. Coumel P: Junctional reciprocating tachycardias. The permanent and paroxysmal forms of A-V nodal reciprocating tachycardias. *J Electrocardiol* **8**:79-90, 1975.
90. Coumel P, Attuel P, Motte G, et al.: Paroxysmal junctional tachycardia. Determination of the inferior point of junction of the reentry circuit. Dissociation of the intra-nodal reciprocal rhythms. *Arch Mal Coeur Vaiss* **68**:1255-68, 1975.
91. Gallagher JJ, Sealy WC: The permanent form of junctional reciprocating tachycardia: further elucidation of the underlying mechanism. *Eur J Cardiol* **8**:413-30, 1978.

92. Gallagher JJ, Smith WM, Kerr CR: Etiology of long P-R tachycardia in 33 cases of supraventricular tachycardia (Abstract). *Circulation* **64(Suppl IV)**:IV-145, 1981.

93. Farre J, Ross D, Wiener I, et al.: Reciprocal tachycardias using accessory pathways with long conduction times. *Am J Cardiol* **44**:1099-109, 1979.

94. Epstein ML, Stone FM, Benditt DG: Incessant atrial tachycardia in childhood: association with rate-dependent conduction in an accessory atrioventricular pathway. *Am J Cardiol* **44**:498-504, 1979.

95. Denes P, Kehoe R, Rosen KM: Multiple reentrant tachycardias due to retrograde conduction of dual atrioventricular bundles with atrioventricular nodal-like properties. *Am J Cardiol* **44**:162-70, 1979.

96. Sung RJ, Styperek JL, Myerburg RJ, Castellanos A: Initiation of two distinct forms of atrioventricular nodal reentrant tachycardia during programmed ventricular stimulation in man. *Am J Cardiol* **42**:404-15, 1978.

97. Wu D, Denes P, et al.: An unusual variety of atrioventricular nodal re-entry due to retrograde dual atrioventricular nodal pathways. *Circulation* **56**:50-9, 1977.

98. Tai DY, Chang MS, Svinarich JT, et al.: Mechanisms of verapamil-induced conduction block in anomalous atrioventricular bypass tracts. *J Am Coll Cardiol* **5**:311-7, 1985.

99. Lev M, Leffler WB, Langendorf R, Pick A: Anatomic findings in a case of ventricular preexcitation (Wolff-Parkinson-White syndrome) terminating in complete atrioventricular block. *Circulation* **34**:718-33, 1966.

100. Brechenmacher C, Laham J, Iris L, et al.: Etude histologique des voies anormales de conduction dans un syndrome de Wolff-Parkinson-White et dans un syndrome de Lown-Ganong-Levine. *Arch Mal Coeur* **67**:507, 1974.

101. James TN: Morphology of the human atrioventricular node, with remarks pertinent to its electrophysiology. *Am Heart J* **62**:756-771, 1961.

102. Castellanos A, Jr., Castillo CA, Agha AS, Tesslef M: His bundle electrograms in patients with short P-R intervals, narrow QRS complexes, and paroxysmal tachycardias. *Circulation* **43**:667-78, 1971.

103. Caracta AR, Damato AN, Gallagher JJ, et al.: Electrophysiologic studies in the syndrome of short P-R interval, normal QRS complex. *Am J Cardiol* **31**:245-53, 1973.

104. Castellanos A, Zaman L, Moleiro F, et al.: The Lown-Ganong-Levine syndrome. *Pacing Clin Electrophysiol* **5**:715-40, 1982.

105. Benditt DG, Epstein ML, Arentzen CE, et al.: Enhanced atrioventricular conduction in patients without preexcitation syndrome: relation to heart rate in paroxysmal reciprocating tachycardia. *Circulation* **65**:1474-9, 1982.

106. Bauernfeind RA, Ayres BF, Wyndham CC, et al.: Cycle length in atrioventricular nodal reentrant paroxysmal tachycardia with observations on the Lown-Ganong-Levine syndrome. *Am J Cardiol* **45**:1148-53, 1980.

107. Josephson ME, Kastor JA: Supraventricular tachycardia in Lown-Ganong-Levine syndrome: atrionodal versus intranodal reentry. *Am J Cardiol* **40**:521-7, 1977.

108. Lown B, Ganong WF, Levine SA: The syndrome of short P-R interval, normal QRS complex and paroxysmal rapid heart action. *Circulation* **5**:693, 1952.

109. Blanc JJ, Fontaliran F, Gerbeaux A, et al.: Atrial flutter with 1-1 atrioventricular conduction: Electrophysiologic and histologic correlations. *Am Heart J* **107**:1044, 1984.

110. Shen EN, Keung E, Huycke E, et al.: Intravenous propafenone for termination of reentrant supraventricular tachycardia. A placebo-controlled, randomized, double-blind, crossover study. *Ann Intern Med* **105**:655-61, 1986.

111. Shen EN: Propafenone: A promising new antiarrhythmic agent. *Chest* **98**:434-41, 1990.

112. Sung RJ, Tan HL, Karagounis L, et al.: Intravenous sotalol for the termination of supraventricular tachycardia and atrial fibrillation and flutter: a multicenter, randomized, double-blind, placebo-controlled study. Sotalol Multicenter Study Group. *Am Heart J* **129**:739-48, 1995.

113. Rosenbaum MB, Chiale PA, Ryba D, Elizari MV: Control of tachyarrhythmias associated with Wolff-Parkinson-White syndrome by amiodarone hydrochloride. *Am J Cardiol* **34**:215-23, 1974.

114. Sellers TD, Jr., Bashore TM, Gallagher JJ: Digitalis in the pre-excitation syndrome. Analysis during atrial fibrillation. *Circulation* **56**:260-7, 1977.

115. Gulamhusein S, Ko P, Klein GJ: Ventricular fibrillation following verapamil in the Wolff-Parkinson-White syndrome. *Am Heart J* **106**:145-7, 1983.

116. Gulamhusein S, Ko P, Carruthers SG, Klein GJ: Acceleration of the ventricular response during atrial fibrillation in the Wolff-Parkinson-White syndrome after verapamil. *Circulation* **65**:348-54, 1982.

117. Sung RJ, Elser B, McAllister RG, Jr.: Intravenous verapamil for termination of re-entrant supraventricular tachycardias: intracardiac studies correlated with plasma verapamil concentrations. *Ann Intern Med* **93**:682-9, 1980.

118. Svinarich JT, Tai DY, Sung RJ: Is beta-adrenergic blockade contraindicated in Wolff-Parkinson-White patients prone to atrial fibrillation? (Abstract). *Circulation* **70**:II-251, 1984.

119. Clemo HF, Belardinelli L: Effect of adenosine on atrioventricular conduction. II: Modulation of atrioventricular node transmission by adenosine in hypoxic isolated guinea pig hearts. *Circ Res* **59**:437-46, 1986.

120. Clemo HF, Belardinelli L: Effect of adenosine on atrioventricular conduction. I: Site and characterization of adenosine action in the guinea pig atrioventricular node. *Circ Res* **59**:427-36, 1986.

121. Lerman BB, Belardinelli L: Cardiac electrophysiology of adenosine. Basic and clinical concepts. *Circulation* **83**:1499-509, 1991.

122. Lerman BB, Greenberg M, Overholt ED, et al.: Differential electrophysiologic properties of decremental retrograde pathways in long RP' tachycardia. *Circulation* **76**:21-31, 1987.

123. Ellenbogen KA, Rogers R, Old W: Pharmacological characterization of conduction over a Mahaim fiber: evidence for adenosine sensitive conduction. *Pacing Clin Electrophysiol* **12**:1396-404, 1989.

124. Sung RJ: Can alteration of dual atrioventricular nodal pathway physiology be related to sinus node dysfunction? *J Cardiovasc Electrophysiol* **9**:479-80, 1998.

125. Keim S, Curtis AB, Belardinelli L, et al.: Adenosine-induced atrioventricular block: a rapid and reliable method to assess surgical and radiofrequency catheter ablation of accessory atrioventricular pathways. *J Am Coll Cardiol* **19**:1005-12, 1992.

126. Souza JJ, Zivin A, Flemming M, et al.: Differential effect of adenosine on anterograde and retrograde fast pathway conduction in patients with atrioventricular nodal reentrant tachycardia. *J Cardiovasc Electrophysiol* **9**:820-4, 1998.

127. Borggrefe M, Budde T, Podczeck A, Breithardt G: High frequency alternating current ablation of an accessory pathway in humans. *J Am Coll Cardiol* **10**:576-582, 1987.

128. Jackman WM, Wang X, Friday KJ, et al.: Catheter ablation of accessory atrioventricular pathways (Wolff-Parkinson-White syndrome) by radiofrequency current. *New Engl J Med* **324**:1605-1611, 1991.

129. Brugada J, Martinez-Sanchez J, Kuzmicic B, et al.: Radiofrequency catheter ablation of atriofascicular accessory pathways guided by discrete electrical potentials recorded at the tricuspid annulus. *Pacing Clin Electrophysiol* **18**:1388-94, 1995.

130. Heald SC, Davies DW, Ward DE, et al.: Radiofrequency catheter ablation of Mahaim tachycardia by targeting Mahaim potentials at the tricuspid annulus. *Br Heart J* **73**:250-257, 1995.

131. Klein LS, Hackett FK, Zipes DP, Miles WM: Radiofrequency catheter ablation of Mahaim fibers at the tricuspid annulus. *Circulation* **87**:738-747, 1993.

132. McClelland JH, Wang X, Beckman KJ, et al.: Radiofrequency catheter ablation of right atriofascicular (Mahaim) accessory pathways guided by accessory pathway activation potentials. *Circulation* **89**:2655-66, 1994.

133. Mounsey JP, Griffith MJ, McComb JM: Radiofrequency ablation of Mahaim fiber following localization of Mahaim pathway potentials. *J Cardiovasc Electrophysiol* **5**:432-437, 1994.

134. Okishige K, Strickberger SA, Walsh EP, et al.: Catheter ablation of the atrial origin of a decrementally conducting atriofascicular accessory pathway by radiofrequency current. *Journal of Cardiovascular Electrophysiology* **2**:564-575, 1991.

135. Okishige K, Goseki Y, Itoh A, et al.: New electrophysiologic features and catheter ablation of atrioventricular and atriofascicular accessory pathways: evidence of decremental conduction and the anatomic structure of the Mahaim pathway. *J Cardiovasc Electrophysiol* **9**:22-33, 1998.

136. Sealy WC, Hattler BG, Jr., Blumenschein SD, Cobb FR: Surgical treatment of Wolff-Parkinson-White syndrome. *Ann Thorac Surg* **8**:1-11, 1969.

137. Sealy WC, Wallace AJ, Ramming KP, et al.: An improved operation for the definitive treatment of the Wolff-Parkinson-White syndrome. *Ann Thorac Surg* **17**:107-13, 1974.

138. Sealy WC, Gallagher JJ, Wallace AG: The surgical treatment of Wolff-Parkinson-White Syndrome: evolution of improved methods for identification and interruption of the Kent Bundle. *Ann Thorac Surg* **22**:443-57, 1976.

139. Sealy WC, Anderson RW, Gallagher JJ: Surgical treatment of supraventricular tachyarrhythmias. *J Thorac Cardiovasc Surg* **73**:511-22, 1977.

140. Sealy WC, Gallagher JJ, Pritchett EL: The surgical anatomy of Kent bundles based on electrophysiological mapping and surgical exploration. *J Thorac Cardiovasc Surg* **76**:804-15, 1978.

141. Sealy WC, Gallagher JJ, Pritchett EL: The surgical approach to supraventricular arrhythmias. *Cardiovasc Clin* **11**:365-80, 1981.

142. Sealy WC, Gallagher JJ: Surgical treatment of left free wall accessory pathways of atrioventricular conduction of the Kent type. *J Thorac Cardiovasc Surg* **81**:698-706, 1981.

143. Sealy WC, Gallagher JJ: Surgical problems with multiple accessory pathways of atrioventricular conduction. *J Thorac Cardiovasc Surg* **81**:707-12, 1981.

144. Gaita F, Haissaguerre M, Giustetto C, et al.: Catheter ablation of permanent junctional reciprocating tachycardia with radiofrequency current. *J Am Coll Cardiol* **25**:648-54, 1995.

145. Kuo CT, Lauer MR, Young C, et al.: Role of atrial extrastimulation in the diagnosis of atrioventricular node reentrant tachycardia with antegrade atrioventricular conduction via bystander accessory connection. *Am Heart J* **131**:839-42, 1996.

146. Young C, Lauer MR, Liem LB, Sung RJ: A characteristic electrocardiographic pattern indicative of manifest left-sided posterior septal/paraseptal accessory atrioventricular connections. *Am J Cardiol* **72**:471-5, 1993.

147. Lee KL, Lauer MR, Young C, et al.: Characteristic electrocardiographic features of manifest left anterior paraseptal accessory atrioventricular connection. *Am Heart J* **131**:814-8, 1996.

148. Huycke EC, Nguyen NX, et al.: Spontaneous conversion of atrial flutter to antidromic atrioventricular reciprocating tachycardia in the Wolff-Parkinson-White syndrome. *Am Heart J* **115**:917-9, 1988.

149. Lai WT, Huycke EC, Keung EC, et al.: Electrophysiologic manifestations of the excitable gap of orthodromic atrioventricular reciprocating tachycardia demonstrated by single extrastimulation. *Am J Cardiol* **63**:545-55, 1989.

CHAPTER 13

ATRIAL TACHYCARDIAS AND ATRIAL FLUTTER

Atrial tachyarrhythmias are defined as supraventricular tachyarrhythmias that do not require the AV node or ventricular tissue for initiation and maintenance. Therefore, this definition excludes AV junctional tachycardia, AV nodal reentrant tachycardia, and AV reciprocating tachycardia involving an accessory AV connection. These arrhythmias are discussed in detail elsewhere ("Atrioventricular Nodal Reentrant Tachycardia" on page 487 and "Ventricular Preexcitation Syndromes: The Wolff-Parkinson-White Syndrome and Variants" on page 539). The main focus of this chapter is on focal and macroreentrant atrial tachycardias including atrial flutter. Although atrial fibrillation is briefly discussed here, it is reviewed in more detail in Chapter 14.

13.1 Classification of Atrial Tachycardias

There has been numerous classification schemes proposed for atrial tachyarrhythmias. They have been classified by their presumed cellular mechanism, their rate or surface ECG features, their presumed substrate of origin, their sensitivity to specific pharmacological agents, or their clinical presentation and clinical course [1]. Often the classification is merely arbitrary, using such terms as "type I", "classic", "type A", or "common". All of these classification schemes have problems. For example, the use of pharmacological sensitivity is notoriously inconsistent. In the past, termination of a supraventricular tachycardia by adenosine or verapamil was used as evidence that the tachycardia was either AV nodal reentrant tachycardia or AV reciprocating tachycardia. However, it is now clear that many atrial tachycardias may be terminated by these agents [2,3]. In addition, termination by adenosine and verapamil has been used as evidence that the mechanism of the arrhythmia is triggered activity. However, reentrant arrhythmias that utilize a critical area of slow conduction may also be terminated by these agents.

Because of these and other limitations, another classification system has been proposed based upon endocardial mapping data from electrophysiology studies [1]. This classification scheme is useful to the interventional electrophysiologist because it attempts to classify atrial tachycardias based on potential target tissues for electrode catheter ablation (Table 13-1.) By this classification scheme, atrial tachyarrhythmias are divided into four general groups. *Macroreentrant atrial tachycardias* utilize a macroscopic reentrant circuit, the critical portion of which is a protected isthmus created between two or more functional, fixed anatomic, or surgically-produced barriers. These atrial tachycardias can be cured by transection of the isthmus with radiofrequency (RF) lesions, thereby eliminating the possibility of electrical conduction through the critical isthmus region. *Focal atrial tachycardias* arise from a focal area of atrial tissue, do not require the presence of fixed barriers for initiation or maintenance of the arrhythmia, and may result from either microreentry, triggered activity, or automaticity. Focal atrial tachycardias have an anatomic preference for the crista terminalis, ostium of the coronary sinus, atrial septum, and pulmonary veins. The so-called "sinoatrial" or "sinus node reentrant tachycardia" is a form of "cristal" atrial tachycardia (see below). Focal tachycardias can be eliminated by *focal* application of RF energy. *Inappropriate sinus tachycardia* is a unique form of atrial tachycardia that is neither clearly focal in origin nor generated by a macroscopic reentrant circuit. Finally, *atrial fibrillation* is a disorganized, chaotic atrial tachyarrhythmia which may be triggered by closely-coupled atrial premature depolarizations, or a rapid atrial tachycardia, often originating within the pulmonary veins.

TABLE 13-1. Classification of atrial tachyarrhythmias

Focal Atrial Tachycardia
Cristal atrial tachycardia
Atrial tachycardia of pulmonary venous origin
Other focal atrial tachycardias (atrial septum, coronary sinus, orifice of atrial appendages, multifocal)
Inappropriate Sinus Tachycardia
Macroreentrant Atrial Tachycardia
Typical atrial flutter
Clockwise atrial flutter
Counterclockwise atrial flutter
Atypical atrial flutter
Other macroreentrant atrial tachycardias (e.g., incisional)
Atrial Fibrillation
Adapted from [1].

13.2 Focal Atrial Tachycardia

The sites of origin of focal atrial tachycardias are not randomly distributed within the right and left atria. Focal atrial tachycardias preferentially originate from a focal region within the: 1) crista terminalis (cristal atrial tachycardias); 2) atrial septum (but clearly outside the AV node); 3) pulmonary veins; 4) the ostium of the coronary sinus; 5) orifices of the right or left atrial appendages (Figure 13-1).

Focal atrial tachycardias may be caused by abnormal automaticity, triggered activity, and microreentry. *In vitro* evidence suggests that triggered activity related to delayed afterdepolarizations may play an important arrhythmogenic role in patients with atrial tachycardias resulting from digitalis intoxication [4]. Regardless of the mechanism, the defining characteristic of a focal tachycardia is the ability to successfully eliminate the arrhythmia by *focal* application of RF energy. This distinguishes these tachyarrhythmias

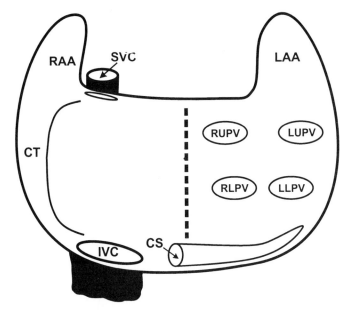

FIGURE 13-1. Schematic of the right and left atria summarizing the typical sites of origin of focal atrial tachycardias. Preferential sites include the orifice of the right (RAA) or left (LAA) atrial appendages, crista terminalis (CT), the ostium of the coronary sinus (CS), and the pulmonary veins, including the right upper (RUPV). right lower (RLPV), left upper (LUPV), and left lower (LLPV). The pulmonary veins are also preferential sites of origin (>95%) for the focal triggers of atrial fibrillation, especially the upper pulmonary veins (LUPV > RUPV). The CT is an uncommon origin for atrial fibrillation triggers. IVC, inferior vena cava; SVC, superior vena cava.

from macroreentrant atrial tachycardias that depend upon a protected isthmus and require transection of the isthmus with a series of RF lesions for ablative cure.

13.2.1 CLINICAL AND ELECTROCARDIOGRAPHIC PRESENTATION

Patients with focal atrial tachycardia usually present with paroxysmal sustained atrial tachycardia if reentry is the underlying mechanism, but with repetitive atrial tachycardia or continuous tachycardia if it is caused by abnormal automaticity. Frequently, focal atrial tachycardias due to automaticity or triggered activity may exhibit a "warm-up" phenomenon, during which the atrial rate gradually accelerates from a slower initial rate to the faster rate maintained throughout most of the duration of the tachycardia. Unlike patients with paroxysmal supraventricular tachycardia due to AV nodal reentry or AV reciprocation utilizing an accessory AV connection, patients with a focal atrial tachycardia often have underlying structural heart disease, most often coronary artery disease [5-8]. Patients with a reentrant mechanism are typically older and are more likely to have an underlying cardiac disease as compared to patients having a focal atrial tachycardia with automaticity as the underlying mechanism.

Analysis of the P-wave morphology may assist in localization of a focal atrial tachycardia. However, a common problem that frequently complicates P-wave analysis is superimposition of the QRS complex and T-wave. Atrioventricular block may be spontaneously present during atrial tachycardia (Figure 13-2), or it may be induced by carotid sinus massage (Figure 13-3). Transient production of AV block (with adenosine or carotid sinus massage) allows visualization of the P-wave morphology during atrial tachycardia. Electrocardiographic leads aVL and V_1 were most helpful for distinguishing right atrial foci from left atrial foci [9,10]: the sensitivity and specificity of using a posi-

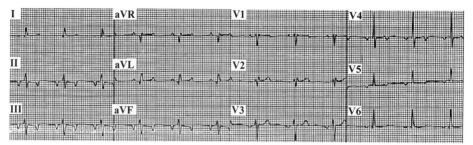

FIGURE 13-2. Focal atrial tachycardia with 2:1 AV conduction block. Note long R-P interval and the negative P-waves in ECG leads II, III, and aVF. Activation mapping localized the tachycardia to the region near
the ostium of the coronary sinus. The tachycardia was successfully eliminated with RF ablation (not shown).

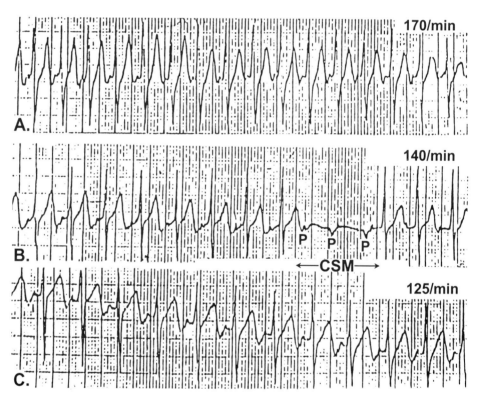

FIGURE 13-3. Electrocardiographic rhythm strips showing slowing of atrial tachycardia after intravenous
infusion of procainamide. Panel A: Baseline atrial tachycardia (1:1 AV conduction) before procainamide
infusion. Panel B: After administration of procainamide, 500-mg; carotid sinus massage (CSM) exposes P
waves of atrial tachycardia. Panel C: After infusion of procainamide, 1000 mg, atrial tachycardia rate has
further decreased and continues to conduct to the ventricles in a 1:1 fashion. ECG lead II shown. Paper
speed 25 mm/sec. From [79] with permission.

tive or biphasic P-wave in lead aVL to predict a right atrial focus are 88% and 79%, respectively. The sensitivity and specificity of a positive P-wave in lead V_1 in predicting a left atrial focus are 93% and 88%, respectively. Furthermore, ECG leads II, III, and aVF are helpful for providing clues for differentiating superior from inferior foci. If the site of atrial tachycardia origin is close to the inter-atrial septum, the atrium of origin may be difficult to establish. Atrial tachycardias with a right pulmonary vein origin may be easily confused with those having a right atrial origin. However, a monophasic, positive P-waves in lead V_1, along with a markedly inferiorly directed P-wave axis, suggestive of a left atrial origin.

Atrial tachycardia often exhibits a variable RP interval with intermittent AV block, (with or without carotid sinus massage or intravenous administration of adenosine) (Figure 13-3). However, the RP interval is dependent upon the tachycardia rate and AV conduction properties; consequently, AV block may not be observed. Adenosine may cause tachycardia termination before blocking conduction within the AV node. Unlike sinus tachycardia, during focal atrial tachycardia the AV nodal conduction delay may be substantial, and the RP-to-PR ratio may be less than one so that the P-wave appears to follow the QRS complex [5,11]. Because the AV node is not part of the reentrant circuit, AH interval prolongation and 2:1 and 3:1 AV conduction may occur without termination of the tachycardia. Atrioventricular block is particularly common in the case of a focal atrial tachycardia resulting from digitalis intoxication (Figure 13-4).

While atrial cardiomyopathy may be the cause of atrial tachycardia, continuous atrial tachycardia may itself cause a tachycardia-induced cardiomyopathy. Heart failure is not infrequently the first manifestation of an incessant atrial tachycardia due to a tachycardia-induced cardiomyopathy, especially in children. Typically, the impaired left ventricular function improves and often returns to normal following successful treatment of the arrhythmia, emphasizing the importance of early diagnosis and curative or suppressive therapy.

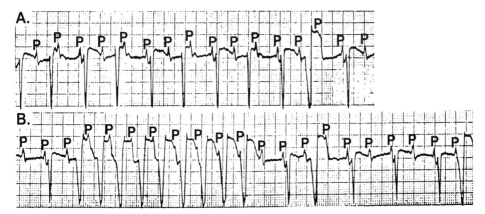

FIGURE 13-4. ECG rhythm strips showing atrial tachycardia with AV block (3:2 AV Wenckebach in panel A and 2:1 AV block in panel B) due to digoxin intoxication (serum digoxin level of 4.6 ng/dl). Ventricular premature depolarizations and a short run of ventricular tachycardia presumably caused by digitalis-induced automaticity or triggered activity is also noted. Paper speed 25 mm/sec. From [79] with permission.

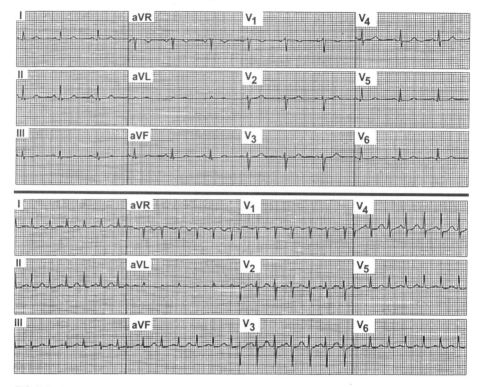

FIGURE 13-5. Cristal tachycardia localized to the high right atrium near the sinus node. Upper panel: 12-lead ECG showing baseline sinus rhythm. Lower panel: 12-lead ECG showing atrial tachycardia. The tachycardia was induced by programmed atrial extrastimulation, mapped to the high crista terminalis, and successfully ablated using RF energy (not shown). Note the similarity of the P-wave morphology during tachycardia compared with that recorded during sinus rhythm.

Functional dissociation within the region of the sinus node and reentry-mediated echo impulses have been demonstrated in animal heart preparations [12-14]. In man, reentry within this area of the atrium may include the sinoatrial node, the perinodal zone, and atrial tissue adjacent to the sinus node [11,15] in the crista terminalis. *Cristal atrial tachycardia* is defined as a focal atrial tachycardia that arises along the crista terminalis. Included in this definition is the so-called "sinoatrial reentrant tachycardia" (Figure 13-5). Unless the tachycardia originates from the most superior aspect of the crista terminalis, the P-wave morphology and axis during tachycardia will differ from that seen during sinus rhythm. As previously discussed (see "Functional Anatomy of the Conduction System" on page 1), the sinoatrial node is a diffuse region that occupies the superior aspect of the crista terminalis. Since the entire length of the crista can act as the substrate for atrial tachycardia, it is expected that some focal atrial tachycardias will have an activation sequence similar to that seen during sinus rhythm. However, there is neither evidence that "sinoatrial reentrant tachycardia" behaves differently from focal tachycardias arising from other regions of the crista, nor that it involves the histological sinus node [1]. Furthermore, *in vivo* electrophysiological mapping of the crista terminalis confirms

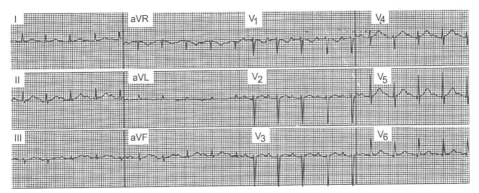

FIGURE 13-6. Paroxysmal focal atrial tachycardia localized to atrial septum superior and posterior to the compact AV node. The tachycardia was inducible by programmed atrial extrastimulation and rapid atrial burst pacing. The tachycardia was insensitive to adenosine and the patient did not exhibit dual AV nodal pathway physiology. After mapping, the tachycardia was successfully ablated with a single application of RF energy.

that there is no single activation sequence generated by the sinus node; the earliest activation and P-wave axis vary with changes in autonomic tone. Thus, sinoatrial reentrant tachycardia may not represent a specific atrial tachycardia, but instead may be a form of cristal atrial tachycardia.

In addition to the crista terminalis, focal atrial tachycardias may originate near the ostium of the coronary sinus (Figure 13-2), the atrial septum (outside the AV node) (Figure 13-6), and the pulmonary veins and present as a stable, organized atrial tachycardia (Figures 13-7 & 13-8), or may be rapid enough to degenerate into atrial fibrillation (Figure 13-9).

Focal atrial tachycardias, especially those arising within the pulmonary veins, may trigger atrial fibrillation. Attempts have been made to cure paroxysmal and persistent atrial fibrillation with RF catheter ablation, based on the surgical Maze procedure. While these early attempts had low success and high complication rates, they nevertheless revealed that an underlying focus of a rapid atrial tachycardia was frequently unmasked after creation of the linear endocardial lesions. Furthermore, if the rapidly firing focus – frequently located within one of the pulmonary veins – could be abolished with focal application of RF energy, the result was no further episodes of atrial fibrillation.

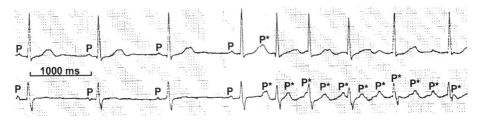

FIGURE 13-7. Organized atrial tachycardia originating in a left pulmonary vein in a patient with paroxysmal atrial tachycardia and fibrillation. This pulmonary vein focus (cycle length approximately 280-msec) was successfully ablated with RF energy. P, sinus P-wave; P*, P-wave inscribed during atrial tachycardia (best seen in lower ECG tracing).

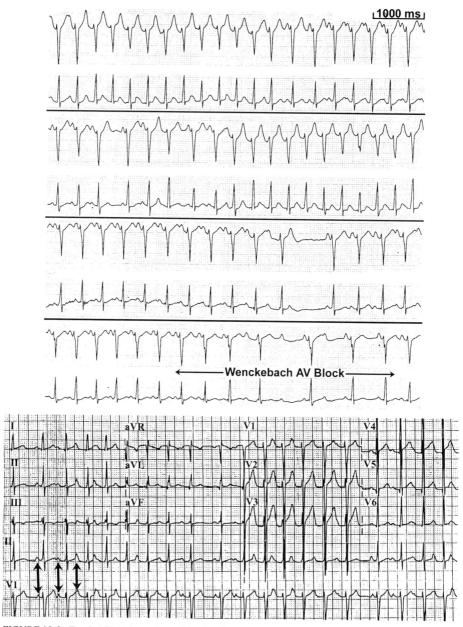

FIGURE 13-8. Focal atrial tachycardias originating in the pulmonary veins of a 28-year old man with incessant supraventricular tachycardia (ambulatory ECG in upper panel) and mild left ventricular dysfunction on echocardiogram. The patient was asymptomatic but was found to have a rapid pulse during a routine examination. At least three different P-wave morphologies are observed on the 12-lead ECG (lower panel, arrows). Note the variable PR intervals during tachycardia and Wenckebach-type AV block. Three different foci were ablated in the right and left upper, and right lower pulmonary veins, eliminating the tachycardias. Follow-up ambulatory ECG monitoring showed sinus rhythm with normal rate variation. Pulmonary vein atrial tachycardias can exhibit P-waves with morphologies very similar to that seen during sinus rhythm.

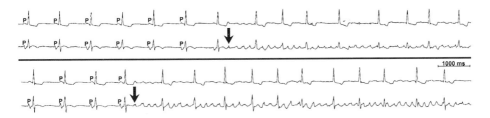

FIGURE 13-9. Electrocardiographic rhythm strips recorded from a patient with rapid atrial tachycardia originating within the ostia of a pulmonary vein. The onset of the atrial tachycardia (arrows) degenerates into atrial fibrillation. Catheter ablation was successful at eliminating this triggering focus.

These initial findings have been extended to a larger number of patients, thus providing a causative link between atrial tachycardia and atrial fibrillation. This observation is important because it suggests that paroxysmal atrial fibrillation may be curable by focal application of RF energy.

The prevalence of a rapidly firing focus in the general population of patients with paroxysmal atrial fibrillation is unknown. Even for patients with focally triggered atrial fibrillation, the mechanism of maintenance of the tachyarrhythmia has yet to be determined. The focal trigger may be essential only for the initiation of atrial fibrillation. Multiple reentrant wavelets, facilitated by short- and long-term electrical remodeling, may be necessary for maintenance of the arrhythmia. It is possible, at least in some patients with structurally normal hearts, that the rapid focal activity is essential for both the initiation *and* maintenance of atrial fibrillation.

A number of factors such as stretch, fibrosis, ischemia, variations in autonomic tone, or atrial remodeling induced by atrial fibrillation itself may further influence the propensity for the firing of the focal trigger. While the relevance of a focal trigger has been clearly demonstrated for a subset of patients with very frequent paroxysms of atrial fibrillation, it is not clear if patients with less frequent paroxysmal atrial fibrillation, or even those with persistent or chronic atrial fibrillation, may have a focal trigger.

The patient history, the 12-lead EGG, and the finding of multiple paroxysms of atrial fibrillation and frequent atrial premature beats during ambulatory ECG monitoring are very suggestive of a focal trigger for atrial fibrillation (Figures 13-7 & 13-9). Patients with paroxysmal atrial fibrillation who have a documented underlying focal atrial trigger usually have frequent (more than once a week) episodes of atrial fibrillation as well as frequent atrial ectopic beats documented during ambulatory ECG recording. Often, the P-wave morphology of the isolated atrial premature depolarizations is similar or identical to that of the atrial premature depolarizations triggering atrial fibrillation.

Multifocal atrial tachycardia appears to be a special type of atrial tachycardia in which atrial activation originates from multiple atrial foci. Focal atrial tachycardias with multiple origins may arise from the pulmonary veins and may occur in young, healthy subjects with no structural heart disease (Figure 13-8). Typically, however, multifocal atrial tachycardia is observed in patients with exacerbations of chronic obstructive pulmonary disease (especially with cor pulmonale), acute illnesses (pneumonia, pulmonary thromboembolism, sepsis) or exacerbations of congestive heart failure in patients with atherosclerotic coronary artery disease [16-19]. Furthermore, it may be observed after general surgery and a complicated course in the intensive care unit, often in association with non-pulmonary infections, diabetes mellitus, and lung carcinoma.

Multifocal atrial tachycardia is often associated hypoxemia, α- or β-adrenergic stimulation, or treatment with theophylline, sometimes in the setting of hypokalemia and digoxin therapy. Therefore, multifocal atrial tachycardia may be due to abnormal automaticity of several atrial foci, or triggered activity due to delayed afterdepolarizations [20-22].

The ECG criteria required to diagnose multifocal atrial tachycardia (Figure 13-10) include the following: 1) atrial rate greater than 100 beats/min; 2) well-organized, discrete P-waves of at least three morphologic types without a dominant pacemaker; 3) irregular variation in the P-P interval; and 4) an isoelectric baseline between P-waves [17]. The atrial rate during multifocal atrial tachycardia is generally less than 150 beats/min and typically exhibits 1:1 AV conduction. The P-waves are sometimes inconspicuous on the electrocardiogram making differentiation from atrial fibrillation difficult. Indeed, patients with multifocal atrial tachycardia may eventually develop atrial fibrillation or atrial flutter [16]. Multifocal atrial tachycardia is distinguished from sinus tachycardia with frequent premature atrial depolarizations by the absence of a dominant sinus pacemaker. No significant electrophysiologic data are available on the mechanism of multifocal atrial tachycardia, although some cases may result from multiple triggering foci in the pulmonary veins.

13.2.2 ELECTROPHYSIOLOGIC CHARACTERISTICS AND DIAGNOSIS

Intracardiac electrophysiology testing may be required to establish the diagnosis of focal atrial tachycardia, often by excluding other tachycardia mechanisms. In the laboratory, localization of the origin of a focal atrial tachycardia is achieved using multisite endocardial mapping performed with steerable pacing and recording catheters. Generally, one catheter is positioned in the right ventricular apex in order to perform programmed ventricular stimulation and assess retrograde ventriculoatrial conduction. A second multipo-

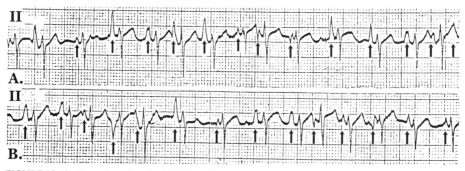

FIGURE 13-10. Recording of surface ECG lead II showing multifocal atrial tachycardia. Panels A and B are from a continuous recording. Note the presence of discrete P-waves with at least three different morphologic patterns, irregular P-P intervals, and an isoelectric baseline between most of the P-waves. Paper speed 25 mm/sec. From [79] with permission.

lar catheter is positioned at the His bundle region. Right atrial pacing and recording can be performed using a 10- or 20-pole catheter draped along the lateral, superior, and septal portions of the right atrium (Figure 13-11). Alternatively, the catheter tip can be placed in ostium of the coronary sinus with the remaining proximal catheter electrodes allowed to lie along the floor of the right atrium, laterally, and then continue superiorly parallel to crista terminalis to the high right atrium near the junction of the superior vena cava (see "Typical Clockwise & Counterclockwise Atrial Flutters" on page 627). In this way, the right atrial activation sequence can be evaluated during tachycardia (i.e., from high to low right atrium, or from the low to high right atrium). As a surrogate for the left atrial activation, a multipolar catheter is usually inserted into the coronary sinus. After establishing that the tachycardia is confined to the atria, the ventricular catheter is often removed and replaced by a large-tip quadripolar mapping/ablating catheter.

Focal atrial tachycardia due to microreentry may be initiated with atrial premature beats (Figure 13-12) or by achievement of a critical atrial rate (Figure 13-13), presumably because of the development of block in one limb of the reentrant pathway. Focal atrial tachycardias due to reentry can be initiated over a well-defined reproducible echo zone by premature atrial extrastimulation (Figure 13-14). Atrial extrastimulation can also reproducibly terminate the tachycardia. A high-to-low sequence of atrial activation is seen during a cristal atrial tachycardia originating in the superior aspect of the crista terminalis. A low-to-high activation sequence is observed when the atrial tachycardia originates in the posterior or inferior regions of the atria (Figure 13-12). Focal atrial tachycardias due to abnormal automaticity cannot be initiated or terminated by atrial extra-

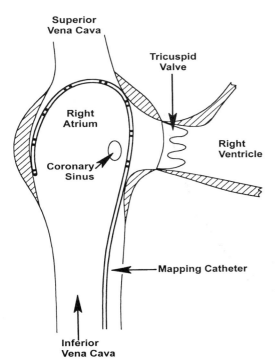

FIGURE 13-11. Schematic diagram depicting right anterior oblique fluoroscopic view of heart and possible multipolar electrode catheter position for initial mapping of right atrial tachycardia. Catheter re-positioning may be necessary based on initial mapping data. In particular, the electrodes may have to be positioned to the area within the isthmus between the inferior vena cava and tricuspid annulus with the catheter tip near the ostium of the coronary sinus. This allows mapping of atrial tachycardias originating within the isthmus (inferior crista terminalis) or near the ostium of the coronary sinus. If mapping studies suggest the tachycardia is in the left atrium, a trans-septal catheterization must be performed.

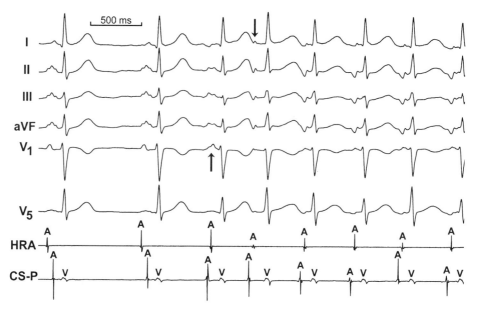

FIGURE 13-12. Onset of paroxysmal focal atrial tachycardia by spontaneous atrial premature depolarization (APD). The triggering APD (upward arrow) has a different morphology than the first and subsequent beats of the atrial tachycardia (downward arrow). Note also the change in the right atrial activation sequence. During sinus rhythm, endocardial activation of the high right atrium (HRA) precedes activation near the ostium of the coronary sinus (CS-P) (high-to-low sequence). However, the activation sequence during the APD and the tachycardia is early in the region of the CS-P than the HRA (low-to-high sequence). See text for additional discussion.

stimuli [23,24], but may occur spontaneously or be provoked during the intravenous administration of catecholamines.

Atrial tachycardia is definitively excluded (and AV reciprocation or AV nodal reentry is included) if ventricular pacing terminates the tachycardia without retrograde atrial activation. If there are more atrial activations than ventricular activations, the diagnosis of atrial tachycardia is reasonably assured. (This assumes that AV nodal reentrant tachycardia with 2:1 AV conduction is ruled-out). If there is an identical number of atrial and ventricular activations, other criteria and maneuvers must be employed. For a long RP

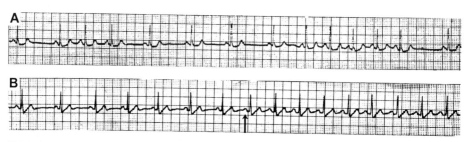

FIGURE 13-13. Cristal atrial tachycardia with P-wave morphology and axis similar to that seen during sinus rhythm. Panel A: onset of non-sustained atrial tachycardia (3rd and 9th P-waves). Panel B: onset of sustained cristal tachycardia (arrow) resulting from acceleration of sinus rate

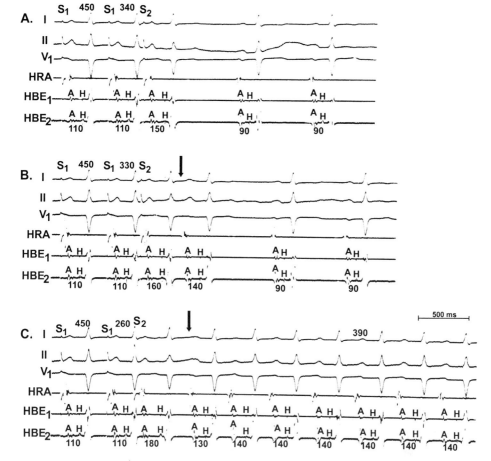

FIGURE 13-14. Initiation of high cristal atrial tachycardia ("sinoatrial reentrant tachycardia") with atrial extrastimulation. Surface ECG leads I, II, and V, are simultaneously displayed with endocardial recordings from the high right atrium (HRA) and His bundle (HBE). Panel A: High high right atrial pacing (S_1-S_1 = 450-msec) with delivery of an atrial premature depolarization (S_2) at a coupling interval (S_1-S_2) of 340-msec fails to induce the atrial arrhythmia. Panel B: Reducing of the coupling interval (S_1-S_2) to 330-msec provokes an atrial echo (arrow) due to intra-atrial reentry. Note the atrial echo depolarization exhibits a high-to-low atrial activation sequence. Panel C: Further shortening of the premature coupling interval (S_1-S_2) to 260-msec) initiates (arrow) sustained atrial tachycardia having a cycle length of 390-msec. Again, note the high-to-low atrial activation sequence during tachycardia. A, atrial electrogram; H, His-bundle electrogram. From [79] with permission.

tachycardia, the main differential diagnosis is either an atypical (fast-slow or slow-slow) AV nodal reentrant tachycardia or the permanent form of junctional reentrant tachycardia involving a slowly conducting retrograde accessory AV connection. For a short RP tachycardia, an accessory AV connection and typical AV nodal reentrant tachycardia must be excluded. In order to exclude an accessory AV connection, the atrial activation must be dissociated from the ventricular activation. Therefore, the first maneuver consists of introducing progressively earlier premature ventricular beats during tachycardia. If a

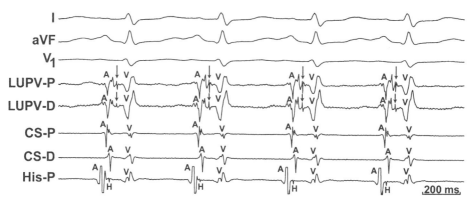

FIGURE 13-15. High-frequency "spike" electrograms recorded in a pulmonary vein during sinus rhythm. The patient's atrial tachycardia, induced by isoproterenol, was mapped to the left upper pulmonary vein. Intracardiac recordings are shown from distal and proximal electrodes in an upper branch of the left upper pulmonary vein (LUPV-D, and LUPV-P) and the coronary sinus (CS-D and CS-P), and the proximal His bundle region (His-P). During sinus rhythm, note the locally-recorded "spike" electrograms (arrows) that are inscribed after the recording of the far-field global left atrial activation.

premature ventricular depolarizations advances the next atrial activation at a time of anterograde His bundle activation, an accessory AV connection is present (although this maneuver does not necessarily prove that the accessory connection is part of the tachycardia circuit (i.e., it may be a "bystander pathway"). Sometimes, atrial extrastimuli, double ventricular extrastimuli, or ventricular overdrive pacing must be performed in addition to single ventricular extrastimuli in order to differentiate atrial tachycardia from AV nodal reentry. Atrioventricular reciprocating tachycardia using an accessory AV connection or AV nodal reentrant tachycardia is favored if ventricular overdrive pacing resets the tachycardia, or if it resumes after termination of ventricular pacing with an equal number of atrial and ventricular activations. Atrial tachycardia is suggested if ventricular pacing or ventricular extrastimuli cause transient AV conduction block, dissociating atrial from ventricular activation.

Focal atrial tachycardias of pulmonary venous origin display a number of unique electrophysiological characteristics. For mapping of an atrial tachycardia originating within the left atrium or pulmonary veins, the transseptal approach is preferred to the retrograde trans-aortic, trans-mitral approach because of the ease with which the mapping catheter can be manipulated in the left atrium. Patients with focal pulmonary vein triggers often exhibit high-frequency "spike" electrograms, even during sinus rhythm (Figure 13-15). Electrophysiology study and mapping of focal atrial tachycardias originating within the pulmonary veins can be difficult, primarily because of the inability to reliably induce the tachyarrhythmias. Programmed extrastimulation rarely provokes the arrhythmias. A variety of pharmacological agents, including isoproterenol, epinephrine, adenosine, α-adrenergic agonists, and vagotonic agents have been evaluated. In general, the intravenous infusion of isoproterenol (or "washout" phase) has proved most successful at triggering these tachyarrhythmias (Figure 13-16).

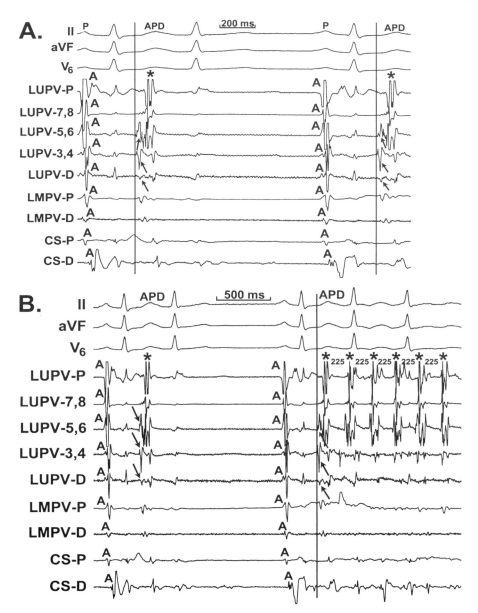

FIGURE 13-16. Intracardiac recordings from a pulmonary vein in a patient with paroxysmal atrial tachycardia and fibrillation. Note different paper speeds in panels A and B. A steerable decapolar catheter is positioned in the upper branch of the left upper pulmonary vein (LUPV), and a steerable quadripolar catheter is placed in the orifice of a middle branch of the left upper pulmonary vein (LMPV). Electrogram recordings are arranged from proximal (P) to distal (D). Recordings are also obtained from the proximal (CS-P) and distal (CS-D) coronary sinus. Panel A: atrial premature depolarizations (APD) occur spontaneously. The earliest activation (approximately 75-msec before the surface P-wave) is recorded in the LUPV. Note the high-frequency "spike" electrogram seen at the onset of the earliest atrial electrogram (arrows). Panel B: after discontinuation of an isoproterenol infusion, an atrial tachycardia develops (cycle length = 225-msec) with an electrogram activation sequence identical to that of the APDs. The "spike" electrogram is also seen at onset of the earliest atrial electrograms during the tachycardia (arrows). A, atrial electrogram during sinus rhythm.

13.3   Inappropriate Sinus Tachycardia

Inappropriate sinus tachycardia [25-27] is an uncommon, ill-defined clinical syndrome, most commonly found in young women, characterized by an abnormally elevated resting heart rate accompanied by an exaggerated increase in heart rate with minimal exertion or postural change (Table 13-2.) The excessive sinus rate must be correlated with symptoms and is usually associated with hypersensitivity to adrenergic stimulation. The resting heart rate is generally greater than 100 beats/min or, if less, the heart rate increases above 100 beats/min with minimal exertion. The morphology of the P-wave must be consistent with a sinus origin. The most common symptoms associated with inappropriate sinus tachycardia including: palpitations, dizziness, shortness of breath, fatigue, presyncope, and rarely, frank syncope. Compared to patients with AV nodal reentrant tachycardia, patients with inappropriate sinus tachycardia may have symptom amplification profiles similar to those seen in patients with hypochondriasis [28]. Inappropriate sinus tachycardia remains a diagnosis of exclusion; a secondary cause of sinus tachycardia must be ruled-out, as must *paroxysmal* atrial tachycardias. Patients with inappropriate sinus tachycardia usually do not have associated cardiac disease.

Inappropriate sinus tachycardia may be caused by a primary abnormality of the sinus node with enhanced automaticity, hypersensitivity to sympathetic tone, or a deficiency of vagal influence on the heart [25,26,29]. Patients usually exhibit a marked reduction in the resting atrial rate after the administration of β-adrenergic blocking agents such as propranolol, atenolol and metoprolol. This response suggests hypersensitivity to sympathetic tone as the underlying mechanism of inappropriate sinus tachycardia. However, in contrast, some patients may exhibit small increments in sinus rate after atropine administration, a finding that suggests a deficient vagal influence on the resting heart rate.

Interestingly, inappropriate sinus tachycardia has also been noted to develop acutely in some patients who have recently undergone RF catheter ablation for a wide variety of supraventricular tachycardias [30,31]. Most commonly, this condition arises after AV node modification or ablation of accessory AV pathways; it generally resolves within a few weeks or months. The mechanism appears to be a loss of parasympathetic influence on the sinoatrial node.

TABLE 13-2.   Diagnosis of inappropriate sinus tachycardia

Document inappropriate tachycardia using ECG, ambulatory ECG recording; or exercise stress test

Correlation of symptoms with ECG rhythm recording of tachycardia.

Exclusion of secondary causes including orthostatic hypotension, fever, anemia, physical deconditioning, congestive heart failure, drugs, hypoxemia, hyperthyroidism or other endocrine or metabolic disorders.

Electrophysiology testing to rule-out atrial tachycardia.

The diagnosis of the syndrome of inappropriate sinus tachycardia must be made on clinical grounds. However, autonomic and electrophysiology testing may be required in selected patients to clarify the mechanism and rule out a focal atrial tachycardia. Atrial extrastimulation and incremental atrial pacing do not terminate inappropriate sinus tachycardia, a finding that may distinguishes this arrhythmia form most focal atrial tachycardias, including the so-called "sinoatrial reentrant tachycardia" (cristal tachycardia originating in the high right atrium). Although commonly viewed as a focal structure, in reality the sinus node is poorly-defined, distributed structure located at the most superiomedial aspect of the crista terminalis. Inappropriate sinus tachycardia can be distinguished from a focal atrial tachycardia originating near the superior aspect of the crista terminalis using endocardial activation mapping. The activation sequence in a small region of the superior crista terminalis can be recorded using multipolar catheters with closely spaced electrodes (1-2 mm). Although the rate of a focal atrial tachycardia originating within this area may increase with the infusion of catecholamines, the site of earliest activation will not be affected. However, in the case of inappropriate sinus tachycardia, the locus of earliest activation will actually migrate superiorly and inferiorly along the crista terminalis as the rate increases or decreases, respectively, in response to a catecholamine infusion [1].

Initial treatment for patients with inappropriate sinus tachycardia is medical therapy, typically β-adrenergic blocking agents. In severe cases, class IA and IC drugs, or even amiodarone have been recommended. However, the risk profile of these drugs generally makes their use in young patients unpalatable.

Catheter ablative therapies, including sinus node modification, sinus node ablation, or total AV junctional ablation coupled with permanent pacemaker implantation should be reserved for patients with severe, medically-refractory, debilitating symptoms, in whom other reversible conditions and atrial tachycardias have been excluded. In addition, patients must be subjected to an extensive discussion of the potential benefits and risks. It is important to also counsel patients that many symptoms related to the syndrome of inappropriate sinus tachycardia including fatigue, depression, lethargy will not be affected by any ablation procedure; only symptoms clearly related to a rapid heart rate will be relieved by a successful ablation.

Some investigators have achieved modification of the sinus node rate response using radiofrequency energy [27,32-34]. Activation mapping of the crista terminalis is performed using multipolar catheters as described above during the intravenous infusion of isoproterenol. Under the influence of catecholamines, the increase in heart rate is associated with a superior shift in earliest sinus node activation. Radiofrequency energy is applied during isoproterenol infusion to produce a series of lesions along the superio-medial aspect of the crista terminalis extending inferiorly 1- to 2-cm. Successful ablation is marked by a progressive inferior shift in sinus node activation associated with a significant reduction (at least 10%) in sinus rate. While immediate success in the electrophysiology laboratory is relatively high, a durable long-term maintenance of sinus rate reduction occurs in less than 50% of patients [35].

13.4   Macroreentrant Atrial Tachycardia

The first description of atrial flutter was in the early 1900s. Both Lewis and Scherf initially proposed that atrial flutter was caused by a single rapidly firing focus. On the basis
of studies in experimental animals and vector analysis of the ECGs in humans, Lewis
and colleagues later concluded that atrial flutter was the result of circus movement in the
atria. Their experimental studies included very limited mapping of induced atrial flutter
in the normal canine atria. From these latter studies, Lewis concluded that atrial flutter
was due to reentry around the great veins.

Major advances in understanding the mechanism of atrial flutter occurred when improved mapping techniques became available, including the use of simultaneous multisite recordings. The initial catheter mapping studies in the 1950s and 1960s supported
the theory that atrial flutter is an intra-atrial reentrant rhythm with an activation wavefront traveling in a caudo-cranial direction in the left atrium and in a cranio-caudal direction in the right atrium. However, subsequent mapping studies indicated that the entire
duration of the atrial flutter cycle length could be explained by reentrant activation of the
right atrium alone, with the reentrant wavefront traveling up the atrial septum and down
the right atrial free wall. The demonstration of transient entrainment and interruption of
atrial flutter in humans has provided strong additional evidence that atrial flutter is an intra-atrial reentrant rhythm with an excitable gap. Thus, data indicate that the reentrant
circuit in atrial flutter in humans involves reentrant excitation in the right atrium, with
the impulse traveling in a caudo-cranial direction in the inter-atrial septum and a cranio-
caudal direction in the right atrial free wall (*counterclockwise atrial flutter*) (Figure 13-
17). *Clockwise atrial flutter* has been shown to be due to activation of the same reentrant
circuit, but in the opposite direction from that just described. Concealed entrainment
pacing techniques, intra-atrial echocardiography, and three-dimensional mapping tech-

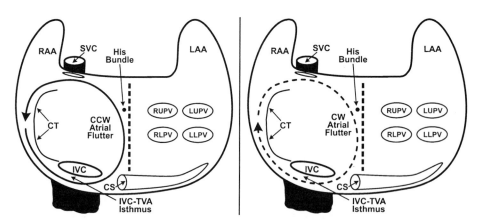

FIGURE 13-17. Schematic diagrams illustrating the reentry circuits responsible for counterclockwise
(CCW) (left panel) and clockwise (CW) (right panel) atrial flutters. The critical portion of the reentry circuit
for both flutters is the isthmus lying between the tricuspid valve annulus (TVA), ostium of the coronary sinus,
inferior vena cava (IVC) and the eustachian ridge. As is discussed later in this chapter, elimination of conduction within the IVC-TVA isthmus can cure both the CW and CCW forms of atrial flutter. For other abbreviations see Figure 13-1. See text for additional discussion.

niques, have better defined and characterized the atrial flutter reentry circuit. Several boundaries, whether fixed or functional, have been identified in the right atrium. These are the orifice of the superior vena cava, the crista terminalis, the orifice of the inferior vena cava, the eustachian ridge, the coronary sinus orifice, and the tricuspid annulus. The arrangement of these boundaries seems prone to a certain reentrant circuit. During counterclockwise and clockwise atrial flutters, conduction proceeds through a protected isthmus between the tricuspid valve annulus and the coronary sinus ostium, with the boundary of this region also including the Eustachian ridge. Another boundary includes the superior vena cava, the inferior vena cava, and a line of block located between them in the region of the crista terminalis. Functional or fixed block in this area can be demonstrated in patients with inducible atrial flutter.

Although the most common form of macroreentrant atrial tachycardia is the typical counterclockwise and clockwise forms of atrial flutter, macroreentrant atrial tachycardias can also occur in association with surgical scars (*incisional atrial tachycardia*) resulting most commonly from repair of congenital heart conditions, especially repairs of atrial septal defects [36-47]. Patients with significant structural heart disease or a history of previous cardiac surgery or catheter ablation may also exhibit any number of truly atypical atrial flutters. Macroreentrant atrial tachycardias also may be confined to the left atrium, although most of these remain unexplored at the present time. The common denominator for all these tachyarrhythmias is that they conduct within a macroreentrant circuit that involves an isthmus (which may be difficult to localize and define) protected by two or more barriers.

13.4.1 Typical Clockwise & Counterclockwise Atrial Flutters

Clinical and electrocardiographic presentation
Counterclockwise atrial flutter has the classic negative sawtooth flutter waves in ECG leads II, III, and aVF (Figure 13-18, upper panel), while clockwise atrial flutter is described as exhibiting positive flutter waves in these same leads, although the P-waves may often be flat and poorly-visualized (Figure 13-18, lower panel). As discussed above, clockwise and counterclockwise atrial flutters share the same right atrial reentrant circuit, although the reentrant wavefront travels in opposite directions to support the two different tachycardias. In this type of atrial flutter, the reentrant circuit courses across the floor of the right atrium through an isthmus bounded by the tricuspid annulus as its anterior barrier and the inferior vena cava with crista terminalis (and its medial continuation, the eustachian ridge) as the posterior barrier. Typically, the atrial rate during these tachyarrhythmias is 280-300 beats/min. Normally there is 2:1 or 3:1 AV conduction, yielding ventricular rates of 90-150 beats/min. The flutter waves can be readily visualized by producing AV block with carotid sinus massage or intravenous adenosine (Figure 13-19). Rarely, atrial flutter may exhibit 1:1 AV conduction (Figure 13-20), especially during high catecholamine states. Atrial flutter with ventricular rates of 280-300 beats/min are at high risk of degenerating into ventricular fibrillation.

Atrial flutter often is seen in patients who also have atrial fibrillation, and not uncommonly the two rhythms may oscillate between each other. Atrial flutter rarely is a

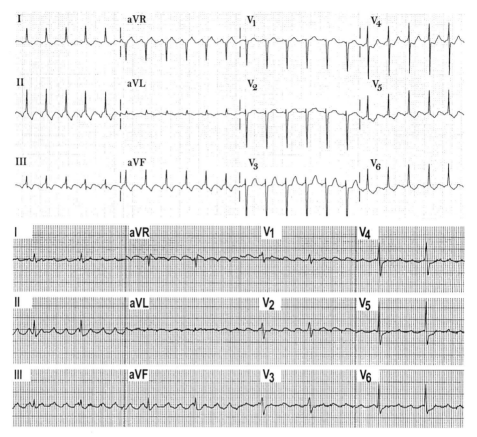

FIGURE 13-18. Counterclockwise atrial flutter (upper panel) with 2:1 AV conduction exhibiting the characteristic negative flutter waves ("sawtooth" pattern) in ECG leads II, III, and aVF. Clockwise atrial flutter (lower panel) with varying AV conduction (4:1 and 5:1) utilizes the same reentry circuit, but with impulse propagation in the opposite direction. Typically, flutter waves during clockwise atrial flutter are positive in ECG leads II, III, and aVF, but in some cases P-wave morphology may be difficult to define.

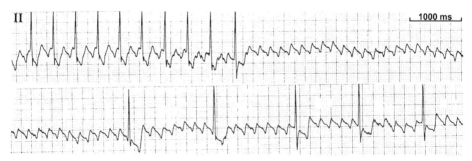

FIGURE 13-19. Continuous ECG recording illustrating the effect of intravenous adenosine (12-mg) on AV conduction in a patient with counterclockwise atrial flutter. Initially, 2:1 AV conduction is present (left half, upper panel). Adenosine produces transient block of AV conduction, allowing easy visualization of flutter waves (ECG lead II). Adenosine does not terminate typical clockwise or counterclockwise atrial flutter.

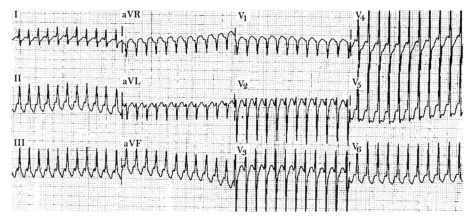

FIGURE 13-20. Counterclockwise atrial flutter exhibiting 1:1 AV conduction at a rate of 270 beats/min (cycle length = 220-msec). Because of the rapid ventricular rate, atrial flutter with 1:1 AV conduction is at high-risk of degenerating into ventricular fibrillation.

persistent rhythm; rather, it is typically paroxysmal, lasting for variable periods of time, usually seconds to hours, but on occasion even a few days. Persistent or chronic atrial flutter is unusual because atrial flutter usually converts to sinus rhythm or degenerates to atrial fibrillation, either spontaneously or as a result of therapy. However, it is not uncommon for atrial fibrillation to organize into clockwise or counterclockwise atrial flutter and, in fact, atrial flutter may only be inducible by first provoking atrial fibrillation that subsequently organizes into clockwise or counterclockwise atrial flutter.

Electrophysiologic characteristics and diagnosis
In general, clockwise or counterclockwise atrial flutter can be provoked either by single premature atrial extrastimuli (Figure 13-21) or by rapid atrial pacing. The initiation of atrial flutter may be preceded by a transitional rhythm of atrial fibrillation. These recordings are made using a 20-pole steerable catheter with the tip in the ostium of the coronary sinus and the proximal segments lying along the isthmus between the inferior vena cava and tricuspid annulus. The more proximal segments then extend to the lateral right atrium and, finally, superiorly to the high right atrium (Figure 13-22). As seen in Figure 13-23, during counterclockwise atrial flutter, activation proceeds from the high right atrium along the right lateral wall (between the crista terminalis and the tricuspid valve annulus, along the floor of the right atrium within the isthmus bordered by the tricuspid valve annulus and the medial extension of the crista terminalis (merging with the eustachian ridge) to the region of the coronary sinus. Finally, it proceeds cephalad back toward the superior right atrium after activating the His bundle region. The clockwise atrial flutter utilizes the identical reentrant circuit, but with propagation in the reverse direction.

Specialized pacing techniques such as entrainment are utilized in the electrophysiology laboratory in order to prove reentry as the underlying mechanism and identify the locations of the reentrant circuit (see "Mapping Using Concealed Entrainment" on page 147). *Manifest entrainment (continuous resetting with fusion)* is observed during a macroreentrant atrial tachycardia if pacing is performed outside of the reentrant circuit. In

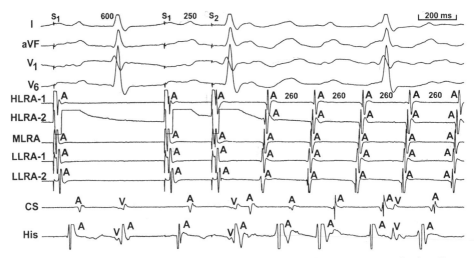

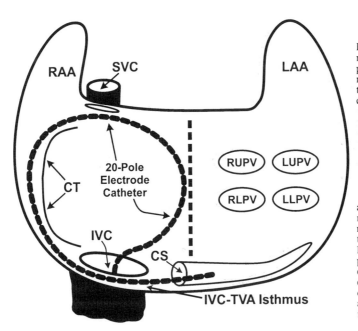

FIGURE 13-21. Induction of typical clockwise atrial flutter by a single premature extrastimulus. Same patient as in lower panel of Figure 13-18. An eight-pulse drive train (S_1-S_1 = 600-msec) is delivered followed by an atrial premature stimulus (S_1-S_2 = 250-msec). The resultant clockwise atrial flutter has a cycle length of 260-msec. CS, ostium of coronary sinus; His, His bundle; HLRA, high lateral right atrium; LLRA, low lateral right atrium; MLRA, mid lateral right atrium.

FIGURE 13-22. Optimal positioning of mapping catheter during mapping and ablation of typical clockwise and counterclockwise atrial flutter. A steerable 20-pole electrode catheter enters the heart through the inferior vena cava. The tip of the catheter is positioned inside the ostium of the coronary sinus with proximal electrodes extending laterally and lying within the isthmus bounded by the inferior vena cava and tricuspid valve annulus. From the isthmus, more proximal segments of the catheter extend to the lateral wall, and then superiorly to the high right atrium. Abbreviations as in Figure 13-1.

this case, the P-wave morphology on the surface EGG exhibits constant fusion and the post-pacing interval after termination of the fixed pacing is greater than ($\geq$ 20-msec) the tachycardia cycle length. However, if fixed cycle length pacing is performed *within the reentrant circuit* (at a cycle length slightly shorter than the tachycardia cycle length),

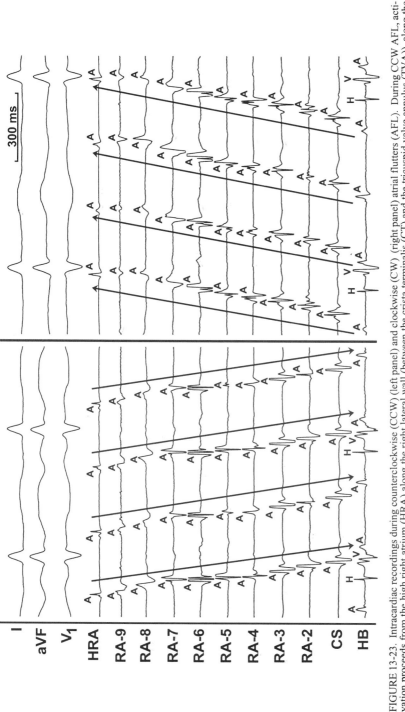

FIGURE 13-23. Intracardiac recordings during counterclockwise (CCW) (left panel) and clockwise (CW) (right panel) atrial flutters (AFL). During CCW AFL, activation proceeds from the high right atrium (HRA) along the right lateral wall (between the crista terminalis (CT) and the tricuspid valve annulus (TVA)), along the floor of the right atrium (RA) within the isthmus bordered by the TVA and the medial extension of the CT (merging with the eustachian ridge) to the region of the coronary sinus (CS). Finally, it proceeds cephalad back toward the superior RA after activating the His bundle (HB) region. The CW AFL utilizes the identical reentrant circuit, but with propagation in the reverse direction. These recordings are made using a 20-pole steerable catheter as shown in Figure 13-22. A, atrial electrogram; H, His bundle electrogram; V, ventricular electrogram.

concealed entrainment can be demonstrated (Figure 13-24). The following criteria must be fulfilled for concealed entrainment to be present: 1) the P-wave morphology recorded on the surface EGG during pacing is identical to that inscribed during spontaneous tachycardia, 2) the interval from the pacing stimulation artifact to the onset of the surface P-wave is equal to interval from the local electrogram to P-wave, and 3) the post-pacing interval is equal to the tachycardia cycle length (±10-msec).

13.4.2 INCISIONAL ATRIAL TACHYCARDIAS

While children with congenital heart disease who have undergone surgical repair have benefited with improved survival rates, it has been at the expense of an increased incidence of cardiac arrhythmias – particularly atrial tachyarrhythmias – in adulthood. Incisional intra-atrial reentrant tachycardia following repair or palliation of congenital heart disease is a common and potentially serious complication. Palliative and corrective cardiac surgeries produce surgical incisions and other conduction barriers, such as conduits and patches for closure of defects. Together with natural anatomic obstacles, such as orifices of great vessels and AV annuli, these conduction barriers may facilitate intra-atrial reentry. The reentrant activation wavefront during tachycardia may circle around conduction barriers and conduct within protected regions of myocardium (isthmus). Ana-

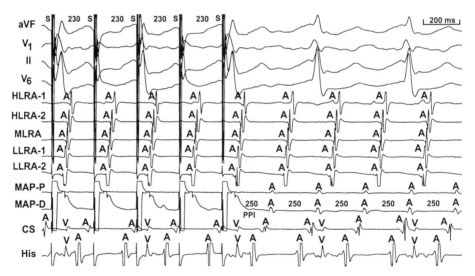

FIGURE 13-24. Demonstration of concealed entrainment in a patient with typical clockwise atrial flutter. A multipolar electrode catheter is positioned as in Figure 13-22. The cycle length of the atrial flutter is 250-msec. Pacing is performed within the isthmus using a quadripolar mapping/recording catheter (MAP-D and MAP-P) between the inferior vena cava and tricuspid valve annulus at a cycle length (S-S) of 230-msec. Note during pacing that the atrial activation sequence in the high- (HLRA), mid- (MLRA), and low-lateral right atrium (LLRA), and isthmus region is identical both during pacing and during the atrial flutter. The P-wave morphology is identical during both the paced activations and the tachycardia on the 12-lead ECG (only leads II, aVF, V₁, and V₆ are shown). The first tachycardia interval recorded at the pacing site (MAP-D) in the isthmus after cessation of pacing – the post-pacing interval (PPI) – is identical to the atrial flutter cycle length (250-msec). These findings indicate that the isthmus is part of the reentry circuit. CS, ostium of coronary sinus; His, His bundle.

tomic barriers, especially scars from surgical incision, may protect the wavefront from lateral collision that would otherwise terminate reentry.

The most common underlying congenital heart disease in these patients and the corrective surgery performed include atrial septal defect repair, the Mustard, Senning, or Rastelli procedure for transposition of the great arteries, or Fontan procedure for tricuspid atresia or double inlet single ventricle. An atrial tachycardia occurring years after complex surgery for congenital heart disease is suggestive of incisional reentry as an underlying mechanism. Incisional intra-atrial reentrant tachycardias are usually sustained atrial arrhythmias with a constant atrial cycle length of more than 200-msec, with sudden onset and termination of the tachycardia, an abnormal P-wave morphology, and episodic Mobitz type I AV block without interruption of the primary tachycardia (Figure 13-25)

As with typical clockwise or counterclockwise atrial flutter, patients with an incisional atrial tachycardia will exhibit concealed entrainment when pacing is performed within the isthmus that is critical for maintenance of the reentrant circuit. Additional techniques of mapping of incisional reentrant atrial tachycardias consist of the following: 1) search for double potentials, which are observed along conduction barriers and may represent surgical suture lines, and 2) search for electrically silent areas, which may represent either scar or conduit or patch material. As with typical atrial flutter, the narrow isthmus of conduction – between, for example, a surgical scar and an anatomic barrier – becomes the target for subsequent RF ablation.

Despite the application of traditional mapping and entrainment techniques for radiofrequency catheter ablation of incisional reentrant tachycardias, the complexity of underlying congenital heart disease and multiple cardiac surgeries remains a considerable challenge. Individual surgical techniques and insufficient imaging modalities, usually based on biplane fluoroscopy, increase the challenge. Electroanatomic mapping (see

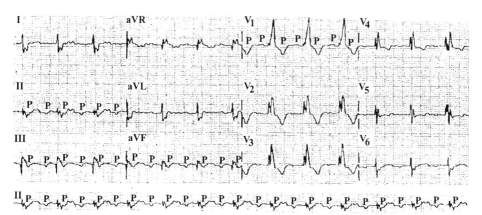

FIGURE 13-25. Incisional atrial tachycardia in patient with surgically-repaired tetralogy of Fallot. There is 2:1 ventricular conduction with a P-P interval of approximately 400-msec (ventricular rate approximately 75 beats/min). During electrophysiology testing, a macroreentrant atrial tachycardia circuit was mapped using concealed entrainment and other specialized mapping techniques. The circuit was located within the low-to-mid anterolateral right atrium in the region of the atriotomy scar. Note that the P-wave morphology is very similar to that seen during typical counterclockwise atrial flutter. However, the reentry circuit responsible for this incisional atrial tachycardia did not involve the isthmus between the inferior vena cava and annulus of the tricuspid valve.

page 146) may be able to overcome some of the limitations of standard techniques. The electroanatomic, non-fluoroscopic mapping technique permits direct association of electrical activity with the underlying anatomic structures to identify the reentrant substrate and to target radiofrequency energy application more effectively. In addition, the ability to record and display features such as silent areas, based on visualization of low-voltage areas, and the ability to display lines of block, based on the delineation of double potentials, provides important adjunctive information to electrical activation display.

13.4.3 ATYPICAL ATRIAL FLUTTERS

Patients with structural heart disease or surgically-repaired congenital heart disease may present with a variety of atypical macroreentrant atrial tachycardias maintained by any number of physiological, anatomical, and pathological barriers. In this cases, extensive mapping procedures may be required, including the use of specialized contact and non-contact mapping technologies (see page 146).

13.5   Pharmacological Therapy for Atrial Tachyarrhythmias

Pharmacological treatment for atrial tachycardias may be directed at either suppression/ prevention of the arrhythmia, or controlling the ventricular response during paroxysms. β-adrenergic blocking agents and Ca^{++} channel blockers may slow the ventricular response during atrial tachycardia by prolonging conduction and refractoriness of the AV node. β-adrenergic blockers may be effective in suppressing both paroxysmal and incessant atrial tachycardias due to enhanced automaticity, which are usually catecholamine-sensitive, but the overall success rates are low. Electrophysiology study may identify a subset group of patients with adenosine- or verapamil-sensitive (Figure 13-26) atrial tachycardia (particularly focal atrial tachycardias) that may be caused by triggered activity related to delayed afterdepolarizations or microreentry involving Ca^{++} channel-dependent slow response tissue as part of the reentrant circuit [48,49]. In this case, verapamil and/or a β-adrenergic blocking agent, used alone or in combination, may be effective for the control of the arrhythmia. Digoxin is frequently used for the treatment of atrial tachycardias, but its predominant effect is to control the ventricular response and it usually does not significantly affect the atrial tachycardia itself (except possibly for high cristal atrial tachycardia).

To terminate or suppress focal or macroreentrant atrial tachycardia, the use of class I antiarrhythmic agents, such as quinidine, procainamide, propafenone or flecainide, may be required, although there overall long-term efficacy may be only 50%. These drugs may convert the arrhythmia to sinus rhythm, but often they merely slow the atrial rate [50] (Figure 13-3). Class IA and IC antiarrhythmic drugs suppress reentrant atrial tachycardia by prolonging refractoriness and slowing conduction within the reentrant circuit [51] (Figure 13-27) and by suppressing premature atrial beats that frequently initiate the arrhythmia.

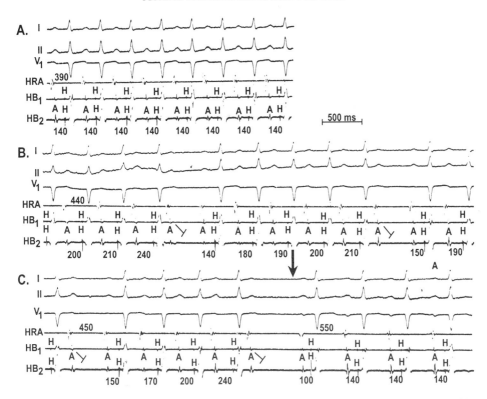

FIGURE 13-26. Termination of a high cristal atrial tachycardia ("sinoatrial reentrant tachycardia") with intravenous verapamil. Same patient as in Figure 13-14. Surface ECG leads I, II, and V_1, are simultaneously displayed with endocardial recordings from the high right atrium (HRA) and His bundle (HB). Panel A: before verapamil administration, the cycle length of the tachycardia is 390-msec and the corresponding AV nodal conduction time is 140-msec. Panel B: after infusion of verapamil of 0.15 mg/kg, the tachycardia cycle gradually lengthens to 440-msec. Note the simultaneous development of atrioventricular nodal Wenckebach phenomenon during tachycardia. Panel C: conversion to sinus rhythm with a sinus cycle length of 550-msec; the arrow identifies the first sinus beat after termination of the tachycardia. A, atrial electrogram; H, His-bundle potential. From [49] with permission.

Compared to class I antiarrhythmic drugs, class III agents such as sotalol and dofetilide are usually ineffective at terminating atrial tachycardias (including atrial flutter and fibrillation); however, class III drugs are often effective at maintaining sinus rhythm after termination of the tachyarrhythmia. The lack of termination efficacy of class III agents appears related to the reverse use-dependence [52] demonstrated by these agents during rapid atrial rates. Amiodarone possesses a multitude of anti-arrhythmic properties, and is, therefore, effective in the treatment of various forms of atrial tachycardias [53]. However, potential serious adverse effects often preclude amiodarone to be chosen as the first line long term antiarrhythmic drug therapy.

Special consideration must be given to the treatment of multifocal atrial tachycardia and atrial tachyarrhythmias due to digitalis intoxication. Multifocal atrial tachycardia is associated with a high mortality rate due to the concomitant cardiac or non-cardiac conditions [16,54]. The primary therapy for multifocal atrial tachycardia is effective treat-

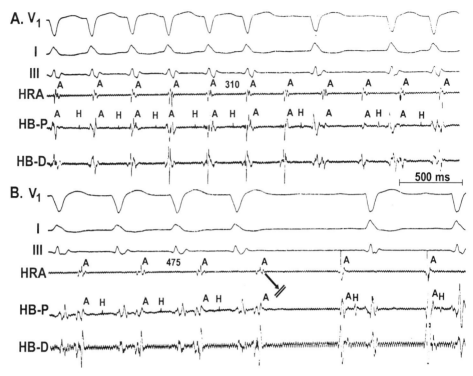

FIGURE 13-27. Termination of reentrant atrial tachycardia with intravenous propafenone. Surface ECG Leads V_1 I, and III are simultaneously displayed with endocardial recordings from the high right atrium (HRA and proximal (HB-P) and distal (HB-D) His bundle region. Panel A: the atrial tachycardia induced by programmed atrial extrastimulation has an atrial cycle length of 310-msec in the control state; intermittent AV block is noted. Panel B: after intravenous infusion of propafenone (2-mg/kg), the atrial cycle length lengthened to 475-msec before conversion (arrow) to sinus rhythm. A, Atrial electrogram; H, His-bundle electrogram; numbers are in milliseconds. From [51] with permission.

ment of the underlying condition. Symptomatic treatment includes improved oxygenation, eliminating or reducing (if possible) the dose of sympathomimetic drugs, theophylline and digoxin, and correction of metabolic and electrolyte abnormalities. Multifocal atrial tachycardia does not generally respond to antiarrhythmic drugs [54]. Digitalis has not been effective in controlling the ventricular response during multifocal atrial tachycardia, and continued increments in digitalis dosage in an attempt to control the ventricular response may result in digitalis intoxication. Specific treatment with verapamil, β-adrenergic blockers, and magnesium may be effective [55]. β-adrenergic blocking agents may reduce the ventricular rate in multifocal atrial tachycardia by prolonging conduction and refractoriness in the AV node [20,54,56,57]. However, the frequent association of multifocal atrial tachycardia with severe pulmonary disease may preclude β-adrenergic blocker therapy. Ca^{2+}-channel blocking agents, such as verapamil, may reduce the heart rate in patients with multifocal atrial tachycardia by slowing the atrial rate [20,56,57].

Digitalis-toxicity often manifests as an atrial tachycardia with AV block with or without associated ventricular arrhythmias (Figure 13-4). Early clinical recognition is essential, as is correction of serum electrolytes (especially K^+) and other metabolic disorders. Intravenous lidocaine or procainamide may be useful for acute suppression of the atrial tachycardia, and treatment with anti-digoxin antibodies may be needed in selected patients with metabolic derangements (e.g., acidosis, hyperkalemia, etc.), congestive heart failure, severe bradycardia or AV block, and recurrent ventricular tachyarrhythmias [58,59]. Electrical cardioversion is contraindicated, as it may potentially provoke fatal ventricular tachyarrhythmias [60,61].

For a complete discussion of the drug treatment for tachyarrhythmias see "Principles of Pharmacotherapy and Antiarrhythmic Drugs" on page 91.

13.6 Catheter Ablation of Atrial Tachyarrhythmias

The limited success of pharmacological treatment has prompted the search for a definitive cure of atrial tachyarrhythmias. The RF catheter ablation technique, which has become a standard treatment for patients with AV nodal reentrant tachycardia or the Wolff-Parkinson-White syndrome, has also emerged as a viable treatment option for patients with atrial tachycardias. Atrial tachycardias are amenable to RF catheter ablation [62-73]. However, the immediate and, especially, long-term success rates are lower compared to those for AV nodal reentrant tachycardia and AV reciprocating tachycardia [68,71,72].

13.6.1 FOCAL ATRIAL TACHYCARDIAS

In the electrophysiology laboratory, localization of the origin of a focal atrial tachycardia is achieved using multisite endocardial mapping performed with steerable pacing and recording catheters. Generally, one quadripolar electrode catheter is positioned in the right ventricular apex in order to perform programmed ventricular stimulation so as to evaluate retrograde ventriculoatrial conduction. A second quadripolar electrode catheter is positioned at the His bundle region. Right atrial pacing and recording can be performed using a 10- or 20-pole electrode catheter with the tip in the ostium of the coronary sinus (Figure 13-22). The remaining proximal catheter electrodes are allowed to lie along the floor of the right atrium, laterally, and then continue superiorly parallel to crista terminalis to the high right atrium near the junction of the superior vena cava. In this way, the right atrial activation sequence can be evaluated during tachycardia (i.e., from high to low right atrium, or from the low to high right atrium). As a surrogate for the left atrial activation, a multipolar catheter is usually inserted into the coronary sinus. After establishing that the tachycardia is confined to the atria, the ventricular catheter is often removed and replaced by a large-tip quadripolar mapping/ablating catheter. For mapping (and ablation) of an atrial tachycardia originating within the left atrium or pulmonary veins, the transseptal approach is preferred to the retrograde transaortic approach because of the ease with which the mapping catheter can be manipulated in the left atrium (Figure 13-28). During left atrial mapping/ablation, heparin should be infused intravenously and the activated clotting time maintained at 250–350-sec in order to prevent thrombus formation in the left atrium.

For a focal atrial tachycardia, activation mapping can be performed to precisely localize the origin of the arrhythmia (see "Activation Mapping" on page 143). Using this technique, the relative timing of the electrogram recorded from the distal electrodes of the mapping/ablating catheter during the atrial tachycardia is compared with the onset of the electrocardiographic P-wave as well as the earliest electrogram recorded from a fixed multipolar electrode catheter (Figures 13-16, 13-29, 13-30, & 13-31). Focal application of RF energy at the origin of these focal arrhythmias results in termination of the arrhythmia (Figures 13-30 & 13-32). Successful ablation of the focal origin of an atrial tachycardia arising within a pulmonary vein is often associated with the elimination of the "spike" electrograms (Figures 13-15 & 13-33).

Special mention should be made concerning the distinction between the RF ablation procedures for a cristal atrial tachycardia localized near the region of the sinus node and inappropriate sinus tachycardia. For high cristal tachycardia, RF energy is delivered at the junction of the superior vena cava and the right atrial appendage (using the fluoroscopic right anterior oblique view) at the site of the earliest atrial electrogram during the tachycardia (which also should precede the onset of electrocardiographic P-wave). A single, or few applications of RF energy, are sufficient to abolish a high cristal atrial tachycardia (Figure 13-32). For patients with inappropriate sinus tachycardia, RF energy

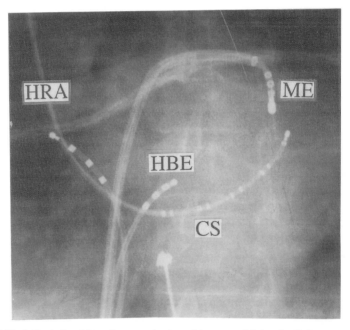

FIGURE 13-28. Left anterior oblique fluoroscopic view of the successful site of radiofrequency catheter ablation in a patient with a focal left atrial tachycardia. CS, coronary sinus; HBE: His bundle electrographic lead; HRA, high right atrium; ME, mapping (ablation) catheter electrode. Note transeptal approach guided by a long intravascular sheath placed from the right femoral vein, into the right atrium, across the inter-atrial septum to reach the left atrium.

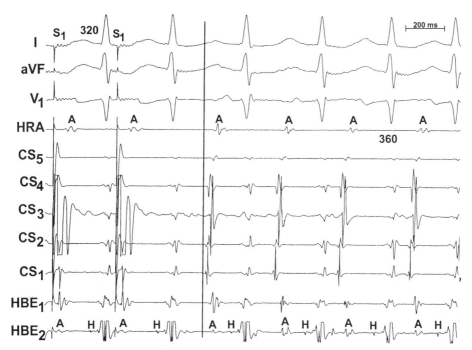

FIGURE 13-29. Atrial tachycardia localized to the lateral left atrium. Same patient as in Figure 13-28. Coronary sinus (CS) pacing at a cycle length (S_1-S_1) of 320-msec induces an atrial tachycardia (cycle length 360-msec) with the earliest onset of atrial activation located at the distal coronary sinus (CS_1) (see vertical line). The arrhythmia is subsequently successfully ablated with the radiofrequency catheter ablation technique targeted at the left lateral atrium site (see Figure 13-28) A: atrial electrogram; H: His bundle potential; HRA: high right atrium; CS_1 to CS_5: distal to proximal coronary sinus; HBE_1, proximal His bundle electrographic lead; HBE_2: distal His bundle electrographic lead.

is delivered during infusion of isoproterenol; catecholamines shift the earliest activation site to the superior aspect of the sinoatrial node region. An effective application of RF energy is signaled by slowing of the rate of sinus tachycardia and by a shifting of the earliest activation site to the middle or inferior aspect of the sinoatrial node region. In contrast to the RF ablation of a focal cristal atrial tachycardia, multiple RF applications are usually required for suppressing inappropriate sinus tachycardia. Clinically, the results of radiofrequency catheter ablation of inappropriate sinus tachycardia are disappointing because of a high recurrence rate.

There are several limitations to the present approach to RF catheter ablation of focal atrial tachycardias, particularly those arising from the pulmonary veins. As mentioned above, it can be very difficult to induce focal sources in the electrophysiology laboratory. In some cases, these focal arrhythmias may respond to chemical alterations in autonomic tone, such as administration of catecholamines. Pacing maneuvers may not be useful at inducing focal atrial tachyarrhythmias, especially those arising within the pulmonary veins. Therefore, despite a characteristic clinical profile and documented frequent atrial tachycardia, the patient may fail to demonstrate adequate spontaneous arrhythmia for mapping during the electrophysiologic study. Pulmonary veins have a

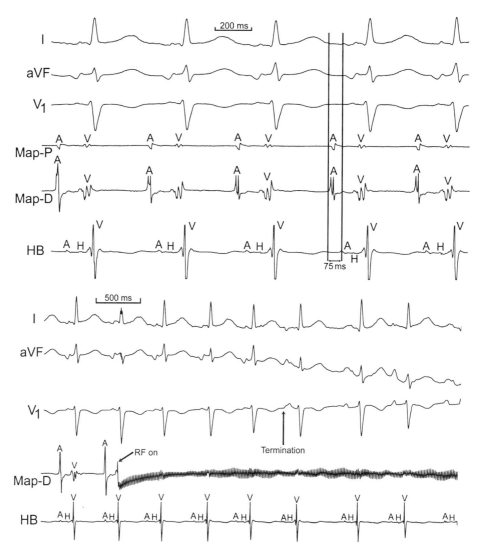

FIGURE 13-30. Activation mapping and ablation of a focal atrial tachycardia localized to the atrial septum. Same patient as in Figure 13-6. Note different recording speeds in upper and lower panels. Upper panel: during atrial tachycardia, the onset of the atrial electrogram recorded by the distal electrodes of the steerable mapping catheter (MAP-D) occurs 75-msec before the onset of the P-wave on the surface ECG and approximately 70-msec before the atrial electrogram recorded at the His bundle region (HB). Lower panel: delivery of radiofrequency (RF) energy at this site resulted in immediate termination of the atrial tachycardia.

complex, three-dimensional branching structure, and the focus responsible for the atrial tachycardia may be found up to 4-cm inside a pulmonary vein. Thus, detailed mapping is frequently difficult, even if the focal arrhythmia is constantly firing (which is generally not the case). Due to the spontaneous variability of firing of the focus, the endpoint in the electrophysiology laboratory may be difficult to determine. In approximately 30% of patients, more than one pulmonary vein focus is present. Newer technologies and tech-

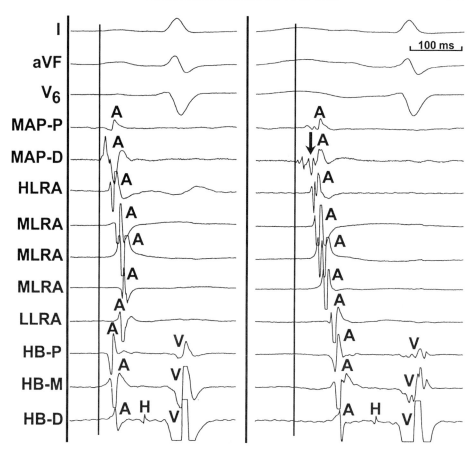

FIGURE 13-31. Activation mapping of a high cristal atrial tachycardia. Left panel: during sinus rhythm the earliest atrial activation at the high right atrium is recorded 16-msec before the onset of the surface P-wave. Right panel: during the atrial tachycardia a fragmented atrial electrogram (downward arrow) is recorded in the region of the high crista terminalis. This electrogram precedes the onset of the surface P-wave by 25-msec and is the successful ablation site (Figure 13-32). HB-D, distal His bundle; HB-M, mid His bundle; HB-P, proximal His bundle; His bundle; HLRA, high lateral right atrium; LLRA, low lateral right atrium; MAP-D, distal mapping electrodes at high right atrium; MAP-P, proximal mapping electrodes at high right atrium; MLRA, mid lateral right atrium.

niques are necessary to streamline the procedure, enhance inducibility, and ease mapping and minimize potential complications including thromboembolic stroke and pulmonary vein stenosis. For an additional discussion regarding the ablation of focal arrhythmias originating within the pulmonary venous system see the discussion of the curative ablation of atrial fibrillation on page 671.

The use of the classic techniques of activation and concealed entrainment mapping to identify the target tissue for RF ablation are limited for a number of reasons (Table 13-3.) Because of the complexity of the three-dimensional structure of both atria and associated diseased atrial tissues with or without surgically-created scars, incision, sutures, patches, conduits, baffles, it is very difficult to perform reliable mapping using electrode

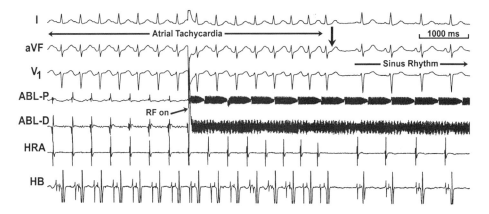

FIGURE 13-32. Successful radiofrequency (RF) ablation of high cristal atrial tachycardia. Same patient as in Figure 13-31. Within 3-sec of the onset of the RF application the tachycardia is terminated and sinus rhythm is restored. ABL-D, distal electrodes on ablation catheter; ABL-P, proximal electrodes on ablation catheter; HB, His bundle; HRA, high right atrium.

catheters under fluoroscopy. In patients with postoperative atrial tachycardias, this is further complicated by structural alteration consequent to long term effects of altered hemodynamics and various surgical procedures such as Mustard/Senning procedure for atrial switch in transposition of the great arteries and palliative Fontan operation for connecting venous atrium to the pulmonary artery in single ventricle physiology (Figure 13-34). Postoperative atrial tachycardias are usually a form of atrial reentry resulting from circus movement of wavefronts around anatomical conduction barriers such as incision, suture lines, conduits, patches, baffles, orifices of great veins and the AV annuli. Although some of postoperative atrial tachycardias may appear to be typical atrial flutter electrocardiographically, they actually have different reentrant paths than the common counterclockwise or clockwise atrial flutter [74]. Finally, despite identification of the areas of entrainment with concealed fusion, a long region of transmural RF lesions may be required to interrupt the reentrant circuit of a macroreentrant atrial tachycardia, especially if it is associated with surgical repair of congenital heart disease.

TABLE 13-3. Limitation of standard techniques for localization and ablation of atrial tachycardias

Inability to reliably and reproducibly manipulate the catheter tip to a desired site using fluoroscopic guidance

Difficult to provoke arrhythmia

Non-sustained arrhythmia

Necessity to map single triggering atrial premature depolarizations that occur only sporadically

Congenital cardiac anomalies or complex anatomy

Surgically-altered cardiac chambers (incisions, shunts, baffles, patches, conduits).

Multiple foci (pulmonary veins)

Failure to completely and permanently eliminate conduction through wide isthmus making up a critical portion of a macroreentrant circuit (must create end-to-end transmural RF lesions)

Very delayed bidirectional isthmus conduction mistaken for true bidirectional isthmus conduction block

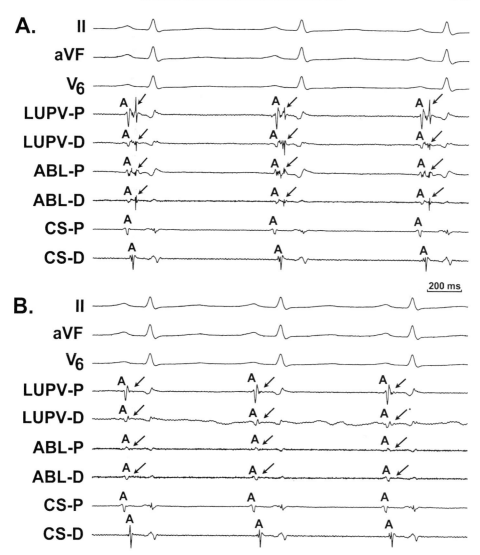

FIGURE 13-33. Effects of radiofrequency (RF) catheter ablation on high-frequency "spike" electrograms in a patient with an atrial tachycardia and atrial fibrillation. Same patient as in Figure 13-15. The patient's atrial tachycardia (which was also the focal trigger for the patient's atrial fibrillation) was induced by isoproterenol and was mapped to the left upper pulmonary vein. Intracardiac recordings are shown from distal and proximal electrodes in an upper branch of the left upper pulmonary vein (LUPV-D, and LUPV-P) and the coronary sinus (CS-D and CS-P). A steerable quadripolar mapping/ablating catheter was also positioned in the LUPV. Panel A: during sinus rhythm, the locally-recorded "spike" electrograms (arrows) were inscribed after the recording of the far-field left atrial activation. During atrial premature depolarizations, or salvos of the atrial tachycardia, inscription of the "spikes" preceded the global left atrial activation (Figure 13-16). At this site a series of RF ablations were performed (30-sec, 30-watts, maximum temperature 50°C) at ABL-D resulting in elimination of the high-frequency electrograms (panel B, arrows). Re-challenge with high dose isoproterenol failed to induce atrial premature depolarizations or the atrial tachycardia.

Because of these limitations, newer mapping and ablation technologies may enhance the success rate during these potentially complex, tedious, and time-consuming procedures. In particular, the non-fluoroscopic electroanatomic mapping system (see page 146) may be of unique benefit for patients with atrial arrhythmias and complex anatomy, such as incisional intra-atrial reentrant tachycardias following corrective surgery of congenital heart disease (Figure 13-35). Surgical conduction barriers such as conduits and patches can be identified as electrically silent areas (very low voltage, far-field signals) using a color-coded voltage map and surgical incisions can be identified as double potentials. Subsequent activation mapping allows demonstration of the reentrant circuit and a protected isthmus.

13.6.2 Typical Clockwise and Counterclockwise Atrial Flutters

Electrophysiologically- and anatomically-guided ablation strategies have been developed for a curative therapy of atrial flutter. Following initial experiences with surgical incisions and DC applications, linear RF current applications have become the established interventional therapy of this arrhythmia. The understanding of atrial flutter as a single boundary-related reentrant circuit has important implications for the ablation therapy. A linear lesion between two opposite barriers bordering a critical isthmus that participates in the reentrant circuit is the fundamental basis for the successful ablation of macroreentrant atrial tachycardias.

As discussed above, during typical clockwise and counterclockwise atrial flutter, conduction proceeds through the isthmus bounded by the inferior vena cava and tricuspid valve annulus (Figures 13-17 & 13-23). Bidirectional conduction can be demonstrat-

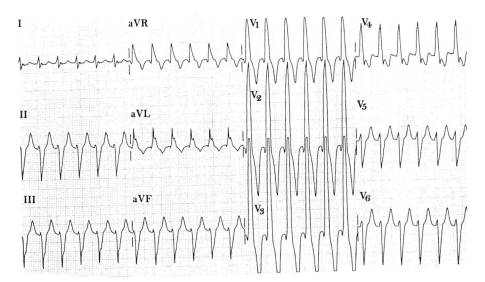

FIGURE 13-34. Electrocardiogram of an atrial tachycardia (confirmed by electrophysiology study) recorded from a 20-year old man who had previously undergone a palliative Fontan procedure for treatment of single ventricle physiology. P-waves are not clearly discernible. The ECG pattern of surgical right bundle branch block and left axis deviation is identical to that seen during sinus rhythm (not shown).

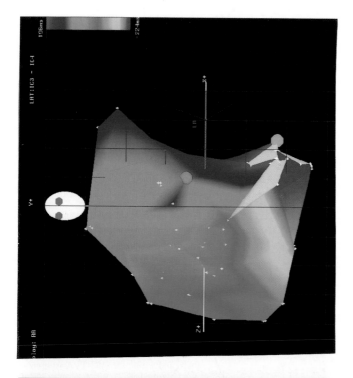

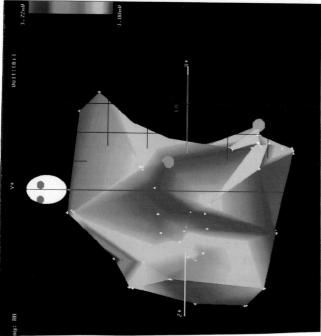

FIGURE 13-35. Magnetic electroanatomical mapping of the atrial tachycardia as shown in Figure 13-34. Left panel: isopotential (voltage) map of the recorded bipolar signals in the right atrium in the left anterior oblique view during the tachycardia. The lowest amplitude signals are designated by the red color. The color range for the signal amplitudes is shown in the top right of the panel. Note the low amplitude signals throughout most of the right atrium representing diffusely diseased atrial tissue. The pink dot depicts the coronary sinus ostium and the orange dot depicts the His bundle recording site. Right panel: activation map of the tachycardia showing the earliest site of activation is located at the low posterior septum near the coronary sinus ostium (the pink dot). The red areas denote sites of early activation and purple denotes late activation. The color range for the activation times is displayed in the top right of the panel. For both panels, the gray areas represent patches or artificial materials. Note activation wavefronts of the tachycardia start at the low posterior interatrial septum near the coronary sinus ostium and rotate in a clockwise rotation. Three applications of radiofrequency energy interrupt the tachycardia and render the tachycardia non-inducible (not shown).

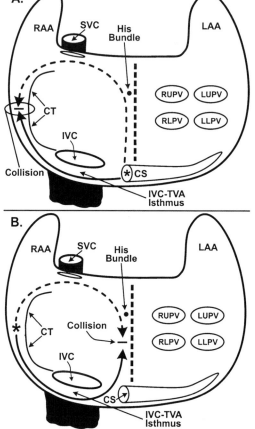

FIGURE 13-36. Schematic diagram illustrating the routes of impulse conduction during electrical pacing from the coronary sinus (CS) and lateral right atrium, in the region of the mid-crista terminalis. Panel A: pacing is performed at the ostium of the CS (★). The depolarization wavefront conducts laterally in a clockwise direction within the isthmus bounded by the inferior vena cava (IVC) and tricuspid valve annulus (TVA). It then proceeds superiorly toward the high right atrium (HRA). Another wavefront conducts counterclockwise from the region of the CS up the atrial septum toward the anteriorly-positioned AV node/His bundle region. Conduction continues to the HRA and then spreads caudally along the crista terminalis. As shown here, these two wavefronts collide in the region of the mid-crista terminalis. Panel B: pacing is performed at the lateral right atrium (★) and spreads caudally in a counterclockwise rotation and cephalad in a clockwise rotation. As shown here, the counterclockwise impulse conducts through the IVC-TVA isthmus and collides with the caudally-directed clockwise impulse in the region of the mid-atrial septum. If recording electrodes are positioned at the His bundle region, as well as along the right lateral atrium anterior to the crista terminalis and within the IVC-TVA isthmus to the CS (Figure 13-22), electrogram recordings similar to those shown in Figure 13-37 can be obtained. Using these catheter positions bidirectional conduction within the IVC-TVA isthmus can be easily documented. Abbreviations as in Figure 13-1.

ed within this isthmus using recording catheter positioned at the His bundle region along with pacing/recording catheter positioned as shown in Figure 13-22. Pacing at the ostium of the coronary sinus and the lateral aspect of the right atrium (Figure 13-36) results in a characteristic activation pattern (Figure 13-37).

Irrespective of the precise location of the reentry circuit, the mechanics of a successful ablation procedure can be divided into five steps: 1) reentry as the mechanism of the arrhythmia must be established; 2) electrophysiological identification must be made of the boundaries defining the reentry circuit; 3) it must be demonstrated that the area between these conduction barriers (i.e., isthmus) is a part of the reentrant circuit; 4) the viable isthmus tissue must be destroyed by connecting the conduction barriers with a linear ablation lesion, thereby creating a line of conduction block through the isthmus; and 5) it should be verified that the line of block is complete.

Reentry can usually be established as the mechanism of the arrhythmia by demonstrating induction by programmed extrastimulation and manifest entrainment. The demonstration of concealed entrainment at a particular pacing site indicates that the pacing site is included within the reentry circuit. Conduction barriers can be identified as areas

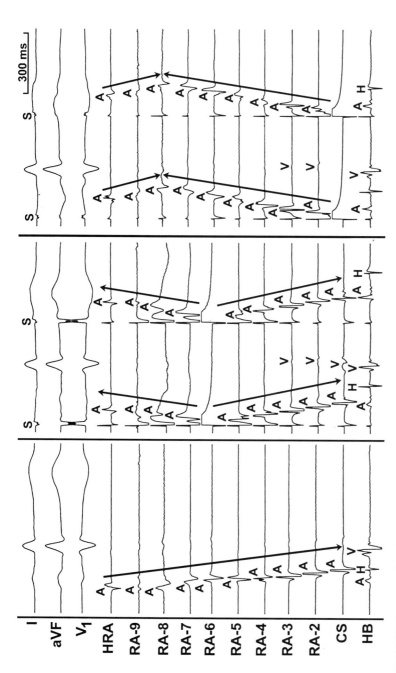

FIGURE 13-37. Demonstration of bidirectional conduction within the atrial isthmus between the tricuspid valve annulus (TVA) and inferior vena cava (IVC) and eustachian ridge. Pacing/recording electrodes were positioned at the His bundle (HB) region and along the crista terminalis from the high right atrium (HRA) to the ostium of the coronary sinus (CS) as shown in Figure 13-22. Recordings were made during sinus rhythm (left panel) and during pacing (120 pulse/min) at the lateral aspect of the isthmus (RA-6) (middle panel) and at the CS (right panel). During lateral isthmus pacing, the conducted wavefront spreads medially across the isthmus to the CS region, as well as superiorly toward the HRA. During CS pacing, the impulse spreads laterally across the isthmus and superiorly up the atrial septum. These separate wavefronts collide in the region of RA-7 and RA-8. Note infra-Hisian block during pacing. A, atrial electrogram, H, His bundle electrogram, V, ventricular electrogram, S, pacing stimulus artifact

that lack electrical activity (such as patches or scars), or may be common anatomic structures such as valve annuli, venous structures such as the inferior vena cava or coronary sinus, or unique right atrial structures such as the eustachian ridge or crista terminalis. After determination of the reentrant circuit and identification of the conduction barriers, conduction within the intervening isthmus (preferably at its narrowest point) must be eliminated by a linear ablation lesion. In typical clockwise or counterclockwise atrial flutter, two ablation approaches have been developed. The established ablation line runs from the medial aspect of the tricuspid annulus toward the inferior vena cava. The alternative approach involves placement of a linear lesion from the septal aspect of the tricuspid annulus toward the coronary sinus orifice and further to the septal end of the eustachian ridge. Presumed advantages of the septal approach are the smooth surface of the atrium in this area and the minor distance between the two barriers. However, using the septal approach, the risk of inadvertent AV block may be increased in some patients due to the close anatomic relation between the septal aspect of the eustachian ridge and the AV node. Either repetitive focal RF applications or a continuous migratory application of RF current ("catheter drag" method) can be used to produce linear lesions. To assist in the creation of a linear lesion, pre-shaped introducer sheaths and catheters that are adapted to the specific anatomic characteristics of the isthmus between the inferior vena cava and the tricuspid annulus have been developed.

Linear RF applications can produce a complete bidirectional conduction block at the ablation line. In patients with typical atrial flutter prior to ablation, pacing from the low lateral right atrium is followed by a simultaneous ascending and descending activation of the inter-atrial septum and pacing from the proximal coronary sinus by simultaneous ascending and descending activation of the lateral right atrial wall (Figures 13-36 & 13-37). Following successful ablation at the isthmus between the inferior vena cava and tricuspid annulus, both the septum and the lateral free wall were activated by a single descending wavefront without evidence of pulse propagation through the isthmus (Figures 13-38, 13-39 & 13-40). In addition, a discontinuity of electrical activity with characteristic double potentials can be found at the ablation site. A complete bidirectional conduction block predicts lower recurrence rates than termination and non-inducibility of atrial flutter and should be the primary endpoint in atrial flutter ablation.

A significant fraction of patients (>50%) with typical clockwise or counterclockwise atrial flutter undergoing ablation between the inferior vena cava and the tricuspid annulus often demonstrate conduction delays or unidirectional conduction block before achieving complete bidirectional conduction block (Figure 13-41). In fact, without demonstrating double atrial potentials and clear line of conduction block (Figures 13-39 & 13-40), extensive conduction delays may mimic a complete conduction block using septal or lateral pacing. Therefore, a continuous recording of the endocardial activation sequence through the isthmus to detect a real discontinuity seems to be superior in identifying a complete conduction block rather than measurements of conduction times during septal or lateral pacing.

As mentioned, if a complete conduction block·within the isthmus is proven following RF ablation, the recurrence rate of the targeted atrial flutter is low. However, following a successful atrial flutter ablation, other atrial tachycardias or flutters, and especially

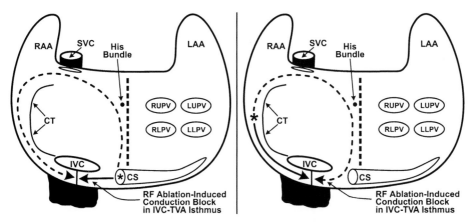

FIGURE 13-38. Schematic diagram to illustrate pacing technique used to demonstrate bidirectional conduction block in the isthmus between the inferior vena cava (IVC) and tricuspid valve annulus (TVA) following RF ablation for clockwise or counterclockwise atrial flutter Pacing (designated by ★) is performed from the region of the coronary sinus (CS) and the lateral isthmus. If there is conduction block within the IVC-TVA isthmus during CS pacing (left panel), then the lateral right atrium and lateral aspects of the IVC-TVA isthmus will only be activated by a single wavefront conducting from a cranial-to-caudal direction with the lateral isthmus activated after the mid- and high right atrium (Figure 13-39). If there is conduction block within the IVC-TVA isthmus during pacing at the lateral isthmus (right panel), then the anterior and posterior atrial septum (CS and His bundle regions) will only be activated by a single wavefront conducting from a cranial-to-caudal direction with His bundle region activated before the region near the CS (Figure 13-40). For abbreviations see Figure 13-1.

atrial fibrillation, are frequent findings. For patients without a history of atrial fibrillation, successful RF ablation of atrial flutter does not appear to be proarrhythmic for atrial fibrillation. The presence of structural heart disease, a history of atrial fibrillation prior to ablation of atrial flutter, inducibility of atrial fibrillation following successful ablation of atrial flutter, and a greater number of failed antiarrhythmic drugs seems to be associated with an occurrence of atrial fibrillation after the atrial flutter ablation procedure.

For patients with an incisional atrial tachycardia, RF catheter ablation in a critical isthmus of conduction, bounded by anatomic barriers, may be curative. As with any macroreentrant tachycardia, however, delineation of the critical isthmus (using activation and entrainment mapping) is critical for successful ablation. Specialized contact and non-contact mapping techniques may be useful in these cases (see page 146 and Figures 13-34 & 13-35).

13.7 Pacemaker Therapy for Atrial Tachyarrhythmias

Total AV nodal ablation with subsequent permanent pacemaker implantation is a therapeutic option in patients with medically uncontrollable atrial tachyarrhythmias with rapid ventricular response, such as atrial flutter or, especially, atrial fibrillation ("Catheter Ablation" on page 671). This procedure ensures ventricular rate control and prevents the possible development of tachycardia-induced cardiomyopathy in patients with chronic rapid ventricular rates.

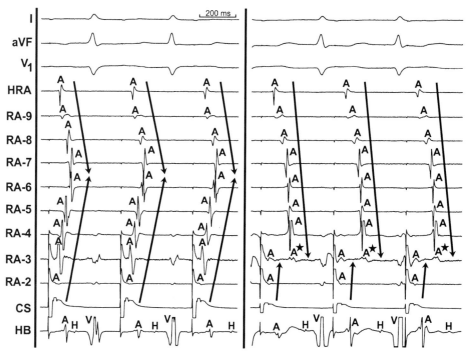

FIGURE 13-39. Demonstration of atrial conduction block within the isthmus bordered by the inferior vena cava and tricuspid valve (IVC-TVA isthmus) following isthmus ablation in a patient with typical counter-clockwise atrial flutter. Pacing is performed at the ostium of the coronary sinus (CS). The position of the 20-pole catheter used to obtain these recordings is as shown in Figure 13-22. Left panel: at baseline before the ablation, pacing at the CS results in lateral conduction within the IVC-TVA isthmus as well as cephalad up the atrial septum to the high right atrium (HRA). Collision of these two wavefronts occurs in the region of the mid-lateral right atrium (at RA-6 or RA-7). Right panel: after a line of RF lesions are applied between the posterior aspect of the TVA and the IVC, pacing is again performed at the CS. Note that the impulse again begins to conduct laterally across the isthmus until it reaches RA-3, thereafter further trans-isthmus conduction is blocked. The next activation is observed at the HRA as the depolarization from the CS proceeds cephalad within the atrial septum to the superior right atrium. Conduction then courses along the lateral RA and crista terminalis to the atrial floor, finally activating the atrial tissue at RA-4. That there is a complete line of conduction block within isthmus at RA-3 is confirmed by the presence of a second atrial activation recorded at this site (denoted by ★). The double atrial potentials inscribed at RA-3 result from activation of atrial tissue on opposite sides of the line of block by two different wavefronts of depolarization. The first atrial activation results from a short segment of clockwise conduction away from the CS, while the second activation is generated by the counterclockwise wavefront traveling superiorly from the CS, caudally along the lateral RA, and then medially within the IVC-TVA isthmus until it reaches the region of RA-3. Only by employing a multipolar catheter with electrodes arrayed along the length of the IVC-TVA isthmus is it possible to document the presence of double atrial potentials thereby verifying the completeness of the RF ablation-induced line of block. If recordings were only available from the ostium of the CS and the lateral isthmus region, it would not be possible to record double potentials straddling the line of block. In this case, slow conduction through an electrically-intact, but damaged, isthmus could not be definitively ruled-out. Abbreviations as in Figure 13-23.

For acute termination, atrial overdrive pacing is effective in terminating reentrant atrial tachycardia and atrial tachycardia caused by triggered activity related to delayed afterdepolarizations [75]. Overdrive atrial pacing is not effective for terminating automatic atrial tachycardia and multifocal atrial tachycardia. While attempting overdrive atrial pacing, it is not uncommon to see inadvertent induction of atrial fibrillation particularly in patients with structural heart disease.

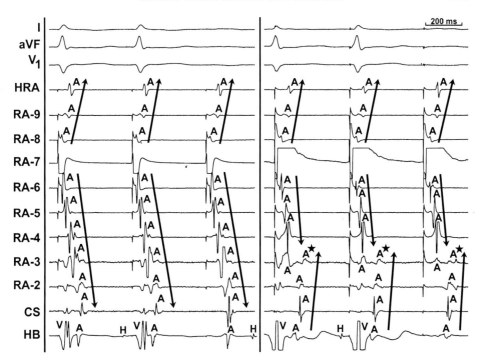

FIGURE 13-40. Demonstration of atrial conduction block within the isthmus bordered by the inferior vena cava and tricuspid valve (IVC-TVA isthmus) following isthmus ablation in a patient with typical counterclockwise atrial flutter. Pacing is performed at the lateral right atrium (RA-7) (region of mid-crista terminalis). The position of the 20-pole catheter used to obtain these recordings is as shown in Figure 13-22. Left panel: at baseline prior to the ablation, lateral pacing results in medial conduction across the IVC-TVA isthmus as well as up the lateral RA to the high right atrium (HRA) and then caudally toward the ostium of the CS. Collision of these two wavefronts occurs in the region of the posterior atrial septum near the CS. Right panel: after a line of RF lesions are applied between the posterior aspect of the TVA and the IVC, pacing is again performed at RA-7. Note that the impulse again begins to conduct medially across the isthmus until it reaches RA-3, thereafter further trans-isthmus conduction is blocked. Activation also proceeds from RA-7 cephalad to the HRA and then caudally to the His bundle region (HB), followed by the CS, and only later reaching the septal - side of the line of block in the isthmus at RA-3. That there is a complete line of conduction block within isthmus at RA-3 is confirmed by the presence of this second atrial activation recorded at this site (denoted by ★). The double atrial potentials inscribed at RA-3 result from activation of atrial tissue on opposite sides of the line of block by two different wavefronts of depolarization. The first atrial activation results from counterclockwise conduction away from the lateral pacing site into the isthmus toward the CS. The second activation is generated by the clockwise wavefront traveling superiorly from RA-7 and then caudally toward the HB and CS. Only by employing a multipolar catheter with electrodes arrayed along the length of the IVC-TVA isthmus is it possible to document the presence of double atrial potentials thereby verifying the completeness of the RF ablation-induced line of block. If recordings were only available from the ostium of the CS and the lateral isthmus region, it would not be possible to record double potentials straddling the line of block. In this case, slow conduction through an electrically-intact, but damaged, isthmus could not be definitively ruled-out. Abbreviations as in Figure 13-23.

The development of curative catheter ablation techniques has largely eliminated the use of permanent pacemaker therapy alone for the treatment of atrial tachycardias and atrial flutter. In patients with a status postsurgical repair of complex congenital heart disease, permanent overdrive atrial pacing has been advocated for chronic management of recurrent reentrant atrial tachycardia [76,77]. Reentrant atrial tachycardia is often observed within the context of tachycardia-bradycardia syndrome in this clinical setting [39]. The pacemaker is programmed to the AAIR pacing mode with a lower pacing rate

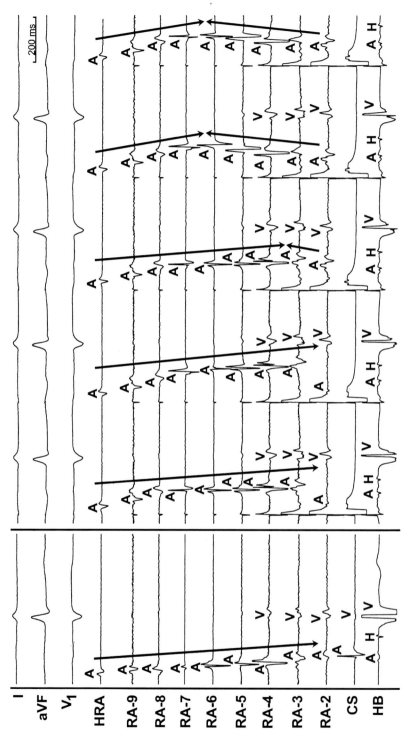

FIGURE 13-41. Intermittent slow trans-isthmus conduction after attempted radiofrequency catheter ablation in a patient with counterclockwise atrial flutter. Catheter recordings as in Figure 13-37 using a 20-pole electrode catheter (Figure 13-22). Recordings are made during sinus rhythm (left panel) and while pacing at 120 pulses/min (right panel) from the region of the coronary sinus. In right panel, the first two beats suggest the presence of conduction block within the isthmus between the inferior vena cava and tricuspid annulus (IVC-TVA). The last two beats show clear evidence of trans-isthmus conduction with collision of two wavefronts at the right lateral atrium (RA-6 and RA-7). The middle beat shows evidence of slow trans-isthmus conduction with collision within the isthmus. Abbreviations as in Figure 13-37.

20% faster than the spontaneous mean daily rate as determined by 24 hour ambulatory ECG recordings. The aim is to achieve a prevalent (>80%) paced rhythm during daily hours. The AAIR pacing mode prevents bradycardia-dependent onset of atrial tachycardia and, in addition, modifies the atrial activation sequence and intraatrial conduction [78]. Alteration of the atrial activation sequence and intraatrial conduction may circumvent electrophysiological parameters for the initiation of intra-atrial reentry. Overall results of permanent overdrive atrial pacing appear effective in suppressing or reducing the arrhythmia recurrence in selected patients; nevertheless, the use of antiarrhythmic drugs may still be necessary.

References

1. Lesh MD, Kalman JM: To fumble flutter or tackle "tach"? Toward updated classifiers for atrial tachyarrhythmias. *J Cardiovasc Electrophysiol* **7**:460-6, 1996.
2. Glatter KA, Cheng J, Dorostkar P, et al.: Electrophysiologic effects of adenosine in patients with supraventricular tachycardia. *Circulation* **99**:1034-40, 1999.
3. Markowitz SM, Stein KM, Mittal S, et al.: Differential effects of adenosine on focal and macroreentrant atrial tachycardia. *J Cardiovasc Electrophysiol* **10**:489-502, 1999.
4. Rosen MR: Cellular electrophysiology of digitalis toxicity. *J Am Coll Cardiol* **5**:22A-34A, 1985.
5. Gomes JA, Hariman RJ, Kang PS, Chowdry IH: Sustained symptomatic sinus node reentrant tachycardia: incidence, clinical significance, electrophysiologic observations and the effects of antiarrhythmic agents. *J Am Coll Cardiol* **5**:45-57, 1985.
6. Curry PV, Callowhill E, Krikler DM: Proceedings: Paroxysmal re-entry sinus tachycardia. *Br Heart J* **38**:311, 1976.
7. Curry PV, Krikler DM. Paroxysmal reciprocating sinus tachycardia. In: Kulbertus HE, ed. *Re-entrant Arrhythmias*. Baltimore, Maryland: University Park Press, 39-62: 1977.
8. Krikler D, Curry P. Atypical initiation of reciprocating tachycardia in the Wolff-Parkinson-White syndrome. In: Kulbertus HE, ed. *Re-entrant Arrhythmias*. Baltimore, Maryland: University Park Press, 144-52: 1977.
9. Tang CW, Scheinman MM, Van Hare GF, et al.: Use of P wave configuration during atrial tachycardia to predict site of origin. *J Am Coll Cardiol* **26**:1315-24, 1995.
10. Man KC, Chan KK, Kovack P, et al.: Spatial resolution of atrial pace mapping as determined by unipolar atrial pacing at adjacent sites. *Circulation* **94**:1357-63, 1996.
11. Wu D, Amat-y-leon F, Denes P, et al.: Demonstration of sustained sinus and atrial re-entry as a mechanism of paroxysmal supraventricular tachycardia. *Circulation* **51**:234-43, 1975.
12. Han J, Malozzi AM, Moe GK: Sino-atrial reciprocation in the isolated rabbit heart. *Circ Res* **22**:355-62, 1968.
13. Allessie MA, Bonke FI. Re-entry within the sinoatrial node as demonstrated by multiple micro- electrode recordings in the isolated rabbit heart. In: Bonke FI, ed. *The Sinus Node*. The Hague: Nijhoff Medical Division, 409-21: 1978.
14. Allessie MA, Bonke FI: Direct demonstration of sinus node reentry in the rabbit heart. *Circ Res* **44**:557-68, 1979.
15. Narula OS: Sinus node re-entry: a mechanism for supraventricular tachycardia. *Circulation* **50**:1114-28, 1974.
16. Lipson MJ, Naimi S: Multifocal atrial tachycardia (chaotic atrial tachycardia). Clinical associations and significance. *Circulation* **42**:397-407, 1970.
17. Shine KI, Kastor JA, Yurchak PM: Multifocal atrial tachycardia. Clinical and electrocardiographic features in 32 patients. *N Engl J Med* **279**:344-9, 1968.
18. Scher D, Arsura E: Multifocal atrial tachycardia: mechanisms, clinical correlates and treatment. *Am Heart J* **118**:574-80, 1989.

19. Phillips J, Spano J, Burch G: Chaotic atrial mechanism. *Am Heart J* **78**:171-79, 1969.

20. Levine JH, Michael JR, Guarnieri T: Treatment of multifocal atrial tachycardia with verapamil. *N Engl J Med* **312**:21-5, 1985.

21. Marchlinski FE, Miller JM: Atrial arrhythmias exacerbated by theophylline. Response to verapamil and evidence for triggered activity in man. *Chest* **88**:931-4, 1985.

22. Lin C, Chuang I, Chenk K, Chiang B: Arrhythmogenic effects of theophylline in human atrial tissue. *Int J Cardiol* **17**:289-97, 1987.

23. Goldreyer BN, Gallagher JJ, Damato AN: The electrophysiologic demonstration of atrial ectopic tachycardia in man. *Am Heart J* **85**:205-15, 1973.

24. Scheinman MM, Basu D, Hollenberg M: Electrophysiologic studies in patients with persistent atrial tachycardia. *Circulation* **50**:266-73, 1974.

25. Krahn AD, Yee R, Klein GJ, Morillo C: Inappropriate sinus tachycardia: evaluation and therapy. *J Cardiovasc Electrophysiol* **6**:1124-8, 1995.

26. Morillo CA, Leitch JW, Yee R, Klein GJ: A placebo-controlled trial of intravenous and oral disopyramide for prevention of neurally mediated syncope induced by head-up tilt. *J Am Coll Cardiol* **22**:1843-8, 1993.

27. Lee RJ, Kalman JM, Fitzpatrick AP, et al.: Radiofrequency catheter modification of the sinus node for "inappropriate" sinus tachycardia. *Circulation* **92**:2919-28, 1995.

28. Zivin A, Glick R, Knight BP, et al.: Psychiatric profile of patients with inappropriate sinus tachycardia. *Pacing Clin Electrophysiol* **21**:923, 1998.

29. Bauernfeind RA, Amat YLF, Dhingra RC, et al.: Chronic non-paroxysmal sinus tachycardia in otherwise healthy persons. *Ann Intern Med* **91**:702-10, 1979.

30. Friedman PL, Stevenson WG, Kocovic DZ: Autonomic dysfunction after catheter ablation. *J Cardiovasc Electrophysiol* **7**:450-9, 1996.

31. Pappone C, Stabile G, Oreto G, et al.: Inappropriate sinus tachycardia after radiofrequency ablation of para-Hisian accessory pathways. *J Cardiovasc Electrophysiol* **8**:1357-65, 1997.

32. Krahn AD, Klein GJ, Norris C, Yee R: The etiology of syncope in patients with negative tilt table and electrophysiological testing. *Circulation* **92**:1819-24, 1995.

33. Jayaprakash S, Sparks PB, Vohra J: Inappropriate sinus tachycardia (IST): management by radiofrequency modification of sinus node. *Aust N Z J Med* **27**:391-7, 1997.

34. Shinbane JS, Lee RJ, Evans JT, et al.: Electrophysiologic & electrocardiographic manifestations of transcatheter radiofrequency sinus node modification in humans. *Pacing Clin Electrophysiol* **19**:594, 1996.

35. Shinbane JS, Lee RJ, Evans JT, et al.: Long-term follow-up after radiofrequency sinus node modification for inappropriate sinus tachycardia. *J Am Coll Cardiol* **29**:199A, 1997.

36. Akhtar M, Caracta AR, Lau SH, et al.: Demonstration of intra-atrial conduction delay, block, gap and reentry: a report of two cases. *Circulation* **58**:947-55, 1978.

37. Haines DE, DiMarco JP: Sustained intraatrial reentrant tachycardia: clinical, electrocardiographic and electrophysiologic characteristics and long- term follow-up. *J Am Coll Cardiol* **15**:1345-54, 1990.

38. Wu D, Denes P, Amat-y-Leon F, et al.: Clinical, electrocardiographic and electrophysiologic observations in patients with paroxysmal supraventricular tachycardia. *Am J Cardiol* **41**:1045-51, 1978.

39. Flinn CJ, Wolff GS, Dick Md, et al.: Cardiac rhythm after the Mustard operation for complete transposition of the great arteries. *N Engl J Med* **310**:1635-8, 1984.

40. Deanfield J, Camm J, Macartney F, et al.: Arrhythmia and late mortality after Mustard and Senning operation for transposition of the great arteries. An eight-year prospective study. *J Thorac Cardiovasc Surg* **96**:569-76, 1988.

41. Martin TC, Smith L, Hernandez A, Weldon CS: Dysrhythmias following the Senning operation for dextro-transposition of the great arteries. *J Thorac Cardiovasc Surg* **85**:928-32, 1983.

42. Hayes CJ, Gersony WM: Arrhythmias after the Mustard operation for transposition of the great arteries: a long-term study. *J Am Coll Cardiol* **7**:133-7, 1986.

43. Janousek J, Paul T, Luhmer I, et al.: Atrial baffle procedures for complete transposition of the great arteries: natural course of sinus node dysfunction and risk factors for dysrhythmias and sudden death. *Z Kardiol* **83**:933-8, 1994.

44. Beerman LB, Neches WH, Fricker FJ, et al.: Arrhythmias in transposition of the great arteries after the Mustard operation. *Am J Cardiol* **51**:1530-4, 1983.

45. Gewillig M, Cullen S, Mertens B, et al.: Risk factors for arrhythmia and death after Mustard operation for simple transposition of the great arteries. *Circulation* **84**:III187-92, 1991.

46. Lesh MD, Kalman JM, Saxon LA, et al.: Electrophysiology of "incisional" reentrant atrial tachycardia complicating surgery for congenital heart disease. *Pacing Clin Electrophysiol* **20**:2107-11, 1997.

47. Kalman JM, VanHare GF, Olgin JE, et al.: Ablation of 'incisional' reentrant atrial tachycardia complicating surgery for congenital heart disease. Use of entrainment to define a critical isthmus of conduction. *Circulation* **93**:502-12, 1996.

48. Tai DY, Chang MS, Svinarich JT, et al.: Mechanisms of verapamil-induced conduction block in anomalous atrioventricular bypass tracts. *J Am Coll Cardiol* **5**:311-7, 1985.

49. Sung RJ, Elser B, McAllister RG, Jr.: Intravenous verapamil for termination of re-entrant supraventricular tachycardias: intracardiac studies correlated with plasma verapamil concentrations. *Ann Intern Med* **93**:682-9, 1980.

50. Kunze KP, Kuck KH, Schluter M, Bleifeld W: Effect of encainide and flecainide on chronic ectopic atrial tachycardia. *J Am Coll Cardiol* **7**:1121-6, 1986.

51. Shen EN, Keung E, Huycke E, et al.: Intravenous propafenone for termination of reentrant supraventricular tachycardia. A placebo-controlled, randomized, double-blind, crossover study. *Ann Intern Med* **105**:655-61, 1986.

52. Sung RJ, Tan HL, Karagounis L, et al.: Intravenous sotalol for the termination of supraventricular tachycardia and atrial fibrillation and flutter: a multicenter, randomized, double-blind, placebo-controlled study. Sotalol Multicenter Study Group. *Am Heart J* **129**:739-48, 1995.

53. Wiener I, Lyons H: Amiodarone for refractory automatic atrial tachycardia: observations on the electrophysiological actions of amiodarone. *Pacing Clin Electrophysiol* **7**:707-9, 1984.

54. Wang K, Goldfarb BL, Gobel FL, Richman HG: Multifocal atrial tachycardia. *Arch Intern Med* **137**:161-4, 1977.

55. Kastor J: Multifocal atrial tachycardia. *N Engl J Med* **322**:1713-17, 1990.

56. Hazard PB, Burnett CR: Verapamil in multifocal atrial tachycardia. Hemodynamic and respiratory changes. *Chest* **91**:68-70, 1987.

57. Hazard PB, Burnett CR: Treatment of multifocal atrial tachycardia with metoprolol. *Crit Care Med* **15**:20-5, 1987.

58. Wenger TL, Butler VP, Jr., Haber E, Smith TW: Treatment of 63 severely digitalis-toxic patients with digoxin-specific antibody fragments. *J Am Coll Cardiol* **5**:118A-123A, 1985.

59. Desantola JR, Marchlinski FE: Response of digoxin toxic atrial tachycardia to digoxin-specific Fab fragments. *Am J Cardiol* **58**:1109-10, 1986.

60. Castellanos A, Jr., Lemberg L, Jude JR, Berkovits BV: Repetitive firing occurring during synchronized electrical stimulation of the heart. *J Thorac Cardiovasc Surg* **51**:334-40, 1966.

61. Castellanos A, Jr., Lemberg L, Budkin A, Brown J: Cardioversion pseudofailures. *Geriatrics* **22**:167-74, 1967.

62. Chiladakis JA, Vassilikos VP, Maounis TN, et al.: Successful radiofrequency catheter ablation of automatic atrial tachycardia with regression of the cardiomyopathy picture. *Pacing Clin Electrophysiol* **20**:953-9, 1997.

63. Feld GK: Catheter ablation for the treatment of atrial tachycardia. *Prog Cardiovasc Dis* **37**:205-24, 1995.

64. Hatala R, Weiss C, Koschyk DH, et al.: Radiofrequency catheter ablation of left atrial tachycardia originating within the pulmonary vein in a patient with dextrocardia. *Pacing Clin Electrophysiol* **19**:999-1002, 1996.

65. Poty H, Saoudi N, Haissaguerre M, et al.: Radiofrequency catheter ablation of atrial tachycardias. *Am Heart J* **131**:481-9, 1996.

66. Mallavarapu C, Schwartzman D, Callans DJ, et al.: Radiofrequency catheter ablation of atrial tachycardia with unusual left atrial sites of origin. *Pacing Clin Electrophysiol* **19**:988-92, 1996.

67. Tracy CM: Catheter ablation for patients with atrial tachycardia. *Cardiol Clin* **15**:607-21, 1997.

68. Goldberger J, Kall J, Ehlert F, et al.: Effectiveness of radiofrequency catheter ablation for treatment of atrial tachycardia. *Am J Cardiol* **72**:787-93, 1993.

69. Sanders WE, Jr., Sorrentino RA, Greenfield RA, et al.: Catheter ablation of sinoatrial node reentrant tachycardia. *J Am Coll Cardiol* **23**:926-34, 1994.

70. Simons GR, Wharton JM: Radiofrequency catheter ablation of atrial tachycardia and atrial flutter. *Coron Artery Dis* **7**:12-9, 1996.

71. Lesh MD, Van Hare GF: Status of ablation in patients with atrial tachycardia and flutter. *Pacing Clin Electrophysiol* **17**:1026-33, 1994.

72. Lesh MD, Van Hare GF, Epstein LM, et al.: Radiofrequency catheter ablation of atrial arrhythmias. Results and mechanisms. *Circulation* **89**:1074-89, 1994.

73. Lesh MD, Kalman JM, Olgin JE: New approaches to treatment of atrial flutter and tachycardia. *J Cardiovasc Electrophysiol* **7**:368-81, 1996.

74. Muller GI, Deal BJ, Strasburger JF, Benson DW, Jr.: Electrocardiographic features of atrial tachycardias after operation for congenital heart disease. *Am J Cardiol* **71**:122-4, 1993.

75. Rosen MR, Reder RF: Does triggered activity have a role in the genesis of cardiac arrhythmias? *Ann Intern Med* **94**:794-801, 1981.

76. Ragonese P, Drago F, Guccione P, et al.: Permanent overdrive atrial pacing in the chronic management of recurrent postoperative atrial reentrant tachycardia in patients with complex congenital heart disease. *Pacing Clin Electrophysiol* **20**:2917-23, 1997.

77. Silka MJ, Manwill JR, Kron J, McAnulty JH: Bradycardia-mediated tachyarrhythmias in congenital heart disease and responses to chronic pacing at physiologic rates. *Am J Cardiol* **65**:488-93, 1990.

78. Rhodes LA, Walsh EP, Gamble WJ, et al.: Benefits and potential risks of atrial antitachycardia pacing after repair of congenital heart disease. *Pacing Clin Electrophysiol* **18**:1005-16, 1995.

79. Sung RJ, Chang MS, Chiang BN: Clinical electrophysiology of supraventricular tachycardia. *Cardiol Clin* **1**:225-51, 1983.

CHAPTER 14

ATRIAL FIBRILLATION

Atrial fibrillation is the most common sustained cardiac arrhythmia encountered in clinical practice. It accounts for more than 300,000 hospital admissions annually in the United States [1]. The prevalence of atrial fibrillation increases with age, (e.g., 0.5% at age 50-59 years and up to 9% at 80-89 years) [2], and, in addition, it increases with the development of cardiac and non-cardiac conditions such as rheumatic heart disease, hypertension, atherosclerotic heart disease, cardiomyopathy, pericarditis, and hyperthyroidism. [3-5]. Atrial fibrillation is also noted to be more prevalent in men than in women [6].

Clinically, atrial fibrillation is often present with a rapid and irregular ventricular response (usually >150/min). The rapid heart rate and the associated loss of atrial contribution to ventricular filling leads to decreased cardiac output, thereby causing dyspnea, fatigue, angina, dizziness, syncope, and/or congestive heart failure [7]. Furthermore, the resulting blood stasis with enhanced platelet aggregation and coagulation [8] predisposes to atrial thrombus formation and subsequent thromboembolism possibly precipitating a cerebrovascular accident. Thus, atrial fibrillation causes significant morbidity and mortality and consumes enormous medical resources for its diagnosis and management of its complications [9-14].

14.1   Pathological Findings

14.1.1   AGING PROCESS

Normally the atrial myocardium contains more connective tissue than the ventricular myocardium. Fatty metamorphosis – an increase in adipose and fibrotic tissues – begins in the third decade. Further degenerative changes cause vacuolization and atrophy of the atrial endocardium that is replaced by collagen and elastic fibers [15-17]. These age-related changes frequently affects the sinoatrial node and its surrounding atrial tissue, and may, thus, cause sinoatrial conduction disturbances (sick sinus syndrome) with advancing age. Atrial dilation due to left ventricular dysfunction can, in addition, facilitate degenerative changes in the atrial tissue. In the ninth decade, amyloid deposits may further compromise the functional properties of the atrium. These age-related degenerative changes may account for electrophysiological inhomogeneity in conduction velocity and refractoriness thereby predisposing to the occurrence of atrial fibrillation.

14.1.2 MYOCARDITIS

Isolated atrial myocarditis may be the cause of atrial fibrillation in certain patients, particularly at a very young age [18]. Lymphocytic infiltration with focal necrosis of adjacent myocytes is the predominant finding. Clinically, it is very difficult to be distinguished from lone atrial fibrillation that is primarily caused by age-related degenerative changes.

14.1.3 RHEUMATIC VALVULAR HEART DISEASE

Both mitral stenosis and mitral regurgitation lead to atrial stretch and enlargement, and therefore, are prone to development of atrial fibrillation [19]. However, no specific atrial changes related to rheumatic heart disease can be found. Clinical studies have noted that advancing age and duration of mitral valve disease are determining factors in the development of atrial fibrillation. The fibrotic degenerative changes are severe and atrial myocytes tend to be separated by thick layers of fibrotic tissue [20].

14.1.4 CORONARY ARTERY DISEASE

Coronary occlusion proximal to the origin of the sinus nodal artery or an atrial branch may cause disturbances in impulse generation of the sinoatrial node and impulse transmission of the atrial tissue as well as nerve injury thereby predisposing to development of atrial fibrillation [21,22]. Nevertheless, the genesis of atrial fibrillation in patients with chronic arteriosclerotic heart disease is usually multifactorial. These include old age, mitral regurgitation, atrial infarction, pericarditis, and congestive heart failure [23,24].

14.1.5 PERICARDITIS

Pericarditis may complicate acute myocardial infarction, uremia, rheumatic fever, lupus erythematosus, pulmonary embolism, etc., and atrial fibrillation may be a clinical manifestation of pericarditis. Inflammatory changes of pericarditis may affect the sinoatrial node and its surrounding nerves, and atrial epicardium [25,26]. Development of atrial premature beats as a result of the changes may trigger an onset of atrial fibrillation.

14.1.6 PRIMARY & SECONDARY CARDIOMYOPATHY

Left ventricular dysfunction due to primary or secondary cardiomyopathy may cause atrial dilation that, in turn, induces and facilitates fibrotic degenerative changes. Rarely, a primary cardiomyopathy may also directly affect the atrial tissue [27], e.g., familial and light-chain associated cardiac amyloidosis [28].

14.1.7 ATRIAL REMODELING & TACHYCARDIA-INDUCED ATRIAL MYOPATHY

Various forms of supraventricular tachyarrhythmias such as atrial tachycardia, atrial flutter, AV reciprocating tachycardia [29], and AV nodal reentrant tachycardia [30] tend to favor the initiation of atrial fibrillation. Loss of synchronous AV contractions may result in atrial stretch which may provoke premature atrial depolarizations and trigger the onset of atrial fibrillation during supraventricular tachycardia [29].

Incessant or repetitive episodes of supraventricular tachycardia and atrial fibrillation can by itself result in altered cellular electrophysiology, a process called "electrical remodeling" [31-34], and eventually cause ultrastructural changes in the atrial tissue [35-37] similar to that of tachycardia-induced cardiomyopathy involving the ventricular myocardium [38]. These changes include loss of myofibrils and fragmentation of sarcoplasmic reticulum resulting in altered cellular Ca^{++} handling with an impaired cytosolic Ca^{++} transient [39,40]. Electrophysiologically, the atrial refractory period is markedly shortened and rate adaptation of the atrial refractory period is reduced or reversed, all of which increases the ease of inducibility and stability of subsequent episodes of atrial fibrillation. Thus, "atrial fibrillation begets atrial fibrillation" [31]. Furthermore, sustained atrial fibrillation can cause "mechanical remodeling" as evidenced by progressive right and left atrial enlargement [32] that accelerates fibrotic degenerative changes in the atrial myocardium.

14.1.8 ATRIAL FIBRILLATION FOLLOWING CARDIAC SURGERY

It is estimated that approximately 30% of patients undergoing cardiac surgery develop atrial fibrillation postoperatively [41]. Although age-related atrial changes, atrial injury, atrial ischemia, perioperative pericarditis are important predisposing factors, a high catecholamine state during the perioperative period potentially provides a triggering mechanism of the onset of atrial fibrillation [42-44].

14.1.9 HYPERTHYROIDISM

No specific anatomic changes in the atria have been described in association with hyperthyroidism. Nevertheless, thyroid hormone tends to increase β-adrenergic receptor density and increase tissue sensitivity to circulating epinephrine and norepinephrine [45]. Thus, it is likely that hyperthyroidism may provide a triggering mechanism for the initiation of atrial fibrillation in patients with preexisting anatomic substrates.

14.2 Electrophysiologic Mechanisms

It has been postulated that atrial fibrillation may be caused by (1) a unifocal or multifocal rapidly discharging foci and (2) a single or multiple reentrant wavelets [46-49]. Observations made in human studies have confirmed that reentry is the predominant mechanism of atrial fibrillation and there are multiple reentrant wavelets. However, a focal origin of atrial fibrillation from left atrial sites close to the pulmonary veins or from the right atrium can be seen in some patients [50].

Focal atrial fibrillation can be exemplified by aconitine-induced atrial fibrillation in a canine model [49], in which removal of a focal atrial tissue can abolish atrial fibrillation. The mechanism of reentry in the atrial tissues can also be demonstrated in various experimental models [51,52]. The wavelength of reentry is the product of conduction velocity and refractory period. To maintain reentry, the circuit length (anatomical path) must exceed the wavelength of reentry to allow a full recovery of excitability (excitable gap) between the "head" and "tail" of the circulating impulse. In atrial fibrillation, there are multiple reentrant wavelets; consequently, there is a tight relationship between the circuit length and the wavelength of reentry such that there is a very short excitable gap [52,53]. This is in contrast to other forms of reentrant tachycardia such as atrial flutter, AV nodal reentrant tachycardia and AV reciprocating tachycardia that are all characterized by the presence of a long excitable gap in the circuit length [54-56].

The complexity of the atrial structure in itself may cause electrophysiological inhomogeneity. First, a myriad of conduction barriers are naturally present, including the AV annuli and various ostia such as the inferior and superior vena cavae and the pulmonary veins. Second, there are variations in fiber orientation, tissue thickness, and characteristics of action potentials with resultant differences in conduction velocity and refractoriness in different parts of the atria [57,58]. In addition, non-uniform distribution of autonomic influences, particularly vagal effects [59,60] in conjunction with aging-induced degenerative changes [15-17], can affect functional properties of the atrium conducive to the genesis of anisotropic reentrant arrhythmias.

Atrial fibrillation of long duration may, by itself, cause gradual atrial stretching leading to atrial enlargement ("mechanical remodeling"). This process can be further accelerated by mitral valvular diseases such as mitral stenosis and mitral regurgitation. Progressive atrial enlargement produces further degenerative changes favoring formation of reentrant circuits.

The altered cellular electrophysiology in the atrial tissue, i.e., "electrical remodeling," associated with recurrent atrial tachyarrhythmias [32,33] has been under extensive investigation. Specifically, shortening and loss of rate adaptation of atrial refractoriness are associated with: 1) intracellular Ca^{++} overload; 2) down-regulation of the L-type Ca^{++} (I_{Ca-L}) channel current; 3) a reduction in the transient outward current (I_{TO}) and; 4) an increase in both the inward rectifier (I_{K1}) and the acetylcholine-sensitive potassium channel ($I_{K(ACH)}$) currents. The fast sodium inward current (I_{Na}), the sustained outward current (I_{SUS}) and the T-type Ca channel (I_{Ca-T}) are not altered [37,61-64]. Of note, experimental studies have demonstrated that during atrial fibrillation there is reduced atrial blood flow as detected by positron emission tomography, and that atrial ischemia can shorten and cause loss of rate adaptation of atrial refractoriness similar to that produced by rapid atrial pacing [65,66]. Moreover, these latter changes can be prevented by blockade of the Na^+/H^+ exchanger. Thus, rapid atrial rate-induced atrial ischemia may play an important role in the genesis of "electrical remodeling" during atrial fibrillation. Activation of Na^+/H^+ exchange induced by atrial ischemia leads to inward Na^+ entry into the cell. Ischemia-induced depression of Na^+/K^+ pump also increases intracellular Na^+ accumulation. The increase in intracellular Na$^+$ concentration promotes reversal of Na$^+$/Ca^{++} exchange, causing intracellular Ca^{++} accumulation followed by a down regulation of I$_{Ca-L}$. This hypothesis explains why verapamil, a blocker of I$_{Ca-L}$, attenuates changes in atrial refractoriness caused by atrial tachycardia, but it doesn't alter the propensity of atrial tachycardia to promote atrial fibrillation [63]. It is tempting to postulate that a specific gene defect linking to an ion channel or channels may be responsible for the genesis of atrial fibrillation in a rare clinical entity of familial atrial fibrillation [67-69], similar to that of congenital long QT syndrome [70].

14.3 Classification of Atrial Fibrillation

To distinguish atrial fibrillation from atrial flutter and other forms of atrial tachycardia can sometimes be difficult. Atrial fibrillation usually has a frequency of irregular atrial impulses between 350 and 600 per minute and tends to exhibit irregular ventricular responses referred to as "irregular irregularity." However, atrial flutter and rapid atrial tachycardia can also exhibit irregular ventricular responses due to conduction delay, concealed conduction [71] and varying degrees of AV block.

There are several ways to classify atrial fibrillation, but very few of them are clinically useful. For instance, atrial fibrillation can be either "fine" or "coarse" based on an arbitrary threshold of 0.1 mV of the "f" waves in lead V$_1$ [72]. Coarse atrial fibrillation may be mistaken for atrial flutter. "Lone atrial fibrillation" depicts atrial fibrillation occurring in an otherwise structurally normal heart in the absence of systemic disease [73-75]. This is in contrast to atrial fibrillation occurring in the presence of structural heart disease such as "rheumatic atrial fibrillation" related to mitral stenosis and "non-rheumatic atrial fibrillation" associated with hypertensive or arteriosclerotic heart disease and primary or secondary cardiomyopathy with or without congestive heart failure [76].

Atrial fibrillation with a rapid ventricular rate is often called "rapid atrial fibrillation." Besides palpitation, "rapid atrial fibrillation" may cause dizziness, angina pectoris, shortness of breath and symptoms of congestive heart failure [77]. All these symptoms may subside following slowing of the ventricular rate with AV nodal depressants. When the ventricular rate is reduced to be between 60-90 beats per minute it is often referred to as "controlled atrial fibrillation." Patients with preexisting AV nodal dysfunction may present with atrial fibrillation with a relatively slow ventricular rate. In this subgroup of patients, treatment with digitalis or other AV nodal depressants may further reduce the ventricular rate thereby causing symptoms of dizziness and/or syncope.

Based on the time course and temporal patterns, atrial fibrillation can be classified as "acute" and "chronic," and "chronic" can be "paroxysmal," "persistent," or "permanent" [78]. The "persistent" but not the "permanent" form can be converted to sinus rhythm by chemical or electrical cardioversion. There is a tendency for atrial fibrillation to evolve from a "paroxysmal" to a "persistent" and then to a "permanent" form.

Clinically, some patients tend to develop atrial fibrillation during a high adrenergic state (sinus tachycardia) while others seem to have onset of atrial fibrillation associated with high vagal tone (sinus bradycardia). The former is referred to as "catecholamine-sensitive" and the latter "vagally-mediated" atrial fibrillation [79-81]. Catecholamine-sensitive atrial fibrillation is usually triggered by exercise, anxiety, emotional upset or surgery and it responds better to β-adrenergic blocking agents. From a therapeutic stand-point, digitalis should be avoided in vagally-mediated atrial fibrillation because digitalis possesses vagal effects. Under this circumstance, an antiarrhythmic agent with vagolytic properties such as disopyramide may be useful for suppression of atrial fibrillation.

Recording of atrial electrograms has also been used to classify atrial fibrillation [82-87]. It appears that some areas of the atria may show organized while others disor-ganized electrical activities (Figure 14-1), and furthermore, in the same area, organized, disorganized, intermediate, and mixed patterns can be interchangeable and continuously variable. These findings have generated continuous interest in research. However, clini-cal usefulness of these findings remains to be determined.

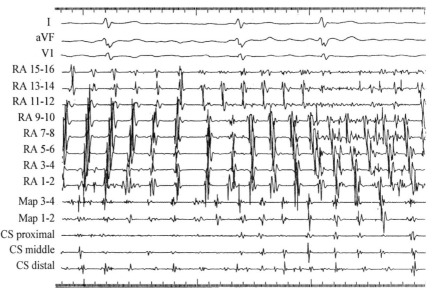

FIGURE 14-1. Intracardiac recordings during atrial fibrillation. ECG leads I, aVF, and V_1 are shown along with intracardiac electrograms from low right atrium (RA 1-2) and at intervening sites cephalad to roof of right atrium (RA 15-16), isthmus region of right atrial floor between the tricuspid valve annulus and inferior vena cava (Map 1-2 & Map 3-4), and proximal to distal coronary sinus (CS). Note relatively organized intracardiac atrial activity in all recordings on the left 2/3 of the figure, while the right 1/3 shows more disorganized atrial activity in all intracardiac leads. Closely adjacent regions can show organized and fragmented activity simultaneously. Paper speed 50 mm/sec

14.4   Pharmacotherapy for Atrial Fibrillation

In general, pharmacologic treatments for atrial fibrillation are directed at either control of ventricular rate or termination and suppression of further episodes of atrial fibrillation and maintenance of sinus rhythm. In the former case, the choice of agents, in general, includes those that primarily exert their effects by inhibiting conduction through the AV node (e.g., β-adrenoceptor blockers, Ca^{++} channel blockers). In the latter case, antiarrhythmic drugs, generally from class IA, IC, or III, are most useful.

14.4.1 TERMINATION OF ATRIAL FIBRILLATION

Because "atrial fibrillation begets atrial fibrillation" [31], new onset atrial fibrillation should be terminated as soon as possible (Table 14-1.) In general, atrial fibrillation lasting for 48 hours or less can be safely cardioverted with electrical or chemical cardioversion without anticoagulation (risk of thromboembolism 0.8%). On the other hand, atrial fibrillation of longer than 48 hours in duration should be anticoagulated with warfarin for 3 to 4 weeks before cardioversion, and continues to be anticoagulated for additional 3 to 4 weeks to prevent thromboembolic complications [88]. The risk of cardioversion-relat-

TABLE 14-1. Acute treatment and termination of atrial fibrillation

Atrial fibrillation duration < 48 hours	Atrial fibrillation duration > 48 hours
Rate control followed by immediate electrical or chemical cardioversion (using ibutilide or procainamide, IV, or oral propafenone or flecainide)	Rate control and anticoagulation (warfarin) for 3-4 weeks followed by electrical or chemical cardioversion with continuation of anticoagulation for an additional 3-4 weeks following successful cardioversion

ed thromboembolism without anticoagulation before cardioversion is about 5% to 7%. The use of 3 to 4 weeks of anticoagulation before cardioversion results in a reduction in the thromboembolic rate to approximately 1.2%. Post-cardioversion anticoagulation serves to inhibit the formation of new thrombi during the subsequent recovery of atrial function regardless of the mode of cardioversion—electrical or chemical [89,90]. Because electrical cardioversion may provoke serious ventricular tachyarrhythmias in patients with hypokalemia or excessive digoxin levels, the serum K$^+$ concentration and digoxin level should be checked prior to the procedure. Chemical cardioversion with ibutilide is contraindicated in patients with hypokalemia or long QT interval (acquired or congenital), for fear of provoking torsade de pointes.

To avoid nearly one month of anticoagulation before cardioversion, alternatively, transesophageal echocardiography can be used to exclude atrial thrombi for early chemical or electrical cardioversion (Figure 14-2). Transesophageal echocardiography is preferred to transthoracic echocardiography because it provides better visualization of the left atrial appendage, which is the major site (90%) of atrial thrombi among patients with atrial fibrillation [91,92]. However, under the circumstance, intravenous heparin should be administered before, during and after cardioversion, and oral anticoagulation with warfarin be maintained for 3 to 4 weeks after successful cardioversion. For patients with atrial thrombi as revealed by the initial transesophageal echocardiography, a follow-up transesophageal echocardiography after 6 weeks anticoagulation with warfarin is recommended to document thrombus resolution before attempted cardioversion. The above transesophageal echocardiography-guided approach appears to have the advantage of accurate exclusion of atrial thrombi before cardioversion and simplified anticoagulation with shorter duration of sustained atrial fibrillation allowing an early recovery of atrial mechanical function [90].

While performing electrical cardioversion, rapid ventricular rate should be slowed with AV nodal depressants (e.g., diltiazem or esmolol) before the delivery of a direct current countershock. This is to reduce the risk of countershock-induced ventricular fibrillation [93] that usually occurs during short RR intervals (≤ 300 ms) with associated overlapping of the ventricular vulnerable period [94]. Electrode pads may be positioned anteriorly and pos-

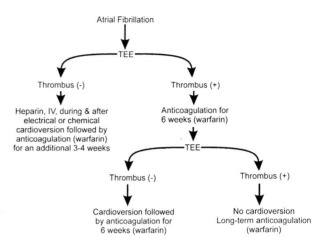

FIGURE 14-2. Suggested algorithm for use of transesophageal echocardiography (TEE) to guide acute treatment and termination of atrial fibrillation. See text for details.

teriorly, near the cardiac apex and at the right upper parasternal border, or posteriorly and at the right lower parasternal border. Compared to the other electrode locations, the posterior–right lower parasternal position seems to provide better anatomic coverage for both atria. The direct current shock should be synchronized to the QRS complex to avoid delivery of the shock during the vulnerable period, potentially triggering ventricular fibrillation. The immediate success rate of electrical cardioversion of atrial fibrillation is approximately 95 %.

In selected patients, internal electrical cardioversion may be required to convert atrial fibrillation to sinus rhythm [95,96]. For internal cardioversion, shocks are delivered through two decapolar electrode catheters positioned, respectively, at the lateral wall of the right atrium and in the coronary sinus (or left pulmonary artery) (Figure 14-3). Also, a quadripolar electrode catheter is placed at the right ventricular apex for sensing and back-up pacing following cardioversion. The internal shock energy required for successful termination of atrial fibrillation ranges from 2–20-J, although occasional patients may require energies over of 30-J.

Atrial fibrillation is often a form of anisotropic reentry with multiple wavelets [82,97]. Therefore, atrial fibrillation may be terminated by drugs (chemical cardioversion) that can increase the wavelength of reentry to reduce the number of wavelets to be maintained in the atria. The indications for chemical cardioversion include: 1) contraindications for conscious sedation or general anesthesia, 2) lack of suitable sites on the patient for placement of electrode pads, and 3) patient refusal of electrical cardioversion. Both class IA and class IC antiarrhythmic agents can be used to terminate atrial fibrillation (e.g., intravenous procainamide 15 mg/kg or oral propafenone 600 mg) [97,98].

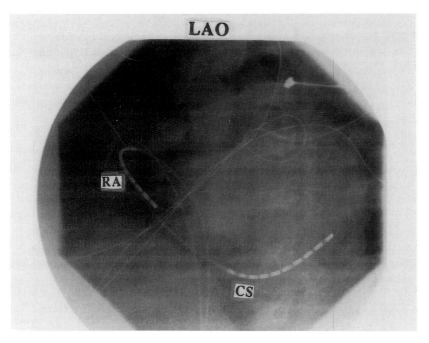

FIGURE 14-3. Fluoroscopic radiograph (left anterior oblique (LAO) view) showing positioning of temporary decapolar electrode catheters in the lateral right atrium (RA) and coronary sinus (CS) for internal cardioversion of atrial fibrillation.

These agents delay recovery of the availability of Na⁺ channels for reexcitation during the phase 3 of the action potential thereby prolonging refractoriness [99,100]. They also possess some K⁺ channel blocking properties that may further prolong refractoriness. The success rate for chemical cardioversion of atrial fibrillation ranges from 30 to 50 %. Class IC agents such as propafenone are relatively contraindicated in patients with reduced left ventricular function (ejection fraction < 40 %), as well as those with significant intraventricular conduction defects (e.g., bifascicular block). Caution should be exercised when using these agents in these patients. Clinically, both class IA and IC antiarrhythmic agents are effective in suppressing atrial premature beats and are also useful for maintaining sinus rhythm and for chronic prophylaxis against atrial fibrillation. By contrast, class IB antiarrhythmic agents (e.g., lidocaine and mexiletine) block inactivated Na⁺ channels during the plateau phase of action potential, and may thereby, abbreviate the duration of action potential and enhance net outward K⁺ current [101,102]. Thus, they are not useful in the treatment of atrial fibrillation.

The class III antiarrhythmic agents (e.g., sotalol, dofetilide and amiodarone) increase action potential duration and prolong refractoriness primarily by blocking outward K⁺ channels that control the process of repolarization. Both sotalol and amiodarone are effective for suppressing the inducibility of atrial fibrillation. They are useful for maintaining sinus rhythm but may not be effective in acutely terminating atrial fibrillation [103]. The relative ineffectiveness of class III agents in terminating atrial fibrillation may be accounted for by: 1) insufficient prolongation of atrial refractoriness and 2) reverse use-dependent effects of class III antiarrhythmic drugs, particularly sotalol and dofetilide, which reduces their therapeutic efficacy at faster rates (shorter cycle lengths). It is postulated that the slow component of the delayed rectifier K^+ channel, I_{Ks} (catecholamine-sensitive channels), which is not disturbed by sotalol and dofetilide, is under less deactivation at shorter cycle lengths. Consequently, the I_{Ks} channel increases its contribution to the repolarizing currents and shorten the action potential duration counteracting the action of class III antiarrhythmic drugs.

Ibutilide is a unique class III antiarrhythmic agent. It not only blocks the rapid component of the delayed rectifier K^+ channel, I_{Kr}, but also activates a slow inward Na^+ current during the plateau phase of the action potential thereby prolonging refractoriness [104,105]. The intravenous form of ibutilide (0.5-1.0 mg/10 minutes administered up to two times 10 minutes apart) has been shown to be effective in terminating atrial flutter and atrial fibrillation [106]. Its therapeutic effectiveness may be related to its more potent increase in atrial refractoriness compared to other antiarrhythmic agents. Probably because atrial fibrillation has a less well-defined reentrant circuit (i.e., multiple wavelets) compared to atrial flutter, the conversion rate of atrial fibrillation by intravenous ibutilide is significantly lower than that for atrial flutter.

14.4.2 MAINTENANCE OF NORMAL SINUS RHYTHM

For those patients in whom chronic antiarrhythmic drug prophylaxis to prevent recurrence of atrial fibrillation is deemed appropriate, the "trigger-substrate" relationship should be considered and a therapeutic strategy individualized (Table 14-2.) Detailed

TABLE 14-2. Maintenance of sinus rhythm

Life-style adjustment (no antiarrhythmic drug therapy)
β-adrenoceptor blocking agents for catecholamine-sensitive atrial fibrillation
Antiarrhythmic agents with vagolytic properties (e.g., disopyramide) for vagally-mediated atrial fibrillation
Class IA (e.g., quinidine), class IC (propafenone, flecainide), or class III (e.g., sotalol, amiodarone)
Correction of associated medical conditions (e.g., hypertension, congestive heart failure, hyperthyroidism, valvular heart disease, etc.)

history taking, physical examination and a complete diagnostic work-up are essential. Rare occurrence of atrial fibrillation in patients with an apparently normal heart may not require antiarrhythmic therapy. Life-style adjustment may be all that is required in some individuals. For instance, abstinence from alcohol ingestion, avoidance of big meals and overexertion, biofeedback maneuvers and psychological counseling for stress reduction may be sufficient to prevent recurrence of atrial fibrillation. β-adrenoceptor blocking agents are the drug of choice for catecholamine-sensitive atrial fibrillation that is triggered by exertion and emotional upset, and antiarrhythmic agents with anticholinergic properties, e.g., disopyramide, are more efficacious for vagally-mediated atrial fibrillation that usually occurs at night or in the early morning hours. In some individuals, a cocktail regimen taking one dose or a few doses of propranolol, disopyramide or procainamide is effective in abating atrial fibrillation. Long-term drug therapy should be reserved for those with frequent, very symptomatic and sustained episodes. The benefits of long-term antiarrhythmic therapy should outweigh potential side effects of antiarrhythmic therapy.

Although antiarrhythmic agents from classes IA, IC, and III have been used for long-term maintenance of sinus rhythm, approximately 50% of patients will have recurrence during a follow-up period of 6 to 36 months [107-115]. Preliminary results from the Canadian Trial of Atrial Fibrillation suggest that oral amiodarone appears to be more effective than other agents, including sotalol and propafenone [116]. However, potential serious side effects of amiodarone have prevented it from being a first line drug therapy, especially in young patients [117].

Concurrent medical conditions that may contribute to the genesis of atrial fibrillation need to be identified and corrected, including hyperthyroidism, pericarditis, active myocardial ischemia, hypertension, and congestive heart failure. In patients with accompanying sinus node dysfunction that requires pacemaker implantation, the maintenance of synchronous AV activation is important in the prevention of atrial fibrillation. Clinical studies have shown that the VVI pacing mode is associated with a higher incidence of atrial fibrillation than either the AAI or DDD pacing modes [118,119]. Pacing using the VVI mode is also associated with an increased incidence of congestive heart failure and thromboembolism [120], compared with AV synchronous pacing. The loss of AV synchronization results in gradual atrial dilation and subsequent clinical complications.

Implantation of a dual chamber (DDD) pacemaker may have a role in the prevention of atrial fibrillation, especially in selected patients with pause-related or vagally-mediated (bradycardia-dependent) atrial fibrillation [121]. A pacing algorithm has also been designed to modulate the pacing rate in response to the atrial premature beat-induced pause, thereby preventing pause-related onset of atrial fibrillation [122]. Moreover, dual site right atrial pacing from the high right atrium and the coronary sinus ostium, or pacing both atria through the right atrium and the coronary sinus to "re-synchronize" atrial activation, may also be used to prevent onset of reentrant atrial fibrillation [123,124]. Although short-term results of these pacing modes appear promising, the progressive nature of the aging and disease processes may reduce their long-term efficacy.

14.4.3 CONTROL OF VENTRICULAR RESPONSE

Maintenance of normal sinus rhythm with class I antiarrhythmic agents is not without risks, particularly in patients with structural heart disease and compromised left ventricular function. In this latter group of patients, the long-term morbidity and mortality may be increased because of adverse effects of these antiarrhythmic agents [125,126]. Therefore, the risk and benefit ratio should be carefully analyzed in these patients and balanced against a treatment strategy designed instead to allow atrial fibrillation to continue while vigorously controlling the ventricular rate and maintaining long-term anticoagulation to reduce the risk of thromboembolism.

In chronic atrial fibrillation, control of the ventricular response is essential in preventing tachycardia-induced cardiomyopathy [75]. Aside from congestive heart failure or significantly compromised left ventricular dysfunction, Ca^{++} channel blockers and β-adrenergic blocking agents have replaced digoxin as the first line agents for reducing the ventricular response in atrial fibrillation. Digoxin has a slower onset of action and is not effective in controlling the ventricular response during high sympathetic tone, e.g., exercise, perioperative period, or acute intercurrent illnesses [127]. Digoxin enhances vagal tone, whereas Ca^{++} channel blockers specifically inhibit the L-type Ca^{++} current which is essential for conduction through the AV node. Clinically, both verapamil and diltiazem, in either oral or intravenous form, have been shown to be effective in reducing the ventricular response of atrial fibrillation in the absence of ventricular preexcitation [128-130]. However, it cannot be overemphasized that intravenous Ca^{++} channel blockers are absolutely contraindicated in patients with atrial fibrillation associated with ventricular preexcitation [131,132].

β-adrenoceptor blocking agents are also very effective in reducing the ventricular response in atrial fibrillation as AV node conduction is under abundant influence of autonomic tone [80,81]. Intravenous esmolol, a very short acting β-adrenergic blocker with a half-life of approximately nine minutes, can be safely used in acute clinical settings, e.g., perioperative period or intensive care unit [133]. Chronic treatment with β-adrenergic blocking drugs is more effective than either digoxin or Ca^{++} channel blocking agents at preventing an abrupt increase in the ventricular rate of atrial fibrillation in response to exercise.

When the ventricular response of atrial fibrillation cannot be controlled with depressants of AV nodal conduction, amiodarone therapy may be instituted. However, if the long-term side effects of amiodarone therapy are of concern, radiofrequency catheter ablation of the AV junction followed by implantation of a permanent pacemaker may be preferred (see "Catheter Ablation" on page 671).

14.4.4 PROARRHYTHMIC EFFECTS OF ANTIARRHYTHMIC DRUGS

Both classes IA and III antiarrhythmic agents may induce QT interval prolongation and polymorphic ventricular tachycardia (torsade de pointes). Risk factors for drug-induced torsade de pointes include female gender, bradycardia, hypokalemia, hypomagnesemia, renal dysfunction, and left ventricular dysfunction. Most episodes of torsade de pointes are self-terminating, but it can cause syncope and can easily degenerate into ventricular fibrillation causing cardiac arrest.

Classes IA, IC, and III antiarrhythmic agents may induce atrial flutter and atrial tachycardia during the course of treatment of atrial fibrillation [134-136]. By the properties of slowing conduction and/or increasing refractoriness of the atrial tissue, a new reentrant circuit can be established as a result of antiarrhythmic therapy. Drug-induced atrial flutter or atrial tachycardia may manifest 1:1 AV conduction resulting in a rapid ventricular response [134-137]. Furthermore, with an increase in refractoriness of the His-Purkinje system and ventricular myocardium, the QRS complex during 1:1 AV conduction can be is markedly aberrant, simulating that of ventricular tachycardia (Figure

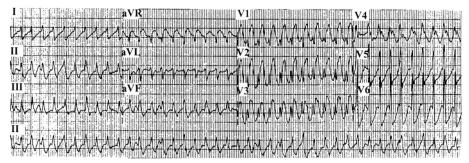

FIGURE 14-4. Illustration of proarrhythmic effects of class I antiarrhythmic agents. After receiving propafenone for one month at a dose of 300 mg three times a day for treatment of paroxysmal atrial fibrillation, this 47 year-old man developed atrial flutter with 1:1 AV conduction at a rate of 250/min. Note marked prolongation of QRS duration (160 ms) with right bundle branch block pattern. ECG during sinus rhythm exhibited normal QRS complex duration (not shown). Paper speed 25 mm/sec.

14-4). Although, atrial flutter and atrial tachycardia may be preexisting arrhythmias that are exposed by antiarrhythmic drugs, catheter ablation of these arrhythmias can be performed effectively if antiarrhythmic therapy appears successful at suppressing atrial fibrillation.

Inherent to properties of antiarrhythmic agents, class IA agents (e.g., quinidine) may provoke torsade de pointes and ventricular fibrillation [138-140]. Moreover, class IC antiarrhythmic agents such as propafenone and flecainide have slower dissociation kinetics [141] compared to class IA antiarrhythmic agents. Clinically they may provoke monomorphic ventricular tachycardia particularly during exercise [140,142-144]. This latter proarrhythmic effect can be accounted for by their use-dependent Na^+ channel blocking effects (Figure 14-5) which create unidirectional block and slow conduction, and thereby provide conditions for reentry, especially in structurally diseased hearts [100,145,146].

Both class IA and IC antiarrhythmic agents also possess negative inotropic and negative chronotropic effects. Potentially they (e.g. disopyramide, flecainide and propafenone) may precipitate congestive heart failure and advanced or complete AV block, particularly in patients with preexisting bifascicular block (complete left bundle branch block or right bundle branch block with right or left axis deviation).

14.5   Non-pharmacological Therapies

The lack of definitive pharmacological therapy for atrial fibrillation has lead to the development of non-pharmacological means in the treatment of this arrhythmia, including surgery, catheter ablation, and implantation of atrial defibrillator.

14.5.1   SURGERY

Among the different types of surgical procedures, the 'maze" operation is curative rather than palliative, as it can more effectively restore sinus rhythm and prevent thromboem-

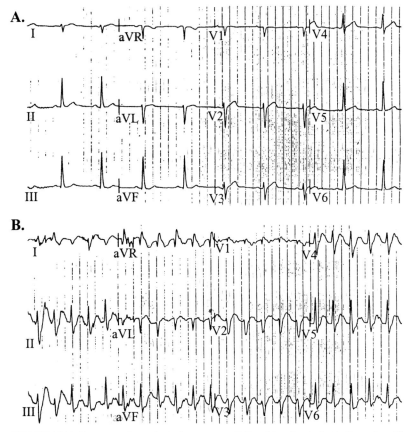

FIGURE 14-5. Frequency-dependent phenomenon of class IA antiarrhythmic drugs in a 52 year-old man receiving propafenone 300 mg three times a day for paroxysmal atrial fibrillation. Panel A, sinus rhythm at 60/min with QRS complex duration measured at 80 ms. Panel B, during stage III of treadmill exercise test, the sinus rate increases to 135/min and the QRS complex duration is 120 ms with a non-specific intraventricular conduction pattern. Paper speed 25 mm/sec.

bolism compared to the "left atrial isolation" and the "corridor" operation (surgical creation of a sinoatrial node – AV node corridor of atrial tissue) [147]. The "maze" operation entails a series of incisions that prevent sufficient space (atrial compartmentalization) for atrial fibrillation to sustain reentry while still allowing transmission of the electrical impulse from the sinoatrial node to the AV node. In the majority of patients (>70%), this surgical procedure can restore sinus rhythm and atrial transport function [148-150]. However, its long term benefit in patients undergoing concomitant mitral valve surgery has been questioned [151]. The surgical "maze" procedure requires extended time for extracorporeal circulation and aortic cross-clamping and thus carries an operative mortality of 2.7% and a high incidence of postoperative complications. The surgical procedure, therefore, is reserved for patients with severe refractory symptoms and those who are undergoing mitral valve surgery. Currently a modified procedure using epicardial and/or endocardial approaches to create linear lesions with a probe electrode catheter during mitral valve surgery is being evaluated [152-154].

14.5.2 CATHETER ABLATION

Radiofrequency catheter ablation has been employed to: 1) create complete AV nodal block (followed by implantation of a permanent pacemaker system) for control of the ventricular rate, 2) modify AV nodal conduction (without producing complete AV block) in order to slow the ventricular response (Figure 14-6), 3) create linear atrial endocardial lesions (mimicking the surgical maze procedure) thereby preventing the development of sustainable atrial fibrillation (Figure 14-7) and, 4) abolish focal atrial premature beats or atrial tachycardia that triggers the onset of atrial fibrillation.

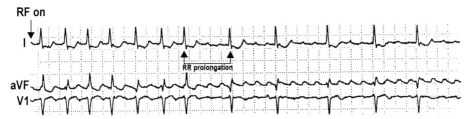

FIGURE 14-6. Modification of the AV nodal conduction with slowing of ventricular rate using the technique of radiofrequency catheter ablation in a patient with medically-refractory atrial fibrillation/flutter. Radiofrequency (RF) energy is delivered to the AV junction anterior to the ostium of the coronary sinus. Note the sudden change in ventricular rate with prolongation of the R-R interval (up arrow) allowing easy visualization of underlying atrial activity. As a result of the RF energy application, the ventricular rate is reduced from 145/min to 75/min. ECG leads I, aVF, and V₁ are simultaneously recorded. Paper speed 25 mm/sec.

The production of complete AV nodal block with subsequent implantation of a permanent pacemaker system (VVIR system if atrial fibrillation is chronic or DDDR system with mode switching if atrial fibrillation is paroxysmal) is the easiest to perform [155,156]. Delivery of radiofrequency energy on the atrial side of the AV junction immediately behind the recording site of the His bundle electrogram will result in AV nodal block.

Modification of AV nodal conduction for the control of the ventricular response during atrial fibrillation has been reported by a number of investigators (Figure 14-6) [157-161]. However, the reproducibility, reliability, and durability of the ablation result remains more "art" than "science". Clinical studies have shown potential risk of inadvertent creation of complete AV block and frequent re-emergence of uncontrolled ventricular rate during long-term follow-up evaluation [160,162].

Based on results of the "maze" operation, the technique of radiofrequency catheter ablation has recently been applied to create linear lesions in both the right and left atria in attempts to cure atrial fibrillation (Figure 14-7) [163-166]. Although the catheter ablation technique appears promising, there are several issues that need to be addressed: 1) What is the proper placement of linear lesions in each atrium? Do they vary according to the type and etiology of atrial fibrillation (e.g., paroxysmal versus chronic, mitral valve

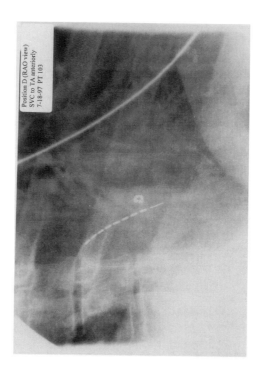

FIGURE 14-7. Fluoroscopic radiogram obtained using right anterior oblique view showing positioning of a multipolar electrode catheter along the anterior wall of the right atrium. This is one of the sites (from superior vena cava anteriorly and caudally to tricuspid valve annulus) where linear lesions are often placed for radiofrequency electrode catheter ablation of atrial fibrillation.

disease versus atherosclerotic coronary artery disease)? 2) What is the minimum number of linear lesions required for prevention of atrial fibrillation? 3) What is the optimum energy, duration of application, and lesion depth necessary for prevention of atrial fibrillation?

Making linear endocardial lesions using the radiofrequency catheter technique is an arduous procedure (>6 hours), subjecting both the patient and the operator to long fluoroscopic exposure. It has a high morbidity with risks of thromboembolism, cardiac perforation, phrenic nerve injury, excessive bleeding, and damage to the sinoatrial and AV nodes. Further refinement of the radiofrequency catheter ablation technique to better mimic the surgical maze procedure remains an ongoing technical challenge.

Since the onset of atrial fibrillation is usually triggered by an atrial premature depolarization or an episode of fast atrial tachycardia (Figure 14-8), radiofrequency catheter ablation may be applied to abolish the culprit atrial premature depolarization or atrial tachycardia. These focal triggering arrhythmias may be located in either the right atrium (especially along the crista terminalis or near the superior vena cava) or left atrium (especially within the pulmonary veins, see below). Successful radiofrequency ablation of the triggering atrial depolarization or tachycardia may entirely prevent recurrence of atrial fibrillation, reduce the frequency of episodes, or improve the response to antiarrhythmic agents. As expected, this "spot" or "focal" ablation does not prevent the emergence of other potentially-triggering atrial premature depolarizations from other locations as a result of the progressive nature of any underlying atrial disease, associated clinical disorders, or the aging process, *per se*.

Recently, the significance of atrial premature depolarizations and non-sustained atrial tachycardias originating within the ostium of the pulmonary veins as a trigger for atrial fibrillation has been appreciated (Figure 14-8) [167]. The regional anatomy of the posterior left atrium and the pulmonary veins is complex (Figure 14-9). Generally, four pulmonary veins insert into the posterior aspect of the left atrium, right and left inferior and superior pulmonary veins. The ostial end of each pulmonary vein is wrapped with a

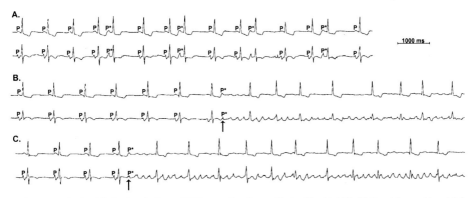

FIGURE 14-8. Double lead ambulatory ECG recording in a patient with atrial fibrillation triggered by atrial ectopic activity originating in the ostium of a pulmonary vein. Panel A: ECG rhythm strip showing normal P waves during sinus rhythm (P) and premature atrial depolarizations (P*). Panels B & C: In the same patient this ectopic activity repeatedly triggered episodes of paroxysmal atrial fibrillation (upward arrow). The ectopic activity was successfully ablated and the patient's atrial fibrillation was eliminated.

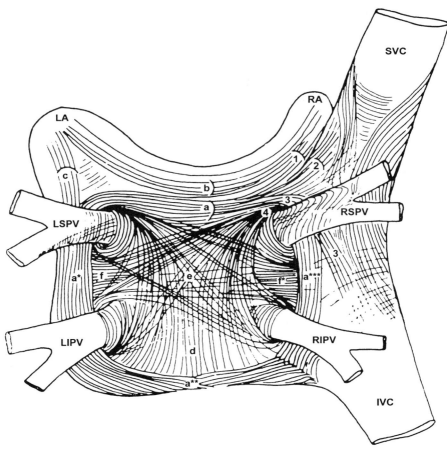

FIGURE 14-9. Schematic diagram of posterior aspect of the left atrium. Generally, there are four pulmonary veins: right (RSPV) and left (LSPV) superior pulmonary veins and right (RIPV) and left (LIPV) inferior pulmonary veins, although the exact number and the precise anatomy may vary dramatically from patient-to-patient. In addition, the pulmonary vein trunks may branch extensively within a few millimeters of their ostial connection with the left atrium. Muscular sleeves of myocardium wrap the veins as they insert into the atrium. These muscular sleeves, which are better developed and more prominent around the superior than inferior veins, normally extend one, two, or possibly even more centimeters backward from the ostial opening. Physiologically these sleeves may act as valves, preventing reflux of left atrial blood into the lungs during atrial systole. These myocardial sleeves are the potential site of origin of atrial tachycardias which may be problematic themselves, or may trigger secondary arrhythmias such as atrial fibrillation or atrial flutter. This illustration shows the typical pattern of the superficial myocardial fibers in the posterior aspect of the left atrium. A main circular fascicle (a, a*, a**, and a***) runs peripherally around the area of the openings of the pulmonary veins. The upper part of this fascicle (a) runs horizontally above the right and left pulmonary veins is formed by fibers descending from the right atrial appendage (1); fibers descending from the wall of the superior vena cava (2); fibers descending from the right atrium (3) and; fibers of the main circular fascicle (a***) extending upward and leftward around the right superior pulmonary vein (4). An interatrial fascicle (b) runs between the right atrium (RA) and left atrium (LA). Some fibers (c) descend from the left atrium into the left part (a*) of the main circular fascicle. Circular fibers leaving the main fascicle turn around the openings of the pulmonary veins, forming sphincter-like structures; other fibers extend over the veins as myocardial sleeves. Loops of fibers coming from the atrium are seen over the RSPV and returning to the atrium. Vertical (d), oblique (e), and transverse (f, f*) fascicles of fibers are also seen in the posterior atrial surface. LA, left atrium; RA, right atrium; SVC, superior vena cava; IVC, inferior vena cava. From [172] with permission.

myocardial sleeve that extends distally from the ostium away from the atrium for a variable distance, possibly a few centimeters. Each muscular sleeve arises as an extension of one or more of the posterior layers of atrial myocardium. These sleeves may act as a muscular sphincter regulating flow into the left atrium or preventing reflux of blood backwards from the left atrium during atrial systole. The myocardial sleeves are better developed around the right and left superior pulmonary veins than the inferior veins. Mapping studies have revealed that ectopic atrial activity originating within the muscular ostia can trigger atrial fibrillation. Radiofrequency catheter ablation of these foci may eliminate the triggered atrial fibrillation [167]. The key to identifying patients with triggering atrial ectopic rhythm is to obtain an EKG recording of the onset of the atrial fibrillation demonstrating the triggering premature atrial depolarizations or atrial tachycardia (Figures 14-8). The superior pulmonary veins are more commonly the site of the triggering premature atrial activity than the inferior veins [167]. Ideally at the time of electrophysiology study the patient will have spontaneous ectopic activity that can be demonstrated to trigger atrial fibrillation. Assuming the triggering activity is frequent (or can be provoked with intravenous medications such as epinephrine, isoproterenol, or adenosine) the foci of the ectopic rhythm may be localized using activation mapping and successfully ablated (Figures 14-10 & 14-11). Access to the left atrium and the pulmonary veins is achieved either through a patent foramen ovale or using the technique of transseptal left heart catheterization (see "Basic Principles of Clinical Cardiac Electrophysiology" on page 21).

Evaluation of the pulmonary vein ablation procedure for treatment of atrial fibrillation is ongoing in clinical centers worldwide. In the Stanford series – as well as that of others – the success rate for prevention of recurrent paroxysmal atrial fibrillation by attempting to *focally* ablate the triggering foci in pulmonary veins is approximately 50% during the follow-up period [168]. In many cases, successful suppression of atrial fibrillation following the procedure requires continuation of the antiarrhythmic drug therapy that had failed to suppress the tachyarrhythmia prior to the ablation [168]. In these patients, the ablation procedure is not a complete cure, but instead enhances the efficacy of previously unsuccessful drug therapy. Presently, progression of underlying cardiac disease and aging, the risk of serious complications, and the relatively low success rate may limit the pulmonary venous ablation procedure to a well-selected group of patients.

However, new techniques, technologies and energy sources are on the horizon and may enhance both the success rate and reduce the risk of complications. As initially developed, the curative ablation procedure for atrial fibrillation resulting from a triggering focus within the pulmonary vein(s) involved identifying the precise location of the focus using activation mapping. Unfortunately, the branching anatomy of the proximal pulmonary veins can be highly complex, making precise localization difficult. In addition, the inability to reliably induce activity from the focal source seriously limits both activation mapping for localization as well as determining if the ablation procedure has been successful (i.e., there can be no reliable endpoint of success if there is no reliable inducibility). For these and other reasons, attempts to target and ablate the triggering *focus* (Figure 14-12) has been associated with a high rate of arrhythmia recurrence. Consequently, clinical practice and research is shifting to an ablation strategy that involves "electrically

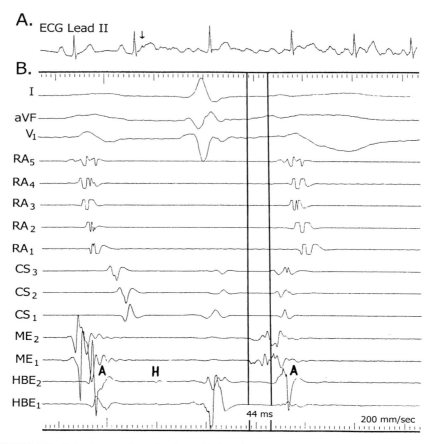

FIGURE 14-10. Activation mapping and catheter ablation of an atrial premature depolarization that triggers atrial fibrillation. Panel A: Spontaneous onset of atrial fibrillation triggered by an atrial premature depolarization (arrow). The atrial premature depolarization occurred frequently and would regularly trigger the onset of atrial fibrillation. Prior event recordings and 12-lead ECGs documented that the atrial premature depolarizations was unifocal in origin (not shown). Panel B: During electrophysiology study, multiple-site electrode mapping localized the earliest onset of atrial activity of the atrial premature depolarization to be in the ostium of the left lower pulmonary vein (44 ms before the atrial activity recorded at the His bundle electrographic lead). Note fragmented low frequency activity recorded at the site (ME_1 & ME_2). Radiofrequency energy delivered at the site abolished the atrial premature depolarization. RA_{1-5}, low to high lateral right atrium; CS_{1-3}, distal to proximal coronary sinus; HBE_{1-2}, distal to proximal His bundle electrographic leads; ME_{1-2}, distal and proximal mapping electrodes; A, atrial electrogram; H, His bundle electrogram. Paper speed 200 mm/sec

isolating" the atrial tissue within the pulmonary vein from the mass of left atrial tissue with which it is in electrical continuity. These pulmonary vein "isolation" procedures involve creating a partial or complete circumferential line of conduction block around the ostium of the vein(s) containing the culprit triggering focus (foci) responsible for the atrial fibrillation. The advantage of this procedure is that precise localization of the triggering focus (foci) within the proximal regions of the branching pulmonary venous system is unnecessary. Rather, by creating an ostial circumferential (or semi-circumferential) lesion with a line of conduction block, tachyarrhythmic activity within

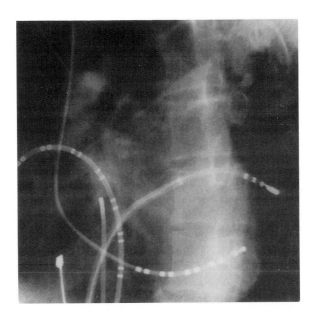

FIGURE 14-11. Left anterior oblique fluoroscopic view showing the position of the ablation catheter tip near the ostium of the left lower pulmonary vein. Application of radiofrequency energy at this site eliminated the atrial premature depolarization responsible for triggering atrial fibrillation as shown in Figure 14-10.

the pulmonary vein(s) may fail to activate the mass of left atrial tissue, preventing induction of atrial fibrillation. Using standard electrode catheter techniques, partial of complete circumferential lesions may be produced using repeated focal applications of RF energy around the ostial tissue, a potentially time-consuming process. Alternatively, new technologies are becoming available that may permit rapid creation of a continuous circumferential ostial line of conduction block using new energy sources, including ultrasound, cryothermia, laser, and enhanced RF (Figure 14-12). It is hoped that these new techniques may increase the long-term success rate, reduce the procedure time, and minimize the potential complications that may include cardiac perforation with pericardial effusion and tamponade, thromboembolic stroke, and pulmonary venous stenosis.

14.5.3 IMPLANTABLE ATRIAL DEFIBRILLATOR

An implantable atrial defibrillator has been developed and has undergone clinical trials [169]. Low energy atrial shocks are delivered between a right atrial lead and a coronary sinus lead after being synchronized to the QRS complex recorded by a right ventricular

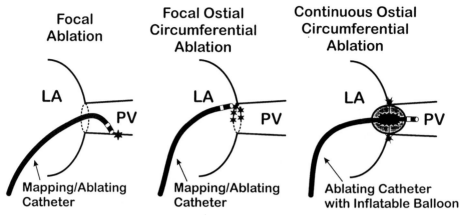

FIGURE 14-12. Summary of ablation techniques for treatment of atrial fibrillation provoked by a triggering focus within a pulmonary vein. Initial attempts to cure atrial fibrillation caused by a focal triggering source within a pulmonary vein (PV) have used activation mapping to precisely localize the focus within the branching venous system combined with delivery of a focal application of RF energy using a standard steerable ablation catheter (left panel). However, attempts to map and ablate the triggering *focus* has been associated with a high rate of arrhythmia recurrence. An alternative ablation strategy involves "electrical isolation" of the atrial tissue within the pulmonary vein from the mass of left atrial (LA) tissue with which it is in electrical continuity. The advantage of this procedure is that it is unnecessary to identify the exact location of the triggering focus (foci) within the proximal regions of the branching pulmonary venous system. Using standard electrode catheter techniques, partial of complete circumferential lesions may be produced using repeated focal applications of RF energy around the ostial tissue (middle panel). Alternatively, special (single and double) balloon-tipped ablation catheters are being designed and evaluated that may allow rapid electrical isolation of pulmonary veins from the LA (right panel). The balloon(s) can be inflated after positioning it in the ostium of the offending pulmonary vein thereby immobilizing the distal segment of the catheter within the pulmonary venous ostium. Thereafter destructive energy can be delivered to the ostial tissue from a probe or transducer integrated into the catheter tip or balloon. There is evidence that creation of partial or complete ostial lesions using RF energy or ultrasound may electrically isolate the triggering focus within the pulmonary vein from the LA [173,174]. Other possible techniques under investigation utilize specialized (tandem balloon) RF delivery systems, cryothermia, or Nd:YAG laser [175-177].

lead. A back-up right ventricular pacing system is also provided. Quick reversion of atrial fibrillation to sinus rhythm is recommended in order to reduce the process of "electrical remodeling." However, there are major issues of concern: (1) safety (QRS synchronized shocks may provoke ventricular fibrillation particularly at short RR intervals) [93,170,171]; (2) patient tolerance of low energy defibrillation shocks; and (3) cost-effectiveness and quality of life issues, especially compared to treatment with one of the ablation options, including curative catheter ablation or AV junctional ablation and implantation of a permanent DDD pacemaker with a mode-switching capability.

References

1. American Heart Association. Heart and Stroke Facts: Statistical Supplement. pg 14, 1996.
2. Vaziri SM, Larson MG, et al.: Echocardiographic predictors of nonrheumatic atrial fibrillation: the Framingham Heart Study. *Circulation* **89**:724-730, 1994.
3. Kannel WB, Abbott RD, Savage DD, McNamara PM: Epidemiologic features of chronic atrial fibrillation: the Framingham study. *N Engl J Med* **306**:1018-22, 1982.
4. Benjamin EJ, Levy D, Vaziri SM, et al.: Independent risk factors for atrial fibrillation in a population-based cohort. The Framingham Heart Study. *JAMA* **271**:840-844, 1994.
5. Wolf PA, Benjamin EJ, Belanger AJ, et al.: Secular trends in the prevalence of atrial fibrillation: The Framingham Study. *Am Heart J* **131**:790-5, 1996.
6. Feinberg WM, Blackshear JL, Laupacis A, et al.: Prevalence, age distribution and gender in patients with atrial fibrillation; analysis and implications. *Arch Intern Med* **155**:469-473, 1995.
7. Pritchett E: Management of atrial fibrillation. *N Engl J Med* **326**:1264-1271, 1992.
8. Sohara H, Amitani S, et al.: Atrial fibrillation activates platelets and coagulation in a time-dependent manner: a study in patients with paroxysmal atrial fibrillation. *J Am Coll Cardiol* **29**:106-12, 1997.
9. Carson PE, Johnson GR, Dunkman WB, et al.: The influence of atrial fibrillation on prognosis in mild to moderate failure. The V-HeFT Studies. The V-HeFT VA Cooperative Studies Group. *Circulation* **87**:VI-102-VI-110, 1993.
10. Middlekauff HR, Stevenson WG, Stevenson LW: Prognostic significance of atrial fibrillation in advanced heart failure. A study of 390 patients. *Circulation* **84**:40-8, 1991.
11. Wolf PA, Kannel WB, McGee DL, et al.: Duration of atrial fibrillation and imminence of stroke: the Framingham study. *Stroke* **14**:664-7, 1983.
12. Wolf PA, Abbott RD, Kannel WB: Atrial fibrillation as an independent risk factor for stroke: the Framingham Study. *Stroke* **22**:983-8, 1991.
13. Wolf PA, Abbott RD, Kannel WB: Atrial fibrillation: a major contributor to stroke in the elderly. The Framingham Study. *Arch Intern Med* **147**:1561-4, 1987.
14. Sherman DG, Goldman L, Whiting RB, et al.: Thromboembolism in patients with atrial fibrillation. *Arch Neurol* **41**:708-710, 1984.
15. Lev M, McMillan JB. Aging changes in the heart. In: Bourne GH, ed. *Structural Aspects of Aging*. London: Pittman Medical, 325-349: 1961.
16. McMillan JB, Lev M: The aging heart: Endocardium. *J Gerontol* **14**:268-283, 1959.
17. McMillan JB, Lev M. The aging heart. Myocardium and epicardium. In: Shock NW, ed. *Biologic Aspects of Aging*. New York, NY: Columbia University Press, 1963-73: 1962.
18. Frustaci A, Chimenti C, Bellocci F, et al.: Histological substrate of atrial biopsies in patients with lone atrial fibrillation. *Circulation* **96**:1180-4, 1997.
19. Probst P, Goldschlager N, Selzer A: Left atrial size and atrial fibrillation in mitral stenosis: factors influencing their relationship. *Circulation* **48**:1282-1287, 1973.
20. Thiedmann KU, Ferrans VJ: Left atrial ultrastructure in mitral valvular disease. *Am J Pathology* **89**:575-604, 1977.
21. Cushing EH, Feil H, Stanton EJ, Wartman WB: Infarction of cardiac auricles (atria): clinical, pathological, and experimental studies. *Br Heart J* **4**:417-34, 1942.
22. Soderstrom N: Myocardial infarction and mural thrombosis in the atria of the heart. *Acta Med Scand Suppl*:217, 1948.
23. Cameron A, Schwartz MJ, Kronmal RA, Kosinski AS: Prevalence and significance of atrial fibrillation in coronary artery disease (CASS registry). *Am J Cardiol* **61**:714-717, 1988.
24. Kannel WB, Abbott RD, Savage DD, McNamara PM: Coronary heart disease and atrial fibrillation: the Framingham Study. *Am Heart J* **106**:389-96, 1983.
25. James TN: Pericarditis and the sinus node. *Arch Intern Med* **110**:305-311, 1962.
26. Spodick DH: Arrhythmias during acute pericarditis; a prospective study in 100 consecutive cases. *JAMA* **5**:39-41, 1976.
27. Ohtani K, Yutani C, Nagatta S, et al.: High prevalence of atrial fibrosis in patients with dilated cardiomyopathy. *J Am Coll Cardiol* **25**:1162-1169, 1995.

28.   Dubrey S, Pollak A, Skinner M, Falk RH: Atrial thrombi occurring during sinus rhythm in cardiac amy-
       loidosis: evidence for atrial electromechanical dissociation. *Br Heart J* **74**:541-544, 1995.

29.   Sung RJ, Castellanos A, et al.: Mechanisms of spontaneous alternation between reciprocating tachycar-
       dia and atrial flutter-fibrillation in the Wolff-Parkinson-White syndrome. *Circulation* **56**:409-16, 1977.

30.   Hurwitz JL, German LD, et al.: Occurrence of atrial fibrillation in patients with paroxysmal supraven-
       tricular tachycardia due to atrioventricular nodal reentry. *Pacing Clin Electrophysiol* **13**:705-10, 1990.

31.   Goette A, Honeycutt C, Langberg JJ: Electrical remodeling in atrial fibrillation. Time course and mech-
       anisms. *Circulation* **94**:2968-2974, 1996.

32.   Sanfilippo AJ, Abascal VM, Sheehan M, et al.: Atrial enlargement as a consequence of atrial fibrilla-
       tion. A prospective echocardiographic study (Abstract). *Circulation* **92**:I-114, 1995.

33.   Wijffels MC, Kirchhof CJ, Dorland R, Allessie MA: Atrial fibrillation begets atrial fibrillation. A study
       in awake chronically instrumented goats. *Circulation* **92**:1954-68, 1995.

34.   Wijffels MC, Kirchhof CJ, Dorland R, et al.: Electrical remodeling due to atrial fibrillation in chronical-
       ly instrumented conscious goats: roles of neurohumoral changes, ischemia, atrial stretch, and high rate
       of electrical activation. *Circulation* **96**:3710-20, 1997.

35.   Morillo CA, Klein GJ, et al.: Chronic rapid atrial pacing. Structural, functional, and electrophysiologi-
       cal characteristics of a new model of sustained atrial fibrillation. *Circulation* **91**:1588-95, 1995.

36.   Sun H, Gaspo R, Leblanc N, Nattel S: Cellular mechanisms of atrial contractile dysfunction caused by
       sustained atrial tachycardia. *Circulation* **98**:719-727, 1998.

37.   Yue L, Feng J, Gaspo R, et al.: Ionic remodeling underlying action potential changes in a dog model of
       atrial fibrillation. *Circulation Research* **81**:512-525, 1997.

38.   Shinbane JS, Wood MA, Jensen DN, et al.: Tachycardia-induced cardiomyopathy: a review of animal
       models and clinical studies. *J Am Coll Cardiol* **29**:709-15, 1997.

39.   Ausma J, Wijffels M, van Eys G, et al.: Dedifferentiation of atrial cardiomyocytes as a result of chronic
       atrial fibrillation. *Am J Pathol* **151**:985-97, 1997.

40.   Ausma J, Wijffels M, Thone F, et al.: Structural changes of atrial myocardium due to sustained atrial fi-
       brillation in the goat. *Circulation* **96**:3157-63, 1997.

41.   Asher CR, Chung MR, Eagle KA, et al.: Atrial fibrillation following cardiac surgery. In: Falk R, Podrid
       P, eds. *Atrial fibrillation mechanisms and management.* 2nd ed: Lippincott-Raven, 183-204.: 1997.

42.   Hogue CW, Domitrovich PP, Stein PK, et al.: RR interval dynamics before atrial fibrillation in patients
       after coronary artery bypass graft surgery. *Circulation* **98**:429-434, 1998.

43.   Andrews TC, Reimold SC, Berlin JA, Antman EM: Prevention of supraventricular arrhythmias after
       coronary artery bypass surgery. *Circulation* **84**:III 236-44, 1991.

44.   Kalman JM, Munawar M, Howes LG, et al.: Atrial fibrillation after coronary artery bypass grafting is
       associated with sympathetic activation. *Ann Thorac Surg* **60**:1707-1715, 1995.

45.   Klein L, Levy GS: New perspectives on thyroid hormone, catecholamines, and the heart. *Am J Med*
       76:167, 1984.

46.   Garrey WE: The nature of fibrillary contraction of the heart - its relation to tissue mass and form. *Am J
       Physiol* **33**:397-414, 1914.

47.   Moe GK, Abildskov JA: Experimental and laboratory reports: Atrial fibrillation as a self-sustaining ar-
       rhythmia independent of focal discharge. *Am Heart J* **58**:59-70, 1959.

48.   Moe GK, Rheinboldt WC, et al.: A computer model of atrial fibrillation. *Am Heart J* **67**:200, 1964.

49.   Scherf D: Studies on auricular tachycardia caused by aconitine administration. *Proc Soc Exp Biol Med*
       64:233-239, 1947.

50.   Jais P, Haissaguerre M, Shah DC, et al.: A focal source of atrial fibrillation treated by discrete radiofre-
       quency ablation. *Circulation* **95**:572-6, 1997.

51.   Mines GR: On dynamic equilibrium in the heart. *J Physiol (London)* **46**:349-383, 1913.

52.   Allessie MA, Bonke FI, Schopman FJ: Circus movement in rabbit atrial muscle as a mechanism of ta-
       chycardia. III. The "leading circle" concept: a new model of circus movement in cardiac tissue without
       the involvement of an anatomical obstacle. *Circ Res* **41**:9-18, 1977.

53.   Task Force of the Working Group on Arrhythmias of the European Society of Cardiology: The Sicilian
       Gambit: A new approach to the classification of antiarrhythmic drugs based on their actions on arrhyth-
       mogenic mechanisms. *Circulation* **84**:1831-1851, 1991.

54. Lai WT, Huycke EC, Keung EC, et al.: Electrophysiologic manifestations of the excitable gap of ortho-dromic atrioventricular reciprocating tachycardia demonstrated by single extrastimulation. *Am J Cardiol* **63**:545-55, 1989.

55. Lai WT, Lee CS, Sheu SH, et al.: Electrophysiological manifestations of the excitable gap of slow-fast AV nodal reentrant tachycardia demonstrated by single extrastimulation. *Circulation* **92**:66-76, 1995.

56. Waldo AL, MacLean WA, Karp RB, et al.: Entrainment and interruption of atrial flutter with atrial pac-ing: studies in man following open heart surgery. *Circulation* **56**:737-45, 1977.

57. Hoffman BF, Cranefield PF: *Electrophysiology of the Heart.* 1st ed. New York: McGraw-Hill, 1960.

58. Spach MS, Starmer CF: Altering the topology of gap junctions as a major therapeutic target for atrial fi-brillation. *Cardiovasc Res* **30**:336-344, 1995.

59. Alessi R, Nusynowitz M, Abildskov JA, Moe GK: Nonuniform distribution of vagal effects on the atrial refractory period. *American Journal of Physiology* **194**:406-410, 1958.

60. Coumel P: Autonomic influences in atrial tachyarrhythmias. *J Cardiovasc Electrophysiol* **7**:999-1007, 1998.

61. Gaspo R, Bosch RF, Bou-Abboud E, Nattel S: Tachycardia-induced changes in Na+ current in a chronic dog model of atrial fibrillation. *Circ Res* **81**:1045-52, 1997.

62. Gaspo R, Bosch RF, Talajic M, Nattel S: Functional mechanisms underlying tachycardia-induced sus-tained atrial fibrillation in a chronic dog model. *Circulation* **96**:4027-35, 1997.

63. Tieleman RG, De Langen C, Van Gelder IC, et al.: Verapamil reduces tachycardia-induced electrical re-modeling of the atria. *Circulation* **95**:1945-53, 1997.

64. Van Wagoner DR, Pond AL, McCarthy PM, et al.: Outward K+ current densities and Kvl.5 expression are reduced in chronic human atrial fibrillation. *Circ Res* **80**:772-781, 1997.

65. Jayachandran V, Zipes DP, Sih HJ, et al: Atrial ischemia mimics electrophysiologic changes of electrical remodeling which are prevented by blockade of the Na+/H+ exchanger with HDE642 (abstract). *Circulation* **98(suppl)**:I-210, 1998.

66. Jayachandran V, Winkle W, Sih HJ, et al: Chronic atrial fibrillation from rapid atrial pacing is associat-ed with reduced atrial blood flow: A positron emission tomography study (abstract). *Circulation* **98(suppl)**:I-209, 1998.

67. Brugada R, Tapscott T, Czernuszewicz GZ, et al.: Identification of a genetic locus for familial atrial fi-brillation. *New Engl J Med* **336**:905-911, 1997.

68. Gould WL: Auricular fibrillation: Report on a familial tendency 1920-1956. *Arch Intern Med* **100**:916-926, 1957.

69. Wolff L: Familial atrial fibrillation. *New Engl J Med* **229**:396-400, 1943.

70. Keating M, Atkinson D, Dunn C, et al.: Linkage of a cardiac arrhythmia, the long QT syndrome, and the Harvey ras-1 gene. *Science* **252**:704-706, 1991.

71. Sung RJ, Myerburg RJ, Castellanos A: Electrophysiological demonstration of concealed conduction in the human atrium. *Circulation* **58**:940-6, 1978.

72. Hewlett AW, Wilson FN: Coarse auricular fibrillation in man. *Arch Intern Med* **15**:786-793, 1915.

73. Evans W, Swann P: Lone auricular fibrillation. *Br Heart J* **16**:189-194, 1954.

74. Friedlander RD, Levine SA: Auricular fibrillation and flutter without evidence of organic heart disease. *New Engl J Med* **211**:624, 1934.

75. Phillips E, Levine SA: Auricular fibrillation without other evidence of heart failure. *Am J Med* **7**:478-489, 1949.

76. Prinzmetal M, Rakita L, Bordaus JL, et al.: The nature of spontaneous auricular fibrillation in man. *JAMA* **157**:1175-1182, 1955.

77. Brill IC: Auricular fibrillation with congestive failure and no other evidence of organic heart disease. *Am Heart J* **13**:175-182, 1937.

78. Flaker GC, Fletcher KA, Rothbart RM, et al.: Clinical and echocardiographic features of intermittent atrial fibrillation that predict recurrent atrial fibrillation. *Am J Cardiol* **76**:355-358, 1995.

79. Coumel P, Attuel P, Lavallee J, et al.: The atrial arrhythmia syndrome of vagal origin. *Arch Mal Coeur Vaiss* **71**:645-56, 1978.

80. Coumel P. Neural aspects of paroxysmal atrial fibrillation. In: Falk RH, Podrid PJ, eds. *Atrial Fibrilla-tion: Mechanisms and Management.* New York, NY: Raven Press, 109-125: 1992.

81. Waxman MB, Cameroon D, Wald RW. Role of the autonomic nervous system in atrial arrhythmias. In: DiMarco JP, Prystowsky EN, eds. *Atrial Arrhythmias: State of the Art*. Armonk, NY: Futura Publishing Co.: 1995.

82. Botteron GW, Smith JM: Quantitative assessment of the spatial organization of atrial fibrillation in the intact human heart. *Circulation* **93**:513-8, 1996.

83. Capucci A, Biffi M, Boriani G, et al.: Dynamic electrophysiological behavior of human atria during paroxysmal atrial fibrillation. *Circulation* **92**:1193-1202, 1995.

84. Huagui L, Hare J, Mughal K, et al.: Distribution of atrial electrogram types during atrial fibrillation: Effect of rapid atrial pacing and intercaval junction ablation. *J Am Coll Cardiol* **27**:1713-1721, 1996.

85. Konings KT, Kirchhof CJ, Smeets JR, et al.: High-density mapping of electrically induced atrial fibrillation in humans. *Circulation* **89**:1665-80, 1994.

86. Kumagai K, Khrestian C, Waldo AL: Simultaneous multisite mapping studies during induced atrial fibrillation in the sterile pericarditis model. Insights into the mechanism of its maintenance. *Circulation* **95**:511-21, 1997.

87. Wells JL, Jr., Karp RB, Kouchoukos NT, et al.: Characterization of atrial fibrillation in man: studies following open heart surgery. *Pacing Clin Electrophysiol* **1**:426-38, 1978.

88. Grimm RA, Stewart WJ, Black IW, et al.: Should all patients undergo transesophageal echocardiography before electrical conversion of atrial fibrillation. *J Am Coll Cardiol* **23**:533-41, 1994.

89. Manning WJ, Silverman DI, et al.: Temporal dependence of the return of atrial mechanical function on the mode of cardioversion of atrial fibrillation to sinus rhythm. *Am J Cardiol* **75**:624-6, 1995.

90. Manning WJ, Silverman DI, Katz SE, et al.: Impaired left atrial mechanical function after cardioversion: relation to the duration of atrial fibrillation. *J Am Coll Cardiol* **23**:1535-40, 1994.

91. Klein AL, Grimm RA, Black IW, et al.: Cardioversion guided by transesophageal echocardiography: the ACUTE pilot study; a randomized controlled trial. *Ann Intern Med* **126**:200-209, 1997.

92. Daniel WG, Erbel R, Kasper W, et al.: Safety of transesophageal echocardiography. A multicenter survey of 10,419 examinations. *Circulation* **83**:817-21, 1991.

93. Ayers GM, Alferness CA, Ilina M, et al.: Ventricular proarrhythmic effects of ventricular cycle length and shock strength in a sheep model of transvenous atrial defibrillation. *Circulation* **89**:413-22, 1994.

94. Hou ZY, Chang MS, Chen CY, et al.: Acute treatment of recent-onset atrial fibrillation and flutter with a tailored dosing regimen of intravenous amiodarone. *Eur Heart J* **16**:521-8, 1995.

95. Santini M, Pandozi C, Gentilucci G, et al.: Intra-atrial defibrillation of human atrial fibrillation. *J Cardiovasc Electrophysiol* **9(suppl)**:S170-S176, 1998.

96. Schmitt C, Alt E, Plewan A, et al: Low-energy intracardiac cardioversion after failed conventional external cardioversion of atrial fibrillation. *J Am Coll Cardiol* **28**:994-999, 1996.

97. Capucci A, Boriani G, Botto GL, et al.: Conversion of recent-onset atrial fibrillation by a single oral loading dose of propafenone or flecainide. *Am J Cardiol* **74**:503-505, 1994.

98. Boriani G, Biffi M, Capucci A, et al.: Oral propafenone to convert recent-onset atrial fibrillation in patients with and without underlying heart disease. *Ann Intern Med* **126**:621-5, 1997.

99. Hondeghem LM, Snyders DJ: Class III antiarrhythmic agents have a lot of potential but a long way to go. Reduced effectiveness and dangers of reverse use dependence. *Circulation* **81**:696-690, 1990.

100. Kirchhof PF, Fabritz L, Franz MR: Postrepolarization refractoriness versus conduction slowing caused by class I antiarrhythmic drugs. *Circulation* **97**:2567-2574, 1998.

101. Noma A: ATP-regulated K^+ channels in cardiac muscle. *Nature* **305**:147-8, 1983.

102. Sakmann B, Noma A, Trautwein W: Acetylcholine activation of single muscarinic K+ channels in isolated pacemaker cells of the mammalian heart. *Nature* **303**:250-3, 1983.

103. Sung RJ, Tan HL, Karagounis L, et al.: Intravenous sotalol for the termination of supraventricular tachycardia and atrial fibrillation and flutter: a multicenter, randomized, double-blind, placebo-controlled study. Sotalol Multicenter Study Group. *Am Heart J* **129**:739-48, 1995.

104. Yang T, Snyders DJ, Roden DM: Ibutilide, a methanesulfonamilide antiarrhythmic, is a potent blocker of the rapidly-activating delayed rectifier K^+ current (I_{kr}) in AT-1 cells: concentration, time-, voltage-, and use dependent effects. *Circulation* **91**:1799-1806, 1995.

105. Lee KS: Ibutilide, a new compound with potent class III antiarrhythmic activity, activates a slow inward Na current in guinea pig ventricular cells. *J Pharmacol Exp Ther* **262**:99-108, 1992.

106. Ellenbogen KA, Stambler BS, Wood MA, et al.: Efficacy of intravenous ibutilide for rapid termination of atrial fibrillation and atrial flutter: a dose-response study. *J Am Coll Cardiol* **28**:130-6, 1996.

107. Anderson JL: Long-term safety and efficacy of flecainide in the treatment of supraventricular tachyarrhythmias: the United States experience. *American Journal of Cardiology* **70**:11A-18A, 1992.

108. Aliot E, Denjoy I, et al.: Comparison of the safety and efficacy of flecainide versus propafenone in hospital out-patients with symptomatic atrial fibrillation/flutter. *American Journal of Cardiology* **77**:66A-71A, 1996.

109. Chun SH, Sager PT, et al.: Long-term efficacy of amiodarone for the maintenance of normal sinus rhythm in patients with refractory atrial fibrillation or flutter. *Am J Cardiol* **76**:47-50, 1995.

110. Szyska A, Paluszkiewicz P, Baszynska H: Prophylactic treatment after electroconversion of atrial fibrillation in patients after cardiac surgery - a controlled two year follow-up study (Abstract). *J Am Coll Cardiol* **21**:A-201, 1993.

111. Crijns HJ, Van Gelder IC, Van Gilst WH, et al.: Serial antiarrhythmic drug treatment to maintain sinus rhythm after electrical cardioversion for chronic atrial fibrillation or atrial flutter. *Am J Cardiol* **68**:335-341, 1991.

112. Gold RL, Haffajee CI, Charos G, et al.: Amiodarone for refractory atrial fibrillation. *Am J Cardiol* **57**:124-127, 1986.

113. Juul-Moller S, Edvardsson AN, Rehnqvist-Ahlberg N: Sotalol versus quinidine for the maintenance of sinus rhythm after direct current cardioversion of atrial fibrillation. *Circulation* **82**:1932-1939, 1990.

114. Middlekauff HR, Wiener I, Stevenson WG: Low-dose amiodarone for atrial fibrillation. *Am J Cardiol* **72**:75F-81F, 1993.

115. Zehender M, Hohnloser S, Muller B: Effects of amiodarone versus quinidine and verapamil in patients with chronic atrial fibrillation: results of a comparative study and a 2 year follow-up. *J Am Coll Cardiol* **19**:1054-1059, 1992.

116. Roy D, Talajic M. The Canadian trial of atrial fibrillation: preliminary results. American College of Cardiology 48th Annual Scientific Sessions. New Orleans, 1999.

117. Sung RJ: Low-dose amiodarone should not be the first-line treatment for atrial fibrillation. *Cardiovasc Drugs Ther* **8**:773-4, 1994.

118. Rosenqvist M: Atrial pacing for sick sinus syndrome. *Clin Cardiol* **13**:43-7, 1990.

119. Rosenqvist M, Brandt J, Schuller H: Long-term pacing in sinus node disease: effects of stimulation mode on cardiovascular morbidity and mortality. *Am Heart J* **116**:16-22, 1988.

120. Andersen HR, Thuesen L, Bagger JP, et al.: Prospective randomised trial of atrial versus ventricular pacing in sick sinus syndrome. *Lancet* **344**:1523-8, 1994.

121. Attuel P, Pellerin D, Mugica J, Coumel P: DDD pacing: an effective treatment modality for recurrent atrial arrhythmias. *Pacing Clin Electrophysiol* **11**:1647-54, 1988.

122. Murgatroyd FD, Nitzsche R, Slade AK, et al.: A new pacing algorithm for overdrive suppression of atrial fibrillation. Chorus Multicentre Study Group. *Pacing Clin Electrophysiol* **17**:1966-73, 1994.

123. Saksena S, Prakash A, Hill M, et al: Prevention of recurrent atrial fibrillation with chronic dual site right atrial pacing. *J Am Coll Cardiol* **28**:687-694, 1996.

124. Saksena S, Delfaut P, Prakash A, et al.: Multisite electrode pacing for prevention of atrial fibrillation. *J Cardiovasc Electrophysiol* **9(suppl)**:S155-S162, 1998.

125. The Cardiac Arrhythmia Suppression Trial (CAST) Investigators: Preliminary report: effect of encainide and flecainide on mortality in a randomized trial of arrhythmia suppression after myocardial infarction. *N Engl J Med* **321**:406-412, 1989.

126. Pritchett EL, Wilkinson WE: Mortality in patients treated with flecainide and encainide for supraventricular arrhythmias. *Am J Cardiol* **67**:976-80, 1991.

127. Goldman S, Probst P, Selzer A, Cohn K: Inefficacy of "therapeutic" serum levels of digoxin in controlling the ventricular rate in atrial fibrillation. *Am J Cardiol* **35**:651-655, 1995.

128. Ellenbogen KA, Dias VC, Plumb VJ, et al.: A placebo-controlled trial of continuous intravenous diltiazem infusion for 24-hour heart rate control during atrial fibrillation and atrial flutter: A multicenter study. *J Am Coll Cardiol* **18**:891-897, 1991.

129. Heywood JT, Graham B, Marais GE, Jutzy KR: Effects of intravenous diltiazem on rapid atrial fibrillation accompanied by congestive heart failure. *Am J Cardiol* **67**:1150-1152, 1991.

130. Waxman HL, Myerburg RJ, Appel R, Sung RJ: Verapamil for control of ventricular rate in paroxysmal supraventricular tachycardia and atrial fibrillation or flutter: a double-blind randomized cross-over study. *Ann Intern Med* **94**:1-6, 1981.

131. Garratt C, Antoniou A, Ward D, Camm AJ: Misuse of verapamil in pre-excited atrial fibrillation. *Lancet* **1**:367-9, 1989.

132. McGovern B, Garan H, Ruskin JN: Precipitation of cardiac arrest by verapamil in patients with Wolff-Parkinson-White syndrome. *Ann Intern Med* **104**:791-4, 1986.

133. Byrd RC, Sung RJ, Marks J, Parmley WW: Safety and efficacy of esmolol (ASL-8052: an ultrashort-acting beta-adrenergic blocking agent) for control of ventricular rate in supraventricular tachycardias. *J Am Coll Cardiol* **3**:394-9, 1984.

134. Feld GK, Chen PS, Nicod P, et al.: Possible atrial proarrhythmic effects of class 1C antiarrhythmic drugs. *Am J Cardiol* **66**:378-83, 1990.

135. Falk RH: Proarrhythmia in patients treated for atrial fibrillation or flutter. *Ann Intern Med* **117**:141-50, 1992.

136. Murdock CJ, Kyles A, Yeung-Lai-Wah JA, et al.: Atrial flutter in patients treated for atrial fibrillation with propafenone. *Am J Cardiol* **66**:755-757, 1990.

137. Crijns HJ, van Gelder IC, Lie KI: Supraventricular tachycardia mimicking ventricular tachycardia during flecainide treatment. *Am J Cardiol* **62**:1303-6, 1988.

138. Minardo JD, Heger JJ, Miles WM, et al.: Clinical characteristics of patients with ventricular fibrillation during antiarrhythmic drug therapy. *N Engl J Med* **319**:257-62, 1988.

139. Ruskin JN, McGovern B, Garan H, et al.: Antiarrhythmic drugs: a possible cause of out-of-hospital cardiac arrest. *N Engl J Med* **309**:1302-6, 1983.

140. Stanton MS, Prystowsky EN, et al.: Arrhythmogenic effects of antiarrhythmic drugs: a study of 506 patients treated for ventricular tachycardia or fibrillation. *J Am Coll Cardiol* **14**:209-15; 1989.

141. Koller BS, Karasik PE, Solomon AJ, Franz MR: Relation between repolarization and refractoriness during programmed electrical stimulation in the human right ventricle. Implications for ventricular tachycardia induction. *Circulation* **91**:2378-84, 1995.

142. Herre JM, Titus C, Oeff M, et al.: Inefficacy and proarrhythmic effects of flecainide and encainide for sustained ventricular tachycardia and ventricular fibrillation. *Ann Intern Med* **113**:671-6, 1990.

143. Josephson ME: Antiarrhythmic agents and the danger of proarrhythmic events. *Ann Intern Med* **111**:101-3, 1989.

144. Morganroth J: Risk factors for the development of proarrhythmic events. *Am J Cardiol* **59**:32E-37E, 1987.

145. Coromilas J, Saltman AE, Waldecker B, et al.: Electrophysiological effects of flecainide on anisotropic conduction and reentry in infarcted canine hearts. *Circulation* **91**:2245-63, 1995.

146. Restivo M, Yin H, Caref EB, et al.: Reentrant arrhythmias in the subacute infarction period: The proarrhythmic effect of flecainide acetate on functional reentrant circuits. *Circulation* **91**:1236-1246, 1995.

147. Wellens HJ, Sie HT, Smeets JLRM, et al.: Surgical treatment of atrial fibrillation. *J Cardiovasc Electrophysiol* **9(suppl)**:S151-S154, 1998.

148. Cox JL, Schuessler RB, Lappas DG: An 8.5 year clinical experience with surgery for atrial fibrillation. *Annals of Surgery* **224**:267-275, 1996.

149. Kawaguchi AT, Kosakai Y, Sasako Y, et al: Risks and benefits of combined maze procedure for atrial fibrillation associated with organic heart disease. *J Am Coll Cardiol* **28**:985-990, 1996.

150. Sandoval N, Velasco VM, Orjuela H, et al: Concomitant mitral valve surgery or atrial septal defect surgery and the modified Cox-maze procedure. *Am J Cardiol* **77**:591-596, 1996.

151. Chua YL, Schaff HV, Orszulak TA, et al: Outcome of mitral valve repair in patients with pre-operative atrial fibrillation: Should the maze procedure be combined with mitral valvuloplasty? *J Thorac Cardiovasc Surg* **107**:408-415, 1994.

152. Beukema WP, Hauw ST, Misier ARR, et al.: Radiofrequency modified maze in patients undergoing valve surgery (abstract). *PACE* **21**:II-869, 1998.

153. Caccitolo JA, Jensen DN, Schaff HV, Mehra R: Can linear radiofrequency ablation lesions replace surgical incisions during open-heart atrial maze procedures? (abstract). *PACE* **21**:III-804, 1998.

154. Melo J, Adragao P, Neves J, et al.: Radiofrequency pulmonary veins isolation during mitral valve surgery to prevent atrial fibrillation: assessment of one year results (abstract). *PACE* **21**:II-88, 1998.

155. Langberg JJ, Chin M, Schamp DJ, et al.: Ablation of the atrioventricular junction with radiofrequency energy using a new electrode catheter. *Am J Cardiol* **67**:142-7, 1991.

156. Fitzpatrick AP, Kourouyan HD, Siu A, et al.: Quality of life and outcomes after radiofrequency His-bundle catheter ablation and permanent pacemaker implantation: impact of treatment in paroxysmal and established atrial fibrillation. *Am Heart J* **131**:499-507, 1996.

157. Feld GK: Radiofrequency catheter ablation versus modification of the AV node for control of rapid ventricular response in atrial fibrillation. *J Cardiovasc Electrophysiol* **6**:217-28, 1995.

158. Fleck RP, Chen PS, Boyce K, et al.: Radiofrequency modification of atrioventricular conduction by selective ablation of the low posterior septal right atrium in a patient with atrial fibrillation and a rapid ventricular response. *Pacing Clin Electrophysiol* **16**:377-81, 1993.

159. Feld GK, Fleck RP, Fujimura O, et al.: Control of rapid ventricular response by radiofrequency catheter modification of the atrioventricular node in patients with medically refractory atrial fibrillation. *Circulation* **90**:2299-307, 1994.

160. Williamson BD, Man KC, Daoud E, et al.: Radiofrequency catheter modification of atrioventricular conduction to control the ventricular rate during atrial fibrillation. *N Engl J Med* **331**:910-7, 1994.

161. Morady F, Hasse C, Strickberger SA, et al.: Long-term follow-up after radiofrequency modification of the atrioventricular node in patients with atrial fibrillation. *J Am Coll Cardiol* **29**:113-21, 1997.

162. Duckeck W, Engelstein ED, et al.: Radiofrequency current therapy in atrial tachyarrhythmias: modulation versus ablation of atrioventricular nodal conduction. *Pacing Clin Electrophysiol* **16**:629-36, 1993.

163. Swartz JF, Pellersels G, Silvers J, et al.: A catheter-based curative approach to atrial fibrillation in humans (abstract). *Circulation* **Suppl**:I-335, 1994.

164. Gaita F, Riccardi R, et al.: Atrial mapping and radiofrequency catheter ablation in patients with idiopathic atrial fibrillation. *Circulation* **97**:2136-2145, 1998.

165. Haissaguerre M, Gencel L, Fischer B, et al.: Successful catheter ablation of atrial fibrillation. *J Cardiovasc Electrophysiol* **5**:1045-52, 1994.

166. Haissaguerre M, Shah DC, Jais P, Clementy J: Role of catheter ablation for atrial fibrillation. *Curr Opin Cardiol* **12**:18-23, 1997.

167. Haissaguerre M, Jais P, Shah DC, et al.: Spontaneous initiation of atrial fibrillation by ectopic beats originating in the pulmonary veins. *N Engl J Med* **339**:659-66, 1998.

168 Young, C, Lauer, MR, et al.: unpublished.

169. Timmermans C, S. L, Tavenier R, and The Worldwide Metrix Investigators: Ambulatory use of the Metrix automatic implantable atrial defibrillator to treat episodes of atrial fibrillation. *PACE* **21**:811, 1998.

170. Ayers GM, Griffin JC: The future role of defibrillators in the management of atrial fibrillation. *Curr Opin Cardiol* **12**:12-7, 1997.

171. Barold HS, Wharton JM: Ventricular fibrillation resulting from synchronized internal atrial defibrillation in a patient with ventricular preexcitation. *J Cardiovasc Electrophysiol* **8**:436-40, 1997.

172. Nathan H, Eliakim M: The junction between the left atrium and the pulmonary veins. An anatomic study of human hearts. *Circulation* **34**:412-422, 1966.

173. Natale A, Pisano E, Santarelli P, et al.: First experience with a novel through-the-balloon ultrasound ablation catheter for pulmonary vein isolation in patients with atrial fibrillation. *Pacing Clin Electrophysiol* **23(Pt II)**:587, 2000.

174. Haissaguerre M, Shah D, Jais P, et al.: Circular multipolar pulmonary vein catheter for mapping guided minimal ablation of atrial fibrillation. *Pacing Clin Electrophysiol* **23(Pt II)**:574, 2000.

175. Roman-Gonzalez J, Asirvatham S, Johnson SB, et al.: Circumferential lesion creation in the pulmonary veins with a novel tandem balloon ablation catheter in dogs: 6-month follow up. *Pacing Clin Electrophysiol* **23(Pt II)**:567, 2000.

176. Fried NM, Lardo AC, Berger RD, et al.: Circumferential lesions in pulmonary veins using an Nd:YAG laser and fiberoptic balloon catheter. *Pacing Clin Electrophysiol* **23(Pt II)**:567, 2000.

177. Matsudaira K, Nakagawa H, Yamanashi WS, et al.: Effect of blood flow lesion size during cryo-catheter ablation. *Pacing Clin Electrophysiol* **23(Pt II)**:741, 2000.

CHAPTER 15

THE SPECTRUM OF MONOMORPHIC VENTRICULAR TACHYCARDIA

It has long been recognized that ventricular tachyarrhythmias generally connote a much worse prognosis compared to supraventricular tachyarrhythmias. This is because ventricular tachyarrhythmias often occur in patients with structural heart disease such as atherosclerotic coronary heart disease with prior myocardial infarction and primary or secondary cardiomyopathy (e.g., dilated cardiomyopathy, sarcoidosis, Chagas' disease, right ventricular dysplasia, etc.) [1]. However, ventricular tachyarrhythmias can also occur in patients without clinical evidence of structural heart disease as a "primary, "idiopathic" or "functional" entity [2-4].

Ventricular fibrillation usually causes immediate circulatory collapse and cardiac arrest, but ventricular tachycardia may present with a variety of symptoms including: palpitations, dyspnea, chest pain, dizziness, syncope, and functional cardiac arrest. Ventricular tachycardia can be either *monomorphic* or *polymorphic* based upon the morphology of the QRS complex recorded by the surface ECG and can be clinically *sustained* or *nonsustained*. A sustained ventricular tachycardia is defined as ventricular tachycardia lasting for 30 seconds or longer, or causing circulatory collapse requiring pharmacologic intervention or resuscitation within that time. Clinically, sustained monomorphic ventricular tachycardia is often inducible by programmed electrical stimulation during an electrophysiology study, thereby allowing delineation of the underlying mechanism.

The electrophysiologic mechanisms of monomorphic ventricular tachycardia depend primarily on anatomical substrates and its clinical presentations [5-9]. Based upon the mode of initiation and termination (electrophysiologic testing), and the responses to pharmacologic agents (pharmacologic testing), recurrent monomorphic ventricular tachycardia can be characterized and subclassified. Characterization of ventricular tachycardia provides a rationale for risk stratification and for planning a proper therapeutic regimen [7,8,10,11].

15.1 Electrophysiologic Mechanisms

Mechanisms of ventricular tachycardia can only be presumptive during electrophysiology study in humans [12,13]. The following electrophysiological principles are applied [14-19] (Table 15-1.)

Reentry requires the presence of a conduction circuit with at least two pathways differing in electrophysiologic properties but electrically-connected both proximally and distally (Figure 15-1). In its simplest form for reentry to occur, a ventricular premature impulse must induce unidirectional conduction block in one pathway (α) and conduct slowly within another, parallel, pathway (β). If conduction within this second pathway is sufficiently slow, the previously blocked α-pathway may recover excitability, allowing the impulse

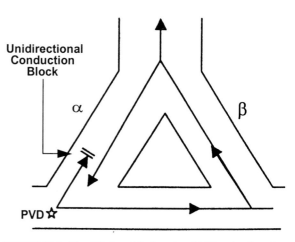

FIGURE 15-1. Simplified model of reentry. Unidirectional conduction block of the premature ventricular depolarization (PVD) occurs in the α pathway with conduction continuing slowly within the parallel β pathway. See text for details.

to conduct within that pathway in the reverse direction (relative to the originally intended direction of conduction within that pathway). Assuming the slow β-pathway has recovered excitability, the impulse may re-excite this conduction pathway thereby initiating a reentrant phenomenon. When this phenomenon is perpetuated, a circus movement (tachycardia) results.

Therefore, ventricular tachycardia due to a reentrant mechanism is suggested by the ability to reproducibly initiate the tachycardia with ventricular extrastimulation and/or rapid ventricular pacing (Figure 15-2). Furthermore, because of the presence of an *excitable gap*, a reentrant ventricular tachycardia may be *reset, entrained* and even terminated by timed extrastimulation and/or overdrive ventricular pacing, assuming the electrical impulses penetrate and alter the refractory periods of the tissues involved [20-24]. This simplified principle of reentry remains valid particularly for bundle branch reentrant ventricular tachycardia [6,25,26]. Using the technique of detailed three dimensional mapping, it has been shown that ventricular tachycardia due to a reentrant mechanism is a form of spiral, vortex-like reentry due to three dimensional anisotropic conduction in the infarcted human heart [27-29].

Automaticity is caused by spontaneous impulse initiation that results from gradual diastolic phase 4 depolarization. This may occur in both normal and partially depolarized fibers. Therefore, ventricular tachycardia resulting from an automatic mechanism should occur spontaneously. Programmed electrical stimulation would not be expected to initiate this arrhythmia, and timed ventricular extrastimulation or overdrive ventricular pacing would not be expected to convert this arrhythmia to a sustained sinus rhythm. Because of limitations of the study technique, normal and abnormal automaticity cannot be distinguished.

TABLE 15-1. Mechanisms of ventricular tachyarrhythmias: electrophysiological and pharmacological classification

Mechanism	Electrophysiological Findings	Pharmacological Findings
Reentry	VT reproducibly provoked with extrastimuli (or, less commonly, rapid fixed cycle length pacing)	VT suppressed, slowed, or terminated by Na$^+$ channel blockers (procainamide); (slow conduction due to depressed Na$^+$ channels, not Ca^{++} channels)
	VT has excitable gap & can be reset by timed extrastimuli & entrained by OD pacing; terminated by OD pacing	Verapamil, adenosine, & β-adrenergic blockers usually fail to alter or affect inducibility
	The interval between the last paced beat & the first beat of the VT increases as the coupling interval of last paced beat decreases	
	Area of slow conduction/continuous fragmented electrical activity	
Automaticity	VT occurs spontaneously, unrelated to PES	VT enhanced/induced by exogenous catecholamines
	VT may show warm-up phenomenon; no resetting or entrainment behavior; not terminated by OD pacing; pacing may accelerate tachycardia	May be suppressed/terminated by β-adrenergic blocking agents & Na$^+$ channel blockers that depress phase 4 diastolic depolarization
	VT usually has LBBB QRS morphology with inferior axis (right ventricular origin); rarely see RBBB QRS morphology	Unaffected by adenosine & verapamil, unless VT is due to Ca^{++} channel-dependent automaticity
Triggered Activity	VT induced by incremental pacing (atrial or ventricular) & often within a critical range of drive cycle lengths (cycle length-dependency)	Often requires infusion of exogenous catecholamines for induction
	First beat of the tachycardia usually occurs late in cardiac cycle	
	Interval between first beat of the VT & the preceding sinus or paced beat decreases as the drive cycle length (sinus or paced) decreases	Verapamil suppresses/terminates the VT; adenosine more likely to terminate VT originating in right ventricle (LBBB QRS morphology) than left ventricular VT (RBBB QRS morphology)
	VT does not exhibit typical resetting and entrainment behavior	Na$^+$ channel blockers (procainamide) may slow but do not suppress VT; β-adrenergic blockers may suppress/terminate tachycardia if VT dependent upon catecholamines for induction

LBBB, left bundle branch block; OD, overdrive pacing; PES, programmed electrical stimulation; RBBB, right bundle branch block; VT, ventricular tachycardia.

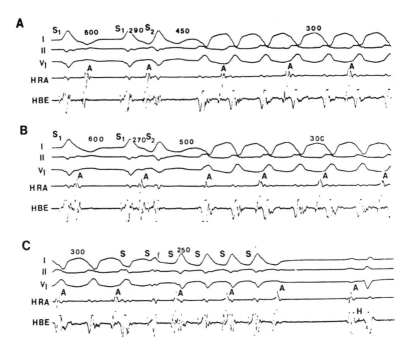

FIGURE 15-2. Induction of reentrant ventricular tachycardia with programmed ventricular extrastimulation in a 64-year-old man with arteriosclerotic coronary heart disease. Ventricular tachycardia cannot be elicited by programmed atrial stimulation, but is readily inducible with programmed right ventricular extrastimulation. (panels A & B) The right ventricle is driven at a cycle length (S1-S1) of 600 ms, ventricular premature beats (S2) with premature coupling intervals of 290 and 270 msec, respectively, provoke an onset of sustained ventricular tachycardia with a right bundle branch block pattern (axis +130°), the cycle length of which is 300 msec. Note that the interval between the initiating ventricular premature beat and the first beat of ventricular tachycardia is inversely related to the premature coupling interval of ventricular premature beats (S2). Panel C: Overdrive right ventricular pacing at a cycle length of 250 msec easily terminates the arrhythmia. The ventricular tachycardia remains inducible and its cycle length remains unchanged after either intravenous verapamil or β-adrenergic blockade with intravenous propranolol (0.2 mg/kg) (not shown). Electrocardiographic leads I, II, and V1 are simultaneously recorded with high right atrial (HRA) and His bundle electrographic (HBE) leads in this and subsequent figures. A, atrial electrogram; f, fusion beat; H, His bundle electrogram; S, stimulus. From [11] with permission.

Triggered activity related to delayed afterdepolarizations does not occur spontaneously and is dependent upon previous depolarizations for its initiation. A delayed afterdepolarization occurs after phase 3 repolarization has restored maximum diastolic potential. The delayed afterdepolarization may reach threshold and initiate an action potential during a critical range of cycle lengths. Generation of a train of such triggered action potentials can thus lead to an arrhythmia. Ventricular tachycardia caused by this mechanism may have some of the following electrophysiologic characteristics: (a) the first beat of tachycardia usually appears late in the cardiac cycle; (b) its initiation is related to a critical range of QRS cycle lengths (usually short rather than long cycle lengths); (c) its onset is more easily triggered by multiple rather than single ventricular depolarizations; and (d) the interval between the first beat of tachycardia and its preceding sinus or paced beat (QRS complex) gradually decreases as the driving cycle length (sinus or paced beats) progressively shortens.

Based on the above-described principles and limitations inherent to the study techniques in humans, electrophysiology study along with pharmacologic testing can be employed to characterize chronic recurrent ventricular tachycardia (Table 15-1.)

15.2   Electrophysiology Study

During incremental atrial and ventricular pacing, the right atrium or right ventricle (apex and outflow tract) are individually paced for 15-20 beats with abrupt cessation. Pacing begins at a cycle length that is 20 ms shorter than the cycle length during sinus rhythm. After each burst of pacing, the cycle length is decreased by 10-20 msec until the shortest pacing cycle length of 250 ms is reached. This stepwise decrease in the pacing cycle length is to examine whether the induction of ventricular tachycardia requires a critical range of cycle lengths [7,8].

During programmed atrial or ventricular extrastimulation, the high right atrium or the right ventricle (apex and outflow tract) are individually paced using a fixed-cycle length train (S_1-S_1). A premature stimuli (S_2) is delivered to the atrium or ventricle (apex, then outflow tract) from late diastole, at progressively shorter coupling intervals (S_1-S_2) after every eighth drive stimulus, until the respective effective refractory periods of the high right atrium, right ventricular apex, or right ventricular outflow tract are encountered. Usually this pacing protocol is performed using two different drive trains (S_1-S_1), e.g., 600 ms and 400 ms. To increase the sensitivity of ventricular tachycardia induction, timed double and triple premature stimuli $(S_3$ and $S_4)$ are delivered to the ventricle if a single premature stimulus (S_2) fails to elicit ventricular tachycardia. The protocol is continued until it provokes ventricular tachycardia or until all extrastimuli $(S_2, S_3$ and $S_4)$ fail to activate the ventricle (refractory period reached) (Figure 15-2). An abrupt long-to-short drive cycle length may also be incorporated into the ventricular extrastimulation protocol in order to facilitate the induction of ventricular tachycardia [30,31]. After the initiation of ventricular tachycardia, short bursts of overdrive ventricular pacing are delivered in an attempt to terminate the arrhythmia (Figure 15-2).

If programmed electrical stimulation is unable to induce ventricular tachycardia, isoproterenol is infused intravenously at 1-5 µg/min until the sinus rate is accelerated to a maximum of 150/min. If isoproterenol does not provoke an onset of ventricular tachycardia, programmed electrical stimulation as described above may be repeated during isoproterenol infusion [32] in selected patients. Isoproterenol should not be administered to patients with angina pectoris associated with atherosclerotic heart disease or hypertrophic cardiomyopathy. During isoproterenol infusion, the patient's tolerance should be closely monitored. Tremor, chest discomfort, and anxiety reaction may preclude further electrophysiology study. In general, programmed electrical stimulation during isoproterenol infusion should only be performed in patients presumed to have the idiopathic variety of ventricular tachycardia with normal cardiac function because the risk of provoking non-clinical ventricular fibrillation is high, particularly in patients with compromised left ventricular function associated with structural heart disease [33].

15.3   Pharmacologic Testing

Pharmacologic testing with intravenous antiarrhythmic agents such as procainamide, propranolol or verapamil can be carried out during electrophysiology study. Electrophysiology study using the above described protocol is performed before and after administration of each drug. The dosage for intravenous verapamil is 0.15 mg/kg of body weight administered over 2 min as a loading dose followed by continuous infusion at 0.005 mg/kg of body weight/min. The dosage for intravenous procainamide is 15 mg/kg delivered as a rapid loading infusion at 50 mg/min followed by a maintenance infusion of 1-3 mg/min. The dosage for intravenous propranolol to achieve significant β-adrenergic blockade is 0.2 mg/kg of body weight at 1 mg/min infusion rate. Programmed electrical stimulation or isoproterenol infusion is repeated 10 minutes after drug administration. Patients with unstable ventricular tachycardia should not undergo pharmacologic testing and those with a history of congestive heart failure or significantly compromised left ventricular function (e.g., left ventricular ejection fraction < 35%) should not receive either verapamil or propranolol for pharmacologic testing.

15.4   Verapamil-nonresponsive Ventricular Tachycardia

Based on the mode of ventricular tachycardia induction and termination, it can be subdivided into two types – one electrically inducible suggestive of reentrant mechanism and the other electrically not inducible but may be provoked with intravenous infusion of isoproterenol suggestive of catecholamine-sensitive enhanced automaticity.

15.4.1   VENTRICULAR TACHYCARDIA RESULTING FROM REENTRY

This form of ventricular tachycardia is usually seen in patients with structural heart disease (e.g., atherosclerotic coronary heart disease with prior myocardial infarction or primary and secondary cardiomyopathy) [5-11].

The QRS morphology of this form of ventricular tachycardia varies greatly among patients because of extensive myocardial involvement of the disease process. As is characteristic of a reentrant arrhythmia, this form of ventricular tachycardia can be elicited by programmed ventricular stimulation with single or multiple extrastimuli and can usually be terminated by ventricular overdrive pacing (Figure 15-2) [7,8,10,11]. During the tachycardia, slow conduction may be identified and an excitable gap demonstrated by ventricular extrastimuli and by overdrive ventricular pacing without termination of the arrhythmia (i.e., resetting and entrainment). These phenomena are in keeping with the presence of a reentrant circuit with an excitable gap [20-24]. Intravenous verapamil, adenosine, and propranolol are not effective in terminating and suppressing this form of ventricular tachycardia [7,8,10,11,34-36]. In fact, both intravenous verapamil and intravenous propranolol may worsen the hemodynamics during the arrhythmia as a result of their hypotensive and negative inotropic effects [37]. The area of slow conduction is probably a consequence of depressed Na^+ channels rather than Ca^{++} channel-dependent slow response [38-40]. This explains the ineffectiveness of Ca^{++} channel blockers, and the comparative effectiveness of class IA antiarrhythmic drugs (e.g., procainamide) in terminating and suppressing the inducibility of this arrhythmia.

15.4.2 VENTRICULAR TACHYCARDIA RESULTING FROM ENHANCED AUTOMATICITY

Ventricular tachycardia of automatic mechanism may be seen in patients with or without clinical evidence of structural heart disease. The morphology of the QRS complex of automatic ventricular tachycardia is often of a complete left bundle branch block pattern associated with a right or left inferior frontal axis. Rarely, an automatic ventricular tachycardia may manifest a complete right bundle branch block pattern, particularly in patients with structural heart disease. Unlike ventricular tachycardia of a reentrant mechanism, the automatic ventricular tachycardia cannot be provoked by programmed electrical stimulation and cannot be converted to a sustained sinus rhythm with overdrive ventricular pacing (Figures 15-3 through 15-6). If the ventricular tachycardia is cate-

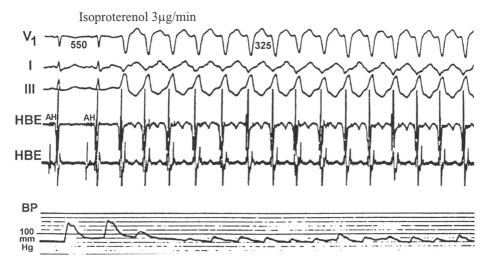

FIGURE 15-3. Induction of a paroxysm of ventricular tachycardia with intravenous infusion of isoproterenol in a 52-year-old man with no clinical evidence of organic heart disease. Following failure of programmed electrical stimulation to induce arrhythmia, isoproterenol infusion at a dosage of 3 μg/min accelerates the sinus rate from 75 to 109 beats/min (cycle length 550 msec) and provokes an onset of ventricular tachycardia with a cycle length of 325 msec. Right femoral arterial pressure is recorded at the bottom. From [7] with permission.

cholamine-sensitive, intravenous infusion of isoproterenol may facilitate its initiation. Neither intravenous verapamil nor adenosine bolus infusion affects this arrhythmia [7,8,10,11,35]. Intravenous propranolol can usually terminate catecholamine-sensitive automatic ventricular tachycardia and suppress its inducibility during isoproterenol infu-

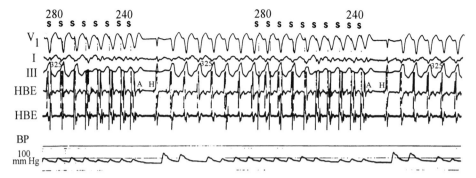

FIGURE 15-4. Response of isoproterenol-induced ventricular tachycardia to overdrive ventricular pacing (same patient as in Figure 15-3). The ventricular tachycardia has a cycle length of 325 msec. Right ventricular overdrive pacing with a cycle length of 280 msec for 7 to 9 beats followed by a ventricular premature beat with a premature coupling interval of 240 msec can only temporarily suppress the ventricular tachycardia as the arrhythmia emerges immediately after each sinus beat. Right femoral arterial pressure is recorded at the bottom. From [7] with permission.

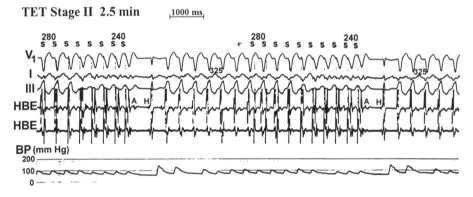

FIGURE 15-5. Provocation of ventricular tachycardia suggestive of catecholamine-sensitive automaticity during treadmill exercise testing. (Left panel) Ventricular tachycardia emerges during stage II of treadmill exercise testing (TET) at which time the sinus rate has accelerated to 150/min (cycle length 400 ms). Note that attainment of comparable cycle lengths during atrial and ventricular pacing cannot provoke onset of ventricular tachycardia as shown in Figure 15-6 (panels A and B). (Right panel) The 12-lead electrocardiogram of the exercise-induced ventricular tachycardia as demonstrated in the left panel. The ventricular tachycardia has an identical QRS morphology to that provoked by isoproterenol infusion as shown in Figure 15-6C. From [10] with permission.

sion (Figure 15-6) [7,8,10,11,41,42]. Intravenous procainamide can also terminate this form of ventricular tachycardia and may also suppress its inducibility by virtue of its depressive action on diastolic phase 4 depolarization.

Two types of automaticity have been shown in cellular electrophysiology [43-47]. Normal automaticity occurs in healthy cells with normal resting potentials. Cardiac Purkinje fibers, with a normal resting potential in the range of −80 to −90 mV, develop normal automaticity due to their inherent diastolic phase 4 depolarization. This type of automaticity can be suppressed by overdrive pacing [48-51], but rarely terminates as a result of pacing. The cellular basis for overdrive suppression appears to be intracellular

A. Control

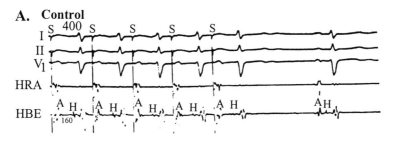

B. Control

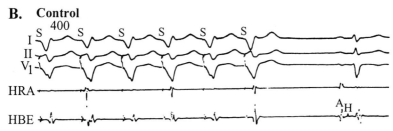

C. Isoproterenol, 4 µg/min, IV

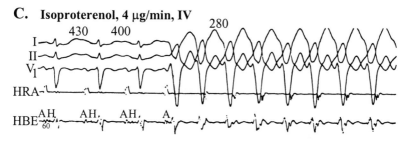

D. Propranolol, 10 mg, IV + Isoproterenol, 4 µg/min, IV

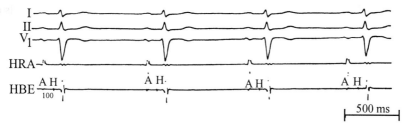

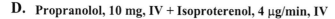

500 ms

FIGURE 15-6. Provocation and suppression of ventricular tachycardia suggestive of catecholamine-sensitive automaticity (same patient as in Figure 15-5). Ventricular tachycardia cannot be elicited by programmed atrial or ventricular stimulation, but is provocable with intravenous infusion of isoproterenol. (A & B) High right atrial (HRA) and right ventricular pacing, respectively, at the cycle length (S-S) of 400 msec (comparable to that which initiates ventricular tachycardia during treadmill exercise testing in this patient, as shown in Figure 15-5) cannot elicit the onset of ventricular tachycardia. (C) Intravenous infusion of isoproterenol (4 µg/min) accelerates the sinus rate (cycle length shortened to 400 msec) and provokes the onset of ventricular tachycardia with a left bundle branch block pattern (frontal axis +120°), the cycle length of which is 280 msec. (D) After β-adrenergic blockade with intravenous propranolol (0.2 mg/kg), infusion of isoproterenol (4 µg/min) can no longer provoke the onset of arrhythmia. From [11] with permission.

Na$^+$ loading and extracellular K$^+$ accumulation during the more frequent action potentials (depolarizations) that activate the electrogenic Na$^+$/K$^+$ pump (net outward current) [52-54], which, in turn, decrease the net rate of diastolic phase 4 depolarization (hyperpolarization) [51].

Abnormal automaticity results from spontaneous activity occurring in cells with abnormal resting potentials in the range of –40 to –60 mV. These abnormally depolarized cells have inactivated fast Na$^+$ channels and exhibit Ca^{++}-dependent slow response action potentials. A variety of pathological conditions are associated with enhanced automaticity at these low levels of resting potential, including high extracellular K$^+$ concentration, [K$^+$]$_o$ catecholamines and low extracellular pH [55-59]. Unlike normal automaticity, this form of automaticity cannot be suppressed by overdrive pacing, and may, in fact, be accelerated by rapid pacing [48-50]. The inability to suppress by overdrive pacing is believed to be due to the lesser degree of Na$^+$ influx required for impulse generation in this case compared to that required for impulse initiation during normal automaticity. In addition, abnormal automaticity is associated with the "warm-up" phenomenon whereby the spontaneous activity exhibits a gradual increase in frequency [49]. Because abnormal automaticity appears to be generated by Ca^{++}-dependent slow response action potentials, it may be suppressed by verapamil [60,61].

If the initiation of this form of ventricular tachycardia initiation is dependent upon exercise or isoproterenol infusion and it cannot be suppressed by intravenous verapamil, the electrophysiological mechanism of the arrhythmia is presumed to be catecholamine-sensitive enhanced automaticity [7,8,10,11].

15.5   Verapamil-Responsive Ventricular Tachycardia

This form of ventricular tachycardia occurs more commonly in young patients who are otherwise healthy although it may be seen in the elderly including those with associated structural heart disease. Its QRS morphology exhibits either a right bundle branch block pattern (usually of a left superior axis) or a left bundle branch block pattern (usually of a right inferior axis). The initiation of this form of ventricular tachycardia depends on the attainment of a critical range of cycle lengths (cycle length-dependency) [7,11] with sinus, atrial-paced, or ventricular-paced rhythm (Figures 15-8 through 15-16). In many patients, programmed ventricular extrastimulation can also trigger an onset of the arrhythmia. However, the development of AV nodal Wenckebach phenomenon may preclude the induction of this arrhythmia from the atrium and the occurrence of entrance block may make it difficult to provoke this arrhythmia from the ventricle. Furthermore, the critical range of cycle lengths for the arrhythmia induction can be as narrow as 10-20 msec and this arrhythmia may also be catecholamine-sensitive, requiring isoproterenol infusion for provocation. Therefore, careful scanning of the pacing cycle length and selection of the pacing site are essential in attempting to provoke this arrhythmia. Intravenous verapamil can easily terminate this arrhythmia and suppress its inducibility (Figures 15-10). In contrast, intravenous propranolol and procainamide can only slow the rate of the arrhythmia and cannot suppress its inducibility. If the arrhythmia is also catecholamine-sensitive, intravenous propranolol (or esmolol) can then terminate the arrhythmia (Figure 15-17) [11,50,62].

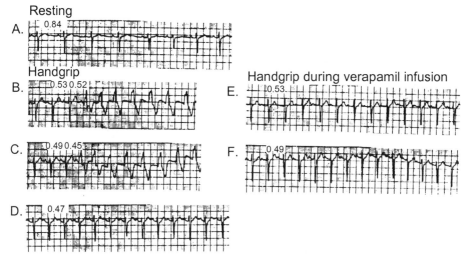

FIGURE 15-7. Cycle length dependency for the initiation of ventricular tachycardia during sinus rhythm in an 18-year-old man with no clinical evidence of organic heart disease. (A) At rest, the cycle length of sinus rhythm is 0.84 sec. The sinus rate then accelerates during handgrip. (B and C) Ventricular tachycardia is initiated when the sinus rhythm attains cycle lengths between 0.53 and 0.49 sec. (D) Further acceleration of the sinus rate (cycle length of 0.48 sec or shorter) initiates no ventricular tachycardia. (B and C) Note that the interval between the first beat of ventricular tachycardia and its preceding sinus beat (QRS complex) shortens (0.52 → 0.45 sec) as the sinus rate accelerates. (E and F) During verapamil infusion, repeated handgrip accelerates the sinus rate with cycle lengths between 0.53 and 0.49 sec but fails to initiate ventricular tachycardia. From [7] with permission.

The maneuver necessary to provoke verapamil-sensitive ventricular tachycardia is highly variable, with induction sometimes possible with rapid atrial or ventricular pacing at a critical cycle length, programmed atrial or ventricular extrastimulation, isoproterenol infusion alone, or isoproterenol infusion in combination with some form of electrical pacing. Apart from its most common electrocardiographic presentation showing a left bundle branch block QRS pattern with an inferior axis or right bundle branch block QRS pattern with a left superior axis, verapamil-sensitive ventricular tachycardia may rarely exhibit a right bundle branch block QRS pattern with a left or right inferior axis. Adenosine can terminate some but not all forms of verapamil-sensitive ventricular tachycardia. Verapamil-sensitive ventricular tachycardia exhibiting a left bundle branch block QRS pattern is more likely to be terminated by adenosine, while less than one third of verapamil-responsive ventricular tachycardias with a right bundle branch block QRS pattern are sensitive to intravenous adenosine [34,35,62,63].

It is tempting to postulate that verapamil-sensitive ventricular tachycardia is probably caused by triggered activity related to delayed afterdepolarizations. Triggered activity related to delayed afterdepolarizations has been demonstrated in isolated tissues and single cells exposed to digitalis, high extracellular Ca^{++}, or catecholamines [64-67]. The mechanism responsible for catecholamine-induced triggered activity is thought to be intracellular Ca^{++} overload and is believed to be mediated by an increase in intracellular cyclic adenosine monophosphate (cAMP) [64,68-71]. β-adrenoceptor blocking agents, verapamil and adenosine should be useful for prevention or termination of some forms of

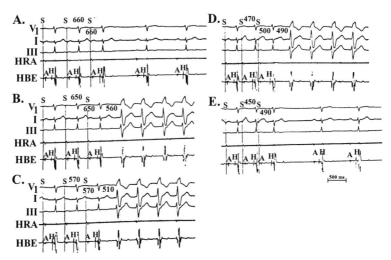

FIGURE 15-8. Induction of ventricular tachycardia during atrial paced rhythms (same patient as in Figure 15-7). (A) HRA pacing at a cycle length (S-S) of 660 msec (corresponding R-R interval, 660 msec) initiates no ventricular tachycardia. (B, C, D) HRA pacing at cycle lengths (S-S) of 650, 570, and 470 msec, respectively (corresponding R-R intervals of 650, 570, and 500 msec, respectively), initiates an onset of ventricular tachycardia. (E) HRA pacing at a cycle length (S-S) of 450 msec (corresponding R-R interval, 490 msec) initiates no ventricular tachycardia. Note that the interval between the first beat of ventricular tachycardia and its preceding atrial paced beat (QRS complex) gradually shortens as the atrial pacing rate progressively increases (B, C, and D). From [7] with permission.

triggered arrhythmias. β-adrenoceptor blocking agents by blocking the catecholamine-induced increase in cAMP, may effectively suppress cAMP-mediated cardiac arrhythmias. Adenosine antagonizes the inotropic and electrophysiologic effects of catecholamines that are mediated through stimulation of the cAMP system [71-75], and consequently, may also suppress triggered activity due to cAMP-mediated delayed afterdepolarizations. Verapamil suppresses delayed afterdepolarizations and triggered activity including digitalis-induced arrhythmia in experimental preparations [74,76-78]. Verapamil suppresses triggered arrhythmias by preventing intracellular Ca++ overload, thereby preventing the initiation of delayed afterdepolarizations and triggered activity.

15.5.1 Reentry Versus Triggered Activity

The mechanism of verapamil-responsive ventricular tachycardia is uncertain and debatable, as differentiation between reentry and triggered activity is difficult. This is because both reentry and triggered activity have similar clinical electrophysiologic manifestations despite having differences in their basic electrophysiologic mechanisms.

Delayed afterdepolarizations do not occur spontaneously. Their occurrence depends on previous depolarizations [16]. Similar to reentry, triggered activity can, therefore, be initiated by programmed electrical stimulation. Both atrial and ventricular pacing may initiate it. In contrast, a reentrant ventricular tachycardia is rarely initiated from the atrium [79,80].

The amplitude of delayed afterdepolarizations increases as the basic driving cycle length shortens [16]. The initiation of an onset of triggered activity is thus a cycle length-dependent phenomenon. Nevertheless, shortening of the basic driving cycle length may induce unidirectional block in one pathway and slow conduction in the other pathway, setting up conditions for reentry to occur [13-16].

Overdrive pacing may penetrate and alter refractoriness of reentrant pathways, thereby terminating a reentrant arrhythmia. On the other hand, overdrive pacing can cause enhancement of electrogenic Na^+ extrusion, which, in turn, hyperpolarizes the membrane potentials and may thereby abolish triggered activity [67].

As the basic driving cycle length shortens, the interval between the last paced (initiating) beat and the first beat of arrhythmia tends to increase in reentry, whereas it tends to decrease in triggered activity. Exceptions to the rule, however, may occur. In reentry, this interval presumably reflects total conduction time in both the anterograde and retrograde limbs of the reentrant circuit. If the retrograde limb conducts rapidly because of early recovery of excitability at shorter cycle lengths, the total conduction time may remain unchanged or even decrease rather than increase. Furthermore, in triggered activi-

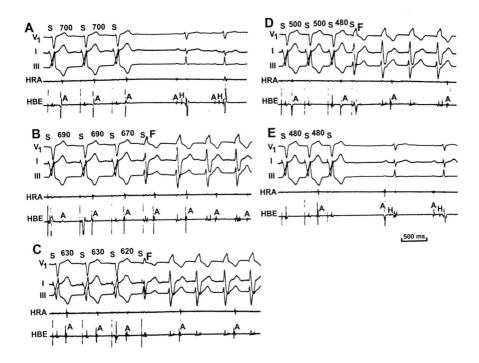

FIGURE 15-9. Induction of ventricular tachycardia during ventricular paced rhythm (same patient as in Figure 15-7). (A) Right ventricular pacing at a cycle length (S-S) of 700 msec initiates no ventricular tachycardia. (B, C, D) Right ventricular pacing at cycle lengths of 690, 630, and 500 msec, respectively, initiates an onset of ventricular tachycardia. (E) Right ventricular pacing at a cycle length of 480 msec initiates no ventricular tachycardia. Note that the interval between the first beat of ventricular tachycardia and its preceding ventricular paced beat gradually shortens as the ventricular pacing rate progressively increases (B, C, and D). F, ventricular fusion. From [7] with permission.

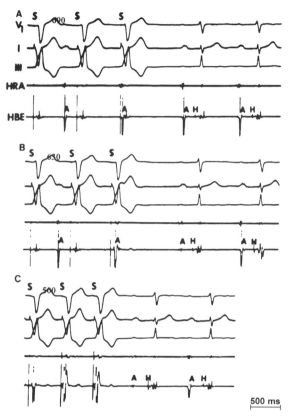

FIGURE 15-10. Suppression of induction of ventricular tachycardia during ventricular paced rhythm with verapamil infusion (same patient as in Figure 15-7). During intravenous infusion of verapamil (0.15 mg/kg followed by 0.005 mg/kg per min), right ventricular pacing at cycle lengths (S-S) of 690 (A), 630 (B), and 500 (C) msec, respectively, initiates no ventricular tachycardia. Note that the ventricular pacing at these cycle lengths initiates onset of ventricular tachycardia before verapamil infusion as shown in Figure 15-9 (B, C, and D). Atrial pacing induces AV nodal Wenckebach at a cycle length of 600 ms but fails to induce ventricular tachycardia during verapamil infusion (not shown). From [7] with permission.

ty, the first delayed afterdepolarization may paradoxically diminish its amplitude and become subthreshold as the basic driving cycle length shortens. The subsequent emergence of the second delayed afterdepolarization may then manifest with an unexpected prolongation of the premature coupling interval [16]. Therefore, the interval between the initiating beat and the first beat of arrhythmia alone may not be a strong indicator for either reentry or triggered activity.

Reentry can be responsible for verapamil-responsive ventricular tachycardia if the genesis of the arrhythmia involves Ca^{++} channel-dependent slow response in the reentrant circuit or is caused by active myocardial ischemia reversible with Ca^{++} channel blocking agents [81,82]. Under these circumstances, β-adrenergic blockade slows the tachycardia rate by decreasing the upstroke of slow response action potentials [83] or by counteracting a high adrenergic state which enhances myocardial conduction [84] consequent to hypotensive effects of sustained tachycardia. However, it has also been shown that the stimulus-evoked transmembrane Ca^{++} entry is generally believed to be via the voltage- and time-dependent channels activated by depolarization and modulated via agonist-β-adrenergic receptor interaction [85]. β-adrenergic stimulation increases the slow inward Ca^{++} current by activating the adenylate cyclase/cyclic adenosine monophosphate (cAMP) system [86-89]. Stimulation of β-adrenergic receptors promotes the conversion

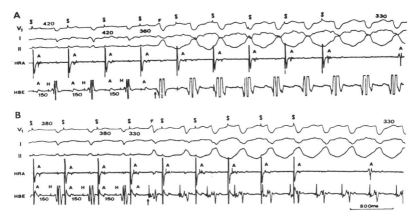

FIGURE 15-11. Induction of ventricular tachycardia with programmed incremental atrial pacing. Ventricular tachycardia can be initiated by pacing either the high right atrium (HRA) or right ventricle or both while attaining a critical range of cycle lengths. (A and B) High right atrial pacing at cycle lengths between 420 and 380 msec triggers paroxysms of ventricular tachycardia of a left bundle branch block pattern (frontal axis +110°) with a cycle length of 330 msec. Note that the QRS interval between the last paced beat and the first beat of ventricular tachycardia decreases when the pacing cycle length is shortened. F, fusion beat. From [11] with permission.

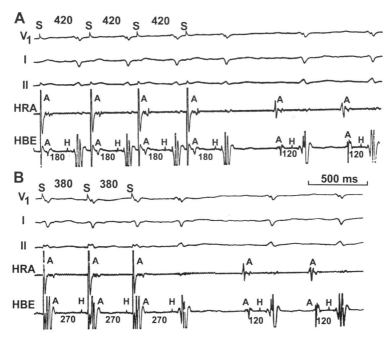

FIGURE 15-12. Suppression of ventricular tachycardia with intravenous infusion of verapamil (same patient as in Figure 15-11). Panels A & B: During intravenous infusion of verapamil (0.15 mg/kg bolus followed by 0.005 mg/kg/min infusion), atrial pacing even within the previously determined critical range of cycle lengths between 420 and 380 msec can no longer trigger the onset of ventricular tachycardia. From [11] with permission.

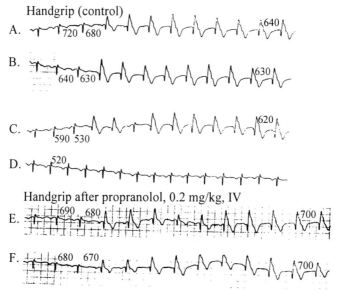

FIGURE 15-13. Effects of β-adrenergic blockade on verapamil-responsive ventricular tachycardia. Same patient as in Figure 15-7. ECG lead V₁ shown. Panels A-C:
At control, repeated handgrips accelerate the sinus rate and trigger an onset of ventricular tachycardia. Note that the ventricular tachycardia starts in late diastole and
that there is a progressive shortening of its coupling interval (680-530 ms) in
response to sinus rate acceleration (cycle length 720-590 ms). Also note that the
QRS complex of ventricular tachycardia has a right bundle branch block pattern.
Panel D: Further acceleration of the sinus rate (cycle length 520 ms) during handgrip
cannot initiate the onset of ventricular tachycardia. Panel E & F: After β-adrenergic
blockade with intravenous propranolol, handgrips continue to trigger the onset of
ventricular tachycardia at a slower rate (cycle length 700 ms). From [11] with permission.

of cytosolic adenosine triphosphate (ATP) to cAMP. Cyclic AMP activates the cAMP-
dependent protein kinase, which phosphorylates protein constituents of the membrane-
bound Ca^{++} channels. Consequently, the availability of functioning slow inward Ca^{++}
channels is increased. Verapamil directly blocks the voltage- and time-dependent slow
inward Ca^{++} channels [85] and may also act as a competitive β-adrenergic receptor antagonist [90]. On the other hand, by competitive inhibition, propranolol circumvents the
stimulatory affects of β-adrenergic agonists on the slow inward Ca^{++} current. The perpetuation of verapamil-responsive ventricular tachycardia may rely principally on the
voltage- and time-dependent Ca^{++} channels with minimal dependence on agonist β-adrenergic receptor interaction. This assumption can explain why verapamil totally suppresses the tachycardia inducibility, and why propranolol only slows the tachycardia rate
(Figures 15-13 through 15-15). Since the onset of triggered activity depends on previous
depolarizations which are Na^+ channel dependent, Na^+ channel blocking agents such as
procainamide may also slow the rate of the arrhythmia without suppressing its inducibility (Figure 15-16).

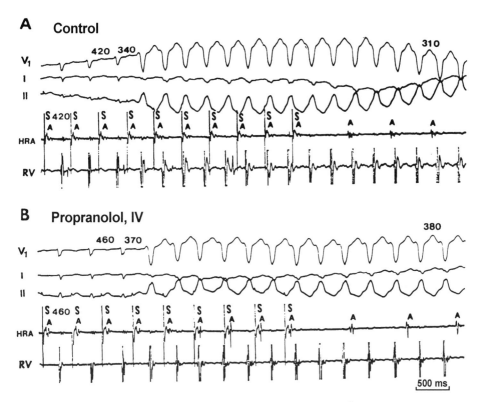

FIGURE 15-14. Effects of β-adrenergic blockade on verapamil-responsive ventricular tachycardia (same patient as in Figure 15-11, study done on separate day). Panel A: At control, high right atrial pacing at a cycle length of 420 msec reproducibly initiates the onset of ventricular tachycardia with a cycle length of 310 msec. Panel B: After β-adrenergic blockade with intravenous propranolol (0.2 mg/kg), the ventricular tachycardia remains inducible during high right atrial pacing at a cycle length of 380 msec. The critical range of cycle lengths at which ventricular tachycardia can be initiated changes from 420-380 to 460-400 msec after β-adrenergic blockade (not shown). From [11] with permission.

15.6   Exercise-induced Ventricular Tachyarrhythmias

Exercise may trigger cardiac arrhythmias in individuals with normal hearts, as well as those with structural heart disease [91]. The etiology of exercise-induced cardiac arrhythmias appears related to a multitude of metabolic, hemodynamic, and electrophysiologic factors, which, either alone or in combination, may facilitate the genesis of arrhythmias by mechanisms of reentry, enhanced automaticity, and triggered activity associated with or without myocardial ischemia [10] (Table 15-2.) While most exercise-induced arrhythmias are unrelated to ischemia, exercise may provoke ventricular tachyarrhythmias secondary to myocardial ischemia due to atherosclerotic coronary heart disease, or, rarely, coronary artery spasm (Table 15-3.) [92,93]. Clinically, exercise-induced ventricular premature beats are usually of no prognostic significance. However, the exercise-related provocation of complex (multiform) ventricular premature beats or

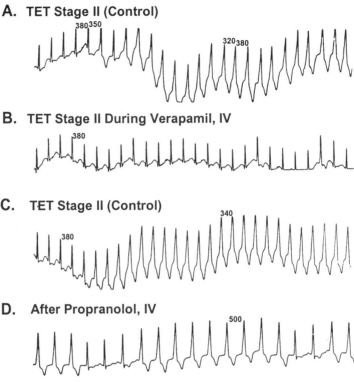

A. TET Stage II (Control)

B. TET Stage II During Verapamil, IV

C. TET Stage II (Control)

D. After Propranolol, IV

FIGURE 15-15. Verapamil-responsive ventricular tachycardia tested with intravenous verapamil and intravenous propranolol (same patient as in Figure 15-11). Panel A: At control during treadmill exercise testing (TET), the sinus rate accelerates (cycle length 380 ms) at stage II and initiates the onset of ventricular tachycardia with cycle lengths ranging from 320 to 380 ms. Panel B: Repeat TET during verapamil infusion can no longer initiate the onset of the arrhythmia. Panel C: At control, ventricular tachycardia is reproduced during TET at stage II with sinus rate acceleration (cycle length 380 ms) (done on a separate day). The cycle length of ventricular tachycardia is 340 ms. Panel D: After β-adrenergic blockade, the ventricular tachycardia slows its rate with a cycle length of 500 ms and becomes continuous requiring intravenous verapamil (5 mg) for termination (not shown). From [11] with permission.

non-sustained or sustained ventricular tachycardia is usually seen in patients with significant structural heart disease and may have a more ominous prognosis. The severity of left ventricular dysfunction generally predicts the clinical outcome in this latter subgroup of patients [94,95].

Ischemic ventricular arrhythmias may manifest as monomorphic or polymorphic ventricular tachycardia or ventricular fibrillation. In some cases, angina pectoris and/or ischemic electrocardiographic ST segment or T wave changes may precede the onset of ventricular tachyarrhythmias during exercise testing. Because of the life-threatening nature of these arrhythmias, repeated exercise testing is not advisable. Coronary arteriography and myocardial radionuclide perfusion imaging are often essential to assess the extent and severity of fixed atherosclerotic coronary heart disease and myocardial ischemia. For patients with significant atherosclerotic coronary heart disease and exer-

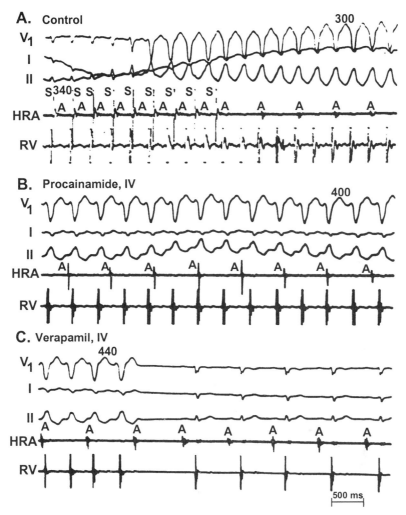

FIGURE 15-16. Effect of intravenous procainamide on verapamil-responsive ventricular tachycardia. Same patient as in Figure 15-11. Panel A: Under control conditions, atrial pacing at a cycle length of 340 ms initiates the onset of ventricular tachycardia with a cycle length of 300 ms. Panel B: After intravenous infusion of procainamide (20 mg/kg), the ventricular tachycardia becomes incessant with a cycle length of 400 ms. Panel C: An intravenous bolus infusion of verapamil (5 mg) terminates the arrhythmia within 3 min.

cise-induced ventricular arrhythmias, coronary artery revascularization either with percutaneous trans-luminal coronary angioplasty/stenting or aortocoronary bypass grafting should be considered as the first line of therapy. Medical therapy and/or implantation of a cardioverter-defibrillator are to be considered for those patients who are not candidates for coronary artery revascularization. Electrophysiologic evaluation is of limited value in the evaluation and management of ischemic ventricular arrhythmias, but post-revascularization electrophysiology study and treadmill exercise testing may be

Isoproterenol, 3 µg/min, IV
Adenosine, 12 mg, IV

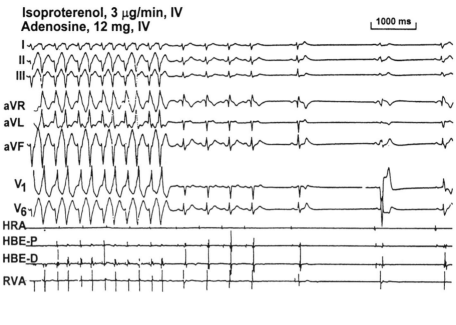

Isoproterenol, 3 µg/min, IV
Esmolol, 70 mg, IV

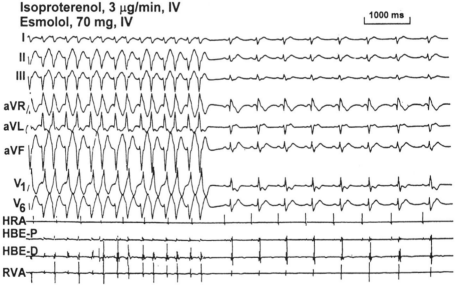

FIGURE 15-17. Termination of catecholamine-dependent verapamil-responsive ventricular tachycardia with intravenous adenosine and esmolol (same patient). Isoproterenol infusion at 3 µg/min is required for tachycardia induction and perpetuation. The ventricular tachycardia shows right bundle branch block-type QRS pattern with a left superior axis (-90°) and marked cycle-length alternans (260 msec and 320 msec). In the upper panel, 12 mg of adenosine, IV, terminates the tachycardia within 10 seconds; in the lower panel, 70 mg of esmolol, IV, terminates the tachycardia within 30 seconds. HRA, high right atrium; HBE-P, His bundle proximal; HBE-D, His bundle distal; RVA, right ventricular apex. From [62] with permission.

TABLE 15-2. Metabolic, hemodynamic, & electrophysiologic effects of exercise

↑Sympathetic Tone, ↓Parasympathetic Tone, & ↑Catecholamines

↑Heart rate

↑Cardiac contractility   ↑ Myocardial oxygen demand

↑Systemic blood pressure

↑Adenylyl cyclase/cAMP system

↑Inositol phospholipid & protein kinase C systems

↑Calmodulin-dependent protein kinase system   ↑Reentry

↑Intracellular Ca^{++} ↑Enhanced automaticity

↑Transmembrane ionic current   ↑Triggered activity

↑Diastolic (phase 4) depolarization

↓Refractory periods of cardiac tissues

useful in selected patients to establish the efficacy of the revascularization procedure in preventing further exercise-related ventricular tachyarrhythmias of an ischemic etiology.

In the subset of patients with coronary artery spasm and variant angina associated with minimal or an absence of gross atherosclerotic coronary artery disease, coronary arteriography with ergonovine challenge is often a useful diagnostic procedure. In these patients, the use of combination drug therapy with nitrates and Ca^{++}-channel blockers is recommended [93]. In such patients, β-adrenoceptor blocking agents are contraindicated

TABLE 15-3. Classification of exercise-induced ventricular tachyarrhythmias

Ischemic (monomorphic VT, polymorphic VT, or VF)

Non-ischemic

 Verapamil-responsive (monomorphic VT)

  Reentry

  Triggered activity

 Verapamil-nonresponsive (monomorphic VT)

  Reentry (electrically inducible)

  Enhanced automaticity (not electrically inducible)

 Idiopathic polymorphic VT

 Idiopathic VF

 Congenital/hereditary long QT syndromes (monomorphic VT or torsade de pointes)

 Proarrhythmic effects of antiarrhythmic drugs (monomorphic VT, polymorphic VT, or torsade de pointes)

because isolated β-adrenergic blockade without concomitant inhibition of α-adrenergic activity may facilitate the development of coronary artery spasm.

Ventricular tachyarrhythmias caused by exercise-induced acute myocardial ischemia may also rarely occur in patients without coronary artery disease or coronary artery spasm. The possibility of having associated hypertrophic cardiomyopathy and anomalous origin of the coronary arteries should be excluded in differential diagnosis [96,97]. Management of ventricular arrhythmias in these patients is addressed by correcting the underlying cardiac disease, including surgical interventions such as myomectomy/myotomy, and repair of the coronary artery abnormality, respectively.

The evaluation and treatment of non-ischemic, exercise-induced ventricular tachyarrhythmias are often effectively pursued with electrophysiology study [7,8,10,11]. These ventricular tachycardias can also be subdivided into verapamil-responsive and verapamil-non-responsive forms. Additionally, exercise may provoke idiopathic polymorphic ventricular tachycardia, idiopathic ventricular fibrillation, torsade de pointes associated with the congenital long QT syndromes, and ventricular arrhythmias due to proarrhythmic effects of antiarrhythmic drugs (Table 15-3.)

Exercise-induced ventricular tachyarrhythmias of various mechanisms may be reproduced during electrophysiology study with or without the use of isoproterenol infusion [7,8,10,11,32]. Similar to effects of exercise, isoproterenol exerts a variety of electrophysiologic effects. It enhances diastolic phase 4 depolarization [14], decreases refractory periods of myocardial tissues [84,98], thereby allowing more degree of ventricular premature stimulation, and potentiates the development of triggered activity by accelerating the sinus rate (shortening of cycle length) and increasing intracellular cAMP [14-16,86-88]. If the initiation of an arrhythmia, regardless of its underlying electrophysiological mechanism is solely dependent on intravenous infusion of isoproterenol, β-adrenergic blockade with intravenous propranolol is extremely effective in terminating and suppressing the arrhythmia.

It appears that the QRS morphology of ventricular tachycardia is not predictive of the underlying mechanism of an exercise-induced ventricular tachycardia as it can be either a right bundle branch block or a left bundle branch block pattern. Furthermore, there is no evidence of excessive secretions of catecholamines at rest or during treadmill exercise testing in this subgroup of patients [11]. It may be that the presence of a low sympathetic threshold and/or an arrhythmia-prone anatomic substrate is responsible for the clinical occurrence of ventricular tachycardia in these patients. The existence of different electrophysiologic mechanisms explains why exercise-induced ventricular tachycardia is not uniformly responsive to β-adrenoceptor blockers [7,8,10,11,42,99-101].

Idiopathic polymorphic ventricular tachycardia associated with a normal QT interval, and torsade de pointes tachycardia associated with the congenital long QT syndromes can be provoked by exertion [102-104] and may be reproducible with exercise testing or with isoproterenol infusion. The usual presenting symptom is recurrent syncope brought on by exercise or emotional stress. Recent studies have implicated different genes affecting Na^+ and K^+ currents responsible for the congenital long QT syndromes [105-109]. Idiopathic ventricular fibrillation is rarely exercise-induced, but may actually develop as a result of degeneration of idiopathic polymorphic ventricular tachycardia or torsade de pointes. β-adrenoceptor blocking agents are often effective in preventing recurrent episodes of symptomatic torsade de pointes associated with the congenital long QT syndromes. However, additional measures include surgical cardiac sympathetic denervation, pacemaker implantation, or implantation of cardioverter-defibrillator should be considered in selected high risk patients with the congenital long QT syndromes [102].

Exercise-induced ventricular tachyarrhythmias may develop secondary to the proarrhythmic effects of antiarrhythmic drugs [110-111]. Antiarrhythmia agents known to be particularly proarrhythmic during exercise are class IA and IC drugs. Sinus tachycardia induced by exercise enhances the use-dependent Na^+ channel blockade of these agents and may thereby induce slow conduction and unidirectional block in Na^+ channel-dependent cardiac tissues, setting the stage for a reentrant arrhythmia to be initiated. In addition, Na^+ channel blocking drugs such as quinidine and procainamide also possess significant K^+ channel blocking effects. In diseased myocardia, these agents may increase dispersion of refractoriness which is also arrhythmogenic. Furthermore, K^+ channel blockade may inhibit repolarizing currents contributing to the development of early afterdepolarizations and precipitate an onset of torsade de pointes. Finally, exercise-induced changes in regional coronary perfusion, regardless of whether there is a component of active myocardial ischemia, may be sufficient to alter local relative antiarrhythmic drug concentrations in normal and diseased myocardia, thereby producing a new arrhythmogenic substrate. Management of drug-induced ventricular tachycardia obviously rests on the identification and elimination of the offending agent.

15.7   Idiopathic Ventricular Tachycardia

Based on results of electrophysiology study and pharmacological testing as described above, the idiopathic variety of ventricular tachycardia can also be divided into verapamil-responsive and verapamil-nonresponsive ventricular tachycardia, either of which can be catecholamine-dependent or catecholamine-independent with respect to the arrhythmia initiation and perpetuation (Table 15-4.)

Certain features differentiate verapamil-responsive ventricular tachycardia of a right bundle branch block pattern from that of a left bundle branch block pattern. In response to overdrive ventricular pacing, entrainment and slow conduction may be demonstrable in the former, suggestive of a reentrant mechanism, but not the latter [62,110]. The former is more likely to exhibit cycle length alternans during tachycardia and the latter is more likely to require isoproterenol infusion for the arrhythmia induction. With regard to the adenosine-sensitivity, only one third of the right bundle branch block pattern and almost all of the left bundle branch block pattern ventricular tachycardia can be terminated by an intravenous bolus of adenosine (Figure 15-17) [62]. Clinically the ventricular tachycardia of a right bundle branch block pattern is more likely to manifest a sustained rhythm, whereas that of the left bundle branch block pattern manifest a repetitive nonsustained form. Also, ventricular tachycardia of a left bundle branch block pattern is more likely to be exertion-related (catecholamine-dependent requiring isoproterenol infusion for induction compared to that of a right bundle branch block pattern). During isoproterenol infusion, repetitive, nonsustained ventricular tachycardia may become sustained [42,113].

TABLE 15-4. Electropharmacologic characteristics of idiopathic ventricular tachycardia

	Verapamil-responsive Catecholamine				Verapamil-nonresponsive Catecholamine	
	Dependent		Independent		Dependent	Independent
QRS pattern	RBBB	LBBB	RBBB	LBBB	LBBB	LBBB
Cycle length dependence	+	+	+	+	–	–
Termination by overdrive pacing	+	+	+	+	–	–
Verapamil	+	+	+	+	–	–
Adenosine	+*	+	–	+	–	–
Esmolol (or propranolol)	+	+	–**	–**	+	–
Procainamide	–**	–**	–**	–**	+	+
Possible mechanism	T,R	T	T,R	T	A	A

+ = yes or responsive; – = no or nonresponsive; * constitutes only a small fraction of verapamil-responsive ventricular tachycardia of RBBB QRS morphology; **slows the rate of ventricular tachycardia without abolishing the tachycardia inducibility; A = automaticity; LBBB = left bundle branch block; RBBB = right bundle branch block; T = triggered rhythmic activity; R = reentry

Both the verapamil-responsive and non-responsive forms of idiopathic ventricular tachycardia arising from the right ventricle (left bundle branch block QRS pattern), should be distinguished from right ventricular tachycardias caused by other pathological conditions, including arrhythmogenic right ventricular dysplasia, bundle branch reentrant tachycardia associated with dilated cardiomyopathy, ventricular tachycardia occurring after surgical repair of ventricular septal defect or tetralogy of Fallot, right-sided antidromic AV reciprocating tachycardia, or ventricular tachycardia associated with atherosclerotic coronary heart disease (usually with prior myocardial infarction) (Table 15-5.) These other varieties of right ventricular tachycardias have reentry as the underlying mechanism they do not usually respond to adenosine and verapamil. Unlike adenosine or verapamil, β-adrenoceptor blocking agents, in general, are not as useful for defining the mechanism of a ventricular tachycardia because — regardless of the underlying electrophysiologic mechanism — any ventricular tachycardia that is catecholamine-dependent is likely to respond to intravenous esmolol or propranolol [11,41,42].

Despite an absence of structural heart disease as determined by clinical evaluation and laboratory testing, a focal myocarditis or subclinical cardiomyopathy cannot be excluded in patients with idiopathic ventricular tachycardia. It has been suggested that abnormal tissue corresponding to the arrhythmogenic focus may be expected to be present in this subgroup of patients [114]. Endomyocardial biopsy and magnetic resonance imaging may be required to rule out such disorders as myocarditis or arrhythmogenic right ventricular dysplasia [115]. Furthermore, incessant or repetitive monomorphic ventricu-

TABLE 15-5. Differential diagnosis of ventricular tachycardia with a QRS morphology of left bundle branch block pattern

	Idiopathic		ARVD		Cardiomyopathy	VSD/TF	Antidromic	ASHD
	TA	A	R	A	BB Reentry	s/p surgery	AVRT	
QRS frontal axis	right inferior		variable		left superior	right inferior / left inferior	left superior/inferior	variable
Initiation & termination by PES	+	−	+	−	+	+	+	+
Adenosine	+	−	−	−	−	−	+	−
Verapamil	+	−	−	−	−	−	+	−

+ = yes or responsive; − = no or nonresponsive; A = automaticity; ARVD = arrhythmogenic right ventricular dysplasia; ASHD = atherosclerotic heart disease; AVRT = atrioventricular reciprocating tachycardia; BB = bundle branch; PES = programmed electrical stimulation; R = reentry; TA = triggered rhythmic activity; TF = tetralogy of Fallot; VSD = ventricular septal defect

lar tachycardia may lead to myocardial dysfunction referred to as tachycardia-induced cardiomyopathy [116]; therefore, determination of whether ventricular tachycardia is the cause or result of the structural heart disease may be difficult in some patients.

15.8   Management of Chronic Recurrent Ventricular Tachycardia

The prognosis of patients with chronic recurrent ventricular tachycardia depends on the presence or absence of structural heart disease [1-4] and if a structural heart disease is present, the long term outcome is determined by the severity of left ventricular dysfunction [115]. The approach to treatment of recurrent ventricular tachycardia is not only influenced by the nature of the heart condition but also by the electrophysiologic mechanism of the arrhythmia [7,8,11]. β-adrenoceptor blocking agents should be considered as the drug of choice in patients with catecholamine-sensitive ventricular tachycardia associated with or without structural heart disease [11,41,42]. Alternatively, catheter ablation of this form of ventricular tachycardia may be considered if the long term treatment with β-adrenoceptor blocking agents is deemed undesirable.

15.8.1   ARTERIOSCLEROTIC HEART DISEASE AND CARDIOMYOPATHY

These patients usually have recurrent monomorphic ventricular tachycardia suggestive of a reentry mechanism [5-8,10,11,118-120]. Antiarrhythmic drug therapy remains the mainstay for the treatment of recurrent monomorphic ventricular tachycardia. However, it alone is usually not satisfactory because most antiarrhythmic drugs exert (1) negative inotropic effects which may precipitate or worsen congestive heart failure; (2) negative chronotropic effects which may cause sinus nodal dysfunction and AV block; and (3) proarrhythmic effects which may worsen the arrhythmia or provoke a new arrhythmia [121]. Otherwise, procainamide, propafenone, sotalol, and amiodarone are common antiarrhythmic drugs used for suppressing chronic recurrent ventricular tachycardia.

   The technique of radiofrequency catheter ablation should also be considered, but the success is often limited by (1) an unstable hemodynamics which precludes detailed mapping of the arrhythmia; (2) the presence of multiple arrhythmogenic foci not easily accessible to radiofrequency energy; (3) a large lesion which is often needed to completely ablate the arrhythmia; (4) the presence of myocardial fibrosis altering the endocardial activation sequence; and (5) the progressive nature of the disease process which promotes development of new ventricular arrhythmias. Even in patients with bundle branch reentrant tachycardia, subsequent emergence of other forms of ventricular arrhythmias is often observed despite successful ablation of bundle branch reentry. The effectiveness in preventing sudden cardiac death along with the ease with which a cardioverter-defibrillator can be transvenously implanted has made the implantation of cardioverter-defibrillator the primary treatment modality in this group of patients. Antiarrhythmic drug therapy or radiofrequency catheter ablation is used only as an adjunctive measure following the implantation of a cardioverter-defibrillator [122]. Prior to the implantation of a cardioverter-defibrillator, it is essential to correct triggering factors such as active ischemic process, congestive heart failure and/or electrolyte imbalance so that the recurrence rate of ventricular tachycardia can be reduced. At times, surgical resection of ventricular aneurysm along with endomyocardial excision of the arrhythmogenic tissue may be needed.

15.8.2 ARRHYTHMOGENIC RIGHT VENTRICULAR DYSPLASIA

Arrhythmogenic right ventricular dysplasia is characterized by fibro-fatty replacement of myocytes with scattered foci of inflammation predominately affecting the right ventricle (the left ventricle can also be involved) [123]. It is a familiar disease and is one of the common causes of sudden cardiac death syndrome in young adults [124]. Clinical identification of this disease include regional hypokinesia and segmental bulging or global hypokinesia of the right ventricle as documented by echocardiography or right ventricular angiography. However, magnetic resonance imaging may be required to unravel the diagnosis [115]. The ventricular tachycardia (a left bundle branch block QRS pattern with a variable frontal axis) associated with this disease is usually of a reentrant mechanism as it can usually be initiated by programmed ventricular extrastimulation, terminated by overdrive ventricular pacing, and is not responsive to intravenous adenosine or verapamil. Potent antiarrhythmic drugs such as sotalol and amiodarone have been advocated for the suppression of ventricular tachycardia associated with right ventricular dysplasia [125]. Because of the progressive nature of the disease, radiofrequency catheter ablation and surgical intervention offer disappointing results, and the implantation of a cardioverter-defibrillator is highly recommended in patients at risk of sudden cardiac death syndrome [126-128].

15.8.3 IDIOPATHIC VENTRICULAR TACHYCARDIA

The prognosis of patients with idiopathic ventricular tachycardia is generally benign [2-4]. However, congestive heart failure and sudden cardiac death have been reported. Echocardiography and magnetic resonance imaging are needed to rule out right ventricular dysplasia, especially in patients with idiopathic right ventricular tachycardia [115]. To avoid tachycardia-induced cardiomyopathy [114], antiarrhythmic drug therapy or radiofrequency catheter ablation [129] is indicated to suppress or abolish the arrhythmia. Treadmill exercise testing [41,42] and electrophysiology study [7,8,10,11] are useful in defining the mechanism and characteristics of idiopathic ventricular tachycardia and in selecting an effective antiarrhythmic regimen, e.g., verapamil or a β-adrenoceptor blocking agent, either alone or in combination, or other antiarrhythmic drugs.

15.9   Radiofrequency Catheter Ablation

The success rate of catheter ablation for ventricular tachycardia depends greatly on the nature of anatomic substrates. A higher success rate and better long-term result are noted for ventricular tachycardia in patients without clinically recognizable structural heart disease (i.e., idiopathic ventricular tachycardia) compared to those with significant structural heart disease such as atherosclerotic heart disease with prior myocardial infarction and primary or secondary cardiomyopathy

15.9.1 IDIOPATHIC VENTRICULAR TACHYCARDIA.

Right ventricular tachycardia usually arises from the outflow tract underneath the pulmonic valve and above the level of the His bundle recording site (complete left bundle branch block/right inferior axis pattern) (Figure 15-18). Ventricular electrograms recorded at the site of ablation should precede the onset of the tachycardia QRS complex. However, ventricular-paced mapping to reproduce a QRS pattern identical or similar to that of the template pattern of the arrhythmia is critical for successful ablation (Figure 15-19 & Figure 15-20) [129]. A right anterior oblique (RAO) followed by a left anterior oblique (LAO) fluoroscopic view should facilitate the mapping procedure before ablation of the arrhythmia (Figure 15-18). Because of the proximity of the arrhythmia focus to the pulmonic valve, valvular movement may make stable positioning of the tip of the ablation catheter difficult to maintain during the application of radiofrequency energy. For the ablation of right ventricular outflow tract ventricular tachycardia, the goal of the radiofrequency application is to achieve a maximum electrode-tissue interface temperature of 60° – 65°C for 30 – 40 sec. Higher temperatures should be avoided. Perforation of the ventricular myocardium is a potentially serious complication.

Idiopathic ventricular tachycardia can also be located at the right ventricular inflow tract or apex. In these cases, the diagnosis of right ventricular dysplasia should be entertained as it is associated with a relatively high recurrence rate of ventricular tachycardia following successful radiofrequency catheter ablation.

Left ventricular tachycardia usually exhibits a right bundle branch block pattern with a superior frontal axis (Figure 15-21). This tachycardia is commonly localized to the posterior or low-mid interventricular septum. The electrograms obtained are often preceded by Purkinje potentials (Figure 15-21) [130-132]. However, these Purkinje potentials are relatively non-specific. Similar to the right ventricular outflow tract tachycardia, it is critical to perform ventricular-paced mapping to match the template QRS pattern of the arrhythmia (Figure 15-22). Less frequently, idiopathic left ventricular tachycardia is located at the left lateral or left anterior wall with a right inferior frontal QRS axis. Likewise, applications of radiofrequency energy that achieve an electrode-tissue interface temperature of 60°-65°C for 30 - 40 sec should suffice for successful elimination of the tachycardia.

15.9.2 VENTRICULAR TACHYCARDIA ASSOCIATED WITH STRUCTURAL HEART DISEASE

Bundle branch reentrant tachycardia accounts for approximately 6% of inducible sustained monomorphic ventricular tachycardia (Figure 15-23) [26]. It occurs more commonly in patients with dilated cardiomyopathy which can be either primary or secondary (e.g., atherosclerotic or valvular heart disease) [133-135]. Typically, there is a combination of nonspecific intraventricular conduction delay of an incomplete left bundle block pattern and a prolonged HV interval at baseline. The tachycardia uses the right bundle

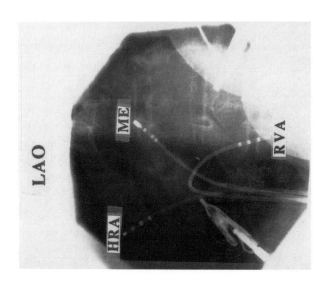

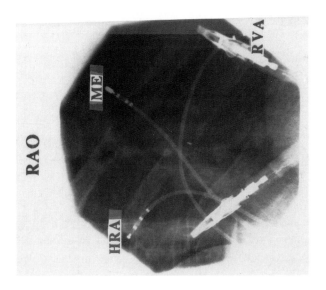

FIGURE 15-18. Fluoroscopic views of a catheter electrode position for ablating idiopathic right ventricular tachycardia arising from the right ventricular outflow tract. LAO, left anterior oblique view; RAO, right anterior oblique view at 30°; HRA, high right atrium; ME, mapping electrode (also ablation electrode); RVA, right ventricular apex.

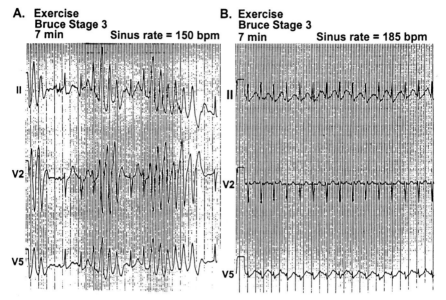

A. Exercise
Bruce Stage 3
7 min   **Sinus rate = 150 bpm**

B. Exercise
Bruce Stage 3
7 min   **Sinus rate = 185 bpm**

FIGURE 15-19. Idiopathic non-sustained ventricular tachycardia provoked by treadmill exercise testing into Stage 3 of the standard Bruce protocol in a 21 year old woman. Panel A: The ventricular tachycardia rate approximated 280 beats per minute. Full 12-lead ECG showed that the ventricular tachycardia had a left bundle branch block QRS pattern with a right inferior frontal plane axis (not shown). Panel B: One year post-catheter ablation, repeat treadmill exercise test to a faster sinus rate failed to provoke ventricular tachycardia. Paper speed 25 mm/sec.

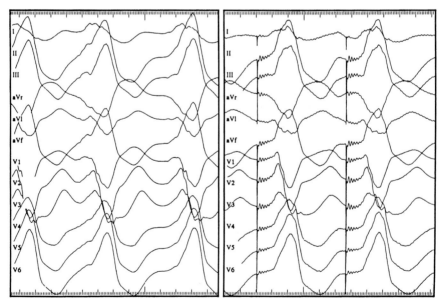

FIGURE 15-20. Ventricular-paced mapping for idiopathic ventricular tachycardia arising from the right ventricular outflow tract. The mapping electrode (ME) is shown in Figure 15-18. Note close similarity of 12 lead QRS morphology between ventricular tachycardia (left panel) and ventricular-paced rhythm (right panel). Paper speed 200 mm/sec

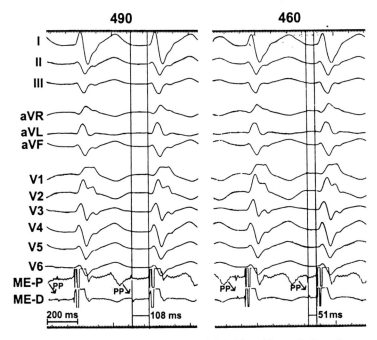

FIGURE 15-21. Recordings of Purkinje potentials in idiopathic ventricular tachycardia arising from the low mid-septum of the left ventricle. Note variable intervals between the Purkinje potential (PP) (arrows) and the onset of QRS complex during ventricular tachycardia. In the left panel, the interval from the PP to local ventricular activation is 108 ms, while in the right panel (recording from different site) this interval measures 51 ms. ME-P, proximal mapping bipolar electrodes; ME-D, distal mapping bipolar electrodes.

branch for anterograde conduction and the left bundle branch for retrograde conduction, thereby manifesting a complete left bundle branch block pattern with a superior frontal axis. Characteristically, there is a constant 1:1 retrograde His bundle potential/ventricular electrogram relationship (Figure 15-23) and spontaneous RR interval variation is preceded by a change in the H-H interval, suggesting that the His-Purkinje system is an integral part of the tachycardia circuit.

Ablation of the proximal right bundle branch is a rather simple procedure and is effective in interrupting the reentrant circuit [133-136]. If there is a preexisting complete left bundle branch block, implantation of a permanent pacemaker is necessary following successful ablation of the arrhythmia. Atypical bundle branch reentrant tachycardia is confined to the left side of the conduction system, not readily amenable to the ablation procedure. Clinically other forms of ventricular tachycardia often emerge following successful ablation of bundle branch reentrant tachycardia, implantation of a cardioverter-defibrillator, with or without concurrent antiarrhythmic drug therapy, is generally needed in this subset group of patients. However, successful ablation of bundle branch reentrant tachycardia serves to reduce the recurrence rate of the arrhythmia, thereby reducing the frequency of intervention from the implanted cardioverter-defibrillator.

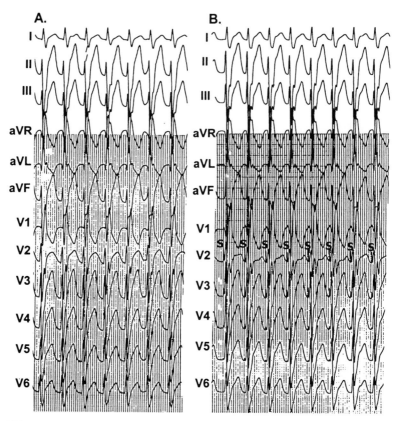

FIGURE 15-22. Ventricular-paced mapping for idiopathic ventricular tachycardia arising from the low mid-septum of the left ventricle. Note close similarity of the QRS morphology (right bundle branch block with a left/superior axis) on 12-lead ECG recording obtained during ventricular tachycardia (Panel A) and ventricular pacing from the successful site of radiofrequency catheter ablation (Panel B). Stimulus artifacts (S) best seen in V_2 or V_3. Paper speed 25 mm/sec.

Aside from bundle branch reentrant tachycardia, the location of ventricular tachycardia cannot usually be predicted from the surface electrocardiogram, and ventricular tachycardia may have variable exits manifesting as ventricular tachycardia with different QRS morphologies. Endocardial mapping is often technically difficult. New technologies are on the horizon. Specialized mapping systems currently available or under investigation include: 1) epicardial mapping through the coronary sinus venous system using a specially-designed system of micro-electrode catheters, 2) a basket catheter with upwards of 32 pairs of electrodes that is placed in the left or right ventricle for computerized mapping of endocardial activation, and 3) a computer-generated color-coded three-dimensional endocardial activation map created using either electromagnetic or high resolution non-contact imaging (Figure 15-24) [137,138].

Useful electrophysiological parameters to guide radiofrequency catheter ablation [139-147] include (1) the earliest site of endocardial activation, (2) mid-diastolic or pre-systolic potentials representing activation via a region of slow conduction, (3) ventricular-paced mapping, and (4) entrainment with concealed fusion along with post-pacing interval from the last stimulus to the following electrogram equal to the ventricular tachycardia cycle length (± ≤30 msec) and the stimulus to the QRS interval equal to the local electrogram to QRS interval during the ventricular tachycardia (Figures 15-25 & 15-26). Of note, in recording mid-diastolic or presystolic potentials, their prevalence is only 8% and artifacts caused by catheter movement in contact with the endocardium should be excluded [148]. Because of the complexity of the anatomic substrate that gives rise to ventricular tachycardia, no single approach has been shown to be reproducibly reliable in predicting the successful site for radiofrequency catheter ablation. Radiofrequency energy is delivered to achieve a temperature of 60–65° for one minute and a series of lesions is applied extending approximately 2–4 cm along the border of the scar tissue [145,146]. Specially-designed radiofrequency ablation catheters that feature cooling of the tip (preventing coagulum formation) may allow creation of larger and deeper endomyocardial lesions. The ability to create larger and deeper lesions may be more effective at eliminating ventricular tachycardia in patients with atherosclerotic coronary artery disease and prior myocardial infarction, or those with a primary or secondary cardiomyopathy [149].

15.9.3 POSTSURGICAL CORRECTION OF TETRALOGY OF FALLOT

The surgical correction procedure of the tetralogy of fallot entails a ventriculotomy in the right ventricular outflow tract through which the ventricular septal defect is repaired, and a patch is placed interposing the incision line of the ventriculotomy to expand the right ventricular outflow tract.

Chronic recurrent monomorphic ventricular tachycardia may occur following surgical correction of the tetralogy of Fallot. The arrhythmia usually occurs between 4 and 12 years after the surgery and characteristically manifests a complete left bundle branch block QRS pattern with a left inferior frontal axis. Antiarrhythmic therapy is often unsuccessful [150]. The mechanism of ventricular tachycardia is of a reentrant mechanism. Electrophysiology study can provoke and terminate the arrhythmia with programmed electrical stimulation and can identify an area of slow conduction along with demonstration of an excitable gap (e.g., entrainment with concealed fusion). The reentrant circuit responsible for the arrhythmia has not been well defined, but it often involves the ventriculotomy scar. Radiofrequency catheter ablation to produce a linear lesion between the scar and the pulmonic valve or between the outflow tract patch and the tricuspid annulus may effectively abolish the arrhythmia [151,152]. Since the scar and the patch are electrically inert areas, the application of the three dimensional anatomic-magnetic imaging technique [137] is expected to provide a useful guide during radiofrequency catheter ablation of the arrhythmia.

15.10   Chemical Ablation of Ventricular Tachycardia

Based on the theory that a "culprit" artery or arteries can be identified, the technique of transcoronary ethyl alcohol infusion was developed for ablating cardiac tachyarrhyth-

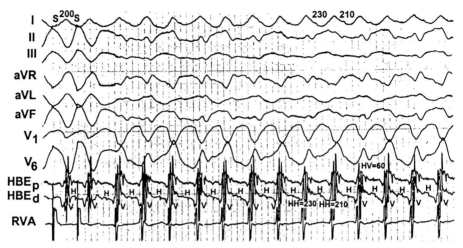

FIGURE 15-23. Induction of bundle branch reentrant ventricular tachycardia in a 64 year-old man with dilated cardiomyopathy. The QRS morphology on the ECG during sinus rhythm showed an incomplete left bundle branch block (LBBB) pattern (not shown). Rapid ventricular pacing at a cycle length of 200 ms provoked the onset of ventricular tachycardia. As seen here, the induced tachycardia exhibits a LBBB QRS morphology. There is a His bundle potential (H) inscribed before each local ventricular electrogram (V) in the distal His bundle recording (HBE$_d$). The HV interval increases from 50 ms during sinus rhythm (not shown) to 60 ms during the tachycardia. Also note that the V-V cycle length alternans is preceded by H-H cycle length alternans (230 and 210 ms) suggesting that the His-Purkinje system is an integral part of the reentrant circuit. Surface ECG leads I, II, III, aVR, aVL, aVF, V$_1$ and V$_6$ are simultaneously recorded. S, stimulus artifact; HBE$_p$, proximal His bundle recording; RVA, right ventricular apex. Paper speed 100 mm/sec.

mias, in particular, ventricular tachycardia [153-156]. The mechanism by which intracoronary infusion of alcohol abolishes ventricular tachyarrhythmias has been primarily ascribed to the interruption of coronary blood supply to the arrhythmogenic substrate.

While transcoronary chemical ablation seems to be effective in destroying the arrhythmia substrate, intracoronary infusion of alcohol can cause coronary arterial spasm and chemical reflux, thus damaging a large volume of myocardium. This may result in worsening of left ventricular function and/or conduction abnormalities, such as sinus arrest or complete atrioventricular block [156-158].

15.11   Surgical Intervention

In selected patients who have failed combined therapy with cardioverter-defibrillator implantation and antiarrhythmic drug therapy, surgical resection of the "culprit" scar tissue may be indicated. Activation mapping and identification of mid-diastolic potential during ventricular tachycardia are used to guide subendocardial resection and application of cryoablation. The success rate of interrupting and/or removing the anatomic substrates of ventricular tachycardia is approximately 90% in experienced hands [159-163].

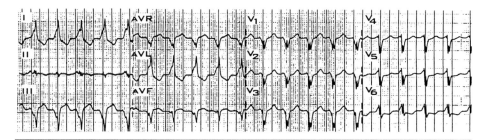

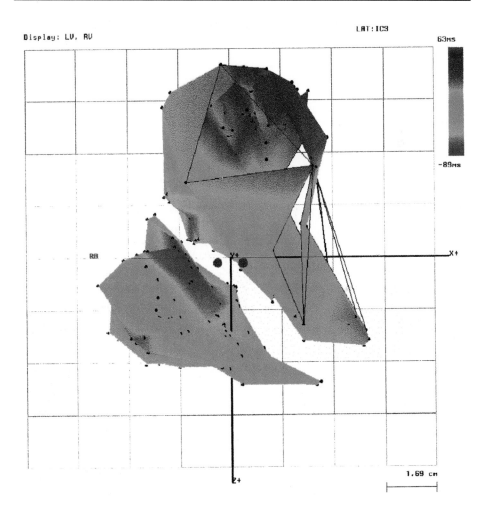

FIGURE 15-24. Ventricular tachycardia in a 45 year-old man with a history of an old inferior wall myocardial infarction. Upper panel: 12 lead ECG of the clinical tachycardia (rate 130/min). The QRS complexes during the ventricular tachycardia exhibited a left bundle branch block pattern with a left superior frontal plane axis. Paper speed 25 mm/sec. Lower panel: coronal view of the anatomic-magnetic map of both the right and left ventricle in this patient during the ventricular tachycardia. Note the earliest site of activation is localized to the basilar portion of the right ventricle directly adjacent to the interventricular septum

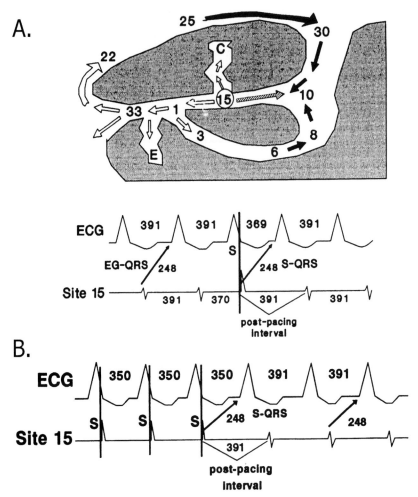

FIGURE 15-25. Schematic diagrams of a figure-eight reentry circuit and tracings of the surface ECG and electrogram timing within the reentrant circuit. Solid arrows indicate non-stimulated tachycardia excitation wave-fronts. Open arrows indicate excitation wave-fronts traveling in an orthodromic direction produced by capturing stimuli. Stimulated antidromic wave-fronts are shown as hatched arrows. All times are given in milliseconds. Panel A, *(upper portion)*: Stimulus capture at site 15 produces an orthodromic wave-front that travels from site 15 to the common pathway exit at site 1 and then to the QRS onset near site 33. A stimulated antidromic wave-front travels from site 15 toward the common pathway entrance at site 10 but collides with the returning non-stimulated orthodromic wave-front from the previous tachycardia beat and is extinguished within the common pathway. The stimulated orthodromic wave-front advances the tachycardia without change in the QRS morphology and then continues through the circuit to reset the tachycardia (entrainment with concealed fusion). The cycle length of this tachycardia is 391 ms. Panel A *(lower portion)*: The effect on the surface ECG of a single stimulus at site 15 is shown. The stimulus artifact is the thick vertical line designated 'S'. The interval from the local electrogram (activation time) during tachycardia at site 15 to the following QRS on the surface ECG is 248 ms (EG-QRS). The interval from the stimulus at site 15 to the advanced QRS (S-QRS) is 248 ms. The post-pacing interval from the stimulus to the succeeding electrogram is 391 ms, which is equal to the tachycardia cycle length. Panel B: The effect of a train of stimuli at site 15 is illustrated. The pacing cycle length of the train is 350 ms. The EG-QRS interval during tachycardia is 248 ms and is equal to the interval from the last stimulus in the train to the last QRS advanced to the pacing cycle length (S-QRS). The post-pacing interval is the interval from the last stimulus to the following electrogram and is equal to the tachycardia cycle length of 391 ms. From [145] with permission.

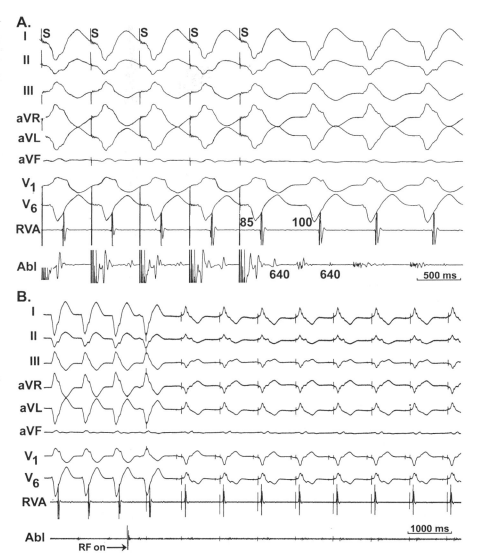

FIGURE 15-26. Entrainment with concealed fusion during ventricular pacing in a 72-year old patient with monomorphic ventricular tachycardia associated with a previous myocardial infarction due to reentry. The findings during programmed electrical stimulation in panel A are consistent with pacing at a reentry circuit site near an "exit" from the infarct scar. From the top of each tracing are surface ECG leads I, II, III, aVR, aVL, aVF, V1, and V6; and bipolar intracardiac recordings from the right ventricular apex (RVA) and ablation (Abl). Panel A: Sustained monomorphic ventricular tachycardia with a cycle length of 640 msec is present. The last five pacing stimuli at a cycle length (S-S) of 560 msec is shown. The ventricular tachycardia is continually reset without an alteration in the QRS morphology consistent with entrainment with concealed fusion. The stimulus-to-QRS (S-QRS) interval is 85 msec. As shown in the last beat of the tracing, the electrogram onset at the recording site occurs 100 msec before the QRS onset. Thus, the S-QRS interval is only 15 msec shorter than the electrogram-to-QRS (EG-QRS) interval. The post-pacing interval matches the ventricular tachycardia cycle length of 640 msec. Panel B: Radiofrequency current is applied to this site during ventricular tachycardia using a temperature-controlled cooled-tip ablation catheter (50 °C for 60 sec). Note that the tachycardia terminates after one beat, with restoration of the patient's baseline rhythm (AV sequential pacing delivered by an implanted pacing-cardioverter-defibrillator).

References

1. Moss AJ: Clinical significance of ventricular arrhythmias in patients with and without coronary artery disease. *Prog Cardiovasc Dis* **23**:33-52, 1980.

2. Adams CW: Functional paroxysmal ventricular tachycardia. *American Journal of Cardiology* **9**:215-222, 1962.

3. Bergdahl DM, Stevenson JG, Kawabori I, Guntheroth WG: Prognosis in primary ventricular tachycardia in the pediatric patient. *Circulation* **62**:897-901, 1980.

4. Vetter VL, Josephson ME, Horowitz LN: Idiopathic recurrent sustained ventricular tachycardia in children and adolescents. *Am J Cardiol* **47**:315-22, 1981.

5. Josephson ME, Horowitz LN, Farshidi A, Kastor JA: Recurrent sustained ventricular tachycardia. 1. Mechanisms. *Circulation* **57**:431-40, 1978.

6. Akhtar M, Gilbert C, Wolf FG, Schmidt DH: Reentry within the His-Purkinje system. Elucidation of re-entrant circuit using right bundle branch and His bundle recordings. *Circulation* **58**:295-304, 1978.

7. Sung RJ, Shapiro WA, Shen EN, et al.: Effects of verapamil on ventricular tachycardias possibly caused by reentry, automaticity, and triggered activity. *J Clin Invest* **72**:350-60, 1983.

8. Sung RJ, Shen EN, Morady F, et al.: Electrophysiologic mechanism of exercise-induced sustained ventricular tachycardia. *Am J Cardiol* **51**:525-30, 1983.

9. Wellens HJ, Duren DR, Lie KI: Observations on mechanisms of ventricular tachycardia in man. *Circulation* **54**:237-44, 1976.

10. Sung RJ, Huycke EC, Lai WT, et al.: Clinical and electrophysiologic mechanisms of exercise-induced ventricular tachyarrhythmias. *Pacing Clin Electrophysiol* **11**:1347-57, 1988.

11. Sung RJ, Keung EC, Nguyen NX, Huycke EC: Effects of beta-adrenergic blockade on verapamil-responsive and verapamil-irresponsive sustained ventricular tachycardias. *J Clin Invest* **81**:688-99, 1988.

12. Wellens HJ: Value and limitations of programmed electrical stimulation of the heart in the study and treatment of tachycardias. *Circulation* **57**:845-53, 1978.

13. Wellens HJJ, Brugada P, Vanagt EJDM, et al.: New studies with triggered automaticity. In: Harrison DC, ed. *Cardiac Arrhythmias, A Decade of Progress.* Boston, MA: G.K. Hall & Co., 601-610: 1981.

14. Hoffman BF, Rosen MR: Cellular mechanisms for cardiac arrhythmias. *Circ Res* **49**:1-15, 1981.

15. Hoffman BF, Dangman, K. Are arrhythmias caused by automatic impulse generation? In: Paes de Carvalho A, Hoffman BF, Liebermann H, eds. *Normal and Abnormal Conduction in the Heart.* Mount Kisco, NY: Futura Publishing, 429-460: 1982.

16. Rosen MR, Reder RF: Does triggered activity have a role in the genesis of cardiac arrhythmias? *Ann Intern Med* **94**:794-801, 1981.

17. Wit AL, Rosen MR, Hoffman BF: Electrophysiology and pharmacology of cardiac arrhythmias. II. Relationship of normal and abnormal electrical activity of cardiac fibers to the genesis of arrhythmias b. Re-entry. Section II. *Am Heart J* **88**:798-806, 1974.

18. Wit AL, Rosen MR, Hoffman BF: Electrophysiology and pharmacology of cardiac arrhythmias. II. Relationship of normal and abnormal electrical activity of cardiac fibers to the genesis of arrhythmias B. Re-entry. Section I. *Am Heart J* **88**:664-70, 1974.

19. Wit AL, Rosen MR, Hoffman BF: Electrophysiology and pharmacology of cardiac arrhythmias. II. Relationship of normal and abnormal electrical activity of cardiac fibers to the genesis of arrhythmias. A Automaticity. *Am Heart J* **88**:515-24, 1974.

20. Almendral JM, Rosenthal ME, Stamato NJ, et al.: Analysis of the resetting phenomenon in sustained uniform ventricular tachycardia: incidence and relation to termination. *J Am Coll Cardiol* **8**:294-300, 1986.

21. Almendral JM, Stamato NJ, Rosenthal ME, et al.: Resetting response patterns during sustained ventricular tachycardia: relationship to the excitable gap. *Circulation* **74**:722-30, 1986.

22. Okumura K, Olshansky B, Henthorn RW, et al.: Demonstration of the presence of slow conduction during sustained ventricular tachycardia in man: use of transient entrainment of the tachycardia. *Circulation* **75**:369-78, 1987.

23. Okumura K, Henthorn RW, et al.: Further observations on transient entrainment: importance of pacing site and properties of the components of the reentry circuit. *Circulation* **72**:1293-307, 1985.

24. Lai WT, Huycke EC, Keung EC, et al.: Electrophysiologic manifestations of the excitable gap of ortho-dromic atrioventricular reciprocating tachycardia demonstrated by single extrastimulation. *Am J Cardiol* **63**:545-55, 1989.

25. Akhtar M, Damato AN, Batsford WP, et al.: Demonstration of re-entry within the His-Purkinje system in man. *Circulation* **50**:1150-62, 1974.

26. Caceres J, Jazayeri M, McKinnie J, et al.: Sustained bundle branch reentry as a mechanism of clinical tachycardia. *Circulation* **79**:256-70, 1989.

27. de Bakker JM, van Capelle FJ, Janse MJ, et al.: Reentry as a cause of ventricular tachycardia in patients with chronic ischemic heart disease: electrophysiologic and anatomic correlation. *Circulation* **77**:589-606, 1988.

28. de Bakker JM, van Capelle FJ, Janse MJ, et al.: Macroreentry in the infarcted human heart: the mecha-nism of ventricular tachycardias with a "focal" activation pattern. *J Am Coll Cardiol* **18**:1005-14, 1991.

29. Pogwizd SM, Hoyt RH, Saffitz JE, et al.: Reentrant and focal mechanisms underlying ventricular tachy-cardia in the human heart. *Circulation* **86**:1872-87, 1992.

30. Denker S, Lehmann M, Mahmud R, et al.: Facilitation of ventricular tachycardia induction with abrupt changes in ventricular cycle length. *Am J Cardiol* **53**:508-15, 1984.

31. Denker S, Lehmann MH, Mahmud R, et al.: Facilitation of macroreentry within the His-Purkinje system with abrupt changes in cycle length. *Circulation* **69**:26-32, 1984.

32. Reddy CP, Gettes LS: Use of isoproterenol as an aid to electrical induction of chronic recurrent ventric-ular tachycardia. *Am J Cardiol* **44**:705-713, 1979.

33. DiCarlo LA, Jr., Morady F, Schwartz AB, et al.: Clinical significance of ventricular fibrillation-flutter induced by ventricular programmed stimulation. *Am Heart J* **109**:959-63, 1985.

34. Lerman BB, Belardinelli L, West GA, et al.: Adenosine-sensitive ventricular tachycardia: evidence sug-gesting cyclic AMP-mediated triggered activity. *Circulation* **74**:270-80, 1986.

35. Lerman BB: Response of nonreentrant catecholamine-mediated ventricular tachycardia to endogenous adenosine and acetylcholine. Evidence for myocardial receptor-mediated effects. *Circulation* **87**:382-90, 1993.

36. Wellens HJ, Bar FW, et al.: Effect of procainamide, propranolol and verapamil on mechanism of tachy-cardia in patients with chronic recurrent ventricular tachycardia. *Am J Cardiol* **40**:579-85, 1977.

37. Stewart RB, Bardy GH, Greene HL: Wide complex tachycardia: misdiagnosis and outcome after emer-gent therapy. *Ann Intern Med* **104**:766-771, 1986.

38. Spear JF, Horowitz LN, Hodess AB, et al.: Cellular electrophysiology of human myocardial infarction. 1. abnormalities of cellular activation. *Circulation* **59**:247-256, 1979.

39. Gilmour RF, Jr., Zipes DP: Cellular basis for cardiac arrhythmias. *Cardiol Clin* **1**:3-11, 1983.

40. Gilmour RF, Jr., Heger JJ, Prystowsky EN, Zipes DP: Cellular electrophysiologic abnormalities of dis-eased human ventricular myocardium. *Am J Cardiol* **51**:137-44, 1983.

41. Sung RJ, Tai DY, Svinarich JT: Beta-adrenoceptor blockade: electrophysiology and antiarrhythmic mechanisms. *Am Heart J* **108**:1115-20, 1984.

42. Sung RJ, Olukotun AY, Baird CL, Huycke EC: Efficacy and safety of oral nadolol for exercise-induced ventricular arrhythmias. *Am J Cardiol* **60**:15D-20D, 1987.

43. Cranefield PF: Action potentials, afterpotentials, and arrhythmias. *Circ Res* **41**:415-23, 1977.

44. Cranefield PF, Wit AL: Cardiac arrhythmias. *Annu Rev Physiol* **41**:459-72, 1979.

45. Cranefield PF: The conduction of the cardiac impulse 1951-1986. *Experientia* **43**:1040-4, 1987.

46. Cranefield PF, Wit AL, Hoffman BF: Conduction of the cardiac impulse. 3. Characteristics of very slow conduction. *J Gen Physiol* **59**:227-46, 1972.

47. Gadsby DC, Cranefield PF: Two levels of resting potential in cardiac Purkinje fibers. *J Gen Physiol* **70**:725-46, 1977.

48. Dangman KH, Hoffman BF: Studies on overdrive stimulation of canine cardiac Purkinje fibers: Maxi-mal diastolic potential as determinant of the response. *J Am Coll Cardiol* **2**:1183-1190, 1983.

49. Johnson NJ, Rosen MR. The distinction between triggered and other cardiac arrhythmias. In: Brugada P, Wellens HJJ, eds. *Cardiac Arrhythmias: Where to Go from Here?* Mount Kisco, NY: Futura Publishing Co., 129-145: 1987.

50. Jalife J, Antzelevitch C: Pacemaker annihilation: diagnostic and therapeutic implications. *Am Heart J* **100**:128-30, 1980.

51. Vassalle M: The relationship among cardiac pacemakers: Overdrive suppression. *Circ Res* **41**:268-277, 1977.

52. Gadsby DC, Cranefield PF: Direct measurement of changes in sodium pump current in canine cardiac Purkinje fibers. *Proc Natl Acad Sci U S A* **76**:1783-7, 1979.

53. Gadsby DC, Cranefield PF: Electrogenic sodium extrusion in cardiac Purkinje fibers. *J Gen Physiol* **73**:819-37, 1979.

54. Gadsby DC: Activation of electrogenic Na+/K+ exchange by extracellular K+ in canine cardiac Purkinje fibers. *J Gen Physiol* **77**:4035-4039, 1980.

55. Coraboeuf E, Deroubaix E, Coulombe A: Acidosis-induced abnormal repolarization and repetitive activity in isolated dog Purkinje fibers. *J Physiol (Paris)* **76**:97-106, 1980.

56. Coulombe A, Coraboeuf E, Deroubaix E: Computer stimulation of acidosis-induced abnormal repolarization and repetitive activity in dog Purkinje fibers. *J Physiol (Paris)* **76**:107-112, 1980.

57. Davis LD, Helmer PR, Ballantyne F, 3rd: Production of slow responses in canine cardiac Purkinje fibers exposed to reduced pH. *J Mol Cell Cardiol* **8**:61-76, 1976.

58. Davis LD, Helmer PR: Electrophysiological effects of norepinephrine on slow responses induced in isolated canine cardiac Purkinje fibers by reduced extracellular pH. *J Pharmacol Exp Ther* **214**:94-100, 1980.

59. Lauer MR, Rusy BF, Davis LD: H+-induced membrane depolarization in canine cardiac Purkinje fibers. *Am J Physiol* **247**:H312-21, 1984.

60. Rosen MR, Wit AL, Hoffman BF. Electrophysiology and pharmacology of cardiac arrhythmias. VI. Cardiac effects of verapamil. *Am Heart J* **89**:665-73, 1975.

61. Zipes DP, Besch HR, Watanabe AM: Role of the slow current in cardiac electrophysiology. *Circulation* **51**:761-6, 1975.

62. Lee KL, Lauer MR, Young C, et al.: Spectrum of electrophysiologic and electropharmacologic characteristics of verapamil-sensitive ventricular tachycardia in patients without structural heart disease. *Am J Cardiol* **77**:967-73, 1996.

63. Sung RJ, Lauer MR. Verapamil, adenosine, and catecholamine-sensitive ventricular tachycardia. In: Zipes DP, Jalife J, eds. *Cardiac Electrophysiology: From Cell to Bedside.* 2nd ed. Philadelphia: W.B. Saunders, 907-919: 1994.

64. Matsuda H, Noma A, Kurachi Y, Irisawa H: Transient depolarization and spontaneous voltage fluctuations in isolated single cells from guinea pig ventricles. Calcium-mediated membrane potential fluctuations. *Circ Res* **51**:142-51, 1982.

65. Moak JP, Rosen MR: Induction and termination of triggered activity by pacing in isolated canine Purkinje fibers. *Circulation* **69**:149-162, 1984.

66. Wit AL, Cranefield PF: Triggered and automatic activity in the canine coronary sinus. *Circ Res* **41**:434-45, 1977.

67. Wit AL, Cranefield PF, Gadsby DC: Electrogenic sodium extrusion can stop triggered activity in the canine coronary sinus. *Circ Res* **49**:1029-42, 1981.

68. Rosen MR, Danilo P, Weiss RM: Actions of adenosine on normal and abnormal impulse initiation in canine ventricle. *Am J Physiol* **244**:H715, 1983.

69. West GA, Isenberg G, Belardinelli L: Antagonism of forskolin effects by adenosine in isolated hearts and ventricular myocytes. *Am J Physiol* **250**:H769-77, 1986.

70. Isenberg G, Belardinelli L: Ionic basis for the antagonism between adenosine and isoproterenol on isolated mammalian ventricular myocytes. *Circ Res* **55**:309-25, 1984.

71. Belardinelli L, Isenberg G: Actions of adenosine and isoproterenol on isolated mammalian ventricular myocytes. *Circ Res* **53**:287-97, 1983.

72. Belardinelli L, Lerman BB: Adenosine: cardiac electrophysiology. *Pacing Clin Electrophysiol* **14**:1672-80, 1991.

73. Lerman BB, Belardinelli L: Cardiac electrophysiology of adenosine. Basic and clinical concepts. *Circulation* **83**:1499-509, 1991.

74. Dobson JG, Schrader J: Role of extracellular and intracellular adenosine in the attenuation of catecholamine evoked responses in guinea pig heart. *J Mol Cell Cardiol* **16**:813, 1984.

75. Rardon DP, Bailey JC: Adenosine attenuation of the electrophysiological effects of isoproterenol on canine cardiac Purkinje fibers. *J Pharmacol Exp Ther* **228**:792-798, 1984.

76. Rodriguez-Pereira E, Viana AP: The actions of verapamil on experimental arrhythmias. *Arzneimitteforschung* **18**:175-179, 1968.

77. Rosen MR, Danilo P: Effects of tetrodotoxin, lidocaine, verapamil, and AHR-2666 on ouabain-induced delayed afterdepolarizations in canine Purkinje fibers. *Circ Res* **46**:117-124, 1980.

78. Melville KI, Shister HE, Hug S: Iproveratril: Experimental data on coronary dilation and antiarrhythmia action. *Can Med Assoc J* **90**:761-770, 1964.

79. Wellens HJ, Bar FW, Farre J, et al.: Initiation and termination of ventricular tachycardia by supraventricular stimuli. Incidence and electrophysiologic determinants as observed during programmed stimulation of the heart. *Am J Cardiol* **46**:576-82, 1980.

80. Zipes DP, Foster PR, Troup PJ, Pedersen DH: Atrial induction of ventricular tachycardia: reentry versus triggered automaticity. *Am J Cardiol* **44**:1-8, 1979.

81. Nguyen NX, Yang PT, Huycke E, Sung RJ: Verapamil and ventricular tachyarrhythmias. *Pacing Clin Electrophysiol* **10**:571-8, 1987.

82. El-Sherif N, Lazzara R: Reentrant ventricular arrhythmias in the late myocardial infarction period. 7. Effect of verapamil and D-600 and the role of "slow channel". *Circulation* **60**:605-615, 1979.

83. Reuter H, Scholz J: The regulation of the calcium conductance of cardiac muscle by adrenaline. *J Physiol (London)* **264**:49-62, 1977.

84. Vargas G, Akhtar M, Damato AN: Electrophysiologic effects of isoproterenol on cardiac conduction system in man. *Am Heart J* **90**:25-34, 1975.

85. Schwartz A, Triggle DJ: Cellular action of calcium channel blocking drugs. *Ann Rev Med* **35**:325-339, 1984.

86. Brum G, Flockerzi V, Hofmann F, et al.: Injection of catalytic subunit of cAMP-dependent protein kinase into isolated cardiac myocytes. *Pflugers Arch* **398**:147-54, 1983.

87. Brum G, Osterrieder W, Trautwein W: Beta-adrenergic increase in the calcium conductance of cardiac myocytes studied with the patch clamp. *Pflugers Arch* **401**:111-8, 1984.

88. Bean BP, Nowycky MC, Tsien RW: Beta-adrenergic modulation of calcium channels in frog ventricular heart cells. *Nature* **307**:371-5, 1984.

89. Kameyama M, Hofmann F, Trautwein W: On the mechanism of beta-adrenergic regulation of the Ca channel in the guinea-pig heart. *Pflugers Arch* **405**:285-93, 1985.

90. Feldman RD, Park GD, Lai CYC: The interaction of verapamil and norverapamil with beta-adrenergic receptors. *Circulation* **72**:547-554, 1985.

91. Jelinek MV, Lown B: Exercise stress testing for exposure of cardiac arrhythmias. *Prog Cardiovasc Dis* **16**:497-522, 1974.

92. Speccia G, Servi SD, Falcone C, et al.: Coronary arterial spasm as a cause of exercise-induced ST-segment elevation inpatients with variant angina. *Circulation* **59**:948-954, 1979.

93. Kugiyama K, Yasue H, Horia Y, et al.: Effects of propranolol and nifedipine on exercise-induced attack in patients with variant angina: assessment by exercise thallium-201 myocardial scintigraphy with quantitative rotational tomography. *Circulation* **74**:374-380, 1986.

94. Califf RM, McKinnis RA, McNeer F, et al.: Prognostic value of ventricular arrhythmias associated with treadmill exercise testing in patients studied with cardiac catheterization for suspected ischemic heart disease. *J Am Coll Cardiol* **2**:1060-1067, 1983.

95. Sami M, Chaitman B, Fisher L, et al.: Significance of exercise-induced ventricular arrhythmias in stable coronary artery disease: A coronary artery surgery study project. *Am J Cardiol* **54**:1182-1187, 1984.

96. Maron BJ, Roberts WC, et al.: Sudden death in young athletes. *Circulation* **62**:218-29, 1980.

97. Northcote RJ, Flannigan C, Ballantyne D: Sudden death and vigorous exercise-a study of 60 deaths associated with squash. *Br Heart J* **55**:198-203, 1986.

98. Han J, de Jalon PG, Moe GK: Adrenergic effects on ventricular vulnerability. *Circ Res* **14**:516-524, 1964.

99. Palileo EV, Ashley WW, Swiryn S, et al.: Exercise provocable right ventricular outflow tract tachycardia. *Am Heart J* **104**:185-93, 1982.

100. Woelfel A, Foster JR, Simpson RJ, Jr., Gettes LS: Reproducibility and treatment of exercise-induced ventricular tachycardia. *Am J Cardiol* **53**:751-6, 1984.

101. Woelfel A, Foster JR, McAllister RG, Jr., et al.: Efficacy of verapamil in exercise-induced ventricular tachycardia. *Am J Cardiol* **56**:292-7, 1985.

102. Tan HL, Hou CJ, Lauer MR, Sung RJ: Electrophysiologic mechanisms of the long QT interval syndromes and torsade de pointes. *Ann Intern Med* **122**:701-14, 1995.

103. de Paola AAV, Horowitz LN, Marques FBR, et al.: Control of multimorphic ventricular tachycardia by propranolol in a child with no identifiable cardiac disease and sudden death. *Am Heart J* **119**:1429-1432, 1990.

104. Coumel P, Fidelle J, V. L, et al.: Catecholamine induced severe ventricular arrhythmias with Adams-Stokes syndrome in children: Report of four cases. *Br Heart J* **40(suppl)**:23-37, 1978.

105. Ackerman MJ: The long QT syndrome: Ion channel diseases of the heart. *Mayo Clin Proc* **73**:250-69, 1998.

106. Wang Q, Chen Q, Li H, Towbin JA: Molecular genetics of long QT syndrome from genes to patients. *Curr Opin Cardiol* **12**:315-320, 1997.

107. Schwartz PJ: The long QT syndrome. *Curr Probl Cardiol* **22**:297-351, 1997.

108. Priori SG, Napolitano C, Paganini V, et al.: Molecular biology of the long QT syndrome: impact on management. *Pacing Clin Electrophysiol* **20**:2052-7, 1997.

109. Moss AJ: The long QT syndrome revisited: current understanding and implications for treatment. *Pacing Clin Electrophysiol* **20**:2879-81, 1997.

110. Anastasiou-Nana MI, Anderson JL, Stewart JR, et al.: Occurrence of exercise-induced and spontaneous wide QRS complex tachycardia during therapy with flecainide for complex ventricular arrhythmias: A probable proarrhythmic effect. *American Heart Journal* **113**:1071-1077, 1987.

111. Kadish AH, Weisman HF, Veltri EP, et al.: Paradoxical effects of exercise on the QT interval in patients with polymorphic ventricular tachycardia receiving type Ia antiarrhythmic agents. *Circulation* **81**:14-9, 1990.

112. Okumura K, Yamabe H, et al.: Characteristics of slow conduction zone demonstrated during entrainment of idiopathic ventricular tachycardia of left ventricular origin. *Am J Cardiol* **77**:379-83, 1996.

113. Lerman BB, Stein K, Engelstein ED, et al.: Mechanism of repetitive monomorphic ventricular tachycardia. *Circulation* **92**:421-9, 1995.

114. Strain JE, Grose RM, Factor SM, Fisher JD: Results of endomyocardial biopsy in patients with spontaneous ventricular tachycardia but without apparent structural heart disease. *Circulation* **68**:1171-1181, 1983.

115. Carlson MD, White RD, Trohman RG, et al.: Right ventricular outflow tract ventricular tachycardia: detection of previously unrecognized anatomic abnormalities using cine magnetic resonance imaging. *J Am Coll Cardiol* **24**:720-7, 1994.

116. Shinbane JS, Wood MA, Jensen DN, et al.: Tachycardia-induced cardiomyopathy: a review of animal models and clinical studies. *J Am Coll Cardiol* **29**:709-15, 1997.

117. Antiarrhythmics Versus Implantable Defibrillators (AVID) Investigators: A comparison of antiarrhythmic drug therapy with implantable defibrillators in patients resuscitated from near-fatal ventricular arrhythmias. *New Engl j Med* **337**:1576-1583, 1997.

118. Josephson ME, Horowitz LN, Farshidi A, et al.: Sustained ventricular tachycardia: evidence for protected localized reentry. *Am J Cardiol* **42**:416-24, 1978.

119. Josephson ME, Horowitz LN, Farshidi A: Continuous local electrical activity. A mechanism of recurrent ventricular tachycardia. *Circulation* **57**:659-65, 1978.

120. Josephson ME, Horowitz LN, Farshidi A, et al.: Recurrent sustained ventricular tachycardia. 2. Endocardial mapping. *Circulation* **57**:440-7, 1978.

121. The CAST Investigators: Preliminary report: effect of encainide and flecainide on mortality in a randomized trial of arrhythmia suppression after myocardial infarction. *N Engl J Med* **321**:406-412, 1989.

122. Strickberger SA, Man KC, Daoud EG, et al.: A prospective evaluation of catheter ablation of ventricular tachycardia as adjuvant therapy in patients with coronary artery disease and an implantable cardioverter-defibrillator. *Circulation* **96**:1525-31, 1997.

123. Burke AP, Farb A, Tashko G, Virmani R: Arrhythmogenic right ventricular cardiomyopathy and fatty replacement of the right ventricular myocardium: are they different diseases? *Circulation* **97**:1571-80, 1998.

124. Thiene G, Nava A, Corrado D, et al.: Right ventricular cardiomyopathy and sudden death in young people. *N Engl J Med* **318**:129-133, 1988.

125. Proclemer A, Crani R, Feruglio GA: Right ventricular tachycardia with ventricular dysplasia: clinical features, diagnostic techniques and current management. *Am Heart J* **103**:415-420, 1989.

126. Breithardt G, Wichter T, Haverkamp W, et al.: Implantable cardioverter defibrillator therapy in patients with arrhythmogenic right ventricular cardiomyopathy, long QT syndrome, or no structural heart disease. *Am Heart J* **127**:1151-8, 1994.

127. Leclercq JF, Chouty F, Cauchemez B, et al.: Results of electrical fulguration in arrhythmogenic right ventricular disease. *Am J Cardiol* **62**:220-4, 1988.

128. Leclercq JF, Coumel P: Characteristics, prognosis and treatment of the ventricular arrhythmias of right ventricular dysplasia. *Eur Heart J* **10 Suppl D**:61-7, 1989.

129. Morady F, Kadish AH, DiCarlo L, et al.: Long-term results of catheter ablation of idiopathic right ventricular tachycardia. *Circulation* **82**:2093-9, 1990.

130. Nishizaki M, Arita M, Sakurada H, et al.: Demonstration of Purkinje potential during idiopathic left ventricular tachycardia: a marker for ablation site by transient entrainment. *Pacing Clin Electrophysiol* **20**:3004-7, 1997.

131. Rodriguez LM, Smeets JL, Timmermans C, Wellens HJ: Predictors for successful ablation of right- and left-sided idiopathic ventricular tachycardia. *Am J Cardiol* **79**:309-14, 1997.

132. Lai LP, Lin JL, Hwang JJ, Huang SK: Entrance site of the slow conduction zone of verapamil-sensitive idiopathic left ventricular tachycardia: evidence supporting macroreentry in the Purkinje system. *J Cardiovasc Electrophysiol* **9**:184-90, 1998.

133. Blanck Z, Dhala A, Deshpande S, et al.: Bundle branch reentrant ventricular tachycardia: cumulative experience in 48 patients. *J Cardiovasc Electrophysiol* **4**:253-62, 1993.

134. Blanck Z, Jazayeri M, Dhala A, et al.: Bundle branch reentry: a mechanism of ventricular tachycardia in the absence of myocardial or valvular dysfunction. *J Am Coll Cardiol* **22**:1718-22, 1993.

135. Blanck Z, Akhtar M: Ventricular tachycardia due to sustained bundle branch reentry: diagnostic and therapeutic considerations. *Clin Cardiol* **16**:619-22, 1993.

136. Tchou P, Jazayeri M, Denker S, et al.: Transcatheter electrical ablation of right bundle branch. A method of treating macroreentrant ventricular tachycardia attributed to bundle branch reentry. *Circulation* **78**:246-57, 1988.

137. Smeets JLRM, Ben-Haim SA, Rodriguez LM, et al.: New method for nonfluoroscopic endocardial mapping in humans. Accuracy assessment and first clinical results. *Circulation* **97**:2426-2432, 1998.

138. Schilling RJ, Peters NS, Davies W: Simultaneous endocardial mapping in the human left ventricle using a noncontact catheter. Comparison of contact and reconstructed electrograms during sinus rhythm. *Circulation* **98**:887-898, 1998.

139. Morady F, Kadish A, Rosenheck S, et al.: Concealed entrainment as a guide for catheter ablation of ventricular tachycardia in patients with prior myocardial infarction. *J Am Coll Cardiol* **17**:678-89, 1991.

140. Stevenson WG, Weiss J, Wiener I, et al.: Localization of slow conduction in a ventricular tachycardia circuit: implications for catheter ablation. *Am Heart J* **114**:1253-8, 1987.

141. Stevenson WG, Weiss JN, Wiener I, et al.: Resetting of ventricular tachycardia: implications for localizing the area of slow conduction. *J Am Coll Cardiol* **11**:522-9, 1988.

142. Stevenson WG, Weiss JN, Wiener I, et al.: Fractionated endocardial electrograms are associated with slow conduction in humans: evidence from pace-mapping. *J Am Coll Cardiol* **13**:369-76, 1989.

143. Stevenson WG, Weiss JN, Wiener I, Nademanee K: Slow conduction in the infarct scar: relevance to the occurrence, detection, and ablation of ventricular reentry circuits resulting from myocardial infarction. *Am Heart J* **117**:452-67, 1989.

144. Stevenson WG, Sager P, Nademanee K, et al.: Identifying sites for catheter ablation of ventricular tachycardia. *Herz* **17**:158-70, 1992.

145. Stevenson WG, Khan H, Sager P, et al.: Identification of reentry circuit sites during catheter mapping and radiofrequency ablation of ventricular tachycardia late after myocardial infarction. *Circulation* **88**:1647-70, 1993.

146. Stevenson WG: Functional approach to site-by-site catheter mapping of ventricular reentry circuits in chronic infarctions. *J Electrocardiol* **27 Suppl**:130-8, 1994.

147. Stevenson WG, Sager PT, Friedman PL: Entrainment techniques for mapping atrial and ventricular tachycardias. *J Cardiovasc Electrophysiol* **6**:201-16, 1995.

148. Waxman HL, Sung RJ: Significance of fragmented ventricular electrograms observed using intracardiac recording techniques in man. *Circulation* **62**:1349-56, 1980.

149. Ruffy R, Imran MA, Santel DJ, Wharton JM: Radiofrequency delivery through a cooled catheter tip allows the creation of larger endomyocardial lesions in the ovine heart. *J Cardiovasc Electrophysiol* **6**:1089-96, 1995.

150. Deal BJ, Scagliotti D, Miller SM, et al.: Electrophysiologic drug testing in symptomatic ventricular arrhythmias after repair of tetralogy of Fallot. *Am J Cardiol* **59**:1380-5, 1987.

151. Chinushi M, Aizawa Y, Kitazawa H, et al.: Successful radiofrequency catheter ablation for macroreentrant ventricular tachycardias in a patient with tetralogy of Fallot after corrective surgery. *Pacing Clin Electrophysiol* **18**:1713-6, 1995.

152. Horton RP, Canby RC, Kessler DJ, et al.: Ablation of ventricular tachycardia associated with tetralogy of Fallot: demonstration of bidirectional block. *J Cardiovasc Electrophysiol* **8**:432-435, 1997.

153. Brugada P, de Swart H, Smeets JL, Wellens HJ: Transcoronary chemical ablation of ventricular tachycardia. *Circulation* **79**:475-82, 1989.

154. Brugada P: Transcoronary techniques and cardiac arrhythmias. *Am J Cardiol* **64**:534-5, 1989.

155. Inoue H, Waller BF, Zipes DP: Intracoronary ethyl alcohol or phenol injection ablates aconitine-induced ventricular tachycardia in dogs. *J Am Coll Cardiol* **10**:1342-9, 1987.

156. Kay GN, Epstein AE, Bubien RS, et al.: Intracoronary ethanol ablation for the treatment of recurrent sustained ventricular tachycardia. *J Am Coll Cardiol* **19**:159-68, 1992.

157. Nellens P, Gursoy S, Andries E, Brugada P: Transcoronary chemical ablation of arrhythmias. *Pacing Clin Electrophysiol* **15**:1368-73, 1992.

158. Okishige K, Andrews TC, Friedman PL: Suppression of incessant polymorphic ventricular tachycardia by selective intracoronary ethanol infusion. *Pacing Clin Electrophys* **14**:188-195, 1991.

159. Haines DE, Lerman BB, Kron IL, DiMarco JP: Surgical ablation of ventricular tachycardia with sequential map-guided subendocardial resection: electrophysiologic assessment and long-term follow-up. *Circulation* **77**:131-41, 1988.

160. Josephson ME, Horowitz LN, et al.: Surgery for recurrent sustained ventricular tachycardia associated with coronary artery disease: the role of subendocardial resection. *Ann N Y Acad Sci* **382**:381-95, 1982.

161. Kienzle MG, Doherty JU, Roy D, et al.: Subendocardial resection for refractory ventricular tachycardia: effects on ambulatory electrocardiogram, programmed stimulation and ejection fraction, and relation to outcome. *J Am Coll Cardiol* **2**:853-8, 1983.

162. Miller JM, Kienzle MG, Harken AH, Josephson ME: Subendocardial resection for ventricular tachycardia: predictors of surgical success. *Circulation* **70**:624-31, 1984.

163. Miller JM, Marchlinski FE, Harken AH, et al.: Subendocardial resection for sustained ventricular tachycardia in the early period after acute myocardial infarction. *Am J Cardiol* **55**:980-4, 1985.

CHAPTER 16

POLYMORPHIC VENTRICULAR TACHYCARDIA AND LONG QT SYNDROMES

Based on the morphological features of the QRS complex, ventricular tachycardia can be classified as monomorphic or polymorphic [1]. Polymorphic ventricular tachycardia is defined as a rapid irregular ventricular tachycardia with alteration of the QRS morphology almost from beat to beat at 150 to 300 beats per minute (Figure 16-1) [2]. Various

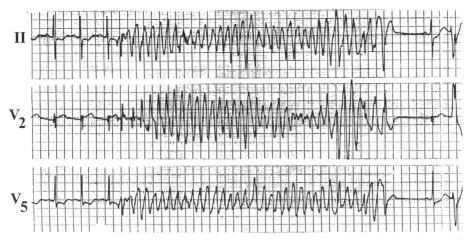

FIGURE 16-1. Polymorphic ventricular tachycardia induced by exercise treadmill testing in a 52 year old man with a history of exertional chest pain. Nonsustained polymorphic ventricular tachycardia developed in stage II of a standard Bruce protocol and was preceded by slight ST-segment elevation in ECG lead V_2 and ST-segment depression in leads II and V_5. Sinus rate is 95/min before the onset of the arrhythmia. Coronary angiography revealed three-vessel coronary artery disease including a 95% stenosis within the proximal portion of the left anterior descending coronary artery. Paper speed 25 mm/sec.

terms have been used to depict this form of ventricular tachycardia. These include "paroxysmal ventricular fibrillation," "transient recurrent ventricular fibrillation," "cardiac ballet," and "atypical ventricular tachycardia" [3-8]. The torsade de pointes tachycardia is also a form of polymorphic ventricular tachycardia that specifically occurs in association with the long QT syndromes [9-17]. During torsade de pointes, the QRS morphology changes its direction simulating a torsion around an imaginary isoelectric line. Classically the onset of torsade de pointes is preceded by a "short-long-short sequence" of RR intervals (Figures 16-2 & 16-3), although the variant form of torsade de pointes can be initiated by a short RR interval [18].

731

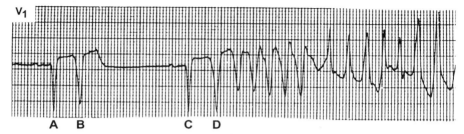

FIGURE 16-2. ECG rhythm strip showing the typical short-long-short R-R interval sequence which triggers an episode of torsade de pointes. A sinus beat (A) is followed by a closely-coupled premature ventricular depolarization (B). After a long pause, a second sinus beat (C) is followed by a second early premature ventricular depolarization (D) which arises during the T-wave of the preceding sinus beat and becomes the first beat of the polymorphic tachycardia. From [17] with permission.

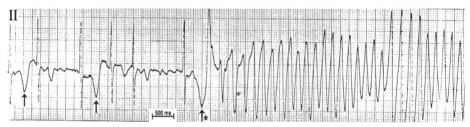

FIGURE 16-3. atrial fibrillation with its highly variable R-R intervals, including short-long-short intervals, can often create the ideal environment in which torsade de pointe can develop. Note the marked QT prolongation and the bizarre deeply inverted T waves (upward arrows) associated with ventricular repolarization following the long R-R intervals. This increasingly abnormal repolarization, most probably due to early afterdepolarizations, eventually triggers the polymorphic ventricular tachycardia (most rightward arrow with asterick).

16.1   Clinical Significance

In the prehospital setting at the emergency room, the prevalence of polymorphic ventricular tachycardia is approximately half (50%) of monomorphic ventricular tachycardia [19]. Similar to monomorphic ventricular tachycardia, polymorphic ventricular tachycardia usually occurs in patients with a structural heart disease such as arteriosclerotic coronary heart disease and primary or secondary cardiomyopathy. There are two major identifiable causes of polymorphic ventricular tachycardia: (1) acute myocardia ischemia resulting from coronary artery occlusion, coronary artery spasm, and aortocoronary bypass grafting; and (2) acquired long QT syndrome due to drug administration (e.g., quinidine, procainamide, sotalol, etc.), electrolyte imbalance (e.g., hypokalemia, hypomagnesemia), myocarditis, and severe bradycardia [20-25].

Polymorphic ventricular tachycardia can also be encountered in subjects without clinical evidence of structural heart disease referred to as an idiopathic entity [26-28]. Idiopathic polymorphic ventricular tachycardia may represent a variant form of the congenital long QT syndrome, in which the ECG marker, i.e., prolongation of the QT interval, is lacking. Idiopathic polymorphic ventricular tachycardia can be either catecholamine-sensitive or catecholamine-non-sensitive. Catecholamine-sensitive (cate-cholaminergic) polymorphic ventricular tachycardia clinically often manifest stress-, or exercise-induced syncope [26,28]. β-adrenergic blocking agents are the drug of choice for catecholamine-sensitive (catecholaminergic) polymorphic ventricular tachycardia; however, implantation of a cardioverter/defibrillator may be indicated in selected cases [27].

Polymorphic ventricular tachycardia may be clinically observed in a subset group of patients without demonstrable structured heat disease prone to sudden cardiac death, in which electrocardiograms show right bundle branch block and ST-segment elevation in leads V_1 through V_3 [29,30]. Clinically this subgroup of patients manifest recurrent syncope and/or sudden cardiac death associated with polymorphic ventricular tachycardia and/or ventricular fibrillation, both of which may be reproduced during electrophysiology study. Genetic studies have suggested that mutations of the cardiac Na^+ channel gene (SCN5A) is responsible for the genesis of ventricular tachyarrhythmias in these patients [31]. β-adrenoceptor blocking agents are not effective in preventing sudden cardiac death, and implantation of a cardioverter/defibrillator is recommended to be the treatment of choice in this subset group of patients [32]. Thus, unlike idiopathic monomorphic ventricular tachycardia, which is generally considered as a benign clinical entity, polymorphic ventricular tachycardia can easily degenerate into ventricular fibrillation. Hence, polymorphic ventricular tachycardia connotes a much worse prognosis than monomorphic ventricular tachycardia [27].

16.2   Mechanisms of QRS Complex Polymorphism

Several hypotheses invoking both non-reentrant and reentrant mechanisms have been proposed to explain polymorphism of the QRS complexes during ventricular tachycardia. Non-reentrant mechanisms include triggered activity brought about by early afterdepolarizations [33,34], a single rapidly firing idioventricular focus with Wenckebach patterns of activation due to progressively prolonged ventricular refractoriness [7], presence of two or more arrhythmogenic foci [10,11], changing the site of an arrhythmia focus [35], and an automatic focus migrating through the myocardium [33,34]. Reentrant mechanisms include a reentrant pathway with intermittent conduction block from its exit site [36], a reentrant circuit with varying exit sites [37], two reentrant circuits in close proximity or far apart competing with each other [38], conduction reversal (orthodromic vs. antidromic) of a reentrant circuit [39], and spiral wave activity resulting from non-stationary scroll waves of electrical activity [40-45].

Digitalis toxicity-induced bidirectional ventricular tachycardia is one example of a non-reentrant mechanism in which two arrhythmogenic foci (due to automaticity or triggered activity resulting from delayed afterdepolarizations) arising from two fascicular divisions of the left bundle branch can generate competing wavefronts of depolarization detectable using the surface 12-lead ECG.

Using the technique of either three-dimensional mapping with transmural electrogram recordings or high-resolution optical imaging with a voltage-sensitive dye, spiral reentry with scroll waves of electrical activity can be demonstrated in animal hearts

[35,42-51]. Of note is the observation that polymorphism of the QRS complex during ventricular tachycardia can be caused by a non-stationary vortex-like (spiral) reentrant activity or focal activity of varying origin and propagation patterns (repetitive firing of multiple sites). Furthermore, observations made in isolated cardiac tissue have shown that vortex-like reentrant activity may be responsible for either monomorphic or polymorphic ventricular tachycardia with a reentrant mechanism [41-45]. Depending on the spiral core dynamics, monomorphic and polymorphic QRS complexes during ventricular tachycardia can be formed. Stationary spirals produce a monomorphic ventricular tachycardia whereas drifting (non-stationary) spirals give rise to a polymorphic ventricular tachycardia. Transitions between these two ECG patterns can occur. These findings can be explicitly illustrated by a theoretical model using computed numerical simulation (Figure 16-4) [52]. The rate of ventricular tachycardia relative to the ventricular refrac-

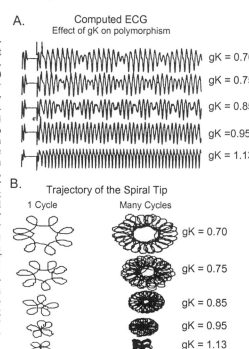

FIGURE 16-4. Computed ECGs and tip trajectories. Panel A: Computed ECGs for different values of K^+ conductance (gK). Panel B: Associated tip trajectories computed from a 40x40 array of excitable cells. Note that as the K^+ conductance (gK) is reduced, the morphology of each complex in the computed ECG gradually shifts from an almost monomorphic ECG (gK = 1.13) to a polymorphic ECG similar to that seen in torsade de pointes (gK = 0.70). In addition, as the size of the flower increases, the degree of amplitude modulation displayed in the ECG is increased. The tip trajectories, shown for a single torsade cycle (left) and for multiple cycles computed over a 50-time unit interval (right) change from a four-petaled flower (gK = 1.13) to an eight-petaled flower (gK = 0.70). Note that the number of reentry complexes within each torsade cycle in the computed ECG is approximately one less than the number of flower petals. The number of petals is determined by the ratio of the spiral rotation frequency to the tip precession frequency. If the ratio is not an integer, then each flower will be rotated from one torsade cycle to the next (as shown on the left), thus introducing another degree of variability in the morphology of the polymorphic ECG. From [52] with permission.

toriness affects the behavior of the spiral center (the rotor) and, subsequently, the ECG manifestation of the arrhythmia. At a slow rate and a relatively shorter ventricular refractory period (e.g., under good K^+ conductance), the spiral center of ventricular tachycardia is stationary and, hence, the ventricular tachycardia is monomorphic. At a faster rate and a relatively long ventricular refractory period (e.g., poor K^+ conductance), the spiral center of ventricular tachycardia is non-stationary and, hence, the ventricular tachycardia is polymorphic.

The fact that a polymorphic ventricular tachycardia is frequently seen in the clinical setting of acute myocardial ischemia (Figure 16-5) is intriguing and may result from ei-

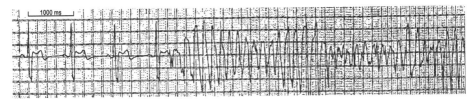

FIGURE 16-5. Development of polymorphic ventricular tachycardia degrading into ventricular fibrillation during the recovery phase following an exercise treadmill test in a 44-year old man. The patient had recently undergone coronary artery bypass surgery for an 80% stenosis of the left main coronary artery. Following resuscitation from this arrhythmia, he underwent repeat coronary angiography that revealed total occlusion of the bypass grafts to the left anterior descending and left circumflex coronary arteries. The patient was referred for repeat coronary bypass surgery.

ther triggered activity or reentry (Figure 16-6). The action potential duration is actually shortened during acute myocardial ischemia because of the activation of ATP-sensitive K^+ channels, $I_{K(ATP)}$, which improves K^+ conductance [53-55]. However, the $I_{K(ATP)}$ activation results in the accumulation of extracellular K^+ concentration, $[K^+]_o$ [56-59]. Consequently, ischemic myocardium often exhibits conduction delay and prolongation of refractoriness beyond repolarization of the action potential, an electrophysiologic phenomenon referred to as post-repolarization refractoriness [60]. Formation of an unexcitable ischemic core surrounded by tissues with slow conduction and dispersion of refractoriness provides an anatomic substrate for the induction of a reentrant arrhythmia. If post-repolarization refractoriness is markedly prolonged, the reentrant arrhythmia may become a non-stationary vortex-like reentrant activity thereby giving rise to a polymorphic form of ventricular tachycardia.

Triggered activity of multifocal origin

Reentry with post-repolarization refractoriness

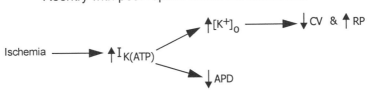

FIGURE 16-6. Mechanism of polymorphic ventricular tachycardia induced by myocardial ischemia. APD, action potential duration, CV, conduction velocity; $[K^+]_o$, extracellular potassium concentration; $I_{K(ATP)}$, adenosine triphosphate-dependent potassium current; RP, refractory period. See text for additional discussion.

16.3   Classification of Long QT Syndromes

Antiarrhythmic drugs that exert their therapeutic effects primarily by delaying cardiac repolarization and prolonging the QT interval have, in recent years, become the favored drug treatment for life-threatening ventricular arrhythmias. Such drugs are presumed to have greater clinical effectiveness and a lower risk profile than more traditional antiarrhythmic drugs, which primarily slow conduction velocity and prolong the QRS duration [61-68]. Although agents that prolong the QT interval may be useful in treating arrhythmias, they may also provoke a unique form of proarrhythmia called torsade de pointes tachycardia (Figure 16-2) [10,11]. Quinidine is the most widely used antiarrhythmic drug that can induce torsade de pointes; the reported incidence of torsade de pointes in patients receiving quinidine is 1% to 8% [33,34]. Often antiarrhythmic drugs such as procainamide, disopyramide, and sotalol may also cause torsade de pointes [69-75]. Torsade de pointes is more than simply an unusual cardiac curiosity as numerous noncardiac agents or conditions may also precipitate it. The acquired and hereditary long QT syndromes and torsade de pointes associated with them have now become a model of the ways in which identifiable cellular and molecular electrophysiologic abnormalities can cause clinical cardiac arrhythmias.

The QT interval recorded on the surface electrocardiogram corresponds to the relatively isoelectric plateau (phase 2) of the action potential (Figure 16-7). The broad T wave is inscribed as a result of rapid repolarization occurring non-simultaneously throughout the ventricles. The QT interval is prolonged by any agent or condition that delays repolarization in the ventricular myocardium. Various agents and conditions cause these long QT syndromes and initiate the torsade de pointes tachycardia (Figure 16-2) (Table 16-1.)

The long QT syndromes have been classified as acquired or hereditary on the basis of the conditions that appear to trigger torsade de pointes. The acquired long QT syndromes are also typically classified as pause-dependent because torsade

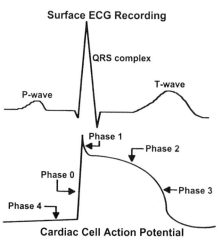

FIGURE 16-7. Relative correspondence of the components of the surface ECG recording and the phases of the ventricular muscle action potential. See text for details.

de pointes associated with them generally occurs at slow heart rates or in response to short-long-short RR interval sequences. The hereditary long QT syndromes are typically considered adrenergic-dependent because torsade de pointes associated with them is generally triggered by adrenergic activation or enhancement of sympathetic tone [33,34]. However, the acquired and hereditary long QT syndromes overlap somewhat. The causes of the acquired long QT syndromes include antiarrhythmic drugs, severe bradycardia, electrolyte disturbances (notably hypokalemia), various non-antiarrhythmic drugs, and numerous non-cardiac disorders (Table 16-1.) The hereditary long QT syndromes include the Jervell and Lange-Nielsen syndrome [76], which is associated with congenital deafness, the Romano-Ward syndrome [77,78], in which hearing is normal.

As mentioned above, the initiation of the acquired, pause-dependent form of torsade de pointes often (although not invariably [18] involves a short-long-short RR interval sequence. As seen in Figure 16-2, a premature ventricular depolarization closely coupled with the last normal QRS complex is followed by a long pause after extrasystole

TABLE 16-1. Classification and causes of the long QT syndromes

---

Acquired long QT syndromes (pause-dependent)

Antiarrhythmic drugs

    Class IA drugs with class III properties

    Class III drugs

Severe bradycardia

    Complete atrioventricular block

    Sinoatrial node dysfunction

Electrolyte disturbances

    Hypokalemia

    Hypomagnesemia

Nonantiarrhythmic drugs

    Psychotropic agents: phenothiazines, haloperidol

    Tricyclic and tetracyclic antidepressants

    Antihypertensive agents: bepridil, lidoflazine, prenylamine, ketanserin

    Antimicrobials: erythromycin, trimethoprim-sulfamethoxazole, pentamidine, amantidine, chloroquine

    Antifungal agents: ketoconazole, itraconazole

    Antihistaminic agents; terfenadine, astemizole

    Other drugs: cocaine, organophosphate insecticides, arsenic, vasopressin

Other conditions

    Cardiac disorders: myocarditis, ventricular tumor

    Endocrine disorders: hypothyroidism, hyperparathyroidism, pheochromocytoma, hyperaldosteronism

    Intracranial disorder: subarachnoid hemorrhage, cerebrovascular accident, encephalitis, head injury

    Nutritional disorders: liquid protein diet, starvation

Hereditary long QT syndromes (adrenergic-dependent)

    Jervell and Lange-Nielsen syndrome

    Romano-Ward syndrome

    Long QT syndrome with syndactyly

Adapted from [17].

---

that precedes another closely coupled premature ventricular depolarization, which constitutes the first beat of the tachycardia. The tachycardia has a rate of 150 to 250 beats/min and is usually self-terminating. It is usually nonsustained and produces either no symptoms or only mild symptoms of presyncope, but it can degenerate into fatal ventricular fibrillation. Although the initiation of torsade de pointes in patients with the hereditary long QT syndromes does not require pauses or bradycardia, adrenergic activation or enhanced sympathetic tone does appear to be necessary to produce the bizarre QT or QTU prolongation characteristic of this form of the disorder.

16.4   Cellular Mechanisms of Long QT Syndromes and Torsade de Pointes

16.4.1 NORMAL CARDIAC ACTION POTENTIAL

For a review of the ionic mechanisms responsible for the generation of the normal action potential, the reader is referred to "Ionic Channels and Transmembrane Currents" on page 105 and "Action Potential Generation in Cardiac Cells" on page 108.

16.4.2 ROLE OF EARLY AFTER-DEPOLARIZATIONS

The study of torsade de pointes in humans is confounded by the transient nature of the condition and its unpredictable of its occurrence and because it generally cannot be induced by programmed electrical stimulation during electrophysiology study [79-81]. Thus, animal studies form the basis for the current understanding of this arrhythmia. It is believed that torsade de pointes is caused by early afterdepolarizations, defined as single or repetitive depolarizations or oscillations of the transmembrane voltage, that occur at low levels of membrane potential because of a failure of normal, complete membrane repolarization. Early afterdepolarizations may occur during the plateau phase (phase 2 early afterdepolarizations) or the early rapid repolarization phase (phase 3 early afterdepolarizations) of the action potential (Figure 16-8 and Figure 16-9) [82-87].

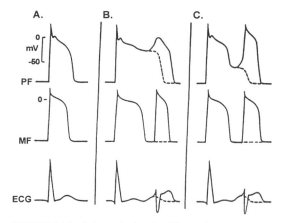

FIGURE 16-8. Schematic drawing illustrating transmembrane action potentials from a Purkinje fiber (PF), a ventricular muscle fiber (MF), and a surface electrocardiogram (ECG). Panel A: Baseline recordings. Panel B: Phase 2 early afterdepolarization. The action potential is more prolonged in the PF than in the MF and shows a flattening of the plateau phase. Because of failure of normal repolarization (dotted line), the PF again depolarizes from its plateau phase potential. The depolarizing potential reaches threshold and is transmitted to the MF. This beat is seen on the surface ECG as a premature ventricular depolarization arising from the end of a prolonged QT interval (or in the midst of a pronounced U wave) (dotted line). The premature ventricular depolarization coincides with the prolonged action potential duration resulting from the early afterdepolarization. Panel C: Phase 3 early afterdepolarization. The sequence is the same except that the early afterdepolarization arises during phase 3 of the PF action potential. From [85] with permission.

Although direct evidence that early afterdepolarizations cause torsade de pointes is lacking, considerable indirect evidence supports this hypothesis. Specifically, conditions that induce early afterdepolarizations initiate torsade de pointes [82-84,88], especially at slow heart rates [89], and conditions that suppress early afterdepolarizations prevent torsade de pointes [90]. Early afterdepolarizations probably arise from the Purkinje fibers rather than from working myocardial cells because interventions that induce early afterdepolarizations do so far more easily in Purkinje fibers than in ventricular myocardial cells [91-93]. In addition, delay of cardiac repolarization with prolongation of the action potential duration—which appears to be necessary for the development of some types of early afterdepolarizations—is more prominent in Purkinje fibers than in ventricular tissue after exposure to antiarrhythmic drugs that delay repolarization [91-94].

Early afterdepolarizations are depolarizing potentials that develop because of a failure of normal repolarization. They do not develop in the absence of a preceding action potential and are, in fact, triggered by it. This is why early afterdepolarizations are called triggered activity. Any imbalance between net inward and outward currents leading to failure of membrane repolarization may suffice to initiate phase 2 or phase 3 early afterdepolarizations [93,95-98]. In general, re-

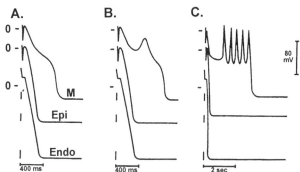

FIGURE 16-9. Quinidine-induced early afterdepolarizations arising from the plateau phase of the action potential. Transmembrane action potentials recorded from single isolated epicardial (Epi), endocardial (Endo), and M (M) cells. Action potential recordings from cells electrically stimulated at various cycle lengths (A = 3.5 sec; B = 5.0 sec; and C = 20 sec). Notice the dramatic prolongation of the action potential duration that occurs (note different time base in panel C) with the development of repetitive early afterdepolarizations during the plateau phase of the action potential. From [245] with permission.

polarization failure and prolongation of the action potential duration and the QT interval may be achieved by reducing net outward current, I_K [88,90-93,99-109] or I_{To} [90], enhancing net inward current, I_{Na} [85,86,110,111] or I_{Ca-L} [102,112-117] or both. In all cases, the generation of early afterdepolarizations appears dependent on, at least, a reduction in net outward current that, in the presence of residual inward currents (such as the "window" currents [96,98,117], delays or prevents normal repolarization. As a result, the membrane potential can oscillate at the plateau phase level (Figure 16-9). If these membrane oscillations, or early afterdepolarizations, conduct from their origin to the ventricular myocardium at large, tachyarrhythmia will result [85].

Some investigators have suggested that a special group of ventricular myocardial cells may play a role in the genesis of early afterdepolarizations [118,119]. Although early afterdepolarizations are usually not inducible in ventricular endomyocardium, they can be elicited in isolated single ventricular cells, termed M cells. These M cells are a distinct type of myocardial cell originating in deep subepicardial or midmyocardial layers. Electrophysiologically, M cells closely resemble Purkinje fibers except for the absence of spontaneous diastolic depolarization. Specifically, these M cells have an action potential longer than that of epicardial and endocardial ventricular cells because of a weaker slow component of the delayed rectifier, I_{Ks} and a more intense late Na$^+$ current, I_{Na} [120,121]. Of note, these cells show a marked prolongation of the action potential duration at slower stimulation rates making them the possible origin of early afterdepolarizations during bradycardia (Figure 16-9).

16.4.3 Intracellular Calcium Overload

The intracellular mechanism responsible for the genesis of early afterdepolarizations remains to be determined. One theory proposes that intracellular Ca++ overload underlies early afterdepolarizations [122]. The role of intracellular Ca++ overload in the genesis of delayed afterdepolarizations, a type of rate-dependent triggered activity, is well recognized [123], for example, in digitalis toxicity. Delayed afterdepolarizations result from the activation of the transient inward current (I_{Ti}) by elevations of cytosolic Ca++ caused by numerous agents or conditions [82,124]. This current is carried by either a non-selective cation channel or the electrogenic Na+-Ca++ exchanger that is stimulated by oscillatory Ca++ release from the sarcoplasmic reticulum. In contrast, the role of Ca++ overload in early afterdepolarizations and torsade de pointes is controversial. In vitro evidence [122] suggests that intracellular Ca++ loading during rapid pre-pause heart rates during a short-long-short sequence may enhance the development of early afterdepolarizations. Indeed, reducing Ca++ overload with flunarizine suppresses experimental sotalol-induced torsade de pointes [125]. However, inhibiting release of Ca++ from the sarcoplasmic reticulum with ryanodine abolished early afterdepolarizations in some studies [125] but not in others [102]. The role of the Na+-Ca++ exchanger in the generation of early afterdepolarizations is also controversial. An in vitro study [127] showed that benzamil and reduced extracellular Na+ concentration abolished early afterdepolarizations induced by isoproterenol, possibly by blocking the Na+-Ca++ exchanger. However, another study [112,113] showed that withdrawing extracellular Na+ failed to abolish both early afterdepolarizations and the inward current associated with them, suggesting that the Na+-Ca++ exchanger does not carry the depolarizing charge for early afterdepolarizations.

16.4.4 Reentry as a Mechanism of Torsade de Pointes

Although torsade de pointes is believed to be initiated by early afterdepolarizations, the mechanism of subsequent beats of the arrhythmia has generated considerable interests for research [35,50,51]. That torsade de pointes is not generally inducible by programmed electrical stimulation has been used as an argument against reentry as the underlying mechanism of the arrhythmia [81]. However, the development of early afterdepolarizations results in the prolongation of the action potential duration. If early afterdepolarization occurs heterogeneously throughout the heart—for example, only in some regions of the Purkinje network—dispersion of the repolarization (QT interval) increases, which may facilitate reentry [128-130]. Thus, reentry may be the mechanism by which torsade de pointes, initiated by an early afterdepolarization, is perpetuated. Of course, the dispersion of repolarization may be an incidental finding that necessarily follows from the spatially non-homogeneous distribution of early afterdepolarizations but that does not by itself lead to reentry. Recently, in animal models with drug-induced long QT interval and torsade de pointes, three dimensional mapping with transmural recordings and high-resolution optical mapping with a voltage-sensitive dye have clearly confirmed that, torsade de pointe, initiated by early afterdepolarizations, can result from either a non-stationary vortex-like reentrant activity or emergence of early afterdepolarizations from different subendocardial foci [50,51].

16.4.5 EFFECT OF ADRENERGIC STIMULATION ON TORSADE DE POINTES

The effects of β_1-adrenergic stimulation on early afterdepolarizations are complex because these effects can both enhance and inhibit these afterdepolarizations. The main effect of β_1-adrenergic activation is to stimulate intracellular adenylyl cyclase activity, which increases cyclic adenosine monophosphate (cAMP) levels [131]. This activates protein kinase A, which phosphorylates Ca^{++} channels and K^+ channels and thereby modulates their function. Phosphorylation of the Ca^{++} channel leads to increased inward current [132-134] that facilitates the development of early afterdepolarizations. Accordingly, early afterdepolarizations can be elicited by administration of isoproterenol to single cells [105,127]. On the other hand, phosphorylation of K^+ channels enhances I_K and I_{TO} [135-137]. This speeds up repolarization, as evidenced by a reduction in the action potential duration [127] and should inhibit the development of early afterdepolarizations.

Other effects of β_1-adrenergic stimulation are also contradictory. For example, the activity of the electrogenic membrane-bound Na^+–K^+ pump is increased [138]. This ion pump extrudes three intracellular Na^+ ions in exchange for two extracellular K^+ ions, generating a net outward repolarizing current. β_1-adrenergic activation of electrogenic Na^+ pumping may thus enhance repolarization and thereby inhibit the development of early afterdepolarizations. However, it also hyperpolarizes the resting membrane potential, thereby counteracting automaticity and decreasing heart rate, both of which may facilitate the development of early afterdepolarizations. To further complicate matters, a β_1-adrenergic-induced positive shift of the activation voltage range of pacemaker currents, I_f, in pacemaker cells [139,140] enhances spontaneous diastolic depolarization and, thus, increases automaticity, accelerates heart rate, and suppresses early afterdepolarizations. Finally, β_1-adrenergic stimulation facilitates conduction of the early afterdepolarizations from Purkinje fibers to the surrounding myocardium [93,100]. The net effect of these β_1-adrenergic effects is unclear, and the role of β_1-adrenergic activation in enhancing or inhibiting early afterdepolarizations remains to be resolved.

The effects of α_1-adrenergic stimulation are even less well clarified. Most hypotheses about the effects of α_1-adrenergic activation on ion currents suggest that this activation should facilitate the development of early afterdepolarizations. Enhancement of I_{Ca-L} secondary to cyclic adenosine monophosphate (cAMP)-independent [133,141] phosphorylation of the Ca^{++} channel by protein kinase C [133,142,143] increases net inward current [132]. In addition, α_1-adrenergic blockade of I_K and I_{TO} delays repolarization and prolongs the action potential duration [136,144]. Finally, α_1-adrenergic stimulation of electrogenic Na^+–K^+ pumping [145] hyperpolarizes the membrane and decreases heart rate. The significance of other effects of α_1-adrenergic stimulation is more speculative. Intracellular Ca^{++} levels increase after enhanced release from cellular stores by the α_1-adrenergic-induced increase in inositol triphosphate [146,147]. This elevation of cytosolic Ca^{++} clearly triggers the development of delayed afterdepolarizations, but its role in early afterdepolarizations is controversial. It is clear that although α_1-adrenergic stimulation alone cannot elicit early afterdepolarizations [99,127], it does facilitate induction of early afterdepolarizations by K^+ channel blockers [100,101,148].

16.5   The Acquired Long QT Syndromes and Torsade de Pointes

16.5.1 TORSADE DE POINTES CAUSED BY ANTIARRHYTHMIC DRUGS

Antiarrhythmic agents are the best studied and most common causes of the acquired long QT syndromes (Figure 16-10). According to the traditional classification of antiarrhythmic drugs (See "Modified Vaughan Williams Classification" on page 113.), only class III drugs block K^+ channels, prolong the action potential duration, and prolong the QT interval. However, in reality, many class IA drugs (primarily Na^+ channel blockers) also show significant K^+ channel blocking behavior. It is best, therefore, to speak in terms of "class III properties" that are found in both class III and many class IA antiarrhythmic drugs. Consequently, both quinidine (class IA) and sotalol (class III) can induce QT prolongation and torsade de pointes because both show significant K^+ channel blocking behavior. Drugs with class III properties block components of I_K and I_{TO}, but I_{K1} appears to be affected only slightly. Inhibition of these transmembrane K^+ currents may delay repolarization, initiate early afterdepolarizations, and precipitate torsade de pointes. Ibutilide, a new class III agent, activates a slow inward Na^+ current in addition to blocking the rapid component of the delayed rectifier, I_{Kr}, [149,150] and thereby prolongs the QT interval which may also lead to development of torsade de pointes.

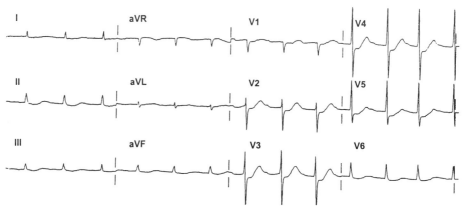

FIGURE 16-10. The acquired long QT syndrome resulting from treatment with a class IA agent. This 12-lead ECG was obtained from an 80-year-old woman treated with quinidine for atrial tachycardia. The maximum uncorrected QT interval measured approximately 600 ms. Within hours of obtaining this ECG the patient suffered a torsade de pointes-related cardiac arrest. Paper speed 25 mm/sec. From [17] with permission.

Patients who develop torsade de pointes when receiving one class IA drug often develop it when receiving other class IA drugs [70]. It is clear that torsade de pointes occurs with normal or low doses of class IA drugs [106,155], but generally with only high doses of class III drugs (especially during slow heart rates). Furthermore, clinical evidence indicates that torsade de pointes rarely occurs during treatment with amiodarone. An understanding of the genesis of early afterdepolarizations can help to explain these differences. At high doses of class IA drugs, blockade of I_{Na} predominates over blockade of I_K [69,81]. This inhibits the depolarizing current required to initiate early afterdepolarizations in excess of the drug-induced reduction in outward repolarizing K^+ currents and is in accordance with studies showing inhibition of early afterdepolarizations by Na^+ channel blocking agents. Because class III agents (except amiodarone) lack significant Na^+ channel blocking properties, higher doses of these agents increase the likelihood of torsade de pointes. A dose-dependent incidence of torsade de pointes has been reported with sotalol [152,153]. The rarity of torsade de pointes during treatment with amiodarone [69,70] may be explained by (1) the drug's additional Ca^{++} channel and Na^+ channel blocking effects [69,154]; (2) its β-adrenergic receptor blocking properties [76,154]; (3) its relative lack of reverse-use dependency; and (4) its resulting reduction of transmural dispersion of repolarization [155]. In fact, amiodarone rarely [156] causes torsade de pointes, even in patients whose previous treatment with other antiarrhythmic drugs has been discontinued because of torsade de pointes [70,76,157]. Finally, a slow heart rate facilitates early afterdepolarizations because it enhances the K^+ channel blocking effect of class IA and class III drugs, a phenomenon called reverse use-dependence [60,158,159]. In contrast, Na^+ channel blockade by class IA drugs is use-dependent; the drugs exert more Na^+ channel blockade at faster heart rates [154].

These explanations do not account for the variations in susceptibility to drug-induced torsade de pointes seen in some patients. Some patients develop torsade de pointes without a marked prolongation of the QT interval, and the duration of the QT interval in these patients does not predict the occurrence of torsade de pointes [70,160]. Additionally, some patients have pronounced prolongation of the QT interval at low doses of class IA drugs; other patients show no significant prolongation of the QT interval even at high doses. These findings suggest that prolongation of the action potential alone does not explain the incidence of torsade de pointes and that other modulatory factors may be involved. Stimulation of adrenergic receptors may play a significant role in various clinical settings. Slow heart rate and hypokalemia [75,161] must also be considered, and ischemia or hypoxia must be ruled out. In addition, genetic differences among patients may play a role: Some phenotypes may possess K^+ channels that are more or less susceptible to blockade.

Bradycardia
Extreme bradycardia as seen during complete or high-grade atrioventricular block may lead to early afterdepolarizations and torsade de pointes [86,162] through prolongation of the action potential duration secondary to both bradycardia-dependent depression of electrogenic Na^+ pumping and more complete inactivation of I_K [118]. Also, slow heart rates are associated with submaximal activation of I_{TO}, which shifts the action potential plateau to a voltage range in which the availability of the Ca^{++} "window" current is increased [114]. Finally, as mentioned above, torsade de pointes caused by class IA and class III antiarrhythmic drugs is enhanced at slow heart rates because these drugs show reverse use-dependence [60,158,159] during which K^+ blockade is increased. Fast heart rates, of course, tend to oppose these actions, preventing early afterdepolarizations and torsade de pointes.

Hypokalemia

Hypokalemia prolongs the cardiac action potential and may cause early afterdepolarizations and torsade de pointes both clinically [163] and experimentally [86]. Because the opening of K^+ channels requires K^+ binding, hypokalemia reduces net outward current by depressing I_K and I_{K1}. In addition, hypokalemia reduces the net outward current generated by electrogenic Na^+ pumping [86,164]. Hypokalemia also enhances the net inward current by increasing I_{Ca-L} which may facilitate the development of early afterdepolarizations and torsade de pointes [86]. Clinically, drug-induced torsade de pointes occurs often in the setting of hypokalemia [161,163,165].

Ischemia and hypoxia

No direct evidence suggests that ischemia and hypoxia are involved in drug-induced torsade de pointes. Clinically, torsade de pointes is usually not associated with electrocardiographic or clinical signs of myocardial ischemia. On the other hand, it is difficult to refute the possibility of this association, given the high incidence of coronary artery disease in patients treated with class IA and class III drugs [166]. Theoretically, ischemia could facilitate torsade de pointes in several ways. Increased dispersion of refractoriness and slow conduction could favor the perpetuation of early afterdepolarizations by a reentrant mechanism. In addition, ischemia-induced increases in numbers of α_1-adrenergic receptors, increased efficiency of effector-receptor coupling [167], and release of norepinephrine from local nerve endings [168] all enhance the net α_1-adrenergic activation, thereby facilitating early afterdepolarizations. Finally, experimental studies have shown that class III drugs prolong the action potential duration and induce early afterdepolarizations more easily in ischemic than in normoxic Purkinje fibers [108].

16.5.2 OTHER CAUSES OF ACQUIRED LONG QT SYNDROMES & TORSADE DE POINTES

Many nonantiarrhythmic drugs and clinical conditions other than those discussed above have been associated with the acquired long QT syndromes and torsade de pointes (Table 16-1.) The underlying mechanisms of this association may involve blockade of I_K (bepridil [169,170], erythromycin [171-174], terfenadine [175], and cocaine [176-178]); stimulation of I_{Ca-L} (prenylamine [179]); or stimulation of I_{Na} (ketanserin [180]). In most instances, however, the mechanism is unclear [169,181-204]. Clinically, it is often unclear whether these agents per se cause torsade de pointes or whether related factors such as hypokalemia or drug-drug interactions are responsible. For example, hypokalemia has been associated with bepridil [169], ketanserin [205,206], hyperparathyroidism [207], hyperaldosteronism [208], and subarachnoid hemorrhage [209,210]; all of these agents and conditions are associated with the acquired long QT syndromes and torsade de pointes. Also, although ketoconazole and itraconazole have not been shown to cause torsade de pointes, concomitant use of these agents with terfenadine has been associated with the arrhythmia. The mechanism responsible appears to involve an increase of terfenadine in the blood to toxic levels; this is caused by the inhibition by itraconazole or ketoconazole of the enzymatic degradation of terfenadine through the cytochrome P-450 system [211,212]. Although it has been suggested that overdoses of tricyclic or tetracyclic antidepressants may prolong the QT interval and may have a proarrhythmic effect, especially in the presence of ischemia, the induction of torsade de pointes by these agents has not been unequivocally shown [183,186].

16.6   The Hereditary Long QT Syndromes

The hereditary (Romano-Ward and Jervell and Lange-Nielsen syndromes) and acquired long QT syndromes share many features, including similar morphologies on surface electrocardiogram, the typical short-long-short initiating sequence, abnormal U-waves, prolongation of the QT or QTU interval, and facilitation by hypokalemia. Clinically, however, hereditary (but not acquired) long QT syndromes are clearly related to adrenergic stimulation or enhancement of sympathetic nervous system tone. Typically, bizarre and dynamic long QT and QTU segments are observed during periods of β_1-adrenergic stimulation or excitement associated with intense sympathetic activation (Figure 16-11).

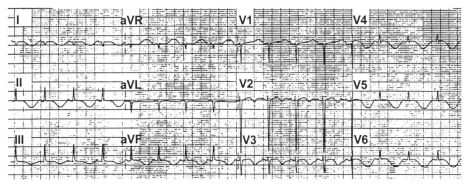

FIGURE 16-11. Example of extreme prolongation of the QT interval in a 21-year-old woman with a history of   recurrent syncope and the hereditary long QT syndrome. This 12-lead electrocardiogram was obtained within 48 hours of the patient suffering a cardiac arrest triggered by exercise. The QT segment is bizarrely inverted in all leads and measured 520 ms even though the RR interval was only 630 ms. From [17] with permission.

Recent molecular genetic studies have linked genetic defects responsible for delayed cardiac repolarization in patients with the hereditary long QT syndrome [117,213-217]. These genetic defects may cause malfunction of some ionic channels reducing outward repolarizing K^+ currents or retarding inactivation of inward Na^+ currents and thereby prolong the action potential duration [215]. These defects may also lead to an inappropriate adaptive response of the action potentials duration to changes in heart rate [117]. It appears that these are various forms of the hereditary long QT syndromes depending on the types of ionic channels (e.g., I_{Ks}, I_{Kr}, I_{Na}) affected (Table 16-2.) Characterization of these gene defects and their resultant functional abnormalities may lead to better clinical distinction among various forms of the hereditary long QT syndrome [218-221]. Consequently, a more specific, targeted therapy with physiological manipulation and pharmacologic treatment can be outlined, and maybe in the future, gene therapy be applied.

It has been shown that patients who develop torsade de pointes while receiving a class IA drug may have a longer QT interval at baseline [166,222] and may respond to drug treatment with a more marked prolongation of the QT interval than patients who do not have drug-induced proarrhythmia. Also, a reduction in pacing rates has been associated with greater prolongation of the QT interval in patients who develop bradycardia-induced torsade de pointes than in patients who do not [222]. It is tempting to speculate that some patients with the acquired long QT syndromes may have a subclinical genetic defect that allows agents that prolong the action potential duration to have an effect on the QT interval that is more pronounced than that in patients who lack this defect [166]. Thus, although it is by no means clear that patients with the acquired long QT syndromes have a genetic defect, some investigators have suggested that the acquired and hereditary long QT syndromes may be different expressions of a shared genetic basis [223,224]. Given the various ionic mechanisms that can cause early after depolarizations and torsade de pointes, some patients may have a genetic defect involving other ion channels. Furthermore, studies show that female sex is an independent risk factor for the development of torsade de pointes and sudden cardiac death in patients with the hereditary [219] and acquired [71] long QT syndromes, suggesting that genetic predisposition is important to this syndrome.

TABLE 16-2. Subtypes of the hereditary long QT syndromes

Subtype	Inheritance	Locus/Gene	Channel Type	Defectors
LQT1	Dominant/ Recessive	11p15.5/KVLQT1	Voltage-gated K$^+$ channel (I_{Ks})	Intragenic deletion Multisense mutations
LQT2	Dominant	7q35-36/HERG	Outwardly rectifying K$^+$ channel (I_{Kr})	Multiple deletions Missense mutations
LQT3	Dominant	3p21-24/SCN5A	Voltage-gated Na$^+$ channel	Missense mutations Intragenic deletions (α-subunit)
LQT4	Dominant	4q25-27/Unknown	Unknown	Unknown
LQT5	Dominant	21q22.1-22.2/ KCNE1(minK)	I_{Ks}	Mutant allele
LQT6	Recessive/X-linked	Unknown	Unknown	Unknown

16.7   Treatment of Polymorphic Ventricular Tachycardia & Long QT Syndromes

Since acute myocardial ischemia may underlie the initiating mechanism of polymorphic ventricular tachycardia, early diagnosis is essential. Coronary angiography is useful and coronary revascularization with percutaneous coronary angioplasty/stenting or aortocoronary artery bypass surgery is indicated in certain patients. In patients with coronary artery spasm, pharmacological treatment with a combination of nitrates and calcium channel blockers is usually effective [225], and rarely transvenous implantation of a cardioverter/defibrillator is indicated

Of drug-induced variety, digitalis toxicity-induced polymorphic or bidirectional tachycardia (Figure 16-12) should be recognized as digitalis should be withheld and treatment with digitalis antibody (Digibind) in addition to correction of electrolyte imbalance and metabolic derangement may be lifesaving. Finally, the acquired form of long QT syndrome should be taken into consideration so that the offending factor(s) can be immediately removed, for example, temporary pacing for bradycardia, correction of hypokalemia, and removal of drugs with class III antiarrhythmic properties, etc.

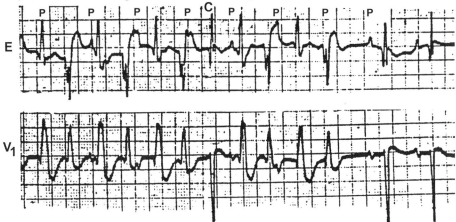

FIGURE 16-12. Bidirectional ventricular tachycardia in a patient with a toxic blood level of digoxin. Esophagael lead (E) and surface ECG lead V_1 are simultaneously recorded. Note the identifiable, regular P wave activity recorded by the E lead unrelated to ventricular activity during the tachycardia (A-V dissociation). Sinus capture beat (C) is also noted. Paper speed 25 mm/sec. (Courtesy of Dr. A. Castellanos, Jr.).

The cornerstone of effective treatment of the acquired and hereditary long QT syndromes and torsade de pointes is the identification and withdrawal of the offending agent or reversal and correction of any underlying predisposing condition (Table 16-3.) After this is done, a rational treatment plan can usually be formulated based on an understanding of the ionic basis for the specific syndrome. In the future, specific tailored therapy, may target the specific ionic currents responsible for the induction of the early afterdepolarizations. For example, if the dominant charge carrier for the early afterdepolarizations is the Na^+ "window" current, Na^+ channel blockade may be more effective. Likewise, Ca^{++} channel blockers may be more effective when the Ca^{++} "window" current is critical [86]. It has been shown experimentally that early afterdepolarizations induced with *Anemonia sulcata* toxin II, or other drugs that delay inactivation of the Na^+ channel, cannot be suppressed with Ca^{++} channel blockers [85]. In contrast, early afterdepolarizations induced by K^+ channel blockers such as clofilium, cesium, and quinidine can be suppressed by K^+ channel openers [91,92,103,104], Ca^{++} channel blockers [93,116], and Na^+ channel blockers [88,90,93,106,107].

Direct extrapolation from experimental studies to bedside management is not yet possible. Therefore, treatment is generally directed at suppressing or preventing early afterdepolarization generation and conduction by increasing the magnitude of repolarizing currents by enhancing outward K^+ currents, decreasing the magnitude of depolariza-

TABLE 16-3. Summary of short- and long-term treatments for torsade de pointes caused by acquired and hereditary long QT syndromes

Treatment	Mechanism	Acquired LQTS* (Pause-Dependent)	Hereditary LQTS* (Adrenergic-Dependent)
Short-term	Remove inciting factors	Withdraw offending agent and correct predisposing conditions, such as hypokalemia, bradycardia, or hypomagnesemia	Correct contributing or predisposing conditions such as hypokalemia, bradycardia, or hypomagnesemia
	Blockade of Na^+ and Ca^{++} current	Lidocaine, magnesium	Lidocaine, magnesium
	Increase heart rate and activate K^+ currents	β_1-adrenergic agonists such as isoproterenol; temporary overdrive electrical pacing	β_1-adrenergic agonists are contraindicated; temporary overdrive electrical pacing
	Inhibit adrenergic and sympathetic activity	Contraindicated because of negative chronotropic effects	β_1-adrenergic antagonists such as propranolol or esmolol
Long-term	Avoid inciting factors	Withhold offending agent (and all similar agents) and prevent predisposing metabolic or electrolyte disturbances	Prevent contributing or predisposing metabolic or electrolyte disturbances
	Inhibit adrenergic and sympathetic activity	Contraindicated because of negative chronotropic effects	β_1-adrenergic blockers such as nadolol Surgical high thoracic left sympathectomy
	Implantable device therapy	Pacemaker implantation for heart block or bradycardia-dependent LQTS Cardioverter-defibrillator not indicated if offending agent can be identified and reliably withheld	Permanent pacemaker implantation with β_1-adrenergic blockers such as nadolol Cardioverter-defibrillator implantation

* LQTS = long QT syndromes. Adapted from [17].

tion currents by enhancing Na$^+$ and Ca^{++} channel blockade, or inhibiting conduction of early afterdepolarizations from their site of origin to the surrounding myocardium. The short- and long-term treatment options for long QT syndromes are summarized below and in Table 16-3.

16.7.1 ENHANCEMENT OF REPOLARIZING CURRENTS

Short-term treatment that appears to be effective includes the enhancement of I_K using overdrive pacing, lidocaine [226,227], or infusion of isoproterenol, although the infusion of isoproterenol is contraindicated in the hereditary long QT syndromes. Experimental studies have suggested that torsade de pointes and early afterdepolarizations can be suppressed by opening K$^+$ channels and thereby shortening the action potential duration. For instance, activating the adenosine triphosphate-sensitive K$^+$ current (I_{K-ATP}) [228] with pinacidil [91,92,116], cromakalim [92], or nicorandil [103] or activating the acetylcholine-sensitive K$^+$ current $I_{K(Ach)}$ [229] with vagal stimulation [104] or administration of acetylcholine [228] may suppress early afterdepolarizations and torsade de pointes. Clinical testing has, indeed, shown that nicorandil can improve repolarization abnormalities in patients with the LQT1 subtype of the hereditary long QT syndrome [230] in which there is a genetic defect affecting the slow component of the delayed rectifier, I_{Ks} (Table 16-2.)

16.7.2 INHIBITION OF DEPOLARIZING CURRENTS

Although torsade de pointes can be induced by class IA drugs that can have both Na$^+$ and K$^+$ blocking properties, it can be suppressed using pure Na$^+$ channel blockade by reducing the depolarizing current (especially the Na$^+$ "window" current). The class IB drug lidocaine and the puffer fish toxin tetrodotoxin suppress early afterdepolarizations and torsade de pointes induced by K$^+$ channel blockers [88,90,93,106,107], Na$^+$ channel agonists [86], Ca^{++} channel agonists [112,113], and hypokalemia [86] in experimental preparations. Case reports [162,231,232] suggest that lidocaine may also be clinically effective, although its effects are inconsistent [70]. Lidocaine is also advantageous because it may enhance outward K$^+$ current [228,229]. The efficacy of Na$^+$ channel blockade may also partially result from the inhibition of conduction of early afterdepolarizations from the Purkinje network to the myocardium. Both clinically and experimentally, mexiletine has been shown to be effective in reducing the QT interval and the dispersion of repolarization in patients with the LQT3 subtype of the long QT syndrome (Table 16-2.) where the genetic defect affects the Na$^+$ channel [233,234].

Verapamil suppresses premature ventricular depolarizations and reduces the amplitude of early afterdepolarizations (as assessed by recordings of the monophasic action potential) in patients with the hereditary long QT syndromes and bradycardia-dependent torsade de pointes [235,236]. In experimental preparations, numerous Ca^{++} channel blockers, including verapamil [93,112,113], D-600 [116], nifedipine [93], nitrendipine [112,113,116], and cadmium [86], suppress early afterdepolarizations and torsade de pointes, but the effect of diltiazem varies [237]. In general, suppression of torsade de pointes and early afterdepolarizations by Ca^{++} channel blockade is not associated with shortening of either the QT interval or the action potential duration. Because clinical experience with Ca^{++} channel blockers has been minimal and because of concern about negative inotropic and chronotropic effects, Ca^{++} channel blockers are not considered first-line therapy for either the hereditary or the acquired long QT syndromes.

16.7.3 MAGNESIUM

Intravenous administration of magnesium is an effective and safe way to clinically suppress torsade de pointes [238]. Although magnesium may inhibit the ischemia-dependent enhancement of $I_{K\text{-}ATP}$ [239], it abolished early afterdepolarizations and torsade de pointes induced by cesium, quinidine, and 4-aminopyridine in experimental studies [88,98,99,237]. The effect of magnesium on early afterdepolarizations and torsade de pointes may be mediated by blockade of Ca^{++} or Na^+ "window" currents [88,98,99,240]. Regardless of the mechanism, the therapeutic effect of magnesium is not associated with a reduction of the action potential duration [162].

16.7.4 ISOPROTERENOL INFUSION AND PACING

As mentioned above, β_1-adrenergic stimulation is contraindicated in torsade de pointes associated with the hereditary long QT syndromes [232]. β_1-adrenergic stimulation may also facilitate induction and propagation of early afterdepolarizations in the acquired long QT syndromes. But, from a clinical standpoint, infusion of isoproterenol usually suppresses early afterdepolarizations and torsade de pointes by enhancing outward K^+ currents, accelerating heart rate and repolarization, thereby shortening the action potential duration and the QT interval [93,135-140,160]. Overdrive temporary or permanent electrical pacing is also an effective treatment for both forms of the long QT syndromes, possibly because it enhances repolarizing K^+ currents or prevents long pauses, either of which may suppress early afterdepolarizations and shorten the QT interval [70,88,110,162,241-244].

16.7.5 β_1-ADRENERGIC BLOCKADE AND SURGICAL SYMPATHECTOMY

All patients with the hereditary, adrenergic-dependent long QT interval syndromes require treatment with β_1-adrenergic receptor blocking agents. Additional treatments may be required in some patients, especially those clinically judged to be at high risk (for example, those who have had cardiac arrest). Some investigators [244] have proposed high thoracic left sympathectomy (surgical removal of the first four or five left-sided thoracic stellate ganglia) as either an initial treatment or adjuvant therapy in patients failing pharmacologic β_1-adrenergic blockade alone. Left sympathectomy is effective because the predominantly left-sided sympathetic innervation of the heart underlies the adrenergic-dependent long QT syndromes [244]. The fact that left sympathectomy is effective in patients in whom β_1-blockade has failed suggests that α_1-adrenergic stimulation may play a role in the genesis of the syndromes [244].

In some experimental models of the acquired drug-induced long QT syndromes, β_1-adrenergic blockade suppresses torsade de pointes [237], possibly by suppressing propagation of early afterdepolarizations from Purkinje fibers to the myocardium. Although it is of experimental interest, β_1-adrenergic inhibition is contraindicated in the acquired forms of the long QT syndromes and torsade de pointes because it decreases heart rate.

16.7.6 IMPLANTABLE CARDIOVERTER-DEFIBRILLATORS

High-risk patients with hereditary long QT syndromes, or patients with an acquired form that cannot be treated effectively by simply withdrawing the offending agent or condition, may require aggressive management with an implantable cardioverter-defibrillator. Designating a patient as "high-risk" requires a clinical judgement, but patients with recurrent episodes of syncope, those who have survived a cardiac arrest, or those that have failed to respond to conventional medical therapy clearly should be viewed as high risk [244].

References

1. Schamroth L. Ventricular rhythms. *The Disorders of Cardiac Rhythm*. Oxford: Blackwell Scientific Publications, 95-111: 1971.
2. Sclarovksy S, Strasberg B, Lewin RF, Agmon J: Polymorphic ventricular tachycardia: Clinical features and treatment. *Am J Cardiol* **44**:339-344, 1979.
3. Loeb HS, Pietras RJ, Gunnar RM, Tobin JR, Jr.: Paroxysmal ventricular fibrillation in two patients with hypomagnesemia. Treatment by transvenous. *Circulation* **37**:210-215, 1968.
4. Meltzer RS, Robert EW, McMorrow M, Martin RP: Atypical ventricular tachycardia as a manifestation of disopryamide toxicity. *Am J Cardiol* **42**:1049-1053, 1978.
5. Ranquin R, Parizel G: Ventricular fibrillo-flutter (torsade de pointes): an established electrocardiographic and clinical entity. *Angiology* **28**:115-118, 1977.
6. Scherf D, Cohen J, Shafiila H: Ectopic ventricular tachycardia, hypokalemia and convulsion in alcoholics. *Cardiologia* **50** 1967.
7. Smirk FH, Ng J: Cardiac ballet repetitions of complex electrocardiographic patterns. *Br Heart J* **31**:426-434, 1969.
8. Tamura K, Tamura T, Yosjida S, et al.: Transient recurrent ventricular fibrillation due to hypopotassemia with special note on the U wave. *Jap Heart J* **8**:652-660, 1967.
9. Dessertenne F: La tachycardie ventriculaire a deux foyers opposes variables. *Arch Mal Coeur* **59**:263-72, 1966.
10. Dessertenne F: Le Complexe electrique ventriculaire a phase lente prolongee. *Sem Hop Paris* **43**:539-41, 1967.
11. Dessertenne F, Coumel P, Fabiato A: Ventricular fibrillation and torsades de pointes. *Cardiovasc Drugs Ther* **4**:1177-82, 1990.
12. Krikler DM, Curry PVL: Torsade de pointes, an atypical ventricular tachycardia. *Br Heart J* **38**:117-120, 1976.
13. Motte G, Coumel P, Abitbol G, et al.: The long QT syndrome and syncope caused by spike torsades. *Arch Mal Coeur Vaiss* **63**:831-53, 1970.
14. Raynaud R, Brochier M, Neel JL, Fauchier JP: Tachycardie ventriculaire a foyer variable et dyskaliemie. *Arch Mal Coeur* **62**:1578-1598, 1969.
15. Singh BN, Gaarder TD, Kanegae T, et al.: Liquid protein diets and torsade de pointes. *JAMA* **240**:115-119, 1978.

16. Slama R, Coumel P, Motte G, et al.: Ventricular tachycardia and "volley of ventricular spikes". Morphological frontiers between ventricular dysrhythmias. *Arch Mal Coeur Vaiss* **66**:1401-11, 1973.

17. Tan HL, Hou CJ, Lauer MR, Sung RJ: Electrophysiologic mechanisms of the long QT interval syndromes and torsade de pointes. *Ann Intern Med* **122**:701-14, 1995.

18. Leenhardt A, Glaser E, et al.: Short-coupled variant of torsade de pointes. A new electrocardiographic entity in the spectrum of idiopathic ventricular tachyarrhythmias. *Circulation* **89**:206-15, 1994.

19. Brady W, Meldon S, DeBehnke D: Comparison of prehospital monomorphic and polymorphic ventricular tachycardia: Prevalence, response to therapy, and outcome. *Ann Emerg Med* **25**:64-70, 1995.

20. Azar RR, Berns E, Seecharran B, et al.: De novo monomorphic and polymorphic ventricular tachycardia following coronary artery bypass grafting. *Am J Cardiol* **80**:76-8, 1997.

21. Brady W, Meldon S, DeBehnke D, et al.: Prehospital polymorphic ventricular tachycardia. *Ann Emerg Med* **22**:1368-1369, 1993.

22. Kelly P, Ruskin JN, Vlahakes GJ, et al.: Surgical coronary revascularization in survivors of prehospital cardiac arrest: Its effect on inducible ventricular arrhythmias and long term survival. *J Am Coll Cardiol* **15**:267-273, 1990.

23. Kelly P, Ruskin JN, Vlahakes GJ, et al.: Surgical coronary revascularization in survivors of prehospital cardiac arrest: its effect on inducible ventricular arrhythmias and long-term survival. *J Am Coll Cardiol* **15**:267-73, 1990.

24. Nishizaki M, Arita M, Sakurada H, et al.: Induction of polymorphic ventricular tachycardia by programmed ventricular stimulation in vasospastic angina pectoris. *Am J Cardiol* **77**:355-60, 1996.

25. Wolfe CL, Nibley C, Bhandari A, et al.: Polymorphous ventricular tachycardia associated with acute myocardial infarction. *Circulation* **84**:1543-51, 1991.

26. Coumel P, Fidelle J, V. L, et al.: Catecholamine induced severe ventricular arrhythmias with Adams-Stokes syndrome in children: Report of four cases. *Br Heart J* **40(suppl)**:23-37, 1978.

27. Eisenberg SJ, Scheinman MM, Dullet NK, et al.: Sudden cardiac death and polymorphous ventricular tachycardia in patients with normal QT intervals and normal systolic cardiac function. *Am J Cardiol* **75**:687-92, 1995.

28. Leenhardt A, Lucet V, Denjoy I, et al.: Catecholaminergic polymorphic ventricular tachycardia in children. A 7-year follow-up of 21 patients. *Circulation* **91**:1512-9, 1995.

29. Brugada P, Brugada J: Right bundle branch block, persistent ST segment elevation and sudden cardiac death: a distinct clinical and electrocardiographic syndrome. A multicenter report. *J Am Coll Cardiol* **20**:1391-6, 1992.

30. Miyazaki T, Mitamura H, Miyoshi S, et al.: Autonomic and antiarrhythmic drug modulation of ST segment elevation in patients with Brugada syndrome. *J Am Coll Cardiol* **27**:1061-1070, 1996.

31. Chen Q, Kirsch GE, Zhang D, et al.: Genetic basis and molecular mechanism for idiopathic ventricular fibrillation. *Nature* **392**:293-6, 1998.

32. Brugada J, Brugada R, Brugada P: Right bundle-branch block and ST-segment elevation in leads V1 through V3: a marker for sudden death in patients without demonstrable structural heart disease. *Circulation* **97**:457-60, 1998.

33. Jackman WM, Clark M, Friday KJ, et al.: Ventricular tachyarrhythmias in the long QT syndromes. *Med Clin North Am* **68**:1079-109, 1984.

34. Jackman WM, Friday KJ, Anderson JL, et al.: The long QT syndromes: a critical review, new clinical observations and a unifying hypothesis. *Prog Cardiovasc Dis* **31**:115-72, 1988.

35. Murakawa Y, Sezaki K, Yamashita T, Kanese Y, Omata M: Three-dimensional activation sequence of cesium-induced ventricular arrhythmias. *Am J Physiol* **273**:H1377-1385, 1997.

36. Inoue H, Murakawa Y, Toda I, et al.: Epicardial activation pattern of torsades de pointes in canine hearts with quinidine-induced long QTU interval but without myocardial infarction. *Am Heart J* **111**:1080-1087, 1986.

37. de Bakker JM, van Capelle FJ, Janse MJ, et al.: Reentry as a cause of ventricular tachycardia in patients with chronic ischemic heart disease: electrophysiologic and anatomic correlation. *Circulation* **77**:589-606, 1988.

38. Downar E, Harris L, Mickleborough LL, et al.: Endocardial mapping of ventricular tachycardia in the intact human ventricle: evidence for reentrant mechanisms. *J Am Coll Cardiol* **11**:783-791, 1988.

39. Kuck KH, Schluter M, Kunze KP, Geiger M: Pleomorphic ventricular tachycardia: demonstration of conduction reversal within the reentry circuit. *Pacing Clin Electrophysiol* **12**:1055-64, 1989.

40. Winfree AT: Electrical instability in cardiac muscle: phase singularities and rotors. *J Theor Biol* **138**:353-405, 1989.

41. Pertsov AM, Davidenko JM, Salomonsz R, et al.: Spiral waves of excitation underlie reentrant activity in isolated cardiac muscle. *Circ Res* **72**:631-50, 1993.

42. Davidenko JM: Spiral wave activity: a possible common mechanism for polymorphic and monomorphic ventricular tachycardias. *J Cardiovasc Electrophysiol* **4**:730-746, 1993.

43. Davidenko JM, Pertsov AV, Salomonsz R, et al.: Stationary and drifting spiral waves of excitation in isolated cardiac muscle. *Nature* **355**:349-51, 1992.

44. Davidenko JM, Pertsov AM, Salomonsz R, et al.: Spatiotemporal irregularities of spiral wave activity in isolated ventricular muscle. *J Electrocardiol* **24 Suppl**:113-22, 1992.

45. Davidenko JM, Kent PF, Chialvo DR, et al.: Sustained vortex-like waves in normal isolated ventricular muscle. *Proc Natl Acad Sci U S A* **87**:8785-9, 1990.

46. Frazier DW, Wolf PD, Wharton JM, et al.: Stimulus-induced critical point. Mechanism for electrical initiation of reentry in normal canine myocardium. *J Clin Invest* **83**:1039-52, 1989.

47. Gray RA, Jalife J, Panfilov A, et al.: Nonstationary vortexlike reentrant activity as a mechanism of polymorphic ventricular tachycardia in the isolated rabbit heart. *Circulation* **91**:2454-69, 1995.

48. Gray RA, Jalife J, Panfilov AV, et al.: Mechanisms of cardiac fibrillation. *Science* **270**:1222-3; discussion 1224-5, 1995.

49. Chen PS, Wolf PD, Dixon EG, et al.: Mechanism of ventricular vulnerability to single premature stimuli in open-chest dogs. *Circ Res* **62**:1191-1209, 1988.

50. El-Sherif N, Caref EB, Yin H, Restivo M: The electrophysiological mechanism of ventricular arrhythmias in the long QT syndrome. Tridimensional mapping of activation and recovery patterns. *Circ Res* **79**:474-492, 1996.

51. Asano Y, Davidenko JM, Baxter WT, et al.: Optical mapping of drug-induced polymorphic arrhythmias and torsade de pointes in the isolated rabbit heart. *J Am Coll Cardiol* **29**:831-42, 1997.

52. Starmer CF, Romashko DN, Reddy RS, et al.: Proarrhythmic response to potassium channel blockade. Numerical studies of polymorphic tachyarrhythmias. *Circulation* **92**:595-605, 1995.

53. Wilde AA, Janse MJ: Electrophysiological effects of ATP sensitive potassium channel modulation: implications for arrhythmogenesis. *Cardiovasc Res* **28**:16-24, 1994.

54. Liu Y, Gao WD, O'Rourke B, Marban E: Synergistic modulation of ATP-dependent K+ currents by protein kinase C and adenosine: implications for ischemic conditioning. *Circ Res* **78**:443-454, 1996.

55. Gross GJ, Auchampach JA: Blockade of ATP-sensitive potassium channels prevents myocardial preconditioning in dogs. *Circ Res* **70**:223-33, 1992.

56. Bekheit SS, Restivo M, Boutjdir M, et al.: Effects of glyburide on ischemia-induced changes in extracellular potassium and local myocardial activation: A potential new approach to the management of ischemia-induced malignant ventricular arrhythmias. *Am Heart J* **119**:1025-33, 1990.

57. Miyoshi S, Miyazaki T, Asanagi M, et al.: Differential role of epicardial and endocardial KATP channels in potassium accumulation during regional ischemia induced by embolization of a coronary artery with latex. *J Cardiovasc Electrophysiol* **9**:292-296, 1998.

58. Mori H, Sakurai K, Miyazaki T, et al.: Local myocardial electrogram and potassium concentration changes in superficial and deep intramyocardium and their relationship with early ischemic ventricular arrhythmias. *Cardiovasc Res* **21**:447-454, 1987.

59. Wilde AA, Escande D, Schumacher CA, et al.: Potassium accumulation in the globally ischemic mammalian heart. A role for the ATP-sensitive potassium channel. *Circ Res* **67**:835-43, 1990.

60. Hondeghem LM, Snyders DJ: Class III antiarrhythmic agents have a lot of potential but a long way to go. Reduced effectiveness and dangers of reverse use dependence. *Circulation* **81**:696-690, 1990.

61. Mason JW: A comparison of seven antiarrhythmic drugs in patients with ventricular tachyarrhythmias. Electrophysiologic Study versus Electrocardiographic Monitoring Investigators. *N Engl J Med* **329**:452-458, 1993.

62. Mason JW: A comparison of electrophysiologic testing with holter monitoring to predict antiarrhythmic-drug efficacy for ventricular tachyarrhythmias. *N Eng J Med* **329**:445-451, 1993.

63.   The Cardiac Arrhythmia Suppression Trial Investigators: Preliminary report: effect of encainide and flecainide on mortality in a randomized trial of arrhythmia suppression after myocardial infarction. *N Engl J Med* **321**:406-412, 1989. .

64.   Ward D, Garratt C, Camm AJ: Cardiac arrhythmia suppression trial and flecainide. *Lancet* **1**:1267-8, 1989.

65.   Ruskin JN: The cardiac arrhythmia suppression trial (CAST). *N Engl J Med* **321**:386-8, 1989.

66.   Akhtar M, Breithardt G, Camm AJ, et al.: CAST and beyond. Implications of the Cardiac Arrhythmia Suppression Trial. Task Force of the Working Group on Arrhythmias of the European Society of Cardiology. *Circulation* **81**:1123-7, 1990.

67.   Greene HL, Roden DM, Katz RJ, et al.: The Cardiac Arrhythmia Suppression Trial: first CAST ... then CAST-II. *J Am Coll Cardiol* **19**:894-8, 1992.

68.   Garratt C, Ward DE, Camm AJ: Lessons from the cardiac arrhythmia suppression trial. *BMJ* **299**:805-6, 1989.

69.   Lazzara R: Amiodarone and torsade de pointes. *Ann Intern Med* **111**:549-51, 1989.

70.   Nguyen PT, Scheinman MM, Seger J: Polymorphous ventricular tachycardia: clinical characterization, therapy, and the QT interval. *Circulation* **74**:340-9, 1986.

71.   Makkar RR, Fromm BS, Steinman RT, et al.: Female gender as a risk factor for torsades de pointes associated with cardiovascular drugs. *JAMA* **270**:2590-7, 1993.

72.   Stevenson WG, Weiss J: Torsades de pointes due to n-acetylprocainamide. *Pacing Clin Electrophysiol* **8**:528-31, 1985.

73.   Haverkamp W, Hordt M, Breithardt G, Borggrefe M: Torsade de pointes secondary to *d,l*-sotalol after catheter ablation of incessant atrioventricular reentrant tachycardia--evidence for a significant contribution of the "cardiac memory". *Clin Cardiol* **21**:55-8, 1998.

74.   Kuck KH, Kunze KP, Roewer N, Bleifeld W: Sotalol-induced torsade de pointes. *Am Heart J* **107**:179-80, 1984.

75.   McKibbin JK, Pocock WA, Barlow JB, et al.: Sotalol, hypokalemia, syncope, and torsade de pointes. *Br Heart J* **51**:157-162, 1984.

76.   Jervell A, Lange-Nielsen F: Congenital deaf-mutism; functional heart disease with prolongation of the QT interval and sudden death. *Am Heart J* **54**:59-68, 1957.

77.   Romano C, Gemme G, Pongiglione R: Aritmie cardiache rare dell' eta pediatrica. *Clin Pediatr (Bologna)* **45**:656-683, 1963.

78.   Ward OC: A new familial cardiac syndrome in children. *J Irish Med Assoc* **54**:103-106, 1964.

79.   Bhandari AK, Shapiro WA, Morady F, et al.: Electrophysiologic testing in patients with the long QT syndrome. *Circulation* **71**:63-71, 1985.

80.   Lazzara R: Mechanisms and management of congenital and acquired long QT syndromes. *Arch Mal Coeur Vaiss* **89 Spec No 1**:51-5, 1996.

81.   Lazzara R, Szabo B, Patterson E, Scherlag BJ. Mechanisms for proarrhythmia with antiarrhythmic drugs. In: Zipes DP, Jalife J, eds. *Cardiac Electrophysiology: From Cell to Bedside*. Philadelphia, PA: W.B. Saunders, 402-407: 1990.

82.   Cranefield PF: Action potentials, afterpotentials, and arrhythmias. *Circ Res* **41**:415-23, 1977.

83.   Cranefield PF, Aronson RS: Torsade de pointes and other pause-induced ventricular tachycardias: the short-long-short sequence and early afterdepolarizations. *Pacing Clin Electrophysiol* **11**:670-8, 1988.

84.   Cranefield PF, Aronson RS: Torsades de pointes and early afterdepolarizations. *Cardiovasc Drugs Ther* **5**:531-7, 1991.

85.   El-Sherif N, Craelius W, Boutjdir M, Gough WB: Early afterdepolarizations and arrhythmogenesis. *J Cardiovasc Electrophysiol* **1**:145-160, 1990.

86.   El-Sherif N, Zeller RH, W. C, Gough WB, Henkin R: QTU prolongation and polymorphic ventricular tachyarrhythmias due to bradycardia-dependent early afterdepolarizations. Afterdepolarizations and ventricular arrhythmias. *Circ Res* **63**:286-305, 1988.

87.   El-Sherif N, Gomes JA, Restivo M, Mehra R: Late potentials and arrhythmogenesis. *Pacing Clin Electrophysiol* **8**:440-62, 1985.

88.   Brachmann J, Scherlag BJ, Rosenshtraukh LV, Lazzara R: Bradycardia-dependent triggered activity: relevance to drug-induced multiform ventricular tachycardia. *Circulation* **68**:846-56, 1983.

89. Priori SG, Napolitano C, Schwartz PJ: Electrophysiologic mechanisms involved in the development of torsades de pointes. *Cardiovasc Drugs Ther* **5**:203-12, 1991.

90. Kaseda S, Gilmour RF, Jr., Zipes DP: Depressant effect of magnesium on early afterdepolarizations and triggered activity induced by cesium, quinidine, and 4-aminopyridine in canine cardiac Purkinje fibers. *Am Heart J* **118**:458-66, 1989.

91. Carlsson L, Abrahamsson C, Drews L, Duker G: Antiarrhythmic effects of potassium channel openers in rhythm abnormalities related to delayed repolarization. *Circulation* **85**:1491-1500, 1992.

92. Fish FA, Prakash C, Roden DM: Suppression of repolarization-related arrhythmias in vitro and in vivo by low-dose potassium channel activators. *Circulation* **82**:1362-1369, 1990.

93. Nattel S, Quantz MA: Pharmacological response of quinidine induced early afterdepolarizations in canine cardiac Purkinje fibres: insights into underlying ionic mechanisms. *Cardiovasc Res* **22**:808-817; 1998.

94. Bursill JA, Wyse KR, Campbell TJ: Quinidine but not disopyramide prolongs cardiac Purkinje fiber action potentials after a pause. *J Cardiovasc Pharmacol* **23**:833-837, 1994.

95. Hoffman BF, Rosen MR: Cellular mechanisms for cardiac arrhythmias. *Circ Res* **49**:1-15, 1981.

96. Tsien RW, Hess P, Lansman JB, Lee KS. Current view of cardiac calcium channels and their response to calcium antagonists and agonists. In: Zipes DP, Jalife J, eds. *Cardiac Electrophysiology and Arrhythmias*. Orlando, FL: Grune & Stratton, 19-29: 1985.

97. Gintant GA, Datyner NB, Cohen IS: Slow inactivation of a tetrodotoxin-sensitive current in canine cardiac Purkinje fibers. *Biophys J* **45**:509-512, 1984.

98. Attwell D, Cohen I, Eisner D, et al.: The steady state TTX-sensitive (window) sodium current in cardiac Purkinje fibers. *Pflügers Archiv* **379**:137-142, 1979.

99. Bailie DS, Inoue H, Kaseda S, et al.: Magnesium suppression of early afterdepolarizations and ventricular tachyarrhythmias induced by cesium in dogs. *Circulation* **77**:1395-402, 1988.

100. Ben-David J, Zipes DP: Alpha-adrenoceptor stimulation and blockade modulates cesium-induced early afterdepolarizations and ventricular tachyarrhythmias in dogs. *Circulation* **82**:225-33, 1990.

101. Kaseda S, Zipes DP: Effects of alpha adrenergic stimulation and blockade on early afterdepolarizations induced by cesium in canine cardiac Purkinje fibers. *J Cardiovasc Electrophysiol* **1**:31-40, 1990.

102. Marban E, Robinson SW, Wier WG: Mechanisms of arrhythmogenic delayed and early afterdepolarizations in ferret ventricular muscle. *J Clin Invest* **78**:1185-1192, 1986.

103. Takahashi N, Ito M, Saikawa T, Arita M: Nicorandil suppresses early afterdepolarisation and ventricular arrhythmias induced by caesium chloride in rabbits in vivo. *Cardiovasc Res* **25**:445-52, 1991.

104. Takahashi N, Ito M, Ishida S, Fujino T, et al.: Effects of vagal stimulation on cesium-induced early afterdepolarizations and ventricular arrhythmias in rabbits. *Circulation* **86**:1987-92, 1992.

105. Song Y, Thedford S, Lerman BB, Belardinelli L: Adenosine-sensitive afterdepolarizations and triggered activity in guinea pig ventricular myocytes. *Circ Res* **70**:743-53, 1992.

106. Roden DM, Woosley RL: QT prolongation and arrhythmia suppression. *Am Heart J* **109**:411-5, 1985.

107. Roden DM, Hoffman BF: Action potential prolongation and induction of abnormal automaticity by low quinidine concentrations in canine Purkinje fibers. Relationship to potassium and cycle length. *Circ Res* **56**:857-867, 1985.

108. Gough WB, et al.: The differential response of normal and ischaemic Purkinje fibres to clofilium, D-sotalol and bretylium. *Cardiovascular Res* **23**:554-559, 1989.

109. Tohse N, Kameyama M, Irasawa I: Intracellular Ca2+ and protein kinase C modulate K+ current in guinea pig heart cells. *Am J Physiol* **253**(5 Pt 2):H1321-H1324, 1987.

110. Hiraoka M, Sunami A, Fan Z, Sawanobori T: Multiple ionic mechanisms of early afterdepolarizations in isolated ventricular myocytes from guinea-pig hearts. *Ann NY Acad Sci* **644**:33-47, 1992.

111. Peper K, Trautwein W: The effect of aconitine on the membrane current in cardiac muscle. *Pflügers Archiv* **296**:328-336, 1967.

112. January CT, Riddle JM: Early afterdepolarizations: mechanism of induction and block. A role for L-type Ca2+ current. *Circ Res* **64**:977-990, 1989.

113. January CT, Shorofsky S: Early afterdepolarizations: newer insights into cellular mechanisms. *J Cardiovasc Electrophysiol* **1**:161-169, 1990.

114. January CT, Moscucci A: Cellular mechanisms of early afterdepolarizations. *Ann NY Acad Sci* **644**:23-32, 1992.

115. January CT, Riddle JM, Salata JJ: A model for early afterdepolarizations: induction with the Ca2+ channel agonist Bay K 8644. *Circ Res* **62**:563-571, 1988.

116. Spinelli W, Sorota S, Siegal M, Hoffman BF: Antiarrhythmic actions of the ATP-regulated K+ current activated by pinacidil. *Circ Res* **68**:1127-1137, 1991.

117. Attwell D, Lee JA: A cellular basis for the primary long Q-T syndromes. *Lancet* **1**:1136-9, 1988.

118. Antzelevitch C, Sicouri S: Clinical relevance of cardiac arrhythmias generated by afterdepolarizations. Role of M cells in the generation of U waves, triggered activity and torsade de pointes. *J Am Coll Cardiol* **23**:259-77, 1994.

119. Antzelevitch C, Nesterenko VV, Yan GX: Role of M cells in acquired long QT syndrome, U waves, and torsade de pointes. *J Electrocardiol* **28 Suppl**:131-8, 1995.

120. Liu DW, Antzelevitch C: Characteristics of the delayed rectifier current (IKr and IKs) in canine ventricular epicardial, midmyocardial, and endocardial myocytes. A weaker IKs contributes to the longer action potential of the M cell. *Circ Res* **76**:351-65, 1995.

121. Sicouri S, Antzelevitch D, Heilmann C, Antzelevitch C: Effects of sodium channel block with mexiletine to reverse action potential prolongation in *in vitro* models of the long term QT syndrome. *J Cardiovasc Electrophysiol* **8**:1280-90, 1997.

122. Jackman WM, Szabo B, Friday KJ, et al.: Ventricular tachyarrhythmias related to early afterdepolarizations and triggered firing: relationship to QT interval prolongation and potential therapeutic role for calcium channel blocking agents. *J Cardiovasc Electrophysiol* **1**:170-195, 1990.

123. Kass RS, Lederer WJ, Tsien RW, Weingart R: Role of calcium ions in transient inward currents and aftercontractions induced by strophanthidin in cardiac Purkinje fibres. *J Physiol (Lond)* **281**:187-208, 1978.

124. Colquhoun D, Neher E, Reuter H, Stevens CF: Inward current channels activated by intracellular Ca in cultured cardiac cells. *Nature* **294**:752-754, 1981.

125. Vos MA, Verduyn C, Lipcsei GE, et al.: Induction of acquired bradycardia dependent torsade de pointes arrhythmias is prevented by flunarizine: a comparison with MgSO4 (Abstract). *Circulation* **86(Suppl I)**:I-560, 1992.

126. Vos MA, Gorgels AP, Verduyn SC, et al.: Ryanodine prevents early afterdepolarizations dependent torsade de pointes arrhythmias in the intact heart (Abstract). *J Am Coll Cardiol* **23**:282A, 1994.

127. Priori SG, Corr PB: Mechanisms underlying early and delayed afterdepolarizations induced by catecholamines. *Am J Physiol* **258**:H1796-805, 1990.

128. Han J, de Jalon PG, Moe GK: Adrenergic effects on ventricular vulnerability. *Circ Res* **14**:516-524, 1964.

129. Kuo CS, Munakata K, Reddy CP, Surawicz B: Characteristics and possible mechanism of ventricular arrhythmia dependent on the dispersion of action potential durations. *Circulation* **67**:1356-1367, 1983.

130. Wiggers CJ: The mechanism and nature of ventricular fibrillation. *Am Heart J* **20**:399-412, 1940.

131. Tsien RW, Giles W, Greengard P: Cyclic AMP mediates the effects of adrenaline on cardiac purkinje fibres. *Nat New Biol* **240**:181-3, 1972.

132. Brucker R, Mugge A, Scholz H: Existence and functional role of alpha1-adrenoceptors in the mammalian heart. *J Mol Cell Cardiol* **17**:639-645, 1985.

133. Lindemann JP, Watanabe AM. Sympathetic control of cardiac electrical activity. In: Zipes DP, Jalife J, eds. *Cardiac Electrophysiology: From Cell to Bedside*. Philadelphia, PA: W.B. Saunders, 277-283: 1990.

134. Reuter H: Calcium channel modulation by neurotransmitters, enzymes and drugs. *Nature* **301**:569-574, 1983.

135. Brum G, Flockerzi V, Hofmann F, et al.: Injection of catalytic subunit of cAMP-dependent protein kinase into isolated cardiac myocytes. *Pflugers Arch* **398**:147-54, 1983.

136. Rosen MR, Jeck CD, Steinberg SF: Autonomic modulation of cellular repolarization and of the electrocardiographic QT interval. *J Cardiovasc Electrophysiol* **3**:487-499, 1992.

137. Walsh KB, Kass RS: Regulation of a heart potassium channel by protein kinase A and C. *Science* **242**:67-69, 1988.

138. Eisner DA. The Na-K pump in cardiac muscle. In: Fozzard HA, Haber E, Jennings RB, eds. *The Heart and Cardiovascular System: Scientific Foundations*. New York, NY: Raven Press, 498-507: 1986.

139. DiFrancesco D, Tromba C: Muscarinic control of the hyperpolarization-activated current (if) in rabbit sino-atrial node myocytes. *J Physiol (Lond)* **405**:493-510, 1988.

140. DiFrancesco D, Tromba C: Inhibition of the hyperpolarization-activated current (if) induced by acetylcholine in rabbit sino-atrial node myocytes. *J Physiol (Lond)* **405**:477-91, 1988.

141. Watanabe AM, Hathaway DR, Besch HR, et al.: alpha-Adrenergic reduction of cyclic adenosine monophosphate concentrations in rat myocardium. *Circ Res* **40**:596-602, 1974.

142. Manalan AS, Jones LR: Characterization of the intrinsic cAMP-dependent protein kinase activity and endogenous substrates in highly purified cardiac sarcolemmal vesicles. *J Biol Chem* **257**:10052-10062, 1982.

143. Nishizuka Y: The role of protein kinase C in cell surface signal transduction and tumour promotion. *Nature* **308**:693-698, 1984.

144. Apkon M, Nerbonne JM: Alpha 1-adrenergic agonists selectively suppress voltage-dependent K+ current in rat ventricular myocytes. *Proc Natl Acad Sci U S A* **85**:8756-60, 1988.

145. Shah A, Cohen IS, Rosen MR: Stimulation of cardiac alpha receptors increases Na/K pump current and decreases gK via a pertussis toxin-sensitive pathway. *Biophys J* **54**:219-225, 1988.

146. Berridge MJ: Inositol triphosphate and diacylglycerol: two interacting second messengers. *Ann Rev Biochem* **56**:159-193, 1987.

147. Brown JH, Buxton AL, Brunton LL: alpha1-Adrenergic and muscarinic cholinergic stimulation of phosphoinositide hydrolysis in adult rat cardiomyocytes. *Circ Res* **57**:532-537, 1985.

148. Carlsson L, Almgren O, Duker G: QTU-prolongation and torsades de pointes induced by putative class III antiarrhythmic agents in the rabbit: etiology and interventions. *J Cardiovasc Pharmacol* **16**:276-285, 1990.

149. Lee KS: Ibutilide, a new compound with potent class III antiarrhythmic activity, activates a slow inward Na current in guinea pig ventricular cells. *J Pharmacol Exp Ther* **262**:99-108, 1992.

150. Yang T, Snyders DJ, Roden DM: Ibutilide, a methanesulfonamilide antiarrhythmic, is a potent blocker of the rapidly-activating delayed rectifier K+ current (Ikr) in AT-1 cells: concentration, time-, voltage-, and use dependent effects. *Circulation* **91**:1799-1806, 1995.

151. Thompson KA, Murray JJ, Blair IA, et al.: Plasma concentrations of quinidine, its major metabolites, and dihydroquinidine in patients with torsades de pointes. *Clin Pharmacol Ther* **43**:636-642, 1988.

152. Hohnloser SH, Singh BN: Proarrhythmia with Class III antiarrhythmic drugs: Definition, electrophysiologic mechanisms, incidence, predisposing factors and clinical implications. *J Cardiovasc Electrophysiol* **6**:920-936, 1995.

153. Hohnloser ST, T. M, Stubbs P, et al.: Efficacy and safety of d-sotalol, a pure class III antiarrhythmic compound, in patients with symptomatic complex ventricular ectopy. Results of a multicenter, randomized, double-blind, placebo-controlled dose-finding study. *Circulation* **92**:1517-1525, 1995.

154. Janse MJ: To prolong refractoriness or to delay conduction (or both)? *Eur Heart J* **13 Suppl F**:14-8, 1992.

155. Sicouri S, Moro S, Litovsky S, et al.: Chronic amiodarone reduces transmural dispersion of repolarization in the canine heart. *J Cardiovasc Electrophysiol* **8**:1269-79, 1997.

156. Bhandari AK, Quock C, Sung RJ: Polymorphous ventricular tachycardia associated with a marked prolongation of the Q-T interval induced by amiodarone. *Pacing Clin Electrophysiol* **7**:341-5, 1984.

157. Mattioni TA, Zheutlin TA, Sarmiento JJ, et al.: Amiodarone in patients with previous drug-mediated torsade de pointes. Long-term safety and efficacy. *Ann Intern Med* **111**:574-580, 1989.

158. Jurkiewicz NK, Sanguinetti MC: Rate-dependent prolongation of cardiac action potentials by a methanesulfonamilide class III antiarrhythmic agent: specific block of rapidly activating delayed rectifier K+ current by dofetilide. *Circ Res* **72**:75-83, 1993.

159. Wang J, Bourne GW, Wang Z, et al.: Comparative mechanisms of antiarrhythmic drug action in experimental atrial fibrillation. Importance of use-dependent effects on refractoriness. *Circulation* **88**:1030-44, 1993.

160. Surawicz B: Electrophysiologic substrate of torsade de pointes: dispersion of repolarization or early afterdepolarizations? *J Am Coll Cardiol* **14**:172-184, 1989.

161. Roden DM, Thompson KA, Hoffman BF, Woosley RL: Clinical features and basic mechanisms of quinidine-induced arrhythmias. *J Am Coll Cardiol* **8(1 Suppl A)**:73A-78A, 1986.

162. Kurita T, Ohe T, Shimizu W, et al.: Early afterdepolarization in a patient with complete atrioventricular block and torsades de pointes. *Pacing Clin Electrophysiol* **16**:33-8, 1993.

163. Kay GN, Plumb VJ, Arciniegas JG, et al.: Torsade de pointes: the long-short initiating sequence and other clinical features: observations in 32 patients. *J Am Coll Cardiol* **2**:806-17, 1983.

164. Noble D: Ionic mechanisms determining the timing of ventricular repolarization: significance for cardiac arrhythmias. *Ann NY Acad Sci* **644**:1-22, 1992.

165. Roden DM, Lazzara R, Rosen M, et al.: Multiple mechanisms in the long-QT syndrome. Current knowledge, gaps, and future directions. The SADS Foundation Task Force on LQTS. *Circulation* **94**:1996-2012, 1996.

166. Bauman JL, Bauernfeind RA, Hoff JV, et al.: Torsade de pointes due to quinidine: observations in 31 patients. *Am Heart J* **107**:425-30, 1984.

167. Priori SG, Corr PB: The importance of alpha-adrenergic stimulation of cardiac tissue and its contribution to arrhythmogenesis during ischemia. *J Cardiovasc Electrophysiol* **1**:529-542, 1990.

168. Schomig A, Dart AM, Dietz R, et al.: Release of endogenous catecholamines in the ischemic myocardium of the rat. Part A: Locally mediated release. *Circ Res* **55**:689-701, 1984.

169. Singh BN: Bepridil therapy: guidelines for patient selection and monitoring of therapy. *Am J Cardiol* **68**:79D-85D, 1992.

170. Nobe S, Aomine M, Arita M: Bepridil prolongs the action potential duration of guinea pig ventricular muscle only at rapid rates of stimulation. *Gen Pharmacol* **24**:1187-96, 1993.

171. Rubart M, Pressler ML, Pride HP, Zipes DP: Electrophysiological mechanisms in a canine model of erythromycin-associated long QT syndrome. *Circulation* **88**:1832-44, 1993.

172. Gitler B, Berger LS, Buffa SD: Torsades de pointes induced by erythromycin. *Chest* **105**:368-372, 1994.

173. Nattel S, Ranger S, Talajic M, et al.: Erythromycin-induced long QT syndrome: concordance with quinidine and underlying cellular electrophysiologic mechanism. *Am J Med* **89**:235-8, 1990.

174. Antzelevitch C, Sun ZQ, Zhang ZQ, Yan GX: Cellular and ionic mechanisms underlying erythromycin-induced long QT intervals and torsade de pointes. *J Am Coll Cardiol* **28**:1836-48, 1996.

175. Chen Y, Gillis RA, Woosley RL: Block of delayed rectifier potassium current IK, by terfenadine in cat ventricular myocytes (Abstract). *J Am Coll Cardiol* **17**:140A, 1991.

176. Chen YW, Follmer CH, Hershkowitz N, et al.: Block of delayed rectifier potassium current, IK, by cocaine in cat ventricular myocytes (Abstract). *J Am Coll Cardiol* **17**:140A, 1991.

177. Schrem SS, Belsky P, Schwartzman D, Slater W: Cocaine-induced torsades de pointes in a patient with the idiopathic long QT syndrome. *Am Heart J* **120**:980-984, 1990.

178. Kimura S, Bassett AL, Xi H, Myerburg RJ: Early afterdepolarizations and triggered activity induced by cocaine. A possible mechanism of cocaine arrhythmogenesis. *Circulation* **85**:2227-2235, 1992.

179. Bayer R, Schwarzmaier J, Pernice R: Basic mechanisms underlying prenylamine-induced 'torsade de pointes': differences between prenylamine and fendiline due to basic actions of the isomers. *Curr Med Res Opin* **11**:254-72, 1988.

180. Zaza A, Malfatto G, Rosen MR: Electrophysiologic effects of ketanserin on canine Purkinje fibers, ventricular myocardium and the intact heart. *J Pharmacol Exp Ther* **250**:397-405, 1989.

181. Kemper AJ, Dunlap R, Pietro DA: Thioridazine-induced torsade de pointes. Successful therapy with isoproterenol. *JAMA* **249**:2931-2934, 1983.

182. Metzger E, Friedman R: Prolongation of the corrected QT and torsades de pointes cardiac arrhythmia associated with intravenous haloperidol in the medically ill. *J Clin Psychopharmacol* **13**:128-132, 1993.

183. Weld FM, Bigger JT, Jr.: Electrophysiological effects of imipramine on ovine cardiac Purkinje and ventricular muscle fibers. *Circ Res* **46**:167-75, 1980.

184. Keren G, Tepper D, Butler B, et al.: Studies on the possible mechanisms of lidoflazine arrhythmogenicity. *J Am Coll Cardiol* **4**:742-7, 1984.

185. Hanley SP, Hampton JR: Ventricular arrhythmias associated with lidoflazine: side-effects observed in a randomized trial. *Eur Heart J* **4**:889-893, 1983.

186. Glassman AH, Roose SP, Bigger JT, Jr.: The safety of tricyclic antidepressants in cardiac patients. Risk-benefit reconsidered. *JAMA* **269**:2673-5, 1993.

187. Lopez JA, Harold JG, Rosenthal MC, et al.: QT prolongation and torsades de pointes after administration of trimethoprim-sulfamethoxazole. *Am J Cardiol* **59**:376-377, 1987.

188. Sartori M, Pratt CM, Young JB: Torsade de pointe. Malignant cardiac arrhythmia induced by amantadine poisoning. *Am J Med* **77**:388-391, 1984.

189. Wharton JM, Demopulos PA, Goldschlager N: Torsade de pointes during administration of pentamidine isethionate. *Am J Med* **83**:571-576, 1987.

190. Goss JE, Ramo BW, Blake K: Torsades de pointes associated with astemizole (Hismanal) therapy. *Arch Intern Med* **153**:2705, 1993.

191. Fauchier JP, Lanfranchi J, Ginies G, Raynaud R: "Syncope par torsades de pointes" au cours d'un traitement par la chloroquine. Etude de l'ectrocardiogramme hisien et traitment par le verapamil. *Ann Cardiol Angeiol (Paris)* **23**:341-46, 1974.

192. Ludomirsky A, Klein HO, Sarelli P, et al.: Q-T prolongation and polymorphous ("torsade de pointes") ventricular arrhythmias associated with organophosphorous insecticide poisoning. *Am J Cardiol* **49**:1654-8, 1982.

193. Ben-Haim SA, Ben-Ami H, Hayam G, et al.: Effect of phosphamidon and obidoxime on the QT-RR relationship of isolated rat heart. *Pharmacol Toxicol* **70**:402-6, 1992.

194. Little RE, Kay GN, Cavender JB, et al.: Torsade de pointes and T-U wave alternans associated with arsenic poisoning. *Pacing Clin Electrophysiol* **13**:164-70, 1990.

195. Mauro VF, Bingle JF, Ginn SM, Jafri FM: Torsade de pointes in a patient receiving intravenous vasopressin. *Crit Care Med* **16**:200-201, 1988.

196. Kumar A, Bhandari AK, Rahimtoola SH: Torsade de pointes and marked QT prolongation in association with hypothyroidism. *Ann Intern Med* **106**:712-713, 1987.

197. Fredlund BO, Olsson SB: Long QT interval and ventricular tachycardia of torsade de pointe type in hypothyroidism. *Acta Med Scand* **213**:231-235, 1983.

198. Sen S, Stober T, Burger L, et al.: Recurrent torsade de pointes type ventricular tachycardia in intracranial hemorrhage. *Intensive Care Med* **10**:263-264, 1984.

199. Shimizu K, Miura Y, Meguro Y, et al.: QT prolongation with torsade de pointes in pheochromocytoma. *Am Heart J* **124**:235-9, 1992.

200. de Keyser J, De Boel S, Ceulemans L, Ebinger G: Torsade pointes as a complication of brainstem encephalitis. *Intensive Care Med* **13**:76-77, 1987.

201. Rotem M, Constantini S, Shir Y, Cotev S: Life-threatening torsade de pointes arrhythmia associated with head injury. *Neurosurgery* **23**:81-92, 1988.

202. Sareli P, Schamroth CL, Passias J, Schamroth L: Torsade de pointes due to coxsackie B3 myocarditis. *Clin Cardiol* **10**:361-362, 1987.

203. Pringle TH, Scobie IN, Murray RG, et al.: Prolongation of the QT interval during therapeutic starvation: a substrate for malignant arrhythmias. *Int J Obes* **7**:253-261, 1983.

204. Bauer MF, Aebert H, Zurbrugg H, et al.: Torsades de pointes arrhythmia in a patient with left ventricular myxoma. *Chest* **105**:1876-8, 1994.

205. Aldariz AE, Romero H, Baroni M, et al.: QT prolongation and torsade de pointes ventricular tachycardia produced by Ketanserin. *PACE Pacing and Clinical Electrophysiology* **9**:836-841, 1986.

206. Zehender M, Meinertz T, Hohnloser S, et al.: Incidence and clinical relevance of QT prolongation caused by the new selective serotonin antagonist ketanserin. Multicenter Ketanserin Research Group. *Clin Physiol* **8(suppl 3)**:90-100, 1990.

207. Kearney P, Reardon M, O'Hare J: Primary hyperparathyroidism presenting as torsades de pointes. *Br Heart J* **70**:473, 1993.

208. Curry P, Fitchett D, Stubbs W, Krikler D: Ventricular arrhythmias and hypokalaemia. *Lancet* **2**:231-233, 1976.

209. Machado C, Baga JJ, Kawasaki R, et al.: Torsade de pointes as a complication of subarachnoid hemorrhage: a critical reappraisal. *J Electrocardiol* **30**:31-7, 1997.

210. Di Pasquale G, Pinelli G, Andreoli A, et al.: Torsade de pointes and ventricular flutter-fibrillation following spontaneous cerebral subarachnoid hemorrhage. *Int J Cardiol* **18**:163-172, 1988.

211. Honig PK, Wortham DC, Zamani K, et al.: Terfenadine-ketoconazole interaction. Pharmacokinetic and electrocardiographic consequences. *JAMA* **269**:1513-1518, 1993.

212. Pohjola-Sintonen S, Viitasalo M, et al.: Itraconazole prevents terfenadine metabolism and increases risk of torsades de pointes ventricular tachycardia. *Eur J Clin Pharmacol* **45**:191-193, 1993.

213. Keating M, Atkinson D, Dunn C, et al.: Linkage of a cardiac arrhythmia, the long QT syndrome, and the Harvey ras-1 gene. *Science* **252**:704-706, 1991.

214. Priori SG, Schwartz PJ, Napolitano C, et al.: A recessive variant of the Romano-Ward long-QT syndrome? *Circulation* **97**:2420-2425, 1998.

215. Roden DM, George AL, Bennett PB: Recent advances in understanding the molecular mechanisms of the long QT syndrome. *J Cardiovasc Electrophysiol* **6**:1023-1031, 1995.

216. Vincent GM: Hypothesis for the molecular physiology of the Romano-Ward long QT syndrome. *J Am Coll Cardiol* **20**:500-503, 1992.

217. Vincent GM: The molecular genetics of the long QT syndrome: genes causing fainting and sudden death. *Annu Rev Med* **49**:263-74, 1998.

218. Moss AJ, Robinson JL: Long QT syndrome. *Heart Dis Stroke* **1**:309-14, 1992.

219. Moss AJ, Schwartz PJ, Crampton RS, et al.: The long QT syndrome. Prospective longitudinal study of 328 families. *Circulation* **84**:1136-44, 1991.

220. Moss AJ: The long QT syndrome revisited: current understanding and implications for treatment. *Pacing Clin Electrophysiol* **20**:2879-81, 1997.

221. Moss AJ: Clinical management of patients with the long QT syndrome: drugs, devices, and gene-specific therapy. *Pacing Clin Electrophysiol* **20**:2058-60, 1997.

222. Ohe T, Kurita T, Aihara N, et al.: Electrocardiographic and electrophysiologic studies in patients with torsades de pointe--role of monophasic action potentials. *Jpn Circ J* **54**:1323-30, 1990.

223. Sanguinetti MC, Jiang C, Curran ME, Keating MT: A mechanistic link between an inherited and an acquired cardiac arrhythmia: HERG encodes the IKr potassium channel. *Cell* **81**:299-307, 1995.

224. Sanguinetti MC, Zou A: Molecular physiology of cardiac delayed rectifier K+ channels. *Heart Vessels* **Suppl 12**:170-2, 1997.

225. Kugiyama K, Yasue H, Horia Y, et al.: Effects of propranolol and nifedipine on exercise-induced attack in patients with variant angina: assessment by exercise thallium-201 myocardial scintigraphy with quantitative rotational tomography. *Circulation* **74**:374-380, 1986.

226. Arnsdorf MF, Bigger JT: The effects of procainamide on components of excitability in long mammalian cardiac Purkinje fibers. *Circulation Research* **38**:115-121, 1976.

227. Carmeliet E, Saikawa T: Shortening of the action potential and reduction in pacemaker activity by lidocaine, quinidine, and procainamide in sheep cardiac Purkinje fibers. An effect on Na or K currents? *Circ Res* **50**:257-272, 1982.

228. Noma A: ATP-regulated K+ channels in cardiac muscle. *Nature* **305**:147-8, 1983.

229. Sakmann B, Noma A, Trautwein W: Acetylcholine activation of single muscarinic K+ channels in isolated pacemaker cells of the mammalian heart. *Nature* **303**:250-3, 1983.

230. Shimizu W, Kurita T, Matsuo K, et al.: Improvement of repolarization abnormalities by a K+ channel opener in the LQT1 form of congenital long-QT syndrome. *Circulation* **97**:1581-8, 1998.

231. Kurita T, Ohe T, Marui N, et al.: Bradycardia-induced abnormal QT prolongation in patients with complete atrioventricular block with torsades de pointes. *Am J Cardiol* **69**:628-33, 1992.

232. Kaplinsky E, Yahino JN, Barzilai J, Neufeld HN: Quinidine syncope: report of a case successfully treated with lidocaine. *Chest* **62**:764-766, 1972.

233. Schwartz PJ, Priori SG, Locati EH, et al.: Long QT syndrome patients with mutations of the SCN5A and HERG genes have differential responses to Na+ channel blockade and to increases in heart rate. Implications for gene-specific therapy. *Circulation* **92**:3381-6, 1995.

234. Shimizu W, Antzelevitch C: Sodium channel block with mexiletine is effective in reducing dispersion of repolarization and preventing torsade des pointes in LQT2 and LQT3 models of the long-QT syndrome. *Circulation* **96**:2038-47, 1997.

235. Shimizu W, Ohe T, Kurita T, et al.: Epinephrine-induced ventricular premature complexes due to early afterdepolarizations and effects of verapamil and propranolol in a patient with congenital long QT syndrome. *J Cardiovasc Electrophys* **5**:438-444, 1994.

236. Cosio FG, Goicolea A, Lopez Gil M, et al.: Suppression of Torsades de Pointes with verapamil in patients with atrio-ventricular block. *Eur Heart J* **12**:635-638, 1991.

237. Nayebpour M, Nattel S: Pharmacologic response of cesium-induced ventricular tachyarrhythmias in anesthetized dogs. *J Cardiovasc Pharmacol* **15**:552-61, 1990.
238. Tzivoni D, Banai S, Schuger C, et al.: Treatment of torsade de pointes with magnesium sulfate. *Circulation* **77**:392-7, 1988.
239. Bethell HW, Vandenberg JI, Camm AJ, Grace AA: Magnesium has concentration and time-dependent effects on action potential duration during myocardial ischemia (Abstract). *Circulation* **90(Pt 2)**:I-524, 1994.
240. Iseri LT, French JH: Magnesium: nature's physiologic calcium blocker. *Am Heart J* **108**:188-193, 1984.
241. Damiano BP, Rosen MR: Effects of pacing on triggered activity induced by early afterdepolarizations. *Circulation* **69**:1013-1025, 1984.
242. DiSegni E, Klein HO, David D, et al.: Overdrive pacing in quinidine syncope and other long QT-interval syndromes. *Arch Intern Med* **140**:1036-1040, 1980.
243. Moss AJ, Liu JE, Gottlieb S, et al.: Efficacy of permanent pacing in the management of high-risk patients with long QT syndrome. *Circulation* **84**:1524-9, 1991.
244. Schwartz PJ, Locati E, Priori SG, Zaza A. The long Q-T syndrome. In: Zipes DP, Jalife J, eds. *Cardiac Electrophysiology: From Cell to Bedside*. Philadelphia, PA: W.B. Saunders, 589-605: 1990.
245. Sicouri S, Antzelevitch C: Drug-induced afterdepolarizations and triggered activity occur in a discrete subpopulation of ventricular muscle cells (M cells) in the canine heart: quinidine and digitalis. *J Cardiovasc Electrophysiol* **4**:48-58, 1993.

CHAPTER 17

VENTRICULAR FIBRILLATION AND SUDDEN CARDIAC DEATH

This final chapter is devoted to a discussion of the broad topic of sudden cardiac death. There are many causes of sudden death including arrhythmia, trauma, intracranial vascular catastrophes, and acute thrombosis or embolism involving the heart or lungs. The present discussion will be restricted to the arrhythmic causes of sudden cardiac death, primarily ventricular fibrillation (Figure 17-1). Not all episodes of ventricular fibrillation lead to death. Ventricular fibrillation may, as with atrial fibrillation, be non-sustained (self-terminating), or the patient may be rescued by bystanders or medical personnel by receiving a direct current countershock before irreversible cellular or organ damage intervenes. It is clear, however, that unlike monomorphic ventricular tachycardia which, depending upon its rate, may continue for many minutes, hours or even days without the patient developing significant hemodynamic compromise, sustained ventricular fibrillation will inevitably lead to death within minutes unless it is terminated. Although some cases of sudden arrhythmic death have been attributed to asystole or electromechanical dissociation, these often represent merely the natural evolution of untreated ventricular fibrillation.

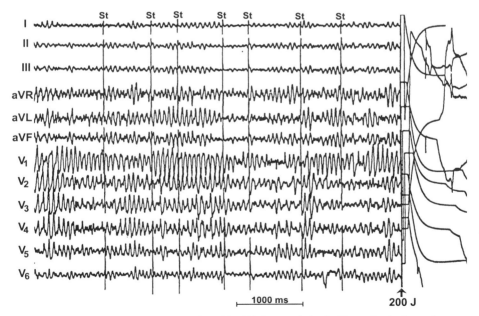

FIGURE 17-1. Ventricular fibrillation terminated by 200-J external shock. The patient's electronic pacemaker continues to deliver pacing stimuli (St) during ventricular fibrillation.

763

17.1   Definition and Epidemiology

Many investigators have grappled with a definition of sudden death. Some suggest that: "Since all death is (eventually) sudden and associated with cardiac arrhythmias, the concept of sudden death is only meaningful if it is unexpected, while arrhythmic death is only meaningful if life could have continued had the arrhythmia been prevented or terminated. Any practical classification of death being sudden or arrhythmic is highly dependent on the quality of available data to ensure that the suddenness was unexpected and that life could have continued if the arrhythmia had been prevented or treated" [1]. Others have defined sudden death as "death which is non-violent or non-traumatic, which is unexpected, which is witnessed, and which is instantaneous or occurs within a few minutes of an abrupt change in previous clinical state" [2]. For present purposes, sudden cardiac death shall be defined as death occurring within minutes from unexpected ventricular fibrillation, or ventricular tachycardia that rapidly (within seconds) accelerates to ventricular fibrillation, and that if prevented or immediately terminated, would allow the patient to return to their previous level of functioning for an indefinite period. Having defined it as such, it will still remain difficult to score any particular patient's unwitnessed death as sudden or non-sudden and, in many cases, the "suddenness," as well as the actual mode of death, may well remain a mystery.

Because of these uncertainties, accurately establishing the scope of the problem of sudden cardiac death remains difficult. Sudden cardiac death is believed to affect up to 400,000 people each year in the United States [3-5], and therefore, is an important public health problem. The survival rate for out-of-hospital cardiac arrest is low, with estimates ranging from 2% to 25% in the United States [6,7]. In addition, prior to the availability of the implantable cardioverter-defibrillator (ICD) or amiodarone, sudden cardiac death survivors had a high rate of mortality after hospital discharge (1 year, 24%; 2 years, 34%; 4 years, 51% mortality rates) compared with an age- and gender-adjusted control group (4 years, 20% mortality) or for a a similar control group discharged after suffering an acute myocardial infarction (4 years, 34% mortality) [8]. Therefore, two issues have confronted clinicians over the years; namely, 1) how best to protect survivors of sudden cardiac death (secondary prevention) and, 2) how to identify, *a priori*, those individuals who have never suffered a cardiac arrest but are at highest risk (primary prevention).

17.2   Type of Arrhythmias Associated with Sudden Cardiac Death

For an out-of-hospital cardiac arrest, the initial rhythm documented by paramedics appears dependent upon the time between collapse and arrival of the emergency medical personnel. When that time is unknown, the initial rhythm is found to be ventricular fibrillation in 40% of patients, asystole in 40%, electromechanical dissociation in 20% and monomorphic ventricular tachycardia in 1% [9]. On the other hand, when the time is known, the proportion of patients with ventricular fibrillation increases while those with asystole decreases as the time between the collapse and the first ECG decreases. For example, if time from collapse to first ECG is 12-16 minutes, the initial rhythm is ventricular fibrillation in 71% of patients and asystole in 29%. At 8-11 minutes after collapse, the first ECG shows ventricular fibrillation in 88% of patients (asystole 12%). At 4-7 minutes, ventricular fibrillation is the initial rhythm 93% of the time (asystole 7%), and if less than 4 minutes elapsed between collapse and first ECG, ventricular fibrillation is the initial arrhythmia documented 95% of the time with asystole seen only 5% of the time [10].

In general, ventricular fibrillation is not commonly precipitated by monomorphic ventricular tachycardia. Firstly, a history of sustained monomorphic ventricular tachycardia is extremely uncommon in survivors of sudden cardiac death [11]. Secondly, in 1287 patients who suffered a cardiac arrest and were treated within 2-3 minutes by an automatic external defibrillator, monomorphic ventricular tachycardia was detected in only 16 patients (1.2%) [9]. Thirdly, patients suffering a cardiac arrest while enrolled in a supervised cardiac rehabilitation program and were resuscitated within 30 sec were found initially with ventricular fibrillation 92% of the time and monomorphic ventricular tachycardia only 8% of the time [12]. Finally, most reports suggesting that monomorphic ventricular tachycardia precedes ventricular fibrillation in cardiac arrest victims comes from Holter monitor tracings. This is already a biased population in that these select patients were undergoing monitoring because they were known to have a recurrent (usually ventricular) tachyarrhythmia (a history very atypical for patients who suffer a cardiac arrest). Often, inspection of these rhythm strips shows that the onset of the tachyarrhythmia is, in reality, ventricular flutter or polymorphic ventricular tachycardia, or simply frank ventricular fibrillation, rather than classic monomorphic ventricular tachycardia [13-16]. Furthermore, because usually only one, or at most two, ECG leads are recorded in these cases, establishing that even the initial beats of the arrhythmia are truly monomorphic is difficult. Even if one grants that the first few beats are monomorphic, virtually all these tracings reveal that the arrhythmia quickly becomes polymorphic, or evolves into frank ventricular fibrillation.

Evidence from the electrophysiology laboratory also supports the conclusion that monomorphic ventricular tachycardia is uncommon in these patients as a presenting arrhythmia. The Seattle investigators found that only 27% of the survivors of a cardiac arrest had monomorphic ventricular tachycardia inducible during electrophysiology testing [17]. In addition, the clinical profile of the out-of-hospital cardiac arrest survivors with coronary artery disease is distinctly different than the profile of patients with a history of coronary artery disease and recurrent monomorphic ventricular tachycardia. Patients in the sudden death group have a lower incidence of remote myocardial infarction and left ventricular aneurysm and a higher ejection fraction than patients in the group with monomorphic ventricular tachycardia [18]. Cardiac arrest survivors with implanted third generation ICDs having the capability to store intracardiac electrograms rarely have non-sustained or sustained monomorphic ventricular tachycardia during long-term follow-up [19]. Finally, patients with a history of recurrent monomorphic ventricular tachycardia only rarely present with ventricular fibrillation during long-term follow-up [18,20-22].

Taken together these data strongly suggest that the sudden collapse of a cardiac arrest is rarely due to monomorphic ventricular tachycardia. Furthermore, finding an individual in asystole or electromechanical dissociation usually indicates that a relatively long time period has passed since the initiating tachyarrhythmia and the recording of the first ECG; prolonged untreated ventricular fibrillation leads eventually to cardiac quiescence. Patients who suffer a cardiac arrest almost certainly present with ventricular fibrillation or a brief run (<15-20 sec) of monomorphic ventricular flutter (ventricular rate >250/min) or polymorphic ventricular tachycardia, either of which quickly degrades into ventricular fibrillation. Finally, the patient population that is at highest risk of having a cardiac arrest appears to be different than those patients at highest risk of suffering recurrent episodes of monomorphic ventricular tachycardia. Consequently, research efforts directed at primary prevention of cardiac arrest should not necessarily target those patients at highest risk of suffering recurrent episodes of monomorphic ventricular tachycardia (e.g., those that have had spontaneous clinical episodes of monomorphic ventricular tachycardia in the past or those that are found to have inducible monomorphic ventricular tachycardia in the electrophysiology laboratory).

17.3   Clinical Profile of Survivors of Sudden Cardiac Death

Coronary artery disease is the most common clinical condition associated with patients who suffer a cardiac arrest (64% to 90% of cases) [23-32]. In the experience of the Seattle investigators, the typical sudden death survivor is a 60 to 70-year old male with a coronary artery disease (78%) and a remote history of a myocardial infarction (45%) [11]. Many other clinical conditions have also been associated with sudden cardiac death and they are outlined in Table 17-1.

17.4   Role of Autonomic Nervous System in Sudden Arrhythmic Death

Enhanced sympathetic tone or increased sensitivity to sympathetic input, possibly in association with a decline in a modulating parasympathetic influence, may play a role in the occurrence of sudden cardiac death.

Clinical studies have shown that administration of β-adrenergic blocking agents to patients in the period following a myocardial infarction results in significant reductions in sudden cardiac death rates, total mortality, and reinfarction rates [33-37] (Figure 17-2). Patients suffering an acute myocardial infarction who received β-adrenergic blockade during and following the acute phase of their infarct also had a reduction in the incidence of early and intermediate-term ventricular fibrillation [38-43].

Animal experiments also suggest an adverse role for the sympathetic nervous system in the occurrence of sudden cardiac death, especially in the setting of acute myocardial ischemia [44,45]. Ischemia-mediated ventricular fibrillation is associated with a marked increase in sympathetic neural traffic to the myocardium following acute arterial occlusion [46], an increase in the number of β-adrenergic receptors, and an increase in cyclic adenosine monophosphate (cAMP) in ischemic, compared with non-ischemic tissues [47-50]. Of possible significance, the rise in cAMP may precede the development of ventricular fibrillation [48,49]. Furthermore, in animals, β-adrenergic blockade appears to protect against ischemia-induced ventricular fibrillation [51-56].

TABLE 17-1. Causes of & conditions associated with sudden cardiac death

Acute myocardial infarction
Atherosclerotic coronary artery disease
Coronary artery spasm
Idiopathic dilated cardiomyopathy
Hypertrophic cardiomyopathy
Left ventricular hypertrophy
Arrhythmogenic right ventricular dysplasia
Congenital heart disease & coronary artery anomalies
Valvular heart disease, primarily aortic stenosis
Congenital and acquired long QT syndromes (torsade de pointes)
Antiarrhythmic drugs
Severe electrolyte abnormalities
Recreational drug use (cocaine, methamphetamine, etc.)
Infiltrative disorders (sarcoidosis, amyloidosis, hemochromatosis, myocarditis, cardiac tumors)
Wolff-Parkinson-White syndrome
Brugada syndrome
East Asian male sudden death syndrome
Complete AV block
Acute myocardial rupture/cardiac tamponade
Massive pulmonary embolism
Idiopathic ventricular fibrillation

Evidence from the canine model of chronic myocardial infarction also suggests that abnormalities of the autonomic nervous system may play a role in triggering sudden death [57]. In this model, sympathetic nerve fibers are interrupted along their course through the infarcted myocardium. Heterogeneous areas of sympathetic denervation subsequently develop in non-infarcted myocardium distal to the region of transmural infarction. Supersensitivity to catecholamines has been noted in some denervated regions with an exaggerated shortening of the effective refractory period in these regions during norepinephrine or isoproterenol infusions [58]. Canine hearts with sympathetic denervation-induced catecholamine supersensitivity have a lower fibrillation threshold, a finding which is reversed by propranolol. These observations in animals have been confirmed in patients [59] with a history of myocardial infarction, ventricular tachycardia, and ventricular fibrillation using a radioactively-labeled analogue of norepinephrine (^{11}C-hydroxyephedrine) and positron emission tomography. Although parasympathetic innervation of the ventricle is sparse, it is important in modulating presynaptic norepinephrine release and activating postsynaptic muscarinic receptors, thereby inhibiting adenylate cyclase activity. As with sympathetic fibers, parasympathetic fibers can be disrupted by myocardial infarction leading to heterogeneous vagal denervation [60]. The significance of these findings relative to sudden cardiac death is yet to be untangled; but

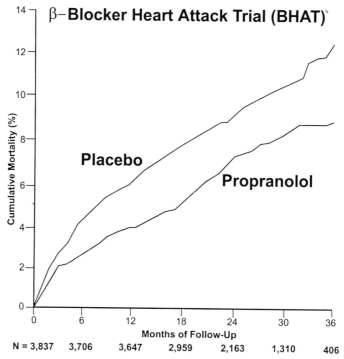

FIGURE 17-2. Data from the β-Blocker Heart Attack Trial (BHAT) showing survival curve for patients who suffered a myocardial infarction and were treated with either a β-adrenergic blocking agent (propranolol) or placebo. Adapted from [33,34].

the role of the autonomic nervous system in triggering ventricular fibrillation in high risk patients remains an intense area of ongoing research.

17.5   Risk Stratification & Predictors of Sudden Arrhythmic Death

The risk factors for sudden cardiac death include:

1. Left ventricular dysfunction, with those patients having the poorest left ventricular ejection fraction having the worst prognosis;
2. Inducibility of monomorphic ventricular tachycardia by programmed electrical stimulation, especially in patients with reduced left ventricular ejection fraction;
3. Ventricular ectopy, including single ventricular premature depolarizations (>10 VPDs/hr) and asymptomatic non-sustained ventricular tachycardia, in the setting of left ventricular dysfunction;
4. Presence of late potentials on the signal-averaged ECG;
5. Reduced heart rate variability;
6. Abnormal baroreceptor sensitivity.

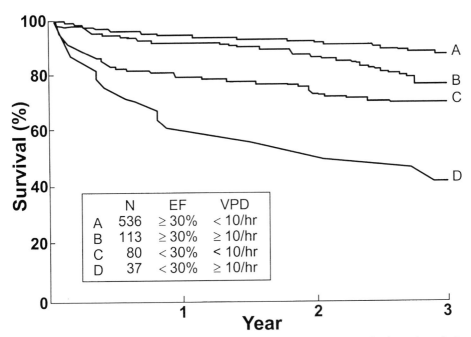

FIGURE 17-3. Survival after an acute myocardial infarction as a function of ejection fraction and ventricular ectopy. Patients with the poorest left ventricular function and the most ventricular ectopy had the worst prognosis. EF, ejection fraction. Adapted from [193].

The severity of left ventricular dysfunction is the single strongest predictor of total cardiac (sudden and non-sudden) mortality. According to the investigators for the Multicenter Investigation of the Limitation of Infarct Size (MILIS) study, a left ventricular ejection fraction < 40% is a sensitive and specific predictor of sudden cardiac death [61]. An ejection fraction <30% is associated with a 3.5-fold increased chance of dying [62-64]. The inducibility of monomorphic ventricular tachycardia by programmed electrical stimulation in the setting of reduced left ventricular function is well established as a powerful predictor for recurrence of sudden cardiac death [17,65-82]. For example, a survivor of sudden cardiac death with an ejection fraction > 30% and found to be non-inducible at electrophysiology study had a risk of recurrence of sudden death or ICD shocks (which were used as a non-fatal equivalent of sudden death) of 2% at one year and 11% at two years, while the risk of recurrent sudden death or ICD shock was 23% at one year and 35% at two years in sudden death survivors with an ejection fraction < 30% [17].

Non-sustained ventricular tachycardia or frequent ventricular premature depolarizations in combination with reduced left ventricular ejection fraction (EF < 40%) identifies a high risk group for sudden cardiac death (Figures 17-3 & 17-4) [61-64,83-90]. However, despite this, the investigators involved in the Cardiac Arrhythmia Suppression Trial (CAST and CAST-II) found that suppression of ventricular ectopy, *per se*, with potent Na⁺ channel blockers not only failed to reduce mortality, but in fact increased mor-

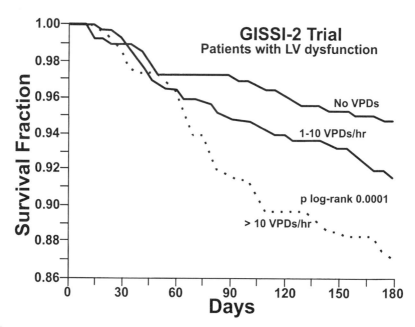

FIGURE 17-4. Survival data from GISSI-2 (Gruppo Italiano per lo Studio della Sopravvivenza nell'Infarto Miocardico) trial of patients with left ventricular (LV) dysfunction and various degrees of ventricular ectopy. Patients with left ventricular dysfunction and > 10 VPDs/hr have a particularly poor prognosis. VPDs, ventricular premature depolarizations. Adapted from [85].

tality in the population they studied [91-93], possibly due to an ischemia-related proarrhythmic mechanism [94].

Other predictors of sudden cardiac death include abnormal heart rate variability [95-104], baroreceptor sensitivity [97,105-108], and signal-averaged ECG [97,100,103,104,109-114]. However, the lack of high predictive accuracy of these tests, even when used in combinations, have made them unsuitable to use as a guide to evaluate which patients should receive aggressive and expensive preventive therapy with, for example, an ICD.

17.6   Evaluation of Patients Surviving a Cardiac Arrest

The main issue to be addressed in the survivor of sudden cardiac death is whether there is any *reliably identifiable* cause for the cardiac arrest (secondary ventricular fibrillation) or whether the cardiac arrest has no specific identifiable precipitant (primary ventricular fibrillation). In the relatively rare case that a reliably identifiable cause can be established, elimination of that inciting influence may be all that is necessary to treat the patient's cardiac arrest. For example, an episode of torsade de pointes leading to ventricular fibrillation may be clearly related to acute QT prolongation secondary to the administration of quinidine or procainamide for treatment of atrial fibrillation. In such a patient, especially if they have normal left ventricular function, probably the only required treatment would be discontinuation of the drug.

The most common identifiable and reversible cause of ventricular fibrillation is acute myocardial ischemia/infarction. For patients who have a cardiac arrest in the setting of a new transmural myocardial infarction, the annual risk of suffering a subsequent cardiac arrest is very low (<2%) [23]. Therefore, these patients usually require no specific treatment directed against the arrhythmia; instead, further diagnostic evaluation and treatment should be directed at the underlying coronary artery disease.

Myocardial ischemia due to fixed coronary artery disease or coronary artery spasm is best diagnosed if there is a history of angina or documented ST elevation or depression prior to the collapse. Unless contraindicated for some reason, all patients who suffer a ventricular fibrillation cardiac arrest should undergo coronary and left ventricular angiography to rule in or out significant coronary artery disease (or coronary anomalies) and assess left ventricular function. Should coronary artery disease be present, establishing that it is physiologically significant using a functional test (e.g., exercise-thallium study or stress-echocardiography test) should also be considered. The finding of high-grade, physiologically-significant proximal coronary artery disease in one or more major vessels (especially in the setting of normal left ventricular function) argues strongly that the patient's cardiac arrest resulted from ischemia and, therefore, treatment should be directed solely at revascularization efforts without treating the arrhythmia, *per se*.

Other identifiable reversible causes of ventricular fibrillation are rare but include recreational drugs, severe electrolyte or acid-base disturbance (e.g. hypokalemia with serum K^+ < 3.0 mEq/L at least, especially in the presence of toxic or near-toxic levels of digoxin), or proarrhythmia from antiarrhythmic drugs (Table 17-1.) In general, however, one should only consider solely attributing a cardiac arrest to these factors if there is no myocardial ischemia/infarction documented and ventricular function is entirely normal. Even focal or mild left ventricular abnormalities may be the cause of a cardiac arrest and therefore, treatment of a primary arrhythmia with an ICD may be necessary in these patients even though some of these secondary factors may have possibly contributed to their cardiac arrest. It is also important to rule out long QT syndromes (congenital or acquired) (see "The Acquired Long QT Syndromes and Torsade de Pointes" on page 742 and "The Hereditary Long QT Syndromes" on page 745). Treatment of survivors of an episode of torsade de pointes due to a congenital or acquired long QT problem may differ significantly from a patient with an old myocardial infarct scar and may range from simply withdrawing an offending agent to implantation of an ICD (see "Treatment of Polymorphic Ventricular Tachycardia & Long QT Syndromes" on page 746).

Other diagnostic studies that are often useful in particular instances include standard transthoracic or transesophagael echocardiography, especially to assess valvular heart disease or evaluate patients for the possibility of right ventricular dysplasia. However, in patients in whom right ventricular dysplasia is suspected, magnetic resonance imaging, right ventricular angiography, or possibly, endomyocardial biopsy may be required to definitively establish a diagnosis. Infiltrative disorders, such as sarcoidosis, amyloidosis, hemochromatosis, or myocarditis, usually require a right ventricular endomyocardial biopsy for diagnosis.

If this assessment of reversible/treatable causes fails to identify any such factors, direction is next focused on an evaluation of the patient's arrhythmic substrate, usually by performing an electrophysiology study. Non-invasive testing such as outpatient ambulatory ECG monitoring, signal-averaged ECG, T-wave alternans, or an assessment of heart rate variability are of little or no value in the evaluation of patients who have already established their risk of sudden cardiac death by actually having a cardiac arrest. On the other hand, an electrophysiology study is often (if not always) performed in these patients even though it may also have limited usefulness in these individuals. It often can provide important information as to whether the patient may have a treatable precipitating arrhythmic cause for their cardiac arrest such as bundle branch reentrant ventricular tachycardia or, especially in young people, the Wolff-Parkinson-White syndrome [115-117]. The purpose of the electrophysiology study is not to prove that ventricular fibrillation is inducible. This is because inducibility of ventricular fibrillation by programmed electrical stimulation is a non-specific finding, regardless of the left ventricular function.

Prior to the development and widespread availability of ICD systems, the best available treatment for survivors of sudden arrhythmic death was revascularization and/or treatment with antiarrhythmic drugs. With the development, validation, and standardization of programmed electrical stimulation as a reliable and reproducible means to induce *monomorphic ventricular tachycardia* in patients having the requisite substrate, this technique had become widely used to evaluate and guide the administration of antiarrhythmic drugs in these patients. Data suggested that patients with inducible ventricular tachycardia that was suppressed by antiarrhythmic drugs had improved survival compared with patients with inducible ventricular tachycardia that was not suppressed by drugs (Figure 17-5). Typically during this procedure a patient with a clinical ventricular tachycardia underwent a baseline electrophysiology study to determine if the monomorphic ventricular tachycardia was reliably and reproducibly provoked using a standardized pacing protocol. If so, the patient remained in the hospital, was loaded with an antiarrhythmic drug, and electrophysiology testing was repeated to determine if the antiarrhythmic drug suppressed the induced monomorphic ventricular tachycardia. This process was repeated until the electrophysiologist judged that the most protective drug had been found. This procedure, termed *electrophysiology-guided drug testing*, is seldom used today. When used, the drugs tested are usually restricted to intravenous procainamide and oral sotalol or amiodarone. In patients who have suffered a cardiac arrest, problems prevent this technique from being widely used today, especially given the success of the ICD in rescuing patients from sudden arrhythmic death. These problems include relatively low inducibility of the clinical ventricular arrhythmia, lack of reliability, reproducibility and significance of any induced arrhythmia, and questionable value and reliability of antiarrhythmic drug suppression in this high risk patient population.

The inducibility of any ventricular tachyarrhythmia in patients who have suffered an out-of-hospital cardiac arrest has been reported to be widely variable, ranging from 45% to 85% [17,65,67,68,70,77,80,82,118-120]. In addition, in a patient who has suffered a cardiac arrest, the significance of inducing monomorphic ventricular tachycardia is unclear at best, and possibly totally irrelevant, especially since monomorphic ventricu-

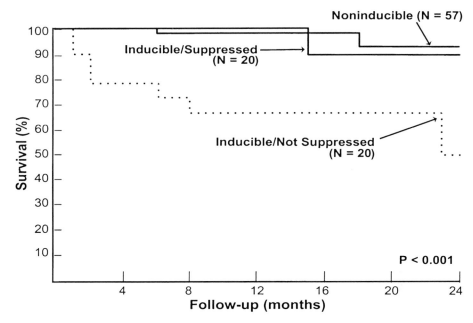

FIGURE 17-5. Survival curves for patients with inducible ventricular tachyarrhythmias and the survival benefit of drug suppression. Electrophysiology-guided drug testing was performed in 97 consecutive patients with a history of coronary artery disease, ejection fraction < 40%, and asymptomatic non-sustained ventricular tachycardia. Adapted from [194].

lar tachycardia appears to be the trigger for a cardiac arrest only rarely (see above "Type of Arrhythmias Associated with Sudden Cardiac Death" on page 764). Furthermore, the induction of ventricular fibrillation, may be a totally non-specific arrhythmia since it can be induced using programmed electrical stimulation in patients with a normal ventricle, who have never suffered cardiac arrest, and have no known clinical factors putting them at risk of having a cardiac arrest. In addition, suppression of induced ventricular tachyarrhythmias is often difficult to achieve with antiarrhythmic drugs with upwards of 66% of these patients still remaining inducible [17,67,68,77,82,118-121]. And finally, the long-term efficacy of antiarrhythmic drugs in this group of patients (even if found to be totally suppressive) is poor, with sudden death rates as high as 31% at two years and 60% at four years [67,68,77,82,118,119,122,123]. Consequently, using electrophysiology-guided drug testing in cardiac arrest survivors may provide these patients with poor intermediate or long-term protection, especially when compared with that provided by an ICD.

17.7 Treatment of Survivors of Sudden Arrhythmic Death

There is no cookbook algorithm that can reliably substitute for clinical judgement when developing the best treatment plan for any individual patient. With this in mind, a consensus has formed around certain treatment principles that can be applied in certain broad groups of patients. However, in practice, the clinician should approach each patient and each patient situation individually, and be aware that over time the standard of care can change.

Surgical revascularization

As alluded to above, patients with a clear ischemic or infarct-related cause for their cardiac arrest may only require a revascularization procedure (coronary artery bypass, angioplasty, coronary stenting, etc.) as their sole treatment. This is particularly true if the patient's collapse occurs during exercise, is preceded by angina, and the patient is subsequently found to have physiologically-significant high-grade proximal coronary artery disease with normal ventricular function and no inducible arrhythmia during electrophysiology testing. Patients with this clinical scenario have been found to do well when treated with coronary revascularization and β-adrenergic blockers alone [124-126]. Even if the cardiac arrest does not occur during exercise and left ventricular function is not absolutely normal, coronary revascularization therapy alone does appear to extol upon cardiac arrest survivors significant protection with one and five year survival of 92% and 82% for surgically treated patients compared to those treated with medical therapy (80% and 51%, respectively) [127-131].

Antiarrhythmic drug therapy

Ever since the CAST (Cardiac Arrhythmia Suppression Trial), the use of antiarrhythmic drugs as a sole treatment for patients with ventricular tachyarrhythmias has become increasingly unpopular. However, the CAST and CAST-II never were designed to address the issue of the use of these agents in the treatment of sudden cardiac death survivors. Rather they were designed to assess the effect of these agents (administered without electrophysiology-guidance and randomly) on the survival of patients believed to be at high risk of sudden cardiac death by virtue of their previous myocardial infarction and baseline ventricular ectopy. However, a variety of other studies, both prospective and retrospective, have tended to support the belief that empiric use of class IA, IB, and IC antiarrhythmic drugs does not provide protection from sudden cardiac death. In fact, these agents may worsen the mortality of patients with ventricular tachyarrhythmias due to a variety of mechanisms, including negative inotropism, increasing incidence of ventricular fibrillation during ischemia, proarrhythmia, or a decrease in heart rate variability [132-143]. A meta-analysis suggests that the only drugs that reduce mortality following a myocardial infarction are β-adrenergic blockers and amiodarone (Figure 17-6) [144]. Taken together, this avalanche of data argues strongly against the routine empiric use of "conventional" (class I) antiarrhythmic drugs as a means of primary prevention in patients at high risk for sudden cardiac death, as well as the use of these agents for electrophysiology-guided suppression of inducible ventricular tachyarrhythmias in patients with a history of, or at high risk for, ventricular arrhythmias or sudden arrhythmic death.

The greatest hope for a safe and effective drug treatment for primary and secondary prevention has fallen upon the class III agents amiodarone and sotalol. In survivors of an out-of-hospital cardiac arrest, both total cardiac mortality and sudden cardiac death are reduced by amiodarone compared with Holter- or electrophysiology-guided antiarrhythmic drug therapy using conventional (class I) antiarrhythmic drugs [118,119,145-147] (Figure 17-7). For patients who have suffered a myocardial infarction and have an ejection fraction < 40% amiodarone does reduce mortality due to ventricular tachyarrhythmias compared to placebo (Figure 17-8), but *does not* reduce total or cardiac mortality in these same patients [148-152]. However, conflicting data from CASCADE (sudden death survivors, Figure 17-7) and GESICA (patients

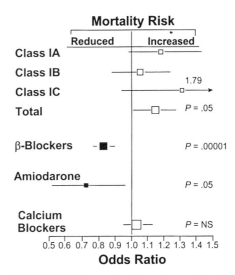

FIGURE 17-6. Meta-analysis showing mortality risk associated with antiarrhythmic drugs, presumably secondary the proarrhythmic effects exerted by these agents. Only β-adrenergic blockers and amiodarone appear to reduce risk. Adapted from [144].

with non-sustained ventricular who are post-myocardial infarction, Figure 17-9) do indicate that amiodarone is, indeed, associated with a decrease in cardiac and total mortality. Unfortunately, recurrent sudden death rates for patients on amiodarone (assessed by documented ventricular fibrillation or syncope with ICD shock) still ranges from 4.5% to 31% at two years [118,119,147,148-152]. *d,l*-Sotalol, a class III drug with β-adrenergic blocking effects has gained some favor, especially after the ESVEM (Electrophysiologic Study Versus Electrocardiographic Monitoring) trial reported that *d,l*-sotalol reduced the

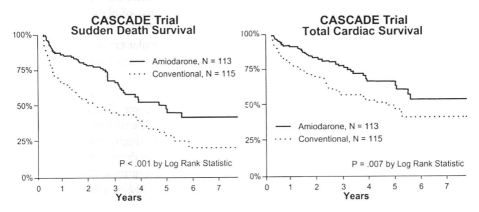

FIGURE 17-7. Sudden cardiac death and total cardiac survival in the CASCADE study. Survivors of an out-of-hospital cardiac arrest were randomized to empiric amiodarone or electrophysiology- or Holter-guided therapy using conventional antiarrhythmic drugs. The endpoints were cardiac arrest from ventricular fibrillation, cardiac mortality, or syncope followed by an ICD shock. Adapted from [119].

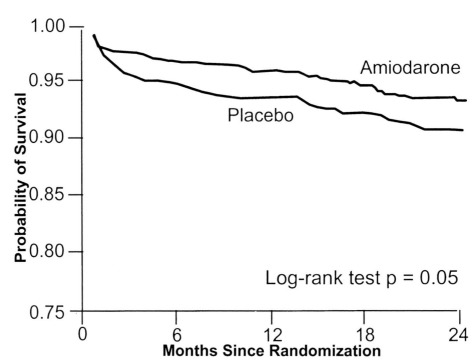

FIGURE 17-8. Prevention of sudden death due to a ventricular tachyarrhythmia (arrhythmic deaths and resuscitated cardiac arrests) by amiodarone. Survival data from EMIAT (European Myocardial Infarction and Amiodarone Trial). Adapted from [148].

recurrence of arrhythmia and overall mortality significantly more than conventional antiarrhythmic drugs [122,123]. However, only about 20% of ESVEM patients were sudden death survivors and the probability of arrhythmia recurrence with sotalol was still 21% at one year and over 40% at four years [122,123]. In addition, the results of the recent SWORD (Survival With Oral *d*-Sotalol) trial [153,154] suggests that it is likely to be the β-adrenergic blocking activity present in racemic *d,l*-sotalol that confers its survival benefit. *d*-Sotalol, which lacks β-adrenergic blocking effects, increases the mortality of patients at high risk for sudden cardiac death [153,154].

Thus, amiodarone appears to be the only drug that has low proarrhythmia and may be effective in reducing arrhythmic mortality in high risk patients. There is conflicting data as to whether amiodarone is associated with a decline in total or cardiac mortality in these patients. However, because patients in these high risk groups, even if receiving amiodarone, still have a mortality risk from sudden cardiac death in excess of those patients who have received an ICD (see "Implantable cardioverter-defibrillators" on page 777) suggests that routine use of amiodarone as a primary preventive treatment in these patients may not be indicated. As a secondary preventive measure for survivors of cardiac arrests, ICD therapy appears to be the preferred option in most patients.

Surgical ablation of ventricular tachycardia

Data from 483 patients who underwent map-directed surgery for elimination of ventricular tachycardia (often with concomitant coronary artery bypass surgery) have been reviewed [155,156]. The major problem with this option is the high operative mortality (6% to 21%), even in those centers with a high patient volume. The low operative mortality of ICD implantation (<1%), the high success rate of these devices at rescuing victims of ventricular fibrillation, and the excellent long-term all-cause survival (75% at 36 months, see "Implantable cardioverter-defibrillators" below) of patients receiving ICDs, has all but eliminated surgery for ventricular tachycardia as a major clinical treatment for sudden cardiac death.

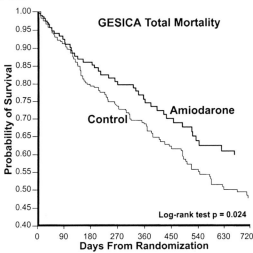

FIGURE 17-9. Data from the GESICA (Grupo de Estudio de la Sobrevida en la Insuficiencia Cardica en Argentina) trial showing that amiodarone reduced total mortality in patients with heart failure and non-sustained ventricular tachycardia but no previous history of sudden cardiac death. Adapted from [195].

Catheter ablation

Patients with severe heart disease and inducible monomorphic ventricular tachycardia may not be adequately protected from sudden cardiac death by ablation of a single (or multiple) target form(s) of ventricular tachycardia (which may be possible 60-70% of the time [157,158]. This is particularly of concern because only about 25% of patients undergoing an acutely successful ablation will remain free of recurrent ventricular tachycardia [159-162]. In addition, as mentioned above, monomorphic ventricular tachycardia is rarely the provoking arrhythmia in victims of sudden cardiac death (see above "Type of Arrhythmias Associated with Sudden Cardiac Death" on page 764). Only in two specific cases does it appear there may be a role for catheter ablation in treating sudden cardiac death survivors – patients with bundle branch reentrant ventricular tachycardia [163] and right ventricular tachycardia due to right ventricular dysplasia [164]. Even in these cases, the electrophysiologist must judge, based possibly upon the inducibility of other forms of ventricular tachycardia, or the severity of the patient's left ventricular dysfunction, whether the catheter ablation procedures provide adequate protection for these patients; additional therapy with an ICD may be indicated.

Implantable cardioverter-defibrillators

Beginning in the late 1980s, a number of studies have shown that ICDs are the most effective treatment in reducing sudden arrhythmic death due to ventricular fibrillation [165-171]. The one and five year sudden death survival in one series of 270 patients who received an ICD was 99% and 96%, respectively, with total survival of 92% and 74% at one and five years, respectively [170]. In the largest retrospective series of cardiac arrest survivors, a total of 331 patients who had received either electrophysiology-guided antiarrhythmic drug therapy or an ICD were followed [172]. In the 150 patients receiving an ICD, the total mortality was 29% versus 62% in the 181 patients without an ICD (Figure 17-10). The effect was most striking in patients with an EF ≤ 40%. This study was also showed that left ventricular function was more important in predicting long-term survival than the presence of an ICD because patients with a high left ventricular ejection fraction (>40%) without a device had a better survival than patients with an ICD and low left ventricular ejection fraction (≤40%) (Figure 17-10). In a prospective study, the Cardiac Arrest Study Hamburg (CASH) investigators found that sudden death survival was significantly better in a a group of cardiac arrest survivors who received an ICD compared with those who received empiric propafenone (196-198) (Figure 17-11).

While ICDs are clearly very effective at reducing sudden death due to ventricular fibrillation, a debate has evolved as to whether amiodarone is equally effective as ICDs at reducing total mortality. Because almost all patients with ventricular tachyarrhythmias or a history of sudden arrhythmic death are elderly, have other chronic diseases, and have poor left ventricular function, this group of patients will have a relatively high total (sudden, cardiac, and non-cardiac) mortality rate. Therefore, as the argument goes, what difference does it make if ICDs reduce sudden death, if these patients will nevertheless die of other diseases or, because of their poor left ventricular function, will die an early cardiac death due to pump failure. In other words, are ICDs simply an expensive

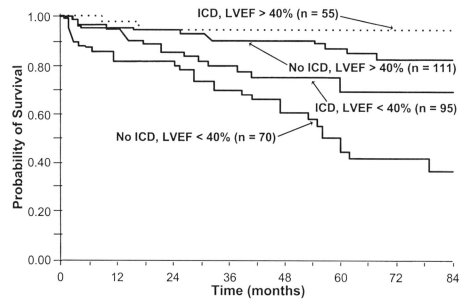

FIGURE 17-10. Survival curves in patients with ICDs as a function of left ventricular ejection fraction. Retrospective study of 331 patients who had suffered an out-of-hospital cardiac arrest and were treated with an ICD. See text for further discussion. Adapted from [172].

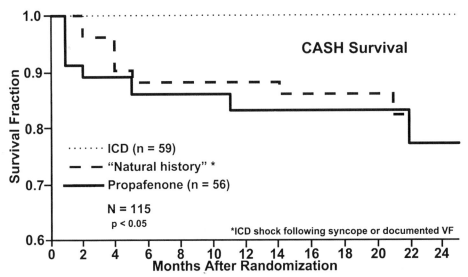

FIGURE 17-11. Sudden death survival curves for patients enrolled in CASH (Cardiac Arrest Study–Hamburg) [196-198]. CASH is a multicenter study in which 230 sudden death survivors were enrolled and randomized to receive either an ICD, empiric amiodarone, empiric propafenone, or metoprolol. The propafenone arm was terminated prematurely when follow-up data indicated that patients receiving empiric propafenone had a far worse survival than the group of patients receiving an ICD. During the two years of follow-up there was no sudden deaths in the ICD group. The "natural history" survival curve estimates the sudden death rate in the ICD group had they not received their ICD. This estimate assumes that the patient would have died at the time they received their first syncopal episode followed by a rescue ICD shock. Adapted from [197].

means to change the *mode of death*, but not the *rate of death* in these patients? Unfortunately, until recently, the best study bearing on this matter is a retrospective study in which patients receiving an ICD were found to have better overall survival than those that received amiodarone [173]. The AVID (Antiarrhythmics Versus Implantable Defibrillators) trial is the first prospective study to address this question [174]. The results of this multicenter study, that included both cardiac arrest survivors and patients who have suffered a sustained or symptomatic episode of ventricular tachycardia, suggest that both sudden and total mortality is significantly reduced in these patients by treatment with ICDs compared with empiric amiodarone or electrophysiology-guided racemic sotalol (Figure 17-12). Viewed one way, ICDs are associated with a 39% decline in overall mortality compared with amiodarone at one year of follow-up, 27% at two years, and 31% at three years of follow-up. However, viewed another way, patients receiving an ICD averaged only 2.1 months longer survival than those in the amiodarone group. While clearly some patients benefit greatly after receiving an ICD, other patients do not benefit at all, compared to their counterparts in the amiodarone treatment group. The AVID trial was terminated prematurely after the follow-up data became available showing the statistically significant survival benefit of ICDs over amiodarone. The Canadian Implantable Defibrillator Study (CIDS), as with AVID, randomized sudden death survivors or patients with symptomatic sustained ventricular tachycardia to receive either amiodarone or an ICD. While the CIDS data showed improved overall survival for

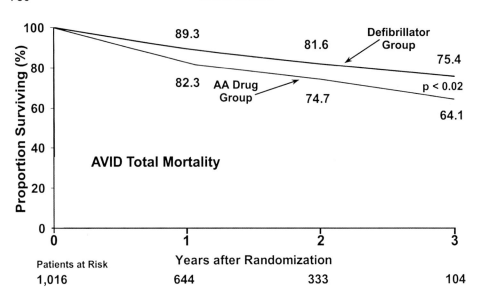

FIGURE 17-12. Total mortality curve from the AVID (Antiarrhythmics Versus Implantable Defibrillators) trial. The trial was terminated prematurely when data indicated that patients who received an ICD had significantly improved total survival compared with those who received either amiodarone or electrophysiology-guided sotalol. AA, antiarrhythmic drug (amiodarone or sotalol) group. Adapted from [174].

the ICD patients compared with the those receiving amiodarone, the difference did not reach statistical significance. [175].

Adjunctive therapy
β-Adrenergic blockers have been demonstrated for decades to reduce total mortality and sudden death mortality after myocardial infarction [33-36,176-178]. More recently, it has been demonstrated that in patients with congestive heart failure, carvedilol reduces the risk of death from 7.8% in untreated patients to 3.2% in the treatment group [179]. Although there is still some debate, the consensus of most investigators is that ACE inhibitors are effective at decreasing total mortality by 18% to 27% in patients with diminished left ventricular ejection fraction and heart failure [180-183].

17.8   Primary Prevention of Sudden Cardiac Death

The widespread and successful use of ICDs in survivors of cardiac arrest has largely addressed the issue of secondary prevention in those patients with no directly treatable cause for their cardiac arrest. However, the task of reliably identifying in advance patients at highest risk of suffering a first cardiac arrest and providing a cost-effective means of primary prevention remains difficult. Addressing this issue is further complicated by establishing an agreed upon definition of "high risk." "High risk" is a relative term with some clinicians considering any patient who has suffered an acute myocardial

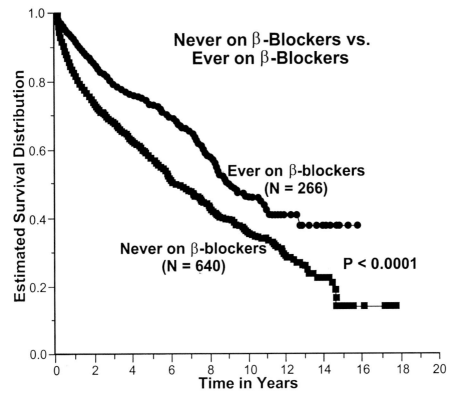

FIGURE 17-13. Survival benefits of ever receiving β-adrenergic blocker therapy in 906 patients who had an out-of-hospital cardiac arrest in the Seattle area between 1970 and 1985. Even part-time treatment with β blocking agents following a cardiac arrest dramatically improved survival compared with a patients that never received these agents or patients that received quinidine or procainamide (not shown). In fact the latter two agents were actually associated with an increased mortality compared to patients that did not receive these class I agents. Adapted from [132].

infarction or who may have abnormal left ventricular function to be "high risk." Clearly, screening all such patients with electrophysiology testing or empirically treating them with ICDs will have a significant economic impact on even the wealthiest society, especially as the proportion of its aged members increase.

The one preventive therapy that all agree should be part of the treatment plan in high risk patients is β-adrenergic blocking agents. The data is so compelling as to their effectiveness that even part-time or occasional use of these agents is associated with a significant reduction in total mortality in these patients (Figure 17-13). The effectiveness of β-adrenergic blockers points to the strong possibility that sympathetic tone, *per se*, or the balance of sympathetic and parasympathetic tone may play a crucial role in precipitating sudden death.

The value of electrophysiology testing to identify patients at high risk of suffering a sudden arrhythmic death has been demonstrated by a meta-analysis [184]. In patients with left ventricular dysfunction and non-sustained ventricular tachycardia, the induc-

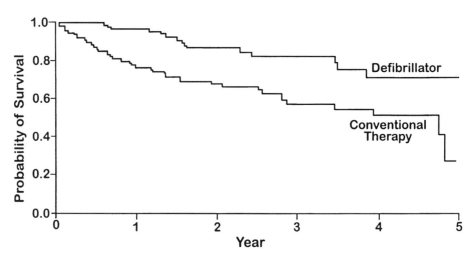

FIGURE 17-14. Survival curves for patients enrolled in MADIT (Multicenter Automatic Defibrillator Implantation Trial). See text for discussion. Adapted from [186].

ibility of sustained ventricular tachycardia is 45% [184]. During a 20 month follow-up period, 18% of the inducible patients, and 7% of the non-inducible patients, had an arrhythmic event, regardless of the type of antiarrhythmic drug therapy they were receiving. The calculated positive predictive accuracy of electrophysiology testing is 18%, while the negative predictive value is 93%. Hence, an electrophysiology study is more able to identify patients with low rather than high risk of sudden cardiac death. Two multicenter randomized controlled trials, the Multicenter Automatic Defibrillator Implantation Trial (MADIT) [185] (Figure 17-14) and the Multicenter Unsustained Tachycardia Trial (MUSTT) [83,186-188] (Figure 17-15) have used electrophysiology testing for risk stratification in patients with significant left ventricular dysfunction after myocardial infarction. The MADIT suggests that high risk patients (those with poor left ventricular function, non-sustained ventricular tachycardia, and inducible sustained ventricular tachycardia not suppressed by intravenous procainamide) were better off receiving an ICD than "conventional medical therapy". The MUSTT study has shown that patients receiving electrophysiology-guided antiarrhythmic treatment have a low rate of sudden cardiac death compared to those receiving no treatment (12% versus 25% in one year, and 18% versus 32% in five years). However, the improved survival rate of patients receiving electrophysiology-guided therapy is seen only in patients receiving an ICD. There is no difference in survival between inducible patients treated exclusively with antiarrhythmic drugs and those inducible patients randomized to receive no antiarrhythmic drug therapy. The MUSTT study has demonstrated that electrophysiology-guided *antiarrhythmic drug* therapy has no value for patients with inducible sustained ventricular tachycardia. Instead, this study suggests that the only effective antiarrhythmic therapy for primary prevention of sudden cardiac death in patients with inducible sustained monomorphic ventricular tachycardia is an ICD.

The recently completed CABG (Coronary Artery Bypass Graft) Patch trial [189,190] randomized patients with coronary artery disease, left ventricular dysfunction,

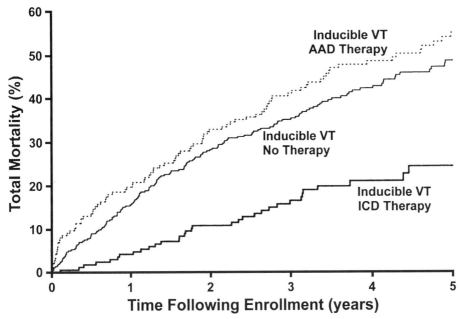

FIGURE 17-15. Survival curves for patients enrolled in MUSTT (Multicenter Unsustained Tachycardia Trial). Survival was statistically improved (P<0.001) in the ICD patients compared with untreated patients or those receiving electrophysiologically-guided drug therapy. AAD, antiarrhythmic drug; ICD, implantable cardioverter-defibrillator; VT, ventricular tachycardia. Adapted from [187].

and a positive signal-averaged ECG who were undergoing elective coronary artery bypass surgery to receive a prophylactic ICD (Figure 17-16). Unlike MADIT, implantation of an ICD failed to confer a survival benefit to this high risk group of patients compared with the control group who received the bypass surgery but no defibrillator. Unlike the MADIT patients, the enrollees in the CABG Patch trial were not screened with an electrophysiology study.

Important multicenter studies that are underway include MADIT-II and SCD-HeFT (Sudden Cardiac Death in Heart Failure Trial) [178,191,192]. SCD-HeFT is designed to determine whether amiodarone or the ICD will decrease overall mortality in patients with coronary artery disease or non-ischemic cardiomyopathy who are in heart failure (New York Heart Association class II or III) and have a left ventricular ejection fraction < 35%. The primary endpoint is total mortality; secondary endpoints include a comparison of arrhythmic and non-arrhythmic mortality and morbidity, as well as quality of life, cost-effectiveness, and incidence of episodes of ventricular tachyarrhythmias. MADIT-II proposes to test the hypothesis that ICDs increase the survival in patients with a history of previous myocardial infarctions and ejection fractions less than 30%. Candidates for this study will never have suffered a cardiac arrest or a symptomatic episode of non-sustained ventricular tachycardia. In fact, MADIT-II participants need not even have asymptomatic non-sustained ventricular tachycardia. They will not be screened with electrophysiology testing; instead they will be randomized to either receive an ICD or not receive an ICD. The endpoint is total mortality. This study may have a significant bear-

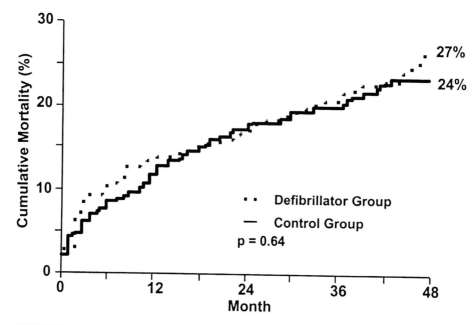

FIGURE 17-16. Total mortality in the CABG Patch trial. See text for discussion. Adapted from [189].

ing on use of ICDs if they are associated with a decline in total mortality in this group of patients. If empiric ICD implantation is viewed as the standard of care in post-myocardial infarction patients with ejection fractions less than 30%, the costs to society will be significant, especially as the population ages.

References

1.   Torp-Pedersen C, Kober L, Elming H, Burchart H: Classification of sudden and arrhythmic death. *Pacing Clin Electrophysiol* **20**:2545-52, 1997.
2.   Roberts WC: Sudden cardiac death: definitions and causes. *Am J Cardiol* **57**:1410-3, 1986.
3.   Myerburg RJ, Demirovic J. Epidemiologic considerations in cardiac arrest and sudden cardiac death: etiology and prehospital and posthospital outcomes. In: Podrid PJ, Kowey PR, eds. *Cardiac Arrhythmia: Mechanisms, Diagnosis, and Management*. Baltimore, MD: Williams & Wilkins, 964-74: 1995.
4.   Gillum RF: Sudden coronary death in the United States: 1980-1985. *Circulation* **79**:756-65, 1989.
5.   Myerburg RJ, Kessler KM, Castellanos A: Sudden cardiac death: epidemiology, transient risk, and intervention assessment. *Ann Intern Med* **119**:1187-97, 1993.
6.   Eisenberg MS, Cummins RO, Damon S, et al.: Survival rates from out-of-hospital cardiac arrest: recommendations for uniform definitions and data to report. *Ann Emerg Med* **19**:1249-59, 1990.
7.   Eisenberg MS, Horwood BT, Cummins RO, et al.: Cardiac arrest and resuscitation: a tale of 29 cities. *Ann Emerg Med* **19**:179-86, 1990.
8.   Eisenberg MS, Hallstrom A, Bergner L: Long-term survival after out-of-hospital cardiac arrest. *N Engl J Med* **306**:1340-3, 1982.
9.   Weaver WD, Hill D, Fahrenbruch CE, et al.: Use of the automatic external defibrillator in the management of out-of- hospital cardiac arrest. *N Engl J Med* **319**:661-6, 1988.
10. Hallstrom AP, Eisenberg MS, Bergner L: The persistence of ventricular fibrillation and its implication for evaluating EMS. *Emerg Health Serv Q* **1**:41-47, 1983.

11. Cobb LA, Weaver WD, Fahrenbruch CE, et al.: Community-based interventions for sudden cardiac death. Impact, limitations, and changes. *Circulation* **85**:I98-102, 1992.

12. Hossack KF, Hartwig R: Cardiac arrest associated with supervised cardiac rehabilitation. *J Cardiac Rehabil* **2**:402-418, 1982.

13. Nikolic G, Bishop RL, Singh JB: Sudden death recorded during Holter monitoring. *Circulation* **66**:218-25, 1982.

14. Pratt CM, Francis MJ, Luck JC, et al.: Analysis of ambulatory electrocardiograms in 15 patients during spontaneous ventricular fibrillation with special reference to preceding arrhythmic events. *J Am Coll Cardiol* **2**:789-97, 1983.

15. Milner PG, Platia EV, Reid PR, Griffith LS: Ambulatory electrocardiographic recordings at the time of fatal cardiac arrest. *Am J Cardiol* **56**:588-92, 1985.

16. Panidid P, Morganroth J: Sudden death in hospitalized patients: Cardiac rhythm disturbances detected by ambulatory electrocardiographic monitoring. *J Am Coll Cardiol* **2**:798-805, 1983.

17. Poole JE, Mathisen TL, Kudenchuk PJ, et al.: Long-term outcome in patients who survive out of hospital ventricular fibrillation and undergo electrophysiologic studies: evaluation by electrophysiologic subgroups. *J Am Coll Cardiol* **16**:657-65, 1990.

18. Adhar GC, Larson LW, Bardy GH, Greene HL: Sustained ventricular arrhythmias: differences between survivors of cardiac arrest and patients with recurrent sustained ventricular tachycardia. *J Am Coll Cardiol* **12**:159-65, 1988.

19. Raitt M, Dolack GL, et al.: Ventricular tachycardia after transvenous defibrillator placement is rare in patients with a history of only ventricular fibrillation. *Pace Clin Electrophysiol* **16**:902A, 1993.

20. Stevenson WG, Brugada P, Waldecker B, et al.: Clinical, angiographic, and electrophysiologic findings in patients with aborted sudden death as compared with patients with sustained ventricular tachycardia after myocardial infarction. *Circulation* **71**:1146-52, 1985.

21. Josephson ME. Recurrent ventricular tachycardia. *Clinical Cardiac Electrophysiology: Techniques and Interpretations*. Philadelphia: Lea & Febiger, 417-615: 1993.

22. Josephson ME. Evaluation of antiarrhythmic drugs. *Clinical Cardiac Electrophysiology: Techniques and Interpretations*. Philadelphia: Lea & Febiger, 630-662: 1993.

23. Cobb LA, Werner JA, Trobaugh GB: Sudden cardiac death. I. A decade's experience with out-of-hospital resuscitation. *Mod Concepts Cardiovasc Dis* **49**:31-6, 1980.

24. Myerburg RJ, Conde CA, Sung RJ, et al.: Clinical, electrophysiologic and hemodynamic profile of patients resuscitated from prehospital cardiac arrest. *Am J Med* **68**:568-76, 1980.

25. Kuller LH: Sudden death--definition and epidemiologic considerations. *Prog Cardiovasc Dis* **23**:1-12, 1980.

26. Kuller L, Cooper M, Perper J: Epidemiology of sudden death. *Arch Intern Med* **129**:714-9, 1972.

27. Bardy GH, Hofer B, Johnson G, et al.: Implantable transvenous cardioverter-defibrillators. *Circulation* **87**:1152-68, 1993.

28. Reichenbach DD, Moss NS, Meyer E: Pathology of the heart in sudden cardiac death. *Am J Cardiol* **39**:865-72, 1977.

29. Warnes CA, Roberts WC: Sudden coronary death: comparison of patients with to those without coronary thrombus at necropsy. *Am J Cardiol* **54**:1206-11, 1984.

30. Warnes CA, Roberts WC: Sudden coronary death: relation of amount and distribution of coronary narrowing at necropsy to previous symptoms of myocardial ischemia, left ventricular scarring and heart weight. *Am J Cardiol* **54**:65-73, 1984.

31. Weaver WD, Lorch GS, Alvarez HA, Cobb LA: Angiographic findings and prognostic indicators in patients resuscitated from sudden cardiac death. *Circulation* **54**:895-900, 1976.

32. Davies MJ: Pathological view of sudden cardiac death. *Br Heart J* **45**:88-96, 1981.

33. BHAT Investigators: The beta-blocker heart attack trial. beta-Blocker Heart Attack Study Group. *JAMA* **246**:2073-4, 1981.

34. BHAT Investigators: A randomized trial of propranolol in patients with acute myocardial infarction. I. Mortality results. *JAMA* **247**:1707-14, 1982.

35. BHAT Investigators: A randomized trial of propranolol in patients with acute myocardial infarction. II. Morbidity results. *JAMA* **250**:2814-9, 1983.

36. Group TS: A multicenter study on timolol in secondary prevention after myocardial infarction. *Acta Med Scand Suppl* **674**:1-129, 1983.

37. Group TS: Timolol-induced reduction in mortality and reinfarction in patients surviving acute myocardial infarction. *N Engl J Med* **304**:801-7, 1981.

38. Herlitz J, Elmfeldt D, Holmberg S, et al.: Goteborg Metoprolol Trial: mortality and causes of death. *Am J Cardiol* **53**:9D-14D, 1984.

39. Herlitz J, Edvardsson N, Holmberg S, et al.: Goteborg Metoprolol Trial: effects on arrhythmias. *Am J Cardiol* **53**:27D-31D, 1984.

40. Herlitz J, Holmberg S, Pennert K, et al.: Goteborg Metoprolol Trial: design, patient characteristics and conduct. *Am J Cardiol* **53**:3D-8D, 1984.

41. Herlitz J, Hartford M, Pennert K, et al.: Goteborg Metoprolol Trial: clinical observations. *Am J Cardiol* **53**:37D-45D, 1984.

42. Herlitz J, Pennert K et al.: Goteborg Metoprolol Trial: tolerance. *Am J Cardiol* **53**:46D-50D, 1984.

43. Hjalmarson A: Acute intervention with metoprolol in myocardial infarction. *Acta Med Scand Suppl* **651**:177-84, 1981.

44. Axelrod PJ, Verrier RL, Lown B: Vulnerability to ventricular fibrillation during acute coronary arterial occlusion and release. *Am J Cardiol* **36**:776-82, 1975.

45. Fisher J, Sonnenblick EH, Kirk ES: Increased ventricular fibrillation threshold with severe myocardial ischemia. *Am Heart J* **103**:966-973, 1982.

46. Lombardi F, Verrier RL, Lown B: Relationship between sympathetic neural activity, coronary dynamics, and vulnerability to ventricular fibrillation during myocardial ischemia and reperfusion. *Am Heart J* **105**:958-65, 1983.

47. Onyanagi M, Matsumori L, Inasake T: Beta-adrenergic receptors in ischemic and non-ischemic canine myocardium: Relation to ventricular fibrillation and effects of pretreatment with propranolol and hexamethonium. *Cardiovasc Pharmacol* **11**:107-114, 1988.

48. Opie LH, Nathan D, Lubbe WF: Biochemical aspects of arrhythmogenesis and ventricular fibrillation. *Am J Cardiol* **43**:131-48, 1979.

49. Opie LH, Muller C: Evidence of role of cyclic AMP as second messenger of arrhythmogenic effects of beta-stimulation. *Adv Cyclic Nucleotide Res* **12**:63-69, 1980.

50. Mukherjee A, Wong TM, Buja LM, et al.: Beta adrenergic and muscarinic cholinergic receptors in canine myocardium. Effects of ischemia. *J Clin Invest* **64**:1423-8, 1979.

51. Anderson JL, Rodier HE, Green LS: Comparative effects of beta-adrenergic blocking drugs on experimental ventricular fibrillation threshold. *Am J Cardiol* **51**:1196-202, 1983.

52. Eller BT, Patterson E, Lucchesi BR: Ventricular fibrillation in a conscious canine model--its prevention by UM-272. *Eur J Pharmacol* **87**:407-13, 1983.

53. Lubbe WF, Muller CA, Worthington M, et al.: Influence of propranolol isomers and atenolol on myocardial cyclic AMP, high energy phosphates and vulnerability to fibrillation after coronary artery ligation in the isolated rat heart. *Cardiovasc Res* **15**:690-9, 1981.

54. Lubbe WF, Podzuweit T, Opie LH: Potential arrhythmogenic role of cycle adenosine monophosphate (AMP) and cytosolic calcium overload: Implications for prophylactic effects of beta-blockers in myocardial infarction and proarrhythmic effects of phosphodiesterase inhibitors. *J Am Coll Cardiol* **19**:1622-1633, 1992.

55. Patterson E, Lynch JJ, Lucchesi BR: Antiarrhythmic and antifibrillatory actions of the beta adrenergic receptor antagonist, *d,l*-sotalol. *J Pharmacol Exp Ther* **230**:519-26, 1984.

56. Patterson E, Lucchesi BR: Antifibrillatory actions of d,l-nadolol in a conscious canine model of sudden coronary death. *J Cardiovasc Pharmacol* **5**:737-44, 1983.

57. Kammerling JJ, Green FJ, Watanabe AM, et al.: Denervation supersensitivity of refractoriness in noninfarcted areas apical to transmural myocardial infarction. *Circulation* **76**:383-93, 1987.

58. Inoue H, Zipes DP: Results of sympathetic denervation in the canine heart: supersensitivity that may be arrhythmogenic. *Circulation* **75**:877-87, 1987.

59. Calkins H, Allman K, Bolling S, et al.: Correlation between scintigraphic evidence of regional sympathetic neuronal dysfunction and ventricular refractoriness in the human heart. *Circulation* **88**:172-9, 1993.

60. Inoue H, Zipes DP: Increased afferent vagal responses produced by epicardial application of nicotine on the canine posterior left ventricle. *Am Heart J* **114**:757-64, 1987.

61. Mukharji J, Rude RE, Poole WK, et al.: Risk factors for sudden death after acute myocardial infarction: two- year follow-up. *Am J Cardiol* **54**:31-6, 1984.

62. Bigger JT, Jr., Fleiss JL, Kleiger R, et al.: The relationships among ventricular arrhythmias, left ventricular dysfunction, and mortality in the 2 years after myocardial infarction. *Circulation* **69**:250-8, 1984.

63. Bigger JT, Jr.: Identification of patients at high risk for sudden cardiac death. *Am J Cardiol* **54**:3D-8D, 1984.

64. Bigger JT, Jr., Weld FM: Analysis of prognostic significance of ventricular arrhythmias after myocardial infarction. Shortcomings of Lown grading system. *Br Heart J* **45**:717-24, 1981.

65. Ruskin JN, DiMarco JP, Garan H: Out-of-hospital cardiac arrest: electrophysiologic observations and selection of long-term antiarrhythmic therapy. *N Engl J Med* **303**:607-13, 1980.

66. Hamer A, Vohra J, Hunt D, Sloman G: Prediction of sudden death by electrophysiologic studies in high risk patients surviving acute myocardial infarction. *Am J Cardiol* **50**:223-9, 1982.

67. Morady F, Scheinman MM, Hess DS, et al.: Electrophysiologic testing in the management of survivors of out-of-hospital cardiac arrest. *Am J Cardiol* **51**:85-9, 1983.

68. Skale BT, Miles WM, Heger JJ, et al.: Survivors of cardiac arrest: prevention of recurrence by drug therapy as predicted by electrophysiologic testing or electrocardiographic monitoring. *Am J Cardiol* **57**:113-9, 1986.

69. Kron J, Kudenchuk PJ, Murphy ES, et al.: Ventricular fibrillation survivors in whom tachyarrhythmia cannot be induced: outcome related to selected therapy. *Pacing Clin Electrophysiol* **10**:1291-300, 1987.

70. Eldar M, Sauve MJ, Scheinman MM: Electrophysiologic testing and follow-up of patients with aborted sudden death. *J Am Coll Cardiol* **10**:291-8, 1987.

71. Freedman RA, Swerdlow CD, Soderholm-Difatte V, Mason JW: Prognostic significance of arrhythmia inducibility or noninducibility at initial electrophysiologic study in survivors of cardiac arrest. *Am J Cardiol* **61**:578-82, 1988.

72. Kehoe R, Tommaso C, Zheutlin T, et al.: Factors determining programmed stimulation responses and long-term arrhythmic outcome in survivors of ventricular fibrillation with ischemic heart disease. *Am Heart J* **116**:355-63, 1988.

73. Marchlinski FE, Gottlieb CD, Sarter B, et al.: ICD data storage: value in arrhythmia management. *Pacing Clin Electrophysiol* **16**:527-34, 1993.

74. Richards DA, Byth K, Ross DL, Uther JB: What is the best predictor of spontaneous ventricular tachycardia and sudden death after myocardial infarction? *Circulation* **83**:756-63, 1991.

75. Waspe LE, Seinfeld D, Ferrick A, et al.: Prediction of sudden death and spontaneous ventricular tachycardia in survivors of complicated myocardial infarction: value of the response to programmed stimulation using a maximum of three ventricular extrastimuli. *J Am Coll Cardiol* **5**:1292-301, 1985.

76. Santarelli P, Bellocci F, Loperfido F, et al.: Ventricular arrhythmia induced by programmed ventricular stimulation after acute myocardial infarction. *Am J Cardiol* **55**:391-4, 1985.

77. Roy D, Marchlinski FE, Doherty JU, et al.: Electrophysiologic testing of survivors of cardiac arrest. *Cardiovasc Clin* **15**:171-7, 1985.

78. Bhandari AK, Rose JS, Kotlewski A, et al.: Frequency and significance of induced sustained ventricular tachycardia or fibrillation two weeks after acute myocardial infarction. *Am J Cardiol* **56**:737-42, 1985.

79. Denniss AR, Richards DA, Cody DV, et al.: Prognostic significance of ventricular tachycardia and fibrillation induced at programmed stimulation and delayed potentials detected on the signal-averaged electrocardiograms of survivors of acute myocardial infarction. *Circulation* **74**:731-45, 1986.

80. Fogoros RN, Elson JJ, Bonnet CA, et al.: Long-term outcome of survivors of cardiac arrest whose therapy is guided by electrophysiologic testing. *J Am Coll Cardiol* **19**:780-8, 1992.

81. Gomes JA, Hariman RI, Kang PS, et al.: Programmed electrical stimulation in patients with high-grade ventricular ectopy: electrophysiologic findings and prognosis for survival. *Circulation* **70**:43-51, 1984.

82. Wilber DJ, Garan H, Finkelstein D, et al.: Out-of-hospital cardiac arrest. Use of electrophysiologic testing in the prediction of long-term outcome. *N Engl J Med* **318**:19-24, 1988.

83. Buxton AE, Fisher JD, Josephson ME, et al.: Prevention of sudden death in patients with coronary artery disease: the Multicenter Unsustained Tachycardia Trial (MUSTT). *Prog Cardiovasc Dis* **36**:215-26, 1993.

84. Kleiger RE, Miller JP, Thanavaro S, et al.: Relationship between clinical features of acute myocardial infarction and ventricular runs 2 weeks to 1 year after infarction. *Circulation* **63**:64-70, 1981.

85. Maggioni AP, Zuanetti G, Franzosi G, et al.: Prevalence and prognostic significance of ventricular arrhythmias after acute myocardial infarction in the fibrinolytic era: GISSI-2 results. *Circulation* **87**:312-322, 1993.

86. Moss AJ: Factors influencing prognosis after myocardial infarction. *Curr Probl Cardiol* **4**:6-53, 1979.

87. Moss AJ, Davis HT, DeCamilla J, Bayer LW: Ventricular ectopic beats and their relation to sudden and nonsudden cardiac death after myocardial infarction. *Circulation* **60**:998-1003, 1979.

88. Ruberman W, Weinblatt E, Goldberg JD, et al.: Ventricular premature beats and mortality after myocardial infarction. *N Engl J Med* **297**:750-757, 1977.

89. Ruberman W, Weinblatt E, Goldberg JD, et al.: Ventricular premature complexes and sudden death after myocardial infarction. *Circulation* **64**:297-305, 1981.

90. Vismara LA, Amsterdam EA, Mason DT: Relation of ventricular arrhythmias in the late hospital phase of acute myocardial infarction to sudden death after hospital discharge. *Am J Med* **59**:6-12, 1975.

91. CAST Investigators: The cardiac arrhythmia suppression trial. *N Engl J Med* **321**:1754-6, 1989.

92. CAST Investigators: Preliminary report: effect of encainide and flecainide on mortality in a randomized trial of arrhythmia suppression after myocardial infarction. *N Engl J Med* **321**:406-412, 1989.

93. CAST Investigators: Effect of the antiarrhythmic agent moricizine on survival after myocardial infarction. The Cardiac Arrhythmia Suppression Trial II Investigators. *N Engl J Med* **327**:227-33, 1992.

94. Anderson JL, Platia EV, Hallstrom A, et al.: Interaction of baseline characteristics with the hazard of encainide, flecainide, and moricizine therapy in patients with myocardial infarction. A possible explanation for increased mortality in the Cardiac Arrhythmia Suppression Trial (CAST). *Circulation* **90**:2843-52, 1994.

95. Kleiger RE, Miller JP, Bigger JT, Jr., Moss AJ: Decreased heart rate variability and its association with increased mortality after acute myocardial infarction. *Am J Cardiol* **59**:256-62, 1987.

96. Vybiral T, Glaeser DH, Goldberger AL, et al.: Conventional heart rate variability analysis of ambulatory electrocardiographic recordings fails to predict imminent ventricular fibrillation. *J Am Coll Cardiol* **22**:557-65, 1993.

97. Barron HV, Lesh MD: Autonomic nervous system and sudden cardiac death. *J Am Coll Cardiol* **27**:1053-60, 1996.

98. Malik M, Farrell T, Cripps T, Camm AJ: Heart rate variability in relation to prognosis after myocardial infarction: selection of optimal processing techniques. *Eur Heart J* **10**:1060-74, 1989.

99. Kautzner J, Camm AJ: Clinical relevance of heart rate variability. *Clin Cardiol* **20**:162-8, 1997.

100. Gomes JA, Winters SL, Ip J, et al.: Identification of patients with high risk of arrhythmic mortality. Role of ambulatory monitoring, signal-averaged ECG, and heart rate variability. *Cardiol Clin* **11**:55-63, 1993.

101. Coumel P: Heart rate variability and the onset of tachyarrhythmias. *G Ital Cardiol* **22**:647-54, 1992.

102. Coumel P: Modifications of heart rate variability preceding the onset of tachyarrhythmias. *Cardiologia* **35**:7-12, 1990.

103. Breithardt G, Borggrefe M, Fetsch T, et al.: Prognosis and risk stratification after myocardial infarction. *Eur Heart J* **16 Suppl G**:10-9, 1995.

104. Farrell TG, Bashir Y, Cripps T, et al.: Risk stratification for arrhythmic events in postinfarction patients based on heart rate variability, ambulatory electrocardiographic variables and the signal-averaged electrocardiogram. *J Am Coll Cardiol* **18**:687-97, 1991.

105. De Ferrari GM, Schwartz PJ: Sudden death after myocardial infarction. Prediction based on the baroreceptor reflex. *Arch Mal Coeur Vaiss* **83**:1521-7, 1990.

106. De Ferrari GM, Vanoli E, Cerati D, Schwartz PJ: Baroreceptor reflexes and sudden cardiac death: experimental findings and background. *G Ital Cardiol* **22**:629-37, 1992.

107. Odemuyiwa O, Farrell T, Staunton A, et al.: Influence of thrombolytic therapy on the evolution of baroreflex sensitivity after myocardial infarction. *Am Heart J* **125**:285-91, 1993.

108. Schwartz PJ, Vanoli E, Stramba-Badiale M, et al.: Autonomic mechanisms and sudden death. New insights from analysis of baroreceptor reflexes in conscious dogs with and without a myocardial infarction. *Circulation* **78**:969-79, 1988.

109. Force AAT: Signal-averaged electrocardiography. *J Am Coll Cardiol* **27**:238-49, 1996.

110. Cripps TR, Camm AJ: The use of the signal-averaged electrocardiogram in predicting arrhythmic events in patients with recent myocardial infarction. *Pacing Clin Electrophysiol* **12**:1956-60, 1989.

111. Denes P, el-Sherif N, Katz R, et al.: Prognostic significance of signal-averaged electrocardiogram after thrombolytic therapy and/or angioplasty during acute myocardial infarction (CAST substudy). Cardiac Arrhythmia Suppression Trial (CAST) SAECG Substudy Investigators. *Am J Cardiol* **74**:216-20, 1994.

112. Gomes JA, Winters SL, et al.: A new noninvasive index to predict sustained ventricular tachycardia and sudden death in the first year after myocardial infarction: based on signal-averaged electrocardiogram, radionuclide ejection fraction and Holter monitoring. *J Am Coll Cardiol* **10**:349-57, 1987.

113. Gomes JA, Winters SL, Martinson M, et al.: The prognostic significance of quantitative signal-averaged variables relative to clinical variables, site of myocardial infarction, ejection fraction and ventricular premature beats: a prospective study. *J Am Coll Cardiol* **13**:377-84, 1989.

114. Gomes JA, Winters SL, Ip J: Post myocardial infarction stratification and the signal-averaged electrocardiogram. *Prog Cardiovasc Dis* **35**:263-70, 1993.

115. Klein GJ, Bashore TM, Sellers TD, et al.: Ventricular fibrillation in the Wolff-Parkinson-White syndrome. *N Engl J Med* **301**:1080-5, 1979.

116. Hays LJ, Lerman BB, DiMarco JP: Nonventricular arrhythmias as precursors of ventricular fibrillation in patients with out-of-hospital cardiac arrest. *Am Heart J* **118**:53-7, 1989.

117. Dubner SJ, Gimeno GM, Elencwajg B, et al.: Ventricular fibrillation with spontaneous reversion on ambulatory ECG in the absence of heart disease. *Am Heart J* **105**:691-3, 1983.

118. CASCADE Investigators: Randomized antiarrhythmic drug therapy in survivors of cardiac of cardiac arrest. *Am J Cardiol* **72**:280-287, 1993.

119. Greene HL: The CASCADE Study--Randomized antiarrhythmic drug therapy in survivors of cardiac arrest in Seattle. *Am J Cardiol* **72**:70F-74F, 1993.

120. Benditt DG, Benson DW, Jr., Klein GJ, Pritzker MR, Kriett JM, Anderson RW: Prevention of recurrent sudden cardiac arrest: role of provocative electropharmacologic testing. *J Am Coll Cardiol* **2**:418-25, 1983.

121. Bigger JT, Jr., Reiffel JA, Livelli FD, Jr., Wang PJ: Sensitivity, specificity, and reproducibility of programmed ventricular stimulation. *Circulation* **73**:II73-8, 1986.

122. Mason JW: A comparison of seven antiarrhythmic drugs in patients with ventricular tachyarrhythmias. Electrophysiologic Study versus Electrocardiographic Monitoring Investigators. *N Engl J Med* **329**:452-458, 1993.

123. Mason JW: A comparison of electrophysiologic testing with holter monitoring to predict antiarrhythmic-drug efficacy for ventricular tachyarrhythmias. *N Engl J Med* **329**:445-451, 1993.

124. Morady F, Scheinman MM: Evaluation of the patient with sudden cardiac death. *Med Clin North Am* **68**:1231-45, 1984.

125. Morady F, DiCarlo L, Winston S, et al.: Clinical features and prognosis of patients with out of hospital cardiac arrest and a normal electrophysiologic study. *J Am Coll Cardiol* **4**:39-44, 1984.

126. Zheutlin TA, Steinman RT, Mattioni TA, Kehoe RF: Long-term arrhythmic outcome in survivors of ventricular fibrillation with absence of inducible ventricular tachycardia. *Am J Cardiol* **62**:1213-7, 1988.

127. Tresch DD, Wetherbee JN, Siegel R, et al.: Long-term follow-up of survivors of prehospital sudden cardiac death treated with coronary bypass surgery. *Am Heart J* **110**:1139-45, 1985.

128. Tresch DD, Grove JR, Keelan MH, Jr., et al.: Long-term follow-up of survivors of prehospital sudden coronary death. *Circulation* **64**:II1-6, 1981.

129. Tresch DD, Keelan MH, Jr., Siegel R, et al.: Long-term survival after prehospital sudden cardiac death. *Am Heart J* **108**:1-5, 1984.

130. Kelly P, Ruskin JN, Vlahakes GJ, et al.: Surgical coronary revascularization in survivors of prehospital cardiac arrest: its effect on inducible ventricular arrhythmias and long-term survival. *J Am Coll Cardiol* **15**:267-73, 1990.

131. Every NR, Fahrenbruch CE, Hallstrom AP, et al.: Influence of coronary bypass surgery on subsequent outcome of patients resuscitated from out of hospital cardiac arrest. *J Am Coll Cardiol* **19**:1435-9, 1992.

132. Hallstrom AP, Cobb LA, Yu BH, et al.: An antiarrhythmic drug experience in 941 patients resuscitated from an initial cardiac arrest between 1970 and 1985. *Am J Cardiol* **68**:1025-31, 1991.

133. Coplen SE, Antman EM, Berlin JA, et al.: Efficacy and safety of quinidine therapy for maintenance of sinus rhythm after cardioversion. A meta-analysis of randomized control trials. *Circulation* **82**:1106-16, 1990.

134. Lynch JJ, DiCarlo LA, Montgomery DG, Lucchesi BR: Effects of flecainide acetate on ventricular tachyarrhythmia and fibrillation in dogs with recent myocardial infarction. *Pharmacology* **35**:181-93, 1987.

135. Stanton MS, Prystowsky EN, et al.: Arrhythmogenic effects of antiarrhythmic drugs: a study of 506 patients treated for ventricular tachycardia or fibrillation. *J Am Coll Cardiol* **14**:209-15; 1989.

136. Levy MN, Wiseman MN: Electrophysiologic mechanisms for ventricular arrhythmias in left ventricular dysfunction: electrolytes, catecholamines and drugs. *J Clin Pharmacol* **31**:1053-60, 1991.

137. Nygaard TW, Sellers TD, Cook TS, DiMarco JP: Adverse reactions to antiarrhythmic drugs during therapy for ventricular arrhythmias. *JAMA* **256**:55-7, 1986.

138. Zuanetti G, Latini R, Neilson JM, et al.: Heart rate variability in patients with ventricular arrhythmias: effect of antiarrhythmic drugs. Antiarrhythmic Drug Evaluation Group (ADEG). *J Am Coll Cardiol* **17**:604-12, 1991.

139. Elharrar V, Gaum WE, Zipes DP: Effect of drugs on conduction delay and incidence of ventricular arrhythmias induced by acute coronary occlusion in dogs. *Am J Cardiol* **39**:544-9, 1977.

140. Pratt CM, Eaton T, Francis M, et al.: The inverse relationship between baseline left ventricular ejection fraction and outcome of antiarrhythmic therapy: a dangerous imbalance in the risk-benefit ratio. *Am Heart J* **118**:433-40, 1989.

141. Packer M: Hemodynamic consequences of antiarrhythmic drug therapy in patients with chronic heart failure. *J Cardiovasc Electrophysiol* **2**:S240-S247, 1991.

142. Gottlieb SS, Kukin ML, Medina N, et al.: Comparative hemodynamic effects of procainamide, tocainide, and encainide in severe chronic heart failure. *Circulation* **81**:860-4, 1990.

143. Mahmarian JJ, Verani MS, Hohmann T, et al.: The hemodynamic effects of sotalol and quinidine: analysis by use of rest and exercise gated radionuclide angiography. *Circulation* **76**:324-31, 1987.

144. Teo KK, Yusuf S, Furberg CD: Effects of prophylactic antiarrhythmic drug therapy in acute myocardial infarction. An overview of results from randomized controlled trials. *JAMA* **270**:1589-95, 1993.

145. Herre JM, Sauve MJ, Scheinman MM: Long-term results of amiodarone therapy. *Clin Cardiol* **10**:121-5, 1987.

146. Herre JM, Sauve MJ, Malone P, et al.: Long-term results of amiodarone therapy in patients with recurrent sustained ventricular tachycardia or ventricular fibrillation. *J Am Coll Cardiol* **13**:442-9, 1989.

147. Fogoros RN, Fiedler SB, Elson JJ: Empiric amiodarone versus "ineffective" drug therapy in patients with refractory ventricular tachyarrhythmias. *Pacing Clin Electrophysiol* **11**:1009-17, 1988.

148. Julian DG, Camm AJ, Frangin G, et al.: Randomised trial of effect of amiodarone on mortality in patients with left-ventricular dysfunction after recent myocardial infarction: EMIAT. European Myocardial Infarct Amiodarone Trial Investigators. *Lancet* **349**:667-74, 1997.

149. Julian DG: The amiodarone trials. *Eur Heart J* **18**:1361-2, 1997.

150. Cairns JA, Connolly SJ, Roberts R, Gent M: Canadian amiodarone myocardial infarction arrhythmia trial(CAMIAT): Rationale and protocol. *Am J Cardiol* **72**:87F-94F, 1993.

151. Cairns JA, Connolly SJ, Roberts R, Gent M: Randomised trial of outcome after myocardial infarction in patients with frequent or repetitive ventricular premature depolarisations: CAMIAT. Canadian Amiodarone Myocardial Infarction Arrhythmia Trial Investigators. *Lancet* **349**:675-82, 1997.

152. Cairns J: Antiarrhythmic therapies for the prevention of ventricular arrhythmias. *Can J Cardiol* **14**:Suppl 1-8, 1998.

153. Waldo AL, Camm AJ, deRuyter H, et al.: Effect of d-sotalol on mortality in patients with left ventricular dysfunction after recent and remote myocardial infarction. The SWORD Investigators. Survival With Oral d-Sotalol. *Lancet* **348**:7-12, 1996.

154. Waldo AL, Camm AJ, deRuyter H, et al.: Survival with oral d-sotalol in patients with left ventricular dysfunction after myocardial infarction: rationale, design, and methods (the SWORD trial). *Am J Cardiol* **75**:1023-7, 1995.

155. Cox JL: Patient selection criteria and results of surgery for refractory ischemic ventricular tachycardia. *Circulation* **79(suppl)**:163-77, 1989.

156. Cox JL: Ventricular tachycardia surgery: a review of the first decade and a suggested contemporary approach. *Semin Thorac Cardiovasc Surg* **1**:97-103, 1989.

157. Blanchard SM, Walcott GP, Wharton JM, Ideker RE: Why is catheter ablation less successful than surgery for treating ventricular tachycardia that results from coronary artery disease? *Pacing Clin Electrophysiol* **17**:2315-35, 1994.

158. Stevenson WG, Khan H, Sager P, et al.: Identification of reentry circuit sites during catheter mapping and radiofrequency ablation of ventricular tachycardia late after myocardial infarction. *Circulation* **88**:1647-70, 1993.

159. Brugada P, de Swart H, Smeets JL, Wellens HJ: Transcoronary chemical ablation of ventricular tachycardia. *Circulation* **79**:475-82, 1989.

160. Evans GT, Jr., Scheinman MM, Zipes DP, et al.: The Percutaneous Cardiac Mapping and Ablation Registry: final summary of results. *Pacing Clin Electrophysiol* **11**:1621-6, 1988.

161. Morady F, Scheinman MM, Di Carlo LA, Jr., et al.: Catheter ablation of ventricular tachycardia with intracardiac shocks: results in 33 patients. *Circulation* **75**:1037-49, 1987.

162. Morady F, Scheinman MM, Griffin JC, et al.: Results of catheter ablation of ventricular tachycardia using direct current shocks. *Pacing Clin Electrophysiol* **12**:252-7, 1989.

163. Tchou P, Jazayeri M, Denker S, et al.: Transcatheter electrical ablation of right bundle branch. A method of treating macroreentrant ventricular tachycardia attributed to bundle branch reentry. *Circulation* **78**:246-57, 1988.

164. Leclercq JF, Chouty F, Cauchemez B, Leenhardt A, Coumel P, Slama R: Results of electrical fulguration in arrhythmogenic right ventricular disease. *Am J Cardiol* **62**:220-4, 1988.

165. Kelly PA, Cannom DS, Garan H, et al.: The automatic implantable cardioverter-defibrillator: efficacy, complications and survival in patients with malignant ventricular arrhythmias. *J Am Coll Cardiol* **11**:1278-86, 1988.

166. Manolis AS, Rastegar H, Estes NA: Automatic implantable cardioverter defibrillator. Current status. *JAMA* **262**:1362-8, 1989.

167. Manolis AS, Tan-DeGuzman W, Lee MA, et al.: Clinical experience in seventy-seven patients with the automatic implantable cardioverter defibrillator. *Am Heart J* **118**:445-50, 1989.

168. Myerburg RJ, Luceri RM, Thurer R, et al.: Time to first shock and clinical outcome in patients receiving an automatic implantable cardioverter-defibrillator. *J Am Coll Cardiol* **14**:508-14, 1989.

169. Tchou PJ, Kadri N, Anderson J, Caceres JA, Jazayeri M, Akhtar M: Automatic implantable cardioverter defibrillators and survival of patients with left ventricular dysfunction and malignant ventricular arrhythmias. *Ann Intern Med* **109**:529-34, 1988.

170. Winkle RA, Mead RH, Ruder MA, et al.: Long-term outcome with the automatic implantable cardioverter- defibrillator. *J Am Coll Cardiol* **13**:1353-61, 1989.

171. Fogoros RN, Elson JJ, Bonnet CA, Fiedler SB, Burkholder JA: Efficacy of the automatic implantable cardioverter-defibrillator in prolonging survival in patients with severe underlying cardiac disease. *J Am Coll Cardiol* **16**:381-6, 1990.

172. Powell AC, Fuchs T, Finkelstein DM, et al.: Influence of implantable cardioverter-defibrillators on the long-term prognosis of survivors of out-of-hospital cardiac arrest. *Circulation* **88**:1083-92, 1993.

173. Newman D, Sauve MJ, Herre J, et al.: Survival after implantation of the cardioverter defibrillator. *Am J Cardiol* **69**:899-903, 1992.

174. Antiarrhythmics Versus Implantable Defibrillators (AVID) Investigators: A comparison of antiarrhythmic drug therapy with implantable defibrillators in patients resuscitated from near-fatal ventricular arrhythmias. *N Engl J Med* **337**:1576-1583, 1997.

175. Connolly SJ, Gent M, Roberts RS, et al.: Canadian Implantable Defibrillator Study (CIDS): study design and organization. CIDS Co-Investigators. *Am J Cardiol* **72**:103F-108F, 1993.

176. Gundersen T, Abrahamsen AM, Kjekshus J, Ronnevik PK: Timolol-related reduction in mortality and reinfarction in patients ages 65-75 years surviving acute myocardial infarction. Prepared for the Norwegian Multicentre Study Group. *Circulation* **66**:1179-84, 1982.

177. Pratt CM, Roberts R: Chronic beta blockade therapy in patients after myocardial infarction. *Am J Cardiol* **52**:661-4, 1983.

178. Domanski MJ, Zipes DP, Schron E: Treatment of sudden cardiac death. Current understandings from randomized trials and future research directions. *Circulation* **95**:2694-9, 1997.

179. Packer M, Bristow MR, Cohn JN, et al.: The effect of carvedilol on morbidity and mortality in patients with chronic heart failure. *N Engl J Med* **334**:1349-55, 1996.

180. Kober L, Torp-Pedersen C, Carlsen JE, et al.: A clinical trial of the angiotensin-converting-enzyme in-hibitor trandolapril in patients with left ventricular dysfunction after myocardial infarction. Trandolapril Cardiac Evaluation (TRACE) Study Group. *N Engl J Med* **333**:1670-6, 1995.

181. Pfeffer MA, Braunwald E, Moye LA, et al.: Effect of captopril on mortality and morbidity in patients with left ventricular dysfunction after myocardial infarction. Results of the survival and ventricular en-largement trial. The SAVE Investigators. *N Engl J Med* **327**:669-77, 1992.

182. Packer M: Do angiotensin-converting enzyme inhibitors prolong life in patients with heart failure treat-ed in clinical practice? *J Am Coll Cardiol* **28**:1323-7, 1996.

183. Visser FC, Visser CA: Current controversies with ACE inhibitor treatment in heart failure. *Cardiology* **87 Suppl** 1:23-8, 1996.

184. Kowey, PR, Taylor, JE, Marinchak, RA, et al.: Does prohgrammed stimulation really help in the evalua-tion of patients with non-sustained ventricular tachycardia? Results of a meta-analysis. *Am Heart J* **123**:481-9, 1993.

185. Moss AJ, Hall WJ, Cannom DS, et al.: Improved survival with an implanted defibrillator in patients with coronary disease at high risk for ventricular arrhythmia. Multicenter Automatic Defibrillator Im-plantation Trial Investigators. *N Engl J Med* **335**:1933-40, 1996.

186. Buxton AE, Lee KL, DiCarlo L, et al.: Nonsustained ventricular tachycardia in coronary artery disease: relation to inducible sustained ventricular tachycardia. MUSTT Investigators. *Ann Intern Med* **125**:35-9, 1996.

187. Buxton AE, Lee KL, Fisher JD, et al.: A randomized study of the prevention of sudden death in patients with coronary artery disease. *New Engl J Med* **341**:1882-90, 1999.

188. Buxton, AE, Hafley, GE, Lehmann, MH, et al.: Prediction of sustained ventricular tachycardia inducible by programmed stimulation in patients with coronary artery disease. Utility of clinical variables. *Circu-lation* **99**:1843-50, 1999.

189. Bigger JT, Jr.: Prophylactic use of implanted cardiac defibrillators in patients at high risk for ventricular arrhythmias after coronary-artery bypass graft surgery. Coronary Artery Bypass Graft (CABG) Patch Trial Investigators. *N Engl J Med* **337**:1569-75, 1997.

190. Bigger JT, Jr., Whang W, Rottman JN, et al.: Mechanisms of death in the CABG Patch trial: a random-ized trial of implantable cardiac defibrillator prophylaxis in patients at high risk of death after coronary artery bypass graft surgery. *Circulation* **99**:1416-21, 1999.

191. Klein H, Auricchio A, Reek S, Geller C: New primary prevention trials of sudden cardiac death in pa-tients with left ventricular dysfunction: SCD-HEFT and MADIT-II. *Am J Cardiol* **83**:91D-97D, 1999.

192. Moss AJ, Cannom DS, Daubert JP, et al.: Multicenter automatic defibrillator implantation trial II (MA-DIT II): design and clinical protocol. *Ann Noninvasive Electrocardiol* **4**:83-91, 1999.

193. Bigger JT, Jr.: Relation between left ventricular dysfunction and ventricular arrhythmias after myocar-dial infarction. *Am J Cardiol* **57**:8B-14B, 1986.

194. Wilber DJ, Olshansky B, Moran JF, Scanlon PJ: Electrophysiological testing and nonsustained ventric-ular tachycardia. Use and limitations in patients with coronary artery disease and impaired ventricular function. *Circulation* **82**:350-8, 1990.

195. Doval HC, Nul DR, Grancelli HO, et al.: Randomised trial of low-dose amiodarone in severe congestive heart failure. Grupo de Estudio de la Sobrevida en la Insuficiencia Cardiaca en Argentina (GESICA). *Lancet* **344**:493-8, 1994.

196. Siebels J, Cappato R, Ruppel R, et al.: Preliminary results of the cardiac arrest study hamburg(CASH). *Am J Cardiol* **72**:109F-113F, 1993.

197. Siebels J, Cappato R, Ruppel R, et al.: ICD versus drugs in cardiac arrest survivors: preliminary results of the Cardiac Arrest Study Hamburg. *Pacing Clin Electrophysiol* **16**:552-8, 1993.

198. Siebels J, Kuck KH: Implantable cardioverter defibrillator compared with antiarrhythmic drug treat-ment in cardiac arrest survivors (the Cardiac Arrest Study Hamburg). *Am Heart J* **127**:1139-44, 1994.

INDEX